Roles of Mitophagy in Cancer Regulation

Ashok Kumar Pandurangan
B.S. Abdur Rahman Crescent Institute of Science and Technology, India

I0894816

IGI Global
Scientific Publishing
Publishing Tomorrow's Research Today

Vice President of Editorial Melissa Wagner
Director of Acquisitions Mikaela Felty
Director of Book Development Jocelynn Hessler
Production Manager Mike Brehm
Cover Design Jose Rosado

Published in the United States of America by
IGI Global Scientific Publishing
701 East Chocolate Avenue
Hershey, PA, 17033, USA
Tel: 717-533-8845
Fax: 717-533-7115
Website: https://www.igi-global.com E-mail: cust@igi-global.com

Library of Congress Cataloging-in-Publication Data

Names: Pandurangan, Ashok Kumar, 1982- editor
Title: Roles of mitophagy in cancer regulation / edited by Ashok Kumar Pandurangan.
Description: Hershey, PA : IGI Global Scientific Publishing, [2025] | Includes bibliographical references and index. | Summary: "The objective of this book is to create a complete archive on Mitophagy in the regulation of cancer. It explores the scientific understanding on how the mitophagy and autophagy signaling is regulated in the early and later stage of cancer"-- Provided by publisher.
Identifiers: LCCN 2024053541 (print) | LCCN 2024053542 (ebook) | ISBN 9798369338360 h/c | ISBN 9798369338377 eISBN
Subjects: LCSH: Cancer cells--Growth--Regulation | Cellular control mechanisms | Autophagic vacuoles | Mitochondrial pathology
Classification: LCC RC269.7 .R65 2025 (print) | LCC RC269.7 (ebook) | DDC 616.99/407--dc23/eng/20250318
LC record available at https://lccn.loc.gov/2024053541
LC ebook record available at https://lccn.loc.gov/2024053542

British Cataloguing in Publication Data
A Cataloguing in Publication record for this book is available from the British Library.

I would like to dedicate this book to my mentor, Professor Sudhandiran Ganapasam.

Table of Contents

Detailed Table of Contents

highlighting successes and challenges. Ongoing research and personalized medicine approaches offer promising avenues for innovative cancer treatments.

Chapter 3

Mitophagy the deliberate breakdown of mitochondria by the autophagic pathway is a crucial component of cell-level mitochondrial quality control. Mitophagy, the act of eliminating damaged or malfunctioning mitochondria, is a crucial part of normal cellular physiology and tissue creation. Shared pathways governing mitophagy, cancer, and cell death could be triggered by a solitary upstream signal convening at the mitochondria. We also discuss the pivotal roles that these processes perform in the cancer microenvironment. Recent studies have contributed to the development of anticancer treatments that either promote or inhibit autophagy, shedding light on the role autophagy and related mechanisms play in the initiation and spread of cancer. In this review paper, we have looked at and investigated the different roles that autophagy and related systems play in the development, maintenance, and expansion of malignancies.

Chapter 4

The second most frequent extracranial malignant tumour in children and the most common solid tumour in infants is neuroblastoma, a cancer of the sympathetic nervous system. Patients' survival rates gradually increase as a result of the most recent developments in neuroblastoma treatment being gradually included into clinical trials and clinical practice guidelines. The capacity to develop treatments for certain molecular targets in neuroblastoma is critical as technologies develop. ALK inhibitors and anti-GD2 treatments are currently the most prominent targeted medicines available for high-risk neuroblastoma; they have both established themselves as cornerstones of treatment in both the upfront and relapsed contexts. Additional molecular targeted therapeutic development has proven difficult and has had mixed results. The identification of possible therapeutic targets keeps up

Preface

INTRODUCTION

Cancer signaling plays a crucial role in the development, progression, and treatment of cancer. It involves complex networks of molecular interactions that regulate cell growth, survival, and metastasis. Dysregulation of these signaling pathways can lead to uncontrolled cell proliferation, evasion of apoptosis, and increased invasiveness. Key pathways implicated in cancer signaling include PI3K/Akt/mTOR, MAPK, Wnt, and Notch. Understanding these signaling mechanisms is essential for developing targeted therapies, identifying biomarkers, and predicting treatment responses. Moreover, cancer signaling often involves crosstalk between multiple pathways, contributing to drug resistance and tumor heterogeneity. Research into cancer signaling continues to reveal new therapeutic targets and improve our understanding of cancer biology, ultimately leading to more effective and personalized treatment strategies.

Mitophagy signaling is a critical cellular process that regulates the selective degradation of damaged or dysfunctional mitochondria. This quality control mechanism is essential for maintaining cellular homeostasis and preventing the accumulation of harmful mitochondria that can lead to oxidative stress and cellular dysfunction. Key components of mitophagy signaling include: 1. PINK1/Parkin pathway: PINK1 accumulates on the outer membrane of damaged mitochondria, recruiting Parkin, an E3 ubiquitin ligase. Parkin then ubiquitinates mitochondrial proteins, marking them for degradation. 2. BNIP3 and NIX: These proteins act as mitochondrial receptors, binding to LC3 on autophagosomes to initiate mitophagy. 3. FUNDC1: A mitochondrial outer membrane protein that interacts with LC3 to promote mitophagy under hypoxic conditions. 4. Mitochondrial dynamics: Fission and fusion processes influence mitophagy, with fission often preceding mitochondrial degradation. 5. Autophagy machinery: General autophagy proteins, such as Atg5, Atg7, and LC3, are essential for mitophagy execution. Mitophagy signaling is implicated in various physiological and pathological processes, including: 1. Cellular stress response 2. Aging 3. Neurodegenerative diseases (e.g., Parkinson's disease) 4. Cancer 5. Cardiovascular diseases Understanding mitophagy signaling mechanisms can provide insights into potential therapeutic targets for diseases associated with mitochondrial dysfunction and oxidative stress.

Mitophagy plays a complex role in cancer regulation, influencing various aspects of tumor development, progression, and treatment response: 1. Tumor suppression: - Mitophagy eliminates damaged mitochondria, reducing oxidative stress and preventing genomic instability. - It helps maintain cellular homeostasis, potentially inhibiting cancer initiation. 2. Metabolic reprogramming: - Cancer cells often exhibit altered mitochondrial function and metabolism. - Mitophagy can modulate these metabolic changes, affecting tumor growth and survival. 3. Cell death regulation: - Mitophagy can promote cancer cell survival by removing dysfunctional mitochondria. - Conversely, excessive mitophagy may lead to cell death in some contexts. 4. Metastasis: - Mitophagy influences cellular energy production and oxidative stress, potentially impacting metastatic potential. 5. Chemoresistance: - Some cancer cells upregulate mitophagy to resist chemotherapy-induced damage. - Targeting mitophagy pathways may enhance treatment efficacy. 6. Tumor microenvironment: - Mitophagy affects the metabolic interactions between cancer cells and stromal cells. 7. Stem cell maintenance: - Mitophagy contributes to cancer stem cell maintenance and self-renewal. 8. Therapeutic implications: - Modulating mitophagy pathways may offer new treatment strategies. - Combining mitophagy inhibitors with existing therapies could enhance anti-cancer effects. Understanding the context-dependent roles of mitophagy in cancer is crucial for developing targeted therapies and improving treatment outcomes. In this book comprised of 12 chapters and each chapter have unique information about mitophagy regulation in cancer.

CHAPTER OVERVIEW

Chapter 1 provides a comprehensive overview of mitophagy and oxidative stress in cancer. It begins by explaining the crucial role of mitochondria in eukaryotic cells, particularly in energy production through aerobic respiration and ATP synthesis. The chapter then delves into the process of mitophagy, a degradation mechanism targeting aged or damaged mitochondria, which is essential for maintaining cellular homeostasis. The four main stages of mitophagy are outlined, emphasizing its importance in preserving mitochondrial quality. It further explores the relationship between mitochondrial damage and various diseases, including cancer. It discusses how disruption of mitochondrial integrity, increased mitochondrial transmembrane potential, oxidative stress, and exposure to toxic agents can lead to mitochondrial dysfunction and homeostatic imbalance. The complex mechanism between cancer cells and mitophagy is highlighted, with particular emphasis on the Warburg effect and the importance of mitochondrial function for cancer cell survival. It also provides an in-depth explanation of the molecular mechanisms of mitophagy, including the ubiquitin-dependent PINK1/Parkin pathway and the ubiquitin-independent receptor-mediated pathway. It also discusses the role of mitophagy in various diseases such as neurodegenerative disorders, cardiovascular diseases, and cancer. The chapter then shifts focus to oxidative stress and its impact on cancer risk, detailing how mitochondria contribute to the production of reactive oxygen species (ROS) and the cellular adaptations to oxidative stress in normal cells. One of the most intriguing aspects of this chapter is its exploration of the dual nature of oxidative stress in cancer cells. While increased ROS production can lead to DNA damage and promote carcinogenesis, cancer cells also develop adaptive mechanisms to combat excessive oxidative stress. The chapter reveals how cancer cells can maintain a delicate balance between increased ROS production (which supports their rapid metabolism) and enhanced antioxidant defenses (which prevent cytotoxic levels of oxidative stress). This balance allows cancer cells to exploit the growth-promoting effects of moderate ROS levels while avoiding the detrimental effects of excessive oxidative damage.

Chapter 2 presents a comprehensive overview of the roles of autophagy and mitophagy in cancer metabolism and their implications for cancer therapy. The key significance and implications of the arguments presented are: These processes can act as both tumor suppressors and promoters, depending on the stage and type of cancer. This dual nature has significant implications for developing targeted cancer therapies. Autophagy and mitophagy play crucial roles in the metabolic remodeling of cancer cells, allowing them to adapt to stressful conditions and maintain their growth. Understanding these mechanisms could lead to new therapeutic strategies that target cancer metabolism.Autophagy and mitophagy can influence the effectiveness of chemotherapy and radiotherapy, sometimes contributing to drug resistance. This insight is crucial for developing more effective combination therapies and overcoming treatment resistance. It highlights the potential of targeting autophagy and mitophagy pathways as a novel approach to cancer treatment. This opens up new avenues for drug development and personalized medicine in oncology. It emphasizes the need for ongoing research to fully understand the complex roles of autophagy and mitophagy in different cancer types and stages. This underscores the importance of continued investment in this field of study. These findings have significant implications for cancer research, drug development, and clinical practice, potentially leading to more effective and personalized cancer treatments in the future.

Chapter 3 explores the role of mitophagy, a selective form of autophagy that targets mitochondria, in cancer development and treatment. The chapter explaining the genetic and epigenetic changes that lead to cancer and highlighting mitophagy as a key target for cancer therapy. The introduction section provides a detailed explanation of autophagy and its regulation by various ATG (autophagy-related) gene products. The authors describe the process of autophagosome formation and the role of key proteins like LC3 in this process. The chapter then focuses on mitophagy, its functions, and its regulators. It discusses how mitophagy is essential for maintaining cellular homeostasis by removing damaged mitochondria. The authors explore the dual role of mitophagy in cancer, noting that it can both suppress and promote tumor growth depending on the context and stage of cancer. The chapter also presents a detailed table of mitophagy regulators and their functions in relation to cancer and other diseases. One of the unique insights from this chapter is the complex and context-dependent role of mitophagy in cancer. While it can act as a tumor suppressor by maintaining cellular homeostasis and preventing the accumulation of damaged mitochondria, it can also promote tumor survival by helping cancer cells adapt to stress conditions. The authors highlight the potential of targeting mitophagy for cancer therapy, suggesting that both inhibition and enhancement of mitophagy could be beneficial depending on the specific cancer context. This dual nature of mitophagy in cancer biology presents both challenges and opportunities for developing targeted cancer therapies, emphasizing the need for a nuanced approach in cancer treatment strategies.

Chapter 4 discusses several molecular targets and treatment approaches for high-risk neuroblastoma (HRNBL). Key targets include GD2, a glycolipid expressed on most neuroblastoma cells, which is targeted by monoclonal antibodies like Dinutuximab and Naxitamab. Anaplastic Lymphoma Kinase (ALK) is another promising target, with ALK inhibitors like Crizotinib showing efficacy in treating ALK-aberrant neuroblastoma. Other potential targets include Aurora Kinase, MDM2, B7-H3, CDK 4/6, RAS-MAPK pathway, and mTOR. The chapter highlights ongoing clinical trials and research efforts to develop and improve targeted therapies for HRNBL. A unique insight from this chapter is the emphasis on the complex interplay between various molecular pathways in neuroblastoma pathogenesis and the potential for combination therapies. The chapter reveals that while some targeted therapies, like anti-GD2 and ALK inhibitors, have shown promise, many others are still in early stages of development or have shown mixed results. This underscores the challenges in developing effective targeted therapies for neuroblastoma and the need for continued research to identify and validate new molecular targets.

This chapter 5 provides a comprehensive overview of natural products modulating mitophagy in breast cancer, exploring their mechanisms and potential therapeutic implications. The introduction highlights the global prevalence of breast cancer and emphasizes the importance of understanding biological mechanisms, particularly mitophagy, in developing effective therapies. Mitophagy, the selective elimination of defective mitochondria, plays a crucial role in maintaining cellular homeostasis and is dysregulated in breast cancer. The chapter delves into the molecular pathways involved in mitophagy, such as AMPK/mTOR, PINK1/Parkin, and BNIP3/NIX pathways, and their roles in breast cancer. It then explores the potential therapeutic implications of modulating mitophagy in breast cancer treatment, including sensitizing cancer cells to apoptosis, overcoming hormone therapy resistance, and targeting cancer stem cells. The chapter extensively discusses various natural products and their effects on breast cancer, including curcumin, resveratrol, green tea extracts, quercetin, berberine, silymarin, ginsenosides, salidroside, catechins, and lycopene. Each of these compounds is analyzed for its potential to modulate mitophagy in breast cancer cells, with detailed explanations of their mechanisms of action and interactions with key mitophagy regulators.

Chapter 6 is a comprehensive review of the regulation of mitophagy in colorectal cancer (CRC) and potential drug interventions. It begins by introducing CRC as a significant global health issue, highlighting its prevalence and the need for improved treatment strategies. The review then delves into the role of mitochondria in cancer cells, emphasizing how mitophagy, the process of selectively removing damaged mitochondria, affects the metabolic environment of cancer cells and enhances their survival capacity. This chapter outlines three important mitophagy pathways: PINK1/Parkin-Mediated Mitophagy, BNIP3/NIX-Mediated Mitophagy, and FUNDC1-Mediated Mitophagy. It then discusses various natural compounds and their potential as anti-cancer agents through modulation of mitophagy in CRC. These compounds include 3-Carboxy proxyl nitroxide (Mito-CP), Mito-Met10, Tanshinone IIA, δ-Valerobetaine, Plasmodium Infection, BH3 mimetic ch282-5, propionate and butyrate, oleanolic acid, adenovirus-based Mst1 overexpression, alpha hederin, 3,4-Dihydroxyphenylethanol (DPE or Hydroxytyrosol), cirsiliol, TEOA (a triterpenoid from Actinidia eriantha), and Aloe gel glucomannan.

Chapter 7 provides a comprehensive overview of mitophagy, its regulatory mechanisms, and its significance in various diseases. It highlights the potential of modulating mitophagy as a therapeutic strategy and discusses both natural and synthetic mitophagy modulators. An interesting insight from the chapter is the emerging role of in-silico approaches in identifying potential mitophagy modulators. The use of machine learning and cross-species workflows for discovering mitophagy inducers, particularly in the context of Alzheimer's disease, represents a novel and promising direction in drug discovery. Additionally, the authors emphasizes the importance of balancing mitophagy modulation, as both insufficient and exfcessive mitophagy can contribute to disease pathology, underscoring the complexity of targeting this process for therapeutic purposes.

Chapter 8 provides a comprehensive overview of Inflammatory Bowel Diseases (IBD), with a specific focus on Colitis-Associated Cancer (CAC). It begins by introducing IBD, including its two main subtypes: Crohn's disease and ulcerative colitis. The chapter highlights the increased risk of colorectal cancer in IBD patients, particularly those with long-standing and severe inflammation. The chapter then delves into the molecular mechanisms of CAC, emphasizing the role of chronic inflammation in promoting tumor growth. It discusses various signaling pathways and immune responses involved in CAC pathogenesis. The chapter also explores the concept of mitophagy, a cellular process involving the selective degradation of damaged mitochondria, and its potential role in CAC development and progression. The chapter outlines current therapeutic approaches for CAC, including surgery, chemotherapy, and targeted therapies. It also discusses the challenges associated with these treatments, such as resistance and adverse effects. The potential of natural products in CAC management is explored, with compounds like curcumin and resveratrol showing promise in preclinical studies.

Chapter 9 is a comprehensive review of the role of mitophagy in cancer drug resistance. Mitophagy, a selective process for removing damaged mitochondria, has emerged as a crucial player in the development of drug resistance across various cancer types. The chapter explores the intricate relationship between mitophagy and cancer drug resistance, discussing the mechanisms involved and their impact on different cancer types. The chapter begins by introducing the concept of cancer drug resistance and its significance in oncology. It then delves into the mechanisms of mitophagy, explaining its role in maintaining cellular homeostasis and energy metabolism. The PINK1-Parkin pathway and receptor-mediated mitophagy are discussed as key mechanisms regulating mitochondrial quality control. The chapter also highlights how mitophagy influences tissue-specific functions and physiological processes, including basal mitophagy, stress-induced mitophagy, and programmed mitophagy.

Chapter 10 provides a comprehensive overview of natural products modulating mitophagy and their implications for cancer therapy. Mitophagy, the selective removal of damaged or dysfunctional mitochondria, plays a crucial role in maintaining cellular homeostasis. The chapter discusses how various natural products, including polyphenols, flavonoids, polyunsaturated fatty acids (PUFAs), alkaloids, and terpenoids, can modulate mitophagy through different mechanisms. The chapter outlines the process of mitophagy, including the recognition of damaged mitochondria, recruitment of mitophagy receptors, formation of autophagosomes, and degradation of mitochondrial components. It then delves into how different classes of natural products interact with these processes. For instance, polyphenols and flavonoids are shown to enhance the AMP-activated protein kinase (AMPK) pathway and trigger mitochondrial fission, promoting the removal of dysfunctional mitochondria. PUFAs, particularly omega-3 fatty acids, are discussed for their potential to promote mitophagy by affecting mitochondrial membrane composition and fluidity. The chapter also explores natural products that inhibit mitophagy, such as certain alkaloids and terpenoids. These compounds are noted for their ability to disrupt mitochondrial dynamics and respiratory chain function, potentially enhancing cancer cells' susceptibility to apoptosis and chemotherapy. The chapter concludes by discussing the challenges and future perspectives in using natural products as modulators of mitophagy, including issues of bioavailability, specificity, and the need for standardization in natural product formulations.

Chapter 11 provides an in-depth exploration of mitophagy and its role in cancer drug resistance. Mitophagy, a selective form of autophagy targeting mitochondria, plays a crucial role in maintaining cellular homeostasis and mitochondrial quality control. In cancer cells, mitophagy acts as both a tumor suppressor and a survival mechanism, enabling cancer cells to withstand metabolic and therapeutic stress. The chapter discusses various pathways involved in mitophagy induction, including the PINK1-Parkin pathway, receptor-mediated pathway, and cardiolipin-driven pathway. The chapter extensively covers how mitophagy contributes to cancer drug resistance through several mechanisms. These include maintaining mitochondrial function and energy production, regulating metabolic flexibility, suppressing apoptosis, modulating cellular signaling pathways, contributing to the cancer stem cell phenotype, and adapting to hypoxic conditions. The chapter also explores strategies to modulate mitophagy for overcoming drug resistance, such as inhibition or induction of mitophagy, dual modulation approaches, genetic and molecular approaches, and combination therapies.

Chapter 12 provides a comprehensive overview of mitophagy, its mechanisms, and its role in cancer development and treatment. Mitophagy is a selective form of autophagy that targets mitochondria for degradation. The chapter begins by introducing the concept of autophagy and its importance in various physiological processes, including cell fate and stress responses. It then delves into the specific mechanisms of mitophagy, highlighting the PINK1/Parkin pathway and the role of mitophagy receptors such as NIX, BNIP3, and FUNDC1.

The chapter explores the relationship between mitophagy and cancer, discussing how dysfunctional mitophagy may contribute to cancer development. It also examines the potential of natural compounds as mitophagic modulators in cancer treatment. Various classes of natural compounds are discussed, including polyphenolic compounds (e.g., quercetin, resveratrol), terpenoid compounds (e.g., docetaxel, β-elemene), saponin compounds (e.g., Paris polyphylla extract, betulinic acid), alkaloid compounds (e.g., camptothecin, berberine), and quinonoid compounds (e.g., thimoquinone, plumbagin). The chapter details how these compounds can influence mitophagy and autophagy pathways, potentially enhancing their anticancer effects.

CONCLUSION

In a nutshell, this book inspires further research and innovation in the field, ultimately leading to the development of novel therapies and interventions that harness the mitophagy signaling. May this edited reference book serve as a catalyst for new discoveries and transformative advancements in the field of mitophagy and cancer.

Ashok Kumar Pandurangan
B.S. Abdur Rahman Crescent Institute of Science and Technology, India

Chapter 1
Mitophagy and Oxidative Stress in Cancer

Fatma Gönül Sezgin
https://orcid.org/0000-0002-9400-5173
Ondokuz Mayıs University, Turkey

Emine İncilay Torunoğlu
https://orcid.org/0000-0003-4641-0067
Necmettin Erbakan University, Turkey

Erdi Can Aytar
https://orcid.org/0000-0001-6045-0183
Usak University, Turkey

ABSTRACT

This chapter highlights mitochondria's central role in eukaryotic cells for energy production via aerobic respiration, synthesizing ATP. Additionally, mitochondria contribute to lipid metabolism, calcium signaling, and ROS production. Mitophagy is crucial for maintaining homeostasis by degrading damaged mitochondria, with its four stages detailed. The link between mitochondrial damage and diseases is explored, along with the significance of mitophagy in cancer cells and potential treatments. This chapter provides insight into mitochondria's biological significance and their role in disease pathogenesis.

DOI: 10.4018/979-8-3693-3836-0.ch001

INTRODUCTION

Mitochondria serve as the energy center in eukaryotic cells, conducting ATP synthesis through aerobic respiration. They also play a role in cellular functions such as lipid metabolism, calcium signaling, and the production and detoxification of reactive oxygen species (ROS). Mitochondria are double-membraned organelles.

Mitochondrial autophagy, known as mitophagy, is crucial for maintaining homeostasis. Mitophagy is a degradation process targeting aged or damaged mitochondria and consists of four main stages: 1) Damaged mitochondria depolarize. 2) Mitochondria are enveloped by autophagosomes, forming mitochondrial autophagosomes. 3) Mitochondrial autophagosomes merge with lysosomes. 4) Mitochondrial contents are broken down by lysosomes.

Mitochondria, responsible for ROS production, serve as organelles that not only produce significant ROS but also act as powerful mitogens. ROS production is a byproduct of oxidative phosphorylation, and its accumulation can impact cellular homeostasis and mitochondrial functions. NADPH is required for the reduction of H_2O_2 and other peroxides produced mitochondrially by peroxidases. Increased mitochondrial ROS production can lead to intracellular toxicity, triggering apoptosis or necrosis. If apoptosis is inhibited, increased ROS production may contribute to neoplastic transformation.

Disruption of mitochondrial integrity, an increase in mitochondrial transmembrane potential (MMP), oxidative stress, hypoxia, and exposure to toxic agents are associated with mitochondrial damage, dysfunction, and disrupted homeostasis. This is linked to various diseases, including neurodegenerative diseases, cancer, and infections. Recent research has focused on mitophagy in understanding the pathogenesis of various diseases.

The mechanism between cancer cells and mitophagy is complex and likely associated with oxidative metabolism and energy homeostasis. The Warburg effect signifies the tendency of cancer cells to use aerobic glycolysis for energy production. The Warburg effect suggests a strong relationship between mitophagy and cancer. Mitochondrial function is crucial for the survival of cancer cells because the elimination of mitochondrial DNA (mtDNA) reduces the growth rate and tumorigenicity of cancer cells.

In conclusion, mitochondria are the central hub for energy production in eukaryotic cells, playing a crucial role in cellular functions, ROS production, and detoxification. Mitophagy is a critical process for maintaining mitochondrial homeostasis, particularly through the degradation of aged or damaged mitochondria. Disruption of mitochondrial integrity and ROS accumulation are linked to various diseases, especially cancer. Understanding mitophagy mechanisms holds potential as a strategy for cancer treatment and prevention.

BACKGROUND

Mitophagy and Oxidative Stress

Mitochondria serve as both the primary source and the primary target of reactive oxygen species (ROS), thereby regulating apoptotic cell death, redox homeostasis, ATP production, energy conversion, cellular communication mechanisms, and immunity (Figure1). Increased mitochondrial ROS under metabolic stress or aging conditions can lead to mitochondrial dysfunction and damage (Pathak & Trebak, 2018). Mitochondria are dynamic organelles constantly undergoing fission and fusion, facilitating the formation of new mitochondria and the removal of damaged ones. The body continuously carries out these processes to maintain the functions and inheritance of mitochondria. However, when facing various challenges such as energy production deficits or encountering oxidative stress, the structure and function of mitochondria can be altered. Accumulation of dysfunctional mitochondria and increased reactive oxygen species can lead to oxidative stress within the cell, negatively impacting its health and functionality. At this point, a process called mitophagy comes into play. Mitophagy is a mechanism that selectively clears damaged or dysfunctional mitochondria, thereby preserving cellular health and restoring the functionality of healthy mitochondria (Wang et al., 2020).

Figure 1. Mitophagy in oxidative stress

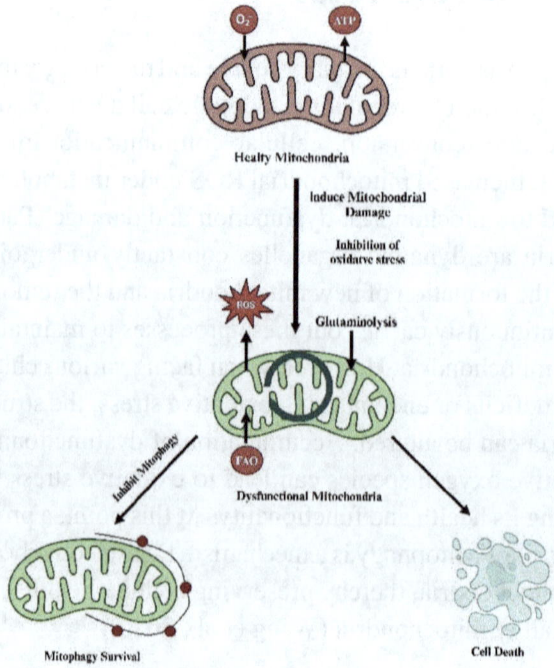

The mitophagy process consists of four main mechanisms: depolarization of damaged mitochondria, which causes loss of their membrane potential, a prerequisite for mitophagy formation; autophagosomes, double-membraned vesicles surrounding mitochondria, which fuse with lysosomes, initiating the process of degradation, with acidic hydrolases from lysosomes entering autophagosomes to degrade mitochondria (Xu et al., 2020).

Various proteins play roles in the mitophagy process. One of the proteins that plays a significant role is PINK-1, synthesized by the PINK-1 gene and consisting of 581 amino acids. Notably, PINK-1 possesses mitochondrial-specific targeting capability and serine/threonine kinase activity. Under normal conditions, the level of PINK-1 protein in a healthy mitochondrion is low. However, when there is a decrease in mitochondrial membrane potential, the proteolysis of PINK-1 is inhibited, leading to an increase in its concentration inside the mitochondrion. In a healthy mitochondrion, due to continuous transfer and rapid removal of PINK-1 protein from the mitochondrial inner membrane, the concentration of PINK-1 is very low and undetectable (Deas et al., 2011)

Another protein, PARKIN, the product of a gene consisting of twelve exons and a member of the E3 ligase family involved in the ubiquitin-proteasome degradation pathway, is translocated selectively to damaged mitochondria in case of a decrease in mitochondrial electrochemical gradient, suppression of mitochondrial fusion, or presence of toxic agents. PARKIN's specific substrates within the mitochondria are Mitofusin 1, 2, and voltage-dependent anion-selective channel protein 1 (VDAC1). Mitofusin 1 and 2 are responsible for initiating the fusion process between healthy and damaged mitochondria. However, they are tagged by Parkin to prevent the fusion of damaged mitochondria with a healthy one, thereby blocking mitochondrial fusion. VDAC1 protein is abundant in the outer mitochondrial membrane. Its amino-terminal acts as a voltage sensor and is also part of a channel that facilitates the passage of substances into the mitochondrion from the outside. Therefore, it is associated with the cell death process known as apoptosis. K27 ubiquitination prevents cell death and supports the mitophagic process, aiding in the clearance of damaged mitochondria (Chen & Chan, 2009; Chu, 2010).

Mitophagy operates through two main molecular mechanisms: the ubiquitin-dependent PINK1/Parkin-mediated pathway and the ubiquitin-independent receptor-mediated pathway (Kazlauskaite et al., 2015).

Ubiquitin-Dependent PINK1/Parkin Pathway

A decrease in mitochondrial membrane potential leads to the accumulation of PINK-1 protein, enabling the selective binding of Parkin, a member of the ubiquitin ligase family, to damaged mitochondria. This binding results in the ubiquitination of two proteins on the outer mitochondrial membrane, triggering the mitophagy process (Youle & Narendra, 2010). The PINK1/Parkin mitophagy pathway is activated under conditions such as oxidative stress, mitochondrial dysfunction, and damage. Following mitochondrial damage, a conformational change in Parkin activates cysteine, revealing its catalytic role and forming an E3 ubiquitin ligase. PINK1 coordinates with Parkin to regulate the mitophagy process, thus preserving mitochondrial quality. Loss of either protein can lead to mitochondrial damage. After mitochondrial damage, the spatial structure of Parkin changes, revealing the catalytic cysteine, leading to the formation of an activated E3 ubiquitin ligase (Riley et al., 2013). PINK1 interacts with Parkin to regulate mitophagy together, ensuring the preservation of mitochondrial quality. Loss of either protein may lead to mitochondrial damage. PINK1 accumulates on the outer mitochondrial membrane and later interacts with a protein called Parkin to regulate the mitophagy process (Kazlauskaite et al., 2015; Lazarou et al., 2015).During this process, the protein Sequestosome-1 (p62/SQSTM1) plays a significant role in the clearance of damaged mitochondria. Studies have shown that the interaction between PINK1/Parkin supports the accumulation of damaged mitochondria. In the absence of this protein, mitochondrial damage may increase. Additionally, it has been observed that while Parkin's translocation to mitochondria is not affected, it influences the destruction of damaged mitochondria. Accumulation of pSer65-Ubiquitin on the outer mitochondrial membrane activates autophagy receptors, initiating mitophagy. Ubiquitin chains assembled by Parkin bind to the TANK-binding kinase 1 (TBK1) complex, activating autophagy receptors. This mechanism ensures an effective mitophagy process and serves as a self-regulating feedback mechanism (Heo et al., 2018). It has been observed that Parkin expression is increased in some cancer cells (breast cancer, prostate cancer). This increase supports cell survival by maintaining mitochondrial homeostasis. Increased Parkin levels make cells more resistant to stress conditions and support tumor development (Ekta et al., 2021). In addition, it has been determined that PINK1-Parkin-mediated mitophagy in colorectal cancer and hepatocellular carcinoma reduces ROS production by clearing damaged mitochondria, ensures genome stability by preventing DNA damage and mutations, and thus suppresses tumor development (Poole & Macleod, 2021)

Ubiquitin-Independent Receptor-Mediated Pathway

In contrast to PINK1/Parkin-mediated mitophagy, a group of proteins located on the outer mitochondrial membrane acts as receptors initiating the autophagy process. These receptors function by directly binding to a protein called LC3 to initiate mitophagy. Among these receptors in mammals are proteins such as NIX/BNIP3L, BNIP3, and FUNDC1. A protein known as BNIP3L or NIX can initiate mitophagy by directly binding to LC3 (Novak et al., 2010). Similarly, BNIP3 is located on the outer mitochondrial membrane and can bind to LC3. Deficiency of BNIP3 significantly affects mitophagy, disrupting the cell's natural death process. BNIP3 and NIX proteins located on the surface of mitochondria are activated under hypoxic conditions and increase mitophagy. Cancer cells that adapt to hypoxia get rid of damaged mitochondria through mitophagy and reduce ROS production. Thus, they survive. This supports tumor growth (Poole & Macleod, 2021). Another protein, FUNDC1, interacts with the outer mitochondrial membrane to initiate mitophagy independently of Parkin(Liu et al., 2012). However, FUNDC1-mediated mitophagy, although independent of Parkin, can be regulated by another mitochondrial protein called MARCH5. The FUNDC1-mediated mitophagy process is controlled through both protein degradation and phosphorylation pathways (Z. Chen et al., 2017). High expression of FUNDC1 may have a tumor suppressive effect in some types of cancer, while it may inhibit cancer development in others. For example, in cervical cancer, FUNDC1 expression is inversely correlated with tumor progression and patient prognosis, suggesting that FUNDC1 plays a tumor suppressive role (Bernardini et.al., 2018).

THE ROLE OF MITOPHAGY IN SOME DISEASES

Cardiovascular diseases, metabolic disorders, neurodegenerative diseases, cancer, congenital immune problems, and some other diseases have been associated with impaired mitophagy function. For instance, neurodegenerative diseases like Alzheimer's disease (AD), Parkinson's disease (PD), Amyotrophic Lateral Sclerosis (ALS), and Huntington's disease (HD) often exhibit dysregulation in mitophagy mechanisms. In AD patients, abnormalities in mitophagy have been detected in the brain, contributing to disease progression by causing calcium accumulation and excessive phosphorylation of Tau protein(Magistretti et al., 2015). In PD, the effects of nitric oxide-mediated S-nitrosylation of Parkin and PINK1 on mitophagy may lead to the accumulation of damaged mitochondria (Rizza et al., 2018). In ALS, damaged mitochondria are believed to contribute to disease onset. In HD, the inability to remove damaged or dead mitochondria may lead to disease progression, and changes in mitochondrial number and size may be observed (Franco-Iborra et al., 2020).

Regarding cardiovascular diseases, there is a close relationship between the function of myocardial cells and mitochondrial quality control. Strengthening mitophagy has been shown to help protect the cardiovascular system by lowering blood pressure. A study demonstrated that increased expression of Parkin, PINK1, and mitochondrial DNA supports mitophagy, thus regulating hypertension (Y. Chen et al., 2020). In terms of cancer, different levels of mitophagy have been observed in various cancer types. High expression of NIX has been found in tumor cells such as lung cancer, breast cancer, cervical cancer, and prostate cancer. Additionally, excessive expression of FUNDC1, which has been shown to prevent hepatocellular carcinoma, is crucial in hepatocytes (Li et al., 2019). A study on metabolic diseases showed that Parkin-mediated mitophagy may preserve pancreatic islet secretion, thereby preventing the onset of type 1 diabetes. Symptoms of type 2 diabetes, such as hyperglycemia and insulin resistance, are often associated with mitochondrial damage because high glucose levels can increase reactive oxygen species production in the mitochondria, leading to oxidative stress (Rovira-Llopis et al., 2017).

The innate immune response provides a rapid response to pathogens or unwanted signals. Recent immunology research has shown that mitochondrial metabolism plays a critical role in innate immune function. Therefore, maintaining the integrity and activity of the mitochondrial network is crucial for a robust immune system (Gkikas et al., 2018).

In conclusion, understanding and regulating the molecular mechanism is crucial for the improvement of many diseases and functional disorders. With the increasing research on mitophagy in recent years, studies to understand how diseases are affected by mitophagy have gained momentum. However, some mechanisms are still not fully elucidated. Therefore, it is necessary to continue research to determine the effects of mitophagy on diseases. Although our understanding of mitophagy has significantly improved, it is essential to focus on developing promising potential therapeutic methods by identifying more specific targets.

OXIDATIVE STRESS INCREASES CANCER RISK

Mitochondria, one of the major sources of reactive oxygen species (ROS) contributing to oxidative stress within cells, play a crucial role in cellular physiology (Figure 2). The electron transport chain (ETC), located on the inner mitochondrial membrane, generates a majority of mitochondrial ROS during the process of oxidative phosphorylation (OXPHOS). Leakage of electrons from complexes I and III of the ETC partially reduces oxygen, leading to the formation of superoxide, which spontaneously dismutates to hydrogen peroxide, collectively considered as mitochondrial ROS (Arfin et al. 2021).

Figure 2. Mitochondria, one of the main sources of reactive oxygen species (ROS), play an important role in cellular physiology.

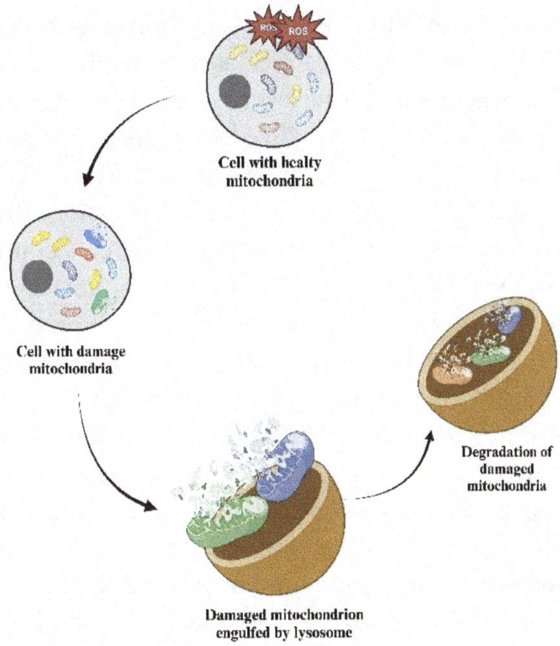

Endogenous modulators such as nitric oxide (NO) and calcium ions (Ca2+), have been observed to regulate mitochondrial ROS production by modulating the metabolic states of mitochondria. Mitochondrial Ca2+ levels enhance electron flow in the ETC, thereby reducing mtROS generation. However, excessive mitochondrial Ca2+ overload increases mtROS production. Additionally, cytokines such as interleukin (IL)-6 and IL-10 regulate gene expression in response to STAT3, a transcription factor that also modulates ETC activity. Therefore, a decrease in STAT3 expression may be associated with an increase in mtROS, particularly at complex I(Feissner et al. 2009; Peng and Jou 2010).

Studies have shown that tumor necrosis factor-alpha (TNF-α) induces an increase in mtROS, dependent on calcium, by triggering shedding of TNF-α receptor-1. Furthermore, various enzymes such as NADPH oxidase, xanthine oxidase, and uncoupled endothelial nitric oxide synthase (eNOS) have been demonstrated to stimulate mtROS production through a process known as "ROS-induced ROS"(Ceylan-Isik et al. 2009).

Another transcription factor, hypoxia-inducible factor 1-alpha (HIF-1α), plays a significant role in reducing ROS through mechanisms including induction of pyruvate dehydrogenase kinase 1 (PKD1) to divert pyruvate away from the mitochondria, triggering mitochondrial selective autophagy, and inducing microRNA-210, which blocks OXPHOS. Low mtROS levels regulate the stability of HIF-1α, leading to hypoxia adaptation, whereas moderate levels of mtROS have been found to regulate the production of proinflammatory cytokines by directly activating mitogen-activated protein kinase (MAPK). However, high levels of mtROS have the capacity to induce apoptosis through mitochondrial pore oxidation and oxidation of autophagy-specific gene 4 (ATG4), which triggers autophagy. Additionally, depending on the tumor cell microenvironment, the c-Myc gene regulates apoptosis by inducing aerobic glycolysis and/or OXPHOS, which are necessary for the activation of specific tumor-suppressor proteins such as Bax and Bak(Gao et al. 2009; Tomiyama et al. 2006; Wise et al. 2008).In summary, mitochondrial ROS production is a complex process with significant regulatory effects on cellular functions and pathophysiological processes.

Cancer cells adapt to meet increased energy demands through the oxygen-independent transport and metabolism of glucose, as well as by regulating the metabolism. Additionally, it has been observed that cancer cells suppress apoptosis by reducing mitochondrial respiration in the presence of oxygen. Under hypoxic conditions, increased production of reactive oxygen species (ROS) occurs as a result of accelerated metabolism; however, this increase is balanced by increased NADPH provided by upregulated glycolysis. NADPH is necessary for the regeneration of the antioxidant glutathione. Therefore, cancer cells both meet their metabolic requirements and keep oxidative stress under control. Transition between isoforms of pyruvate kinase, which is used in glycolysis, has been reported in tumor cells. This transition occurs due to increased production of NADPH by the slow PKM2 isoform. This creates a negative feedback loop by reducing ROS and reinforcing the inhibitory effect of PKM2. Among the genes regulated by ROS are hypoxia-inducible factors (HIF-1α). HIF-1α also regulates the production of the MYC protein, which in turn regulates genes involved in energy production. The condition known as the Warburg effect alters cancer cell metabolism, increasing oxidative stress. Increased oxidative stress is counteracted by its antioxidant effects before reaching cytotoxic levels. Recent studies indicate that tumor cells possess the ability to carry both glycolytic and oxidative phosphorylation (OXPHOS) metabolism, rendering them resistant to oxidative stress. Changes associated with energy metabolism are linked to the expression of specific genes regulated by p53. These changes enable cancer cells to combat oxidative stress by enhancing antioxidant response and detoxification capacity(Arfin et al. 2021; Schmidt et al. 2006; Won et al. 2012).

The protein kinase pathways activated by mitogens (MAPK), including extracellular signal-regulated kinases (ERKs), c-jun NH2-terminal kinases (JNKs), and p38 MAPKs, are regulated by various stimuli through MAPK cascades. The activity of these pathways can be influenced by different stress factors localized within the cell rather than receptor-ligand interactions. For instance, oxidative stress induced by reactive oxygen species (ROS) can activate MAPK pathways such as Proto-Oncogene, Serine/Threonine Kinase (Raf)/MEK/ERK, JNKs, or p38 MAPKs. The Phosphoinositide 3-Kinase (PI3K)/protein kinase B (Akt) pathway targets oxidative stress activation and contributes to a mechanism that upregulates SOD1 gene expression, thereby reducing ROS levels. Inhibition of Akt activation may lead to decreased levels of superoxide and SOD1. Abnormal PI3K/Akt signaling can increase ROS levels through modulation of mitochondrial bioenergetics and activation of NADPH oxidases, potentially contributing to higher ROS levels in cancer cells(Vatner et al. 2020). NADPH oxidases activated by PI3K/Akt can lead to increased ROS production. Heat shock proteins collaborate with the antioxidant system to inhibit or neutralize the cellular effects of ROS. These proteins can provide protection against DNA breaks when cells are exposed to genotoxic effects such as DNA fragmentation. Heat shock proteins may contribute to reducing oxidative stress by increasing the expression of ROS scavenging genes. p53 is a tumor suppressor protein that regulates the expression of genes involved in redox homeostasis(Noshita et al. 2003; Rojo et al. 2004), DNA replication and repair, autophagy, and apoptosis. Additionally, p53 plays a significant role in regulating mitochondrial biogenesis. p53 has dual roles associated with oxidative stress. Under conditions of low oxidative stress, p53 can increase antioxidant defense, while under severe oxidative stress, it can sensitize cells to oxidative stress by upregulating the expression of pro-oxidant genes. NF-κB plays a protective role against oxidative stress by suppressing ROS accumulation. It is known to intersect with a signaling pathway between ROS and cell death. While performing its anti-apoptotic function, NF-κB can contribute to apoptosis through inhibition via the JNK pathway. Additionally, NF-κB has numerous antioxidant targets and can play a pro-oxidant role in inducing NADPH oxidases. These signaling pathways and proteins play a significant role in cancer development and other cellular processes by affecting cells' ability to cope with oxidative stress. Therefore, understanding how oxidative stress is regulated and controlled at the cellular level is important for potenti (Shiber and Ravid 2014)al treatment and prevention strategies (Goh et al. 2011). In the fight against cancer, it is aimed to increase sensitivity to treatment by targeting the energy production, redox balance and cell death pathways of the cells. Cancer cells usually produce high levels of ROS due to metabolic reprogramming and mitochondrial dysfunction. This constitutes both vulnerabilities and treatment targets. Mitochondrial ROS production is closely related to mitophagy and apoptosis. Mitochondria-specific ROS-enhancing compounds (e.g. MitoQ derivatives) can selectively affect cancer cells. For example, MitoTam (tamoxifen targeted to mitochondria) triggers apoptosis by increasing ROS production in mitochondria.

CELLULAR ADAPTATİONS TO OXİDATİVE STRESS İN NORMAL CELLS

Oxidative stress is closely associated with the development of metabolic disorders. It refers to the imbalance between oxidative and antioxidative systems in cells and tissues. This imbalance arises from the excessive production of oxidative free radicals and reactive oxygen species (ROS). Elevated levels of ROS induce changes in the structure and function of cellular proteins and lipids, leading to cellular dysfunction, disturbances in energy metabolism, abnormalities in signal transduction and cell cycle control, impairment of intracellular transport mechanisms, and overall disruption of biological activity (Newsholme et al., 2016).

Living in an oxygen-rich environment is an inevitable consequence of oxidative stress. This results from byproducts of aerobic metabolism and exposure to various toxic substances. However, organisms cope with this stress through low oxygen levels and various defense mechanisms. These include antioxidant defense systems, damage repair and restoration mechanisms. Organisms attempt to minimize oxidative damage with mechanisms such as low tissue oxygen levels and antioxidant defense systems. Adaptation to oxidative stress activates cellular defense mechanisms and protects cells from damage. However, in cases of aging and excessive oxidative stress, cells can eliminate damaged cells through processes such as apoptosis or necrosis (Davies & Percy, 2000).

Over 90% of the oxygen used by living organisms is utilized for energy production through oxidative phosphorylation. This process occurs via the electron transport chain, resulting in the production of ATP and water. Reactive oxygen species (ROS), including superoxide anion (O2−), hydroxyl radical (. OH), hydrogen peroxide (H2O2), and singlet oxygen, are among the reactive species involved. Among these, ROS are the best characterized, while reactive nitrogen species (RNS), such as nitric oxide (.NO) and peroxynitrite (OONO−), are less studied. Other gas compounds such as .NO, carbon monoxide (CO), and hydrogen sulfide (H2S) also serve important regulatory functions (Li & Moore, 2007).

Cellular stress response is a vital mechanism for the body, as cells develop defense responses against damage caused by environmental factors. This response is activated based on macromolecular damage irrespective of the type of stress. There are connections between mechanisms triggered by both DNA and protein damage, sharing common elements. Other cellular responses are specific to the type of stress and are often activated in parallel with the cellular stress response. All organisms utilize stress proteins to cope with stress, forming the minimal stress proteome. Functional analysis of the minimal stress proteome provides insights into the major aspects of cellular stress response, including membrane lipid, protein and DNA damage sensing mechanisms, redox sensing and regulation, cell cycle control, macromolecular stabilization/repair, and energy metabolism control. Additionally, cells can determine stress levels and initiate programmed cell death (apoptosis) if tolerance limits are exceeded (Kültz, 2005).

In nature, plants encounter critical factors that reduce crop yield such as abiotic stresses like salinity, drought, and climate change. Responses to these stresses may lead to the uncontrolled accumulation of reactive oxygen species (ROS) in plant cells, resulting in irreversible metabolic disturbances and even death. Plants have evolved complex mechanisms to detect external signals that provide optimal responses to stressful conditions for survival. In this context, metabolic adaptation is considered a fundamental strategy for protecting and surviving plants under abiotic stress. In this context, the accumulation of proline plays a significant role. Recent proteomic, genomic, and metabolomic studies have shown that proline produced under stressful conditions may play various roles. Proline helps cells adapt to environmental stresses by participating in various biological functions; regulating osmotic balance, scavenging free radicals, chelating metal ions, activating ROS detoxification, maintaining cellular redox balance, regulating cytoplasmic pH balance, functioning as an energy and nutrient source, enhancing membrane stability, and even participating in intercellular signal transduction, thereby increasing cell resilience (Anwar Hossain et al., 2014).

The adaptive response of bacterial antioxidant systems to oxidative stress is coordinated by two main systems, SoxRS and OxyR, which provide stress responses induced by superoxide anions and hydrogen peroxide, respectively. In E. coli cells, a genetic locus known as soxR is responsible for the positive regulation of about nine proteins activated by approximately 40 superoxides. These proteins are induced at the transcriptional level and include important enzymes such as antioxidant manganese-superoxide dismutase, endonuclease IV repairing radical damage in DNA, and glucose-6-phosphate dehydrogenase. Induction of the SoxRS regulon also reduces the level of outer membrane protein (porin) F (OmpF) in bacteria and alters the level of small ribosomal protein S6. Therefore, the identified regulon functions as part of an adaptable protective system against foreign substances. The induction of the SoxRS regulon is also induced by other compounds such as nitric oxide radicals and hypochlorous acid, which can affect the resistance of bacteria to macrophages. OxyR protein serves as a sensor in E. coli cells, functioning in response to an increase in hydrogen peroxide levels and activating the oxidized form of transcription. This activation occurs through a direct oxidation process that activates the OxyR regulon. Reduced and oxidized forms of OxyR have different DNA binding properties and regulate the transcription of different genes depending on their oxidation status (Lushchak, 2011).

The survival of fungal species depends on their ability to detect and respond to changes in the natural environment. Environmental factors such as temperature, water balance, pH, as well as chemical assaults such as reactive oxygen and nitrogen species, disturb cellular balance and cause molecular damage in fungal cells. Therefore, fungi have evolved mechanisms to repair such damage, detoxify chemical assaults, and restore cellular homeostasis. Under stress conditions, fungal cells exhibit various responses. Heat shock increases the synthesis of chaperones that properly fold proteins. Antioxidants are synthesized to cope with oxidative stress. Osmotic levels increase after hyperosmotic shock, which increases water intake into the cell, restoring cellular balance (Brown et al., 2017).

Oxidative stress affects gene expression and directs cellular responses in many mammalian cells. Induction of a set of genes in response to specific oxidative stresses has been identified, including transcription factors, replication proteins, proteases, protease inhibitors, and proteins that affect cell proliferation. Antioxidants such as MnSOD are induced by various cytokines and oxidative stresses. Increased electron flow within mitochondria may require increased levels of MnSOD to maintain normal mitochondrial function following oxidative stress. Changes in cell growth are associated with the pathogenesis of many diseases; some cellular responses lead to cytotoxicity and cytostasis, while others may increase cell proliferation. For example, induction of the gadd genes following oxidative stress is associated with a halt in cell growth, allowing the cell to repair oxidative damage, thereby preventing the fixation of mutations caused by oxidative DNA damage. Increased mRNA expression and activity of ODC in cells exposed to UV or asbestos, on the other hand, increase cell proliferation. Additionally, increased mRNA expression of cellular proto-oncogenes following exposure to oxidants is associated with increased DNA synthesis or proliferation. AOS can interact with many target molecules such as proteins, lipids, and DNA, triggering signals involving activation of transcription factors and regulation of genes or regulons involved in oxidative stress response. Consequently, many proteins are produced, including DNA repair enzymes, antioxidants, protease inhibitors, cytokines, and proteins that affect cell proliferation. These cellular responses can contribute to the restoration of normal cellular functions and adaptation to oxidative stress while also leading to cell death or abnormal proliferation. Therefore, understanding cellular responses to oxidative stress contributes significantly to the understanding of the pathophysiology and treatment of various disease conditions (Hu et al., 2024). In studies conducted on rat gastrocnemius muscle, exercise induced the activation of mitogen-activated protein kinases (MAPKs: p38, ERK 1, and ERK 2) and consequently activated nuclear factor κB (NF-κB). This activation increased the expression of important enzymes for cellular defense (superoxide dismutase) and other enzymes associated with exercise adaptation (eNOS and iNOS). However, when RONS production was inhibited by allopurinol, all these changes were observed to be abolished. These findings provide evidence for the first time that reducing RONS formation significantly affects the MAPK–NF-κB signaling pathway (Gomez-Cabrera et al., 2005).

CONCLUSION

In the fight against cancer, the aim is to increase the sensitivity of cells to treatment by targeting their energy production, redox balance and cell death pathways. Cancer cells usually produce high levels of ROS due to metabolic reprogramming and mitochondrial dysfunction. This constitutes both weaknesses and treatment targets. Mitochondrial ROS production is closely related to mitophagy and apoptosis. Mitochondria-specific ROS-enhancing compounds (e.g. MitoQ derivatives) can selectively affect cancer cells. For example, MitoTam (tamoxifen targeted to mitochondria) triggers apoptosis by increasing ROS production in mitochondria.

Mitophagy plays an important role in the control of oxidative stress. Clearing damaged mitochondria helps reduce ROS production. However, excessive activation or inhibition of mitophagy can lead to an imbalance of ROS levels, affecting the survival of cancer cells or their resistance to treatment. For example, the effect of Parkin on glycolysis may shape the energy production strategies of cancer cells and their response to treatment.

Considering that ROS shed light on mitophagy, the examination of prooxidants becomes important. The knowledge that superoxide can direct Parkin-Pink-mediated mitophagy may lead us to examine the p38 signaling pathway. As a result, the importance of focusing on the mitochondrial microenvironment in order to fully understand the balance of oxidative stress and mitophagy in cancer and to develop targeted therapies emerges. The determination of new agents that will target the redox balance, prooxidant concentration, energy metabolism, Ubiquitin-independent receptor-mediated pathway, Ubiquitin-dependent PINK1/Parkin pathway and signaling pathway molecules in the mitochondrial microenvironment or the adaptation of existing agents to dose changes in this microenvironment will increase the effect on preventing cancer development or tumor suppression.

REFERENCES

Agarwal, E., Goldman, A. R., Tang, H. Y., Kossenkov, A. V., Ghosh, J. C., Languino, L. R., Vaira, V., Speicher, D. W., & Altieri, D. C. (2021). A cancer ubiquitome landscape identifies metabolic reprogramming as target of Parkin tumor suppression. *Science Advances*, *7*(35), eabg7287. DOI: 10.1126/sciadv.abg7287 PMID: 34433563

Anwar Hossain, M., Hoque, M. A., Burritt, D. J., & Fujita, M. (2014). Proline Protects Plants Against Abiotic Oxidative Stress: Biochemical and Molecular Mechanisms. Oxidative Damage to Plants: *Antioxidant Networks and Signaling*, 477–522. DOI: 10.1016/B978-0-12-799963-0.00016-2

Arfin, S., Jha, N. K., Jha, S. K., Kesari, K. K., Ruokolainen, J., Roychoudhury, S., Rathi, B., & Kumar, D. (2021). Oxidative Stress in Cancer Cell Metabolism. *Antioxidants*, *10*(5), 642. DOI: 10.3390/antiox10050642 PMID: 33922139

Bernardini S, Tiezzi A, Laghezza Masci V, Ovidi E. (2018). Natural products for human health: an historical overview of the drug discovery approaches. *Nat Prod Res*. Aug;32(16):1926-1950. .DOI: 10.1080/14786419.2017.1356838

Brown, A. J. P., Cowen, L. E., di Pietro, A., & Quinn, J. (2017). Stress Adaptation. *Microbiology Spectrum*, *5*(4), 5.4.04. Advance online publication. DOI: 10.1128/microbiolspec.FUNK-0048-2016 PMID: 28721857

Ceylan-Isik, A. F., Guo, K. K., Carlson, E. C., Privratsky, J. R., Liao, S. J., Cai, L., Chen, A. F., & Ren, J. (2009). Metallothionein Abrogates GTP Cyclohydrolase I Inhibition-Induced Cardiac Contractile and Morphological Defects Role of Mitochondrial Biogenesis. *Hypertension*, *53*(6), 1023–1031. DOI: 10.1161/HYPERTENSIONAHA.108.123422 PMID: 19398661

Chen, H., & Chan, D. C. (2009). Mitochondrial dynamics–fusion, fission, movement, and mitophagy–in neurodegenerative diseases. *Human Molecular Genetics*, *18*(R2), R169–R176. DOI: 10.1093/hmg/ddp326 PMID: 19808793

Chen, Y., Li, S., Guo, Y., Yu, H., Bao, Y., Xin, X., & Jia, D. (2020). Astaxanthin attenuates hypertensive vascular remodeling by protecting vascular smooth muscle cells from oxidative stress-induced mitochondrial dysfunction. *Oxidative Medicine and Cellular Longevity*, *2020*, 1–19. PMID: 32351673

Chen, Z., Liu, L., Cheng, Q., Li, Y., Wu, H., Zhang, W., Wang, Y., Sehgal, S. A., Siraj, S., Wang, X., Wang, J., Zhu, Y., & Chen, Q. (2017). Mitochondrial E3 ligase MARCH5 regulates FUNDC1 to fine-tune hypoxic mitophagy. *EMBO Reports*, *18*(3), 495–509. DOI: 10.15252/EMBR.201643309/SUPPL_FILE/EMBR201643309-SUP-0009-SDATAEV.ZIP PMID: 28104734

Chu, C. T. (2010). A pivotal role for PINK1 and autophagy in mitochondrial quality control: Implications for Parkinson disease. *Human Molecular Genetics*, *19*(R1), R28–R37. DOI: 10.1093/hmg/ddq143 PMID: 20385539

Davies, K. J. A., & Percy, E. (2000). Oxidative Stress, Antioxidant Defenses, and Damage Removal, Repair, and Replacement Systems. *IUBMB Life*, *50*(4–5), 279–289. DOI: 10.1080/713803728 PMID: 11327322

Deas, E., Plun-Favreau, H., Gandhi, S., Desmond, H., Kjaer, S., Loh, S. H. Y., Renton, A. E. M., Harvey, R. J., Whitworth, A. J., Martins, L. M., Abramov, A. Y., & Wood, N. W. (2011). PINK1 cleavage at position A103 by the mitochondrial protease PARL. *Human Molecular Genetics*, *20*(5), 867–879. DOI: 10.1093/hmg/ddq526 PMID: 21138942

Feissner, R. F., Skalska, J., Gaum, W. E., & Sheu, S. S. (2009). Crosstalk signaling between mitochondrial Ca2+ and ROS. Frontiers in bioscience: a journal and virtual library, 14(4), 1197. DOI: 10.2741/3303

Franco-Iborra, S., Plaza-Zabala, A., Montpeyo, M., Sebastian, D., Vila, M., & Martinez-Vicente, M. (2021). Mutant HTT (huntingtin) impairs mitophagy in a cellular model of Huntington disease. *Autophagy*, *17*(3), 672–689. PMID: 32093570

Gao, P., Tchernyshyov, I., Chang, T. C., Lee, Y. S., Kita, K., Ochi, T., & Dang, C. V. (2009). c-Myc suppression of miR-23a/b enhances mitochondrial glutaminase expression and glutamine metabolism. *Nature*, *458*(7239), 762–765. PMID: 19219026

Gkikas, I., Palikaras, K., & Tavernarakis, N. (2018). The role of mitophagy in innate immunity. *Frontiers in Immunology*, *9*(JUN), 372184. DOI: 10.3389/FIMMU.2018.01283/BIBTEX PMID: 29951054

Goh, J., Enns, L., Fatemie, S., Hopkins, H., Morton, J., Pettan-Brewer, C., & Ladiges, W. (2011). Mitochondrial targeted catalase suppresses invasive breast cancer in mice. *BMC Cancer*, *11*(1), 1–12. DOI: 10.1186/1471-2407-11-191/FIGURES/6 PMID: 21605372

Gomez-Cabrera, M. C., Borrás, C., Pallardo, F. V., Sastre, J., Ji, L. L., & Viña, J. (2005). Decreasing xanthine oxidase-mediated oxidative stress prevents useful cellular adaptations to exercise in rats. *The Journal of Physiology*, *567*(1), 113–120. DOI: 10.1113/jphysiol.2004.080564 PMID: 15932896

Heo, J. M., Ordureau, A., Swarup, S., Paulo, J. A., Shen, K., Sabatini, D. M., & Harper, J. W. (2018). RAB7A phosphorylation by TBK1 promotes mitophagy via the PINK-PARKIN pathway. *Science Advances*, *4*(11), eaav0443. Advance online publication. DOI: 10.1126/sciadv.aav0443 PMID: 30627666

Hu, B., Ouyang, Y., Zhao, T., Wang, Z., Yan, Q., Qian, Q., Wang, W., & Wang, S. (2024). Antioxidant Hydrogels: Antioxidant Mechanisms, Design Strategies, and Applications in the Treatment of Oxidative Stress-Related Diseases. *Advanced Healthcare Materials*, *13*(11), 2303817. DOI: 10.1002/adhm.202303817 PMID: 38166174

Kazlauskaite, A., Martínez-Torres, R. J., Wilkie, S., Kumar, A., Peltier, J., Gonzalez, A., Johnson, C., Zhang, J., Hope, A. G., Peggie, M., Trost, M., van Aalten, D. M., Alessi, D. R., Prescott, A. R., Knebel, A., Walden, H., & Muqit, M. M. (2015). Binding to serine 65-phosphorylated ubiquitin primes Parkin for optimal PINK 1-dependent phosphorylation and activation. *EMBO Reports*, *16*(8), 939–954. DOI: 10.15252/EMBR.201540352/SUPPL_FILE/EMBR201540352.REVIEWER_COMMENTS.PDF PMID: 26116755

Kultz, D. (2005). Molecular and evolutionary basis of the cellular stress response. *Annual Review of Physiology*, *67*(1), 225–257. DOI: 10.1146/ANNUREV.PHYSIOL.67.040403.103635/CITE/REFWORKS PMID: 15709958

Lazarou, M., Sliter, D. A., Kane, L. A., Sarraf, S. A., Wang, C., Burman, J. L., Sideris, D. P., Fogel, A. I., & Youle, R. J. (2015). The ubiquitin kinase PINK1 recruits' autophagy receptors to induce mitophagy. Nature 2015 524:7565, 524(7565), 309–314. DOI: 10.1038/nature14893

Li, L., & Moore, P. K. (2007). An overview of the biological significance of endogenous gases: New roles for old molecules. *Biochemical Society Transactions*, *35*(5), 1138–1141. DOI: 10.1042/BST0351138 PMID: 17956296

Li, W., Li, Y., Siraj, S., Jin, H., Fan, Y., Yang, X., & Chen, Q. (2019). FUN14 Domain-containing 1–mediated mitophagy suppresses hepatocarcinogenesis by inhibition of inflammasome activation in mice. *Hepatology (Baltimore, Md.)*, *69*(2), 604–621. DOI: 10.1002/hep.30191/suppinfo PMID: 30053328

Lushchak, V. I. (2011). Adaptive response to oxidative stress: Bacteria, fungi, plants, and animals. *Comparative Biochemistry and Physiology. Toxicology & Pharmacology : CBP*, *153*(2), 175–190. DOI: 10.1016/j.cbpc.2010.10.004 PMID: 20959147

Magistretti, P. J., & Allaman, I. (2015). A cellular perspective on brain energy metabolism and functional imaging. *Neuron*, *86*(4), 883–901. DOI: 10.1016/j.neuron.2015.03.035 PMID: 25996133

Newsholme, P., Cruzat, V. F., Keane, K. N., Carlessi, R., & De Bittencourt, P. I. H.Jr. (2016). Molecular mechanisms of ROS production and oxidative stress in diabetes. *The Biochemical Journal*, *473*(24), 4527–4550. DOI: 10.1042/BCJ20160503C PMID: 27941030

Noshita, N., Sugawara, T., Lewén, A., Hayashi, T., & Chan, P. H. (2003). Copper-zinc superoxide dismutase affects Akt activation after transient focal cerebral ischemia in mice. *Stroke, 34*(6), 1513–1518. DOI: 10.1161/01.STR.0000072986.46924.F4 PMID: 12738898

Novak, I., Kirkin, V., McEwan, D. G., Zhang, J., Wild, P., Rozenknop, A., Rogov, V., Löhr, F., Popovic, D., Occhipinti, A., Reichert, A. S., Terzic, J., Dötsch, V., Ney, P. A., & Dikic, I. (2010). Nix is a selective autophagy receptor for mitochondrial clearance. *EMBO Reports, 11*(1), 45–51. DOI: 10.1038/embor.2009.256 PMID: 20010802

Pathak, T., & Trebak, M. (2018). Mitochondrial Ca^{2+} signaling. *Pharmacology & Therapeutics, 192*, 112–123. DOI: 10.1016/j.pharmthera.2018.07.001 PMID: 30036491

Peng, T. I., & Jou, M. J. (2010). Oxidative stress caused by mitochondrial calcium overload. *Annals of the New York Academy of Sciences, 1201*(1), 183–188. DOI: 10.1111/j.1749-6632.2010.05634.x PMID: 20649555

Poole LP, Macleod KF. (2021). Mitophagy in tumorigenesis and metastasis. *Cell Mol Life Sci*. Apr;78(8):3817-3851. .DOI: 10.1007/s00018-021-03774-1

Riley, B. E., Lougheed, J. C., Callaway, K., Velasquez, M., Brecht, E., Nguyen, L., Shaler, T., Walker, D., Yang, Y., Regnstrom, K., Diep, L., Zhang, Z., Chiou, S., Bova, M., Artis, D. R., Yao, N., Baker, J., Yednock, T., & Johnston, J. A. (2013). Structure and function of Parkin E3 ubiquitin ligase reveals aspects of RING and HECT ligases. *Nature Communications, 4*(1), 1–9. DOI: 10.1038/ncomms2982 PMID: 23770887

Rizza, S., Cardaci, S., Montagna, C., Di Giacomo, G., De Zio, D., Bordi, M., Maiani, E., Campello, S., Borreca, A., Puca, A. A., Stamler, J. S., Cecconi, F., & Filomeni, G. (2018). S-nitrosylation drives cell senescence and aging in mammals by controlling mitochondrial dynamics and mitophagy. *Proceedings of the National Academy of Sciences of the United States of America, 115*(15), E3388–E3397. DOI: 10.1073/pnas.1722452115 PMID: 29581312

Rojo, A. I., Salinas, M., Martín, D., Perona, R., & Cuadrado, A. (2004). Regulation of Cu/Zn-Superoxide Dismutase Expression via the Phosphatidylinositol 3 Kinase/Akt Pathway and Nuclear Factor-κB. *The Journal of Neuroscience : The Official Journal of the Society for Neuroscience, 24*(33), 7324–7334. DOI: 10.1523/JNEUROSCI.2111-04.2004 PMID: 15317858

Schmidt, M. W., Connolly, J. A. D., Günther, D., & Bogaerts, M. (2006). Element partitioning: The role of melt structure and composition. *Science*, *312*(5780), 1646–1650. DOI: 10.1126/SCIENCE.1126690/SUPPL_FILE/SCHMIDT.SOM.PDF PMID: 16778055

Shiber, A., & Ravid, T. (2014). Chaperoning Proteins for Destruction: Diverse Roles of Hsp70 Chaperones and their Co-Chaperones in Targeting Misfolded Proteins to the Proteasome. *Biomolecules*, *4*(3), 704–724. DOI: 10.3390/biom4030704 PMID: 25036888

Tomiyama, A., Serizawa, S., Tachibana, K., Sakurada, K., Samejima, H., Kuchino, Y., & Kitanaka, C. (2006). Critical Role for Mitochondrial Oxidative Phosphorylation in the Activation of Tumor Suppressors *Bax and Bak.Journal of the National Cancer Institute*, *98*(20), 1462–1473. DOI: 10.1093/jnci/djj395 PMID: 17047195

Vatner, S. F., Zhang, J., Oydanich, M., Berkman, T., Naftalovich, R., & Vatner, D. E. (2020). Healthful aging mediated by inhibition of oxidative stress. *Ageing Research Reviews*, *64*, 101194. DOI: 10.1016/j.arr.2020.101194 PMID: 33091597

Wise, D. R., Deberardinis, R. J., Mancuso, A., Sayed, N., Zhang, X. Y., Pfeiffer, H. K., Nissim, I., Daikhin, E., Yudkoff, M., McMahon, S. B., & Thompson, C. B. (2008). Myc regulates a transcriptional program that stimulates mitochondrial glutaminolysis and leads to glutamine addiction. *Proceedings of the National Academy of Sciences of the United States of America*, *105*(48), 18782–18787. DOI: 10.1073/pnas.0810199105 PMID: 19033189

Won, K. Y., Lim, S. J., Kim, G. Y., Kim, Y. W., Han, S. A., Song, J. Y., & Lee, D. K. (2012). Regulatory role of p53 in cancer metabolism via SCO2 and TIGAR in human breast cancer. *Human Pathology*, *43*(2), 221–228. DOI: 10.1016/j.humpath.2011.04.021 PMID: 21820150

Chapter 2
Autophagy and Mitophagy in Cancer Metabolic Remodeling

Arbab Husain
Mangalayatan University, India

Afreen Khanam
Mangalayatan University, India

Neha Agarwal
https://orcid.org/0009-0000-5079-3959
Aligarh Muslim University, India

Diksha Sharma
https://orcid.org/0009-0009-7772-7973
Mangalayatan University, India

Mohd Farhan
https://orcid.org/0000-0002-1519-9644
King Faisal University, Saudi Arabia

Mohammad Aatif Aatif
King Faisal University, Saudi Arabia

ABSTRACT

Autophagy and mitophagy are vital for cellular homeostasis, especially in cancer metabolic remodeling, where they play complex roles in both tumor suppression and promotion. Autophagy, a recycling mechanism, helps cancer cells survive by recycling nutrients and generating energy, influencing pathways like glycolysis and oxidative phosphorylation, essential for proliferation. Mitophagy, the selective degradation of mitochondria, ensures mitochondrial quality, maintaining energy and regulating ROS levels, aiding adaptation to hypoxic, nutrient-deprived conditions. The chapter also examines the therapeutic potential of targeting autophagy and mitophagy in cancer. While these processes can contribute to resistance against chemotherapy and radiotherapy, emerging strategies aim to modulate them for improved treatment outcomes. Case studies and clinical trials offer insights into current therapies, highlighting successes and challenges. Ongoing research and personalized medicine approaches offer promising avenues for innovative cancer treatments.

DOI: 10.4018/979-8-3693-3836-0.ch002

1. INTRODUCTION

Cancer metabolism is a multifaceted and ever-evolving phenomenon that plays a pivotal role in malignant cells' unrestrained proliferation and persistence. Cancer cells have reprogrammed their metabolic pathways to support their rapid growth and division, particularly emphasizing elevated fatty acid synthesis and altered nutrient utilization. Understanding the intricate interactions within cancer metabolism is crucial for the development of effective therapeutic strategies (Yang et al., 2024; Jang et al., 2013). Targeting specific metabolic pathways that are dysregulated in different cell populations can be pursued by targeting various genes and pathways with a combination of drugs (DeBerardinis and Chandel, 2016). Cancer cells exhibit altered metabolism as compared to normal cells; a phenomenon known as the Warburg effect. The Warburg effect describes the preference of cancer cells for aerobic glycolysis, even in the presence of oxygen (Barba et al., 2024; Vander Heiden et al., 2009). This phenomenon is linked to the activation of oncogenes or the loss of tumor suppressors, thereby advancing cancer progression (Jang et al., 2013). Understanding the mechanisms of aerobic glycolysis may present a new basis for cancer treatment. Thus, targeting the lactate fermentation and/or cancer-promoting sites of other metabolic pathways could provide an interesting strategy to block tumor development. The 'Warburg Effect' or high rates of glycolysis and lactate production observed in cancer cells has additionally shown glucose dependence that suggests an avenue for therapeutic intervention (Jang et al., 2013; Seyfried et al., 2025). A common observation has been that the more aggressive tumors are capable of converting a higher portion of glucose into ATP in glycolysis. Cancer cells inescapably perform high levels of glycolysis and lactate fermentation, which presents a loophole to chemically inhibit glucose utilization for new development. This is what enables cancer cells to make sufficient ATP and the various biomolecules needed for their unabated proliferation (Chen et al., 2025; Yang et al., 2024). It also promotes the accumulation of lactate and acidifies the tumor microenvironment (TME), which can promote tumor progression and invasion. This metabolic reprogramming is driven by oncogenes and tumor suppressor genes, leading to altered expression of metabolic enzymes and transport proteins, as well as changes in signaling pathways (Lee et al., 2023). These alterations in metabolism provide cancer cells with a selective advantage and support their survival and proliferation. Cancer cells also rewire their metabolism to support high rates of nucleotide and lipid synthesis, as well as to adapt to nutrient-poor conditions within the tumour microenvironment. Cancer cells also exhibit increased resistance to cell death, allowing them to evade the normal regulatory processes that would eliminate damaged or abnormal cells. This metabolic flexibility enables cancer cells to survive and thrive in diverse and challenging microenvironments (Martínez-Reyes and Chandel, 2021). In addition, cancer cells often display an increased reliance on glutamine metabolism to support their growth and survival. This metabolic reprogramming is a hallmark of cancer cells (fig. 1), enabling them to adapt to the unfavourable conditions in the tumor microenvironment (TME) characterized by low oxygen, high oxidative stress, acidity, and limited nutrients (Lee et al., 2023). Cancer cells exploit this metabolic reprogramming to produce macromolecules and oncometabolites, leading to the six hallmarks of cancer, including deregulated consumption of glucose and amino acids, alterations of metabolic gene-driven regulations, and glycolysis/tricarboxylic acid (TCA) cycle intermediates being used for macromolecule synthesis (Jacobo-Herrera and Ozsvari., 2023) This metabolic flexibility enables cancer cells to survive and thrive in diverse and challenging microenvironments. In addition to glycolysis, cancer cells also exhibit altered mitochondrial function. Mitochondria are the primary site of energy production in normal cells, but in cancer cells, they are often dysfunctional or altered in their function (Martínez-Reyes and Chandel, 2021). This alteration in mitochondrial function can lead to the production of reactive oxygen species (ROS), which can damage cellular components and contribute to the development of cancer (Jang et al., 2013)._Along with this, cancer cells often display an increased reliance on glutamine metabolism to support their growth and survival. This metabolic adaptation allows cancer cells to maintain high rates of nucleotide and lipid synthesis, as well as to adapt to nutrient-poor conditions within the tumor microenvironment. This reliance on glutamine metabolism provides cancer cells with the necessary building blocks for proliferation and survival (Halama and Suhre, 2022). Glutamine also plays a critical role in replenishing the tricarboxylic acid (TCA) cycle intermediates, which are essential for energy production and biosynthesis. Glutamine is also a precursor for the synthesis of antioxidants that protect cancer cells from oxidative stress. Overall, the increased reliance on glutamine metabolism by cancer cells supports their growth and survival by providing necessary building blocks for proliferation, replenishing TCA cycle intermediates, and synthesizing antioxidants for protection from oxidative stress (Wei et al., 2021). This reliance on glutamine metabolism is a key hallmark of cancer metabolism, allowing cancer cells to thrive in challenging microenvironments and resist cell death. It also provides cancer cells with the necessary resources for survival and proliferation. Glutamine metabolism is a key feature of cancer metabolism, allowing cancer cells to adapt and thrive in diverse and nutrient Glutamine metabolism allows cancer cells to adapt and thrive in diverse and nutrient-poor environments (Cruzat et al., 2018). Research of cancer metabolism is now a broad term that covers several aspects such as glucose, fatty acid, nucleotide, and amino acid biosynthesis. (Yang et al., 2024) demonstrate the reprogramming of cancer cells by increasing the expression of oncogenes and reducing tumor-suppressor gene activity. To survive, cancer cells must reprogram their metabolism and efficiently remodel cellular bioenergetics to the harsh conditions of TME. The pattern of metabolism used by cancer cells is characteristically quite varied because the metabolic behaviour of nutrients in cancer cells depends on different modes and this can be driven to a significant extent, although not always exclusively so; by numerous genetic changes as well as epigenetic modifications that disturb several master gene regulators for key genes controlling energy metabolism. Cancer metabolism is now an area of intense investigation covering a variety of ground-breaking strategies to target metabolic pathways (Rayes and Chandel, 2021).

Cancer cells undergo profound metabolic reprogramming to support rapid proliferation, survival, and adaptation to the tumor microenvironment (TME) (Lee et al., 2023). Metabolic remodelling in cancer progression is a crucial process that allows cancer cells to adapt to the changing microenvironment and sustain their growth and survival. This process involves the reprogramming of cellular metabolism to meet the increased energy and biosynthetic demands of the cancer cells. The shift from oxidative phosphorylation to glycolysis, even in the presence of sufficient oxygen, is a key feature of metabolic reprogramming in cancer cells (Martínez-Reyes and Chandel, 2021). This process is mediated by the activation of oncogenes and the loss of tumor suppressor genes, leading to the upregulation of glycolytic enzymes and the downregulation of mitochondrial biogenesis and function (Jang et al., 2013)

Understanding the mechanisms and implications of cancer metabolism has become a major focus in oncology research. The complex interplay between oncogenic Signaling, the TME, and metabolic reprogramming is crucial for developing effective cancer therapies (Lee et al., 2023). By targeting the unique metabolic features of cancer cells, researchers aim to selectively kill tumor cells while sparing normal tissues, ultimately improving patient outcomes.

Figure 1. The diagram illustrates the ten hallmarks of cancer, representing key biological capabilities acquired during tumor development and progression.

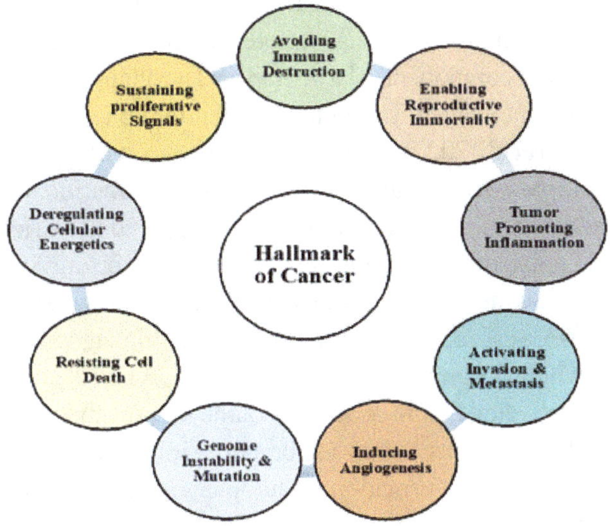

2. AUTOPHAGY: MECHANISM AND SIGNIFICANCE

Autophagy is a vital cellular process that plays a crucial role in maintaining cellular homeostasis and ensuring the survival of cells under various conditions (Voronina et al., 2024; Hippert et al., 2006). Its mechanism involves the formation of autophagosomes, which engulf and digest cellular components, and its significance extends to the regulation of cellular metabolism and energy homeostasis, as well as its role in various diseases (Nakatogawa et al., 2009). It is essential for the removal of misfolded or aggregated proteins, clearing damaged organelles, and eliminating intracellular pathogens (Glick et al., 2010). It helps to maintain the balance between energy production and consumption by removing damaged or dysfunctional organelles and proteins that can impede cellular function (Cao et al., 2021). Furthermore, autophagy has been implicated in various diseases, including cancer, neurodegeneration, cardiomyopathy, diabetes, liver disease, autoimmune diseases, and infections (fig. 2). The dysregulation of autophagy has been linked to the development and progression of these diseases, highlighting its importance in maintaining cellular health (Glick et al., 2010). Autophagy involves the formation of autophagosomes, which are double-membraned vesicles that engulf cellular components and then fuse with lysosomes to form autophagolysosomes (Pyo et al., 2012).

The autophagosomes are formed through the interaction of several key proteins, including the autophagy-related (ATG) genes, which are highly conserved across eukaryotes (Shang et al., 2024; Nakatogawa et al., 2009). The process of autophagy is initiated by the formation of a phagophore, which is a membrane structure that surrounds the cellular component to be degraded. The phagophore then closes, forming an autophagosome, which is then transported to the lysosome for degradation (Ohsumi, 2014; Liu et al., 2024). The molecular pathways of autophagy are complex and involve multiple steps, including the initiation, formation, and maturation of autophagosomes. The initiation of autophagy is triggered by various cellular stress signals, such as nutrient deprivation, oxidative stress, or endoplasmic reticulum stress, which activate the autophagy-related (ATG) proteins (Debnath et al., 2023). The ATG proteins are essential for the generation of autophagosomes and include the ULK complex, which is composed of ULK1, ULK2, ATG13, and RBCC1/FIP200. This complex is activated by the serine-threonine kinase complex and AMPK, and it recruits other ATG proteins to the membranes to initiate autophagy (Kundu et al., 2008; Li et al., 2020). The formation of autophagosomes involves the nucleation and elongation of phagophore membrane, which is mediated by the class III phosphatidylinositol 3-kinase complex and ubiquitin-like conjugation systems (Yu et al., 2018). The phagophore membrane closes further to form an autophagosome, which contains the sequestered cytoplasmic material (Bui et al., 2025). The maturation of autophagosomes involves the fusion of autophagosomes with lysosomes, which is mediated by SNARE proteins, tethering factors, and adaptors (Yu et al., 2018). The autophagosome-lysosome fusion is a critical step in the autophagy process, as it allows the degradation and recycling of the sequestered cytoplasmic material. In addition to the molecular pathways of autophagy, recent studies have also identified new regulators of autophagosome maturation and degradation, including UVRAG, which is involved in the regulation of autophagosome-lysosome fusion (Glick et al., 2010; Liang et al., 2006).

To understand the molecular pathways of autophagy, it is important to look at the key players and regulators involved in this complex process. Several molecular pathways have been identified that govern the process of autophagy (Sabatini, 2006). One of the key players in autophagy is the serine/threonine protein kinase called mTOR (mammalian target of rapamycin) (Glick et al., 2010). mTOR acts as a central regulator for cell growth and metabolism, and it plays a critical role in inhibiting autophagy. mTOR achieves this inhibition through phosphorylation of downstream targets, including the Unc-51-like autophagy activating kinase 1(Shaw., 2009; Glick et al., 2010). Unc-51-like autophagy activating kinase 1 is another essential component in the initiation of autophagy. Upon activation, Unc-51-like autophagy-activating kinase 1 phosphorylates the class III phosphatidylinositol 3-kinase (PI3K) complex, leading to the formation of phosphatidylinositol 3-phosphate (PI3P) on the autophagosomal membrane (Li et al., 2020). This PI3P then recruits effector proteins such as WIPI, which help in the nucleation of autophagosomes. Another crucial regulator of autophagy is the microtubule-associated protein 1 light chain 3. Understanding the molecular mechanisms of autophagy is crucial for the development of therapeutic strategies for various diseases, including cancer, neurodegenerative disorders, and infectious diseases (Ortega et al., 2024; Hippert et al., 2006).

Autophagy plays a multifaceted role in various cellular processes, including the epithelial-mesenchymal transition (EMT) process, metabolic activity, immune response, cancer stem cell (CSC) promotion, cell progression and metastasis, multidrug resistance (MDR) stimulation, cell survival, and cell death. It is involved in modulating EMT, which is critical for cancer metastasis, while also influencing metabolic adaptations under stress. Autophagy affects the immune response by regulating inflammation and antigen presentation. Furthermore, it promotes CSC maintenance, aiding tumor persistence and resistance. By regulating cell progression and metastasis, autophagy contributes to cancer aggressiveness. It also stimulates MDR, enhancing cell survival against chemotherapy. Finally, autophagy plays a dual role in cell fate, promoting survival under stress or triggering cell death when damage is irreparable (Amaravadi et al., 2019; Mizushima & Levine, 2020) (fig. 3).

Figure 2. The figure illustrates the autophagy mechanism, where cells degrade and recycle damaged components to maintain homeostasis and prevent disease.

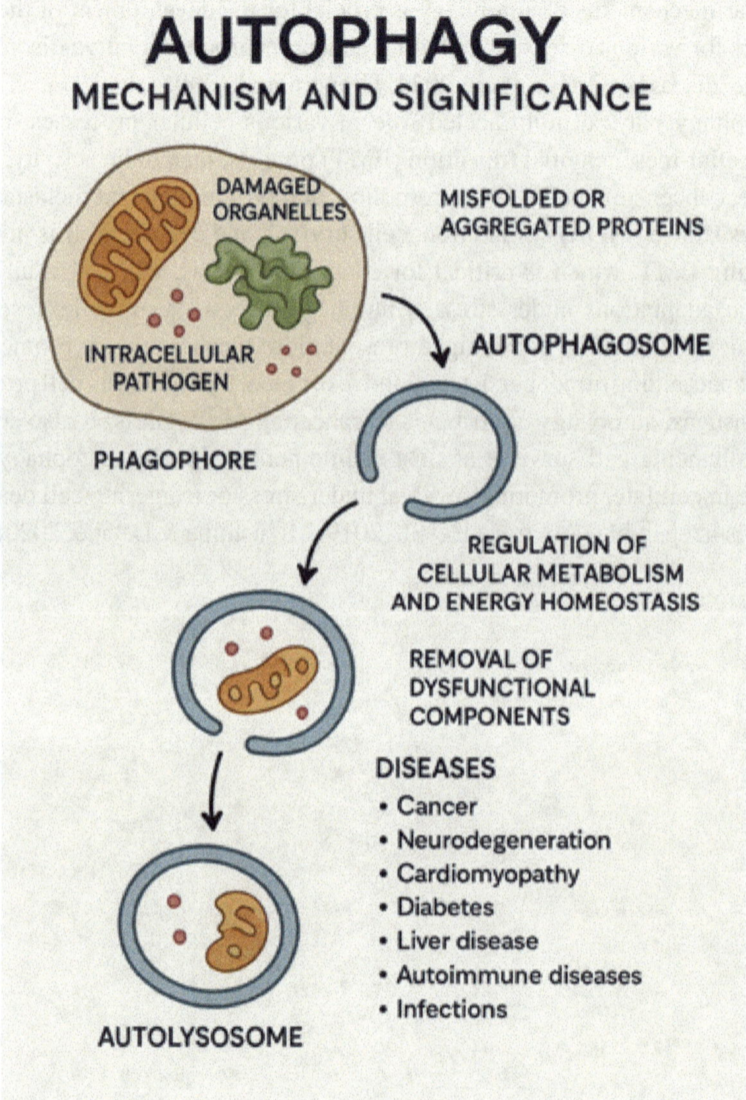

Figure 3. This diagram highlights the diverse roles of autophagy in cancer, including effects on EMT, metabolism, immune response, stem cell regulation, metastasis, drug resistance, cell survival, and cell death.

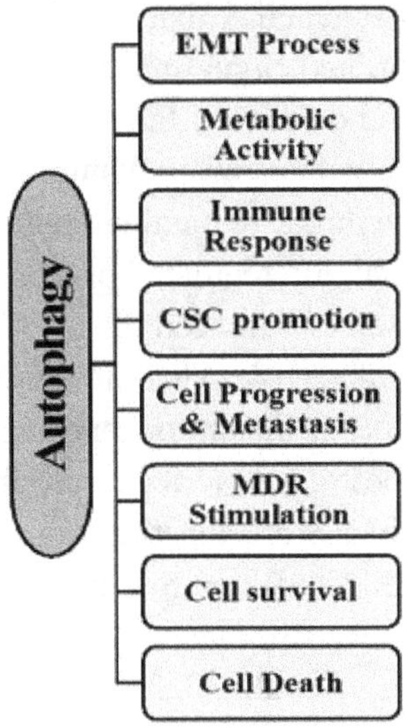

2.1. Mitophagy: Specific Role in Mitochondrial Quality Control

Mitophagy plays a vital role in maintaining mitochondrial quality control by selectively removing damaged or dysfunctional mitochondria from the cell. This process involves the engulfment of mitochondria by autophagosomes and their subsequent degradation within lysosomes, thereby ensuring the removal of defective mitochondria and maintaining the overall health and function of the mitochondrial network (Guan et al., 2021). Mitophagy is an extremely regulated process that is mediated by various mitophagy receptors and adaptors, such as PINK1 and Parkin, which recognize damaged mitochondria and mark them for degradation (Sauve et al., 2022). This process is essential for maintaining mitochondrial homeostasis and preventing the accumulation of damaged mitochondria, which can contribute to various diseases, including neurodegenerative disorders (Lee et al., 2023; Guan et al., 2021). Mitophagy is closely linked to other mitochondrial quality control pathways, such as mitochondrial biogenesis and dynamics, and works together with these pathways to maintain the overall health and function of the mitochondria. Defects in mitophagy have been involved in pathogenesis of several diseases, including neurodegenerative disorders, and enhancing mitophagy is being explored as a potential therapeutic strategy to mitigate these diseases (Antico et al., 2025; Durcan and Fon., 2015). In summary, mitophagy is a critical mechanism for maintaining mitochondrial quality control by selectively removing damaged mitochondria and ensuring the overall health and function of the mitochondrial network (Xu and Hu, 2022).

Mitochondria are essential organelles that play an important role in cellular energy production, metabolism, and Signaling. However, mitochondria can also be a source of cellular stress and damage if they become dysfunctional (Palma et al., 2024; Ney, 2015). Mitophagy, the selective autophagy of mitochondria, is an important mechanism that cells employ to maintain mitochondrial homeostasis and quality control. Mitophagy is a highly regulated process that involves the recognition, engulfment, and degradation of damaged or superfluous mitochondria by the lysosomal system (Palikaras et al., 2018). This process is mediated by specialized mitophagy receptors and adaptors that link mitochondria to the autophagy machinery (Durcan and Fon, 2015). The best-characterized mitophagy pathway involves the PINK1 and Parkin proteins, which work together to mark damaged mitochondria for degradation (Sauve et al., 2022). When mitochondria become depolarized or dysfunctional, PINK1 accumulates on the outer mitochondrial membrane and recruits the E3 ubiquitin ligase Parkin (Lee et al., 2023). Parkin then ubiquitinates various mitochondrial proteins, creating a signal for the autophagy machinery to recognize and engulf the mitochondria (McWilliams and Muqit, 2017). Other mitophagy pathways, such as those mediated by the mitophagy receptors NIX, BNIP3, and FUNDC1, also play important roles in mitochondrial quality control under different cellular conditions. Impaired mitophagy has been involved in the pathogenesis of various diseases, including neurodegenerative disorders, cardiovascular diseases, cancer, and metabolic disorders (Geisler et al., 2010; Ney, 2015). For example, defective mitophagy has been linked to the accumulation of damaged mitochondria and the subsequent induction of oxidative stress, inflammation, and cell death, all of which contribute to disease progression. Conversely, enhancing mitophagy has been proposed as a potential therapeutic strategy for these diseases (Xu and Hu, 2022). Pharmacological modulators of mitophagy, such as small molecules that target the PINK1-Parkin pathway or other mitophagy regulators, are actively being investigated for their therapeutic potential (Sauve et al., 2022). In conclusion, mitophagy is a critical mechanism for maintaining mitochondrial quality control and cellular homeostasis. Understanding the molecular mechanisms and regulation of mitophagy, as well as its role in disease pathogenesis, is an active area of research that holds promise for the development of new therapeutic interventions targeting mitochondrial dysfunction (Palikaras et al., 2018) (Figure 4).

Figure 4. This figure illustrates mitophagy as a selective mechanism for mitochondrial quality control. Damaged mitochondria are recognized by PINK1 and Parkin, ubiquitinated, and engulfed by autophagosomes via receptors like BNIP3, NIX, and FUNDC1. Fusion with lysosomes forms autolysosomes for degradation, reducing oxidative stress, preventing neurodegeneration, and maintaining cellular homeostasis.

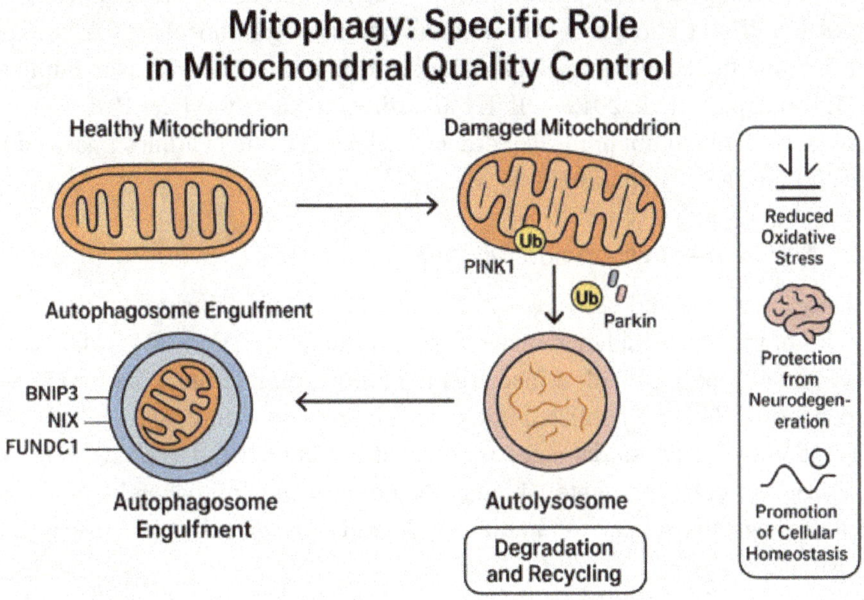

2.2. Mitophagy: Molecular Mechanisms and Pathways

Mitophagy, the selective elimination of mitochondria through autophagy, is a complex process involving multiple molecular mechanisms to ensure the removal of damaged or dysfunctional mitochondria from the cell. The molecular mechanisms of mitophagy can be broadly categorized into two main pathways: the PINK1-Parkin pathway and the NIX/Bnip3 pathway.

The PINK1-Parkin pathway is a key mechanism for mitochondrial quality control that is disrupted in Parkinson's disease (Durcan and Fon, 2015). PINK1 senses mitochondrial damage, recruits and activates Parkin, leading to mitophagy of dysfunctional mitochondria. This pathway is regulated by complex post-translational modifications of PINK1 and Parkin (Sauve et al., 2022) (fig 5).

2.2.1. PINK1 Activation and Recruitment of Parkin

Under normal conditions, the mitochondrial kinase PINK1 (PTEN-induced putative kinase 1) is imported into the inner mitochondrial membrane where it is rapidly degraded. However, when mitochondria are damaged and depolarized, PINK1 accumulates on the outer mitochondrial membrane (Sauve et al., 2022). Accumulated PINK1 phosphorylates ubiquitin at serine 65. Phosphorylated ubiquitin then recruits the E3 ubiquitin ligase Parkin to the mitochondria (Narendra et al., 2024; Kondapalli et al., 2012). PINK1 also directly phosphorylates Parkin at serine 65 in its N-terminal ubiquitin-like domain, which activates Parkin's ligase activity (McWilliams and Muqit, 2017).

2.2.1.1. Parkin Activation and Mitophagy

Once recruited and activated by PINK1, Parkin ubiquitinates multiple outer proteins of mitochondrial membrane proteins (Durcan and Fon, 2015). This creates a feedforward loop, as Parkin-mediated ubiquitination recruits more Parkin to the mitochondria. The ubiquitinated mitochondrial proteins serve as signals for mitophagy, the autophagy of damaged mitochondria (Durcan and Fon, 2015; Kong et al., 2025). Autophagy receptors bind to the ubiquitinated mitochondria and recruit the autophagy machinery to engulf and degrade the mitochondria (McWilliams and Muqit, 2017).

2.2.1.2. Regulation of the Pathway

The PINK1-Parkin pathway is tightly regulated by post-translational modifications. PINK1 itself is regulated by autophosphorylation, which enhances its ability to phosphorylate ubiquitin and Parkin (Mishra et al., 2024; Kondapalli et al., 2012). Parkin is also autoregulated, with its E3 ligase activity suppressed in the cytosol until activated by PINK1-mediated phosphorylation (McWilliams and Muqit, 2017).

2.2.2. NIX/Bnip3 Pathway

The NIX/Bnip3 pathway plays a crucial role in mitophagy by recognizing and targeting mitochondria for degradation by autophagosomes. NIX (BNIP3L) is an outer mitochondrial membrane protein that acts as a mitophagy receptor, recognizing and targeting mitochondria for degradation by autophagosomes (Li et al., 2021). This process is crucial for maintaining cellular homeostasis and is implicated in various biological and pathological processes. The regulation of NIX/Bnip3-mediated mitophagy is complex and involves multiple mechanisms, ensuring precise control over mitochondrial turnover (Palikaras et al., 2018).

2.2.2.1. Mechanism of NIX/Bnip3-Mediated Mitophagy

i. Recognition of Mitochondria:

NIX/Bnip3 binds to the mitochondrial outer membrane, recognizing specific mitochondrial markers such as LC3/GABARAP proteins, which are involved in autophagosome formation (Li et al., 2021).

ii. Autophagosome Recruitment:

NIX/Bnip3 recruits autophagosomes to target mitochondria, enhancing the development of autophagosomes and facilitating the engulfment of mitochondria by autophagosomes (Palikaras et al., 2018; Yamashita et al., 2025).

iii. Dimerization and Activation:

NIX/Bnip3 forms homodimers, which are essential for its mitophagic activity. This dimerization is regulated by phosphorylation events at specific sites, allowing the receptor to switch between proapoptotic and mitophagic functions (Marinkovic and Novak, 2021).

iv. Mitochondrial Elimination:

The autophagosomes containing engulfed mitochondria fuse with lysosomes, leading to the degradation of the mitochondria and the recycling of their components.

v. Biological Functions and Regulation:

- **Developmental Roles**

NIX/Bnip3 plays an essential role in the differentiation of reticulocytes and other cell types, where it regulates the mitochondrial elimination during terminal differentiation (Zhang and Ney, 2009).

- **Pathological Roles**

Dysregulation of NIX/Bnip3-mediated mitophagy has been associated with various human diseases, including cancer, neurological disorders, metabolic disorders, and cardiovascular diseases (Ney, 2015; Liang et al 2024).

- **Regulation**

NIX/Bnip3-mediated mitophagy is regulated at multiple levels, including transcriptional, post-translational, and homodimerization, allowing for precise control over mitochondrial turnover (Zhang and Ney, 2009; Niemi and Friedman, 2024).

2.2.2.2. Other Mechanisms

i. **Atg32 in Yeast**

In yeast, Atg32 is a receptor protein that localizes to the outer membrane of mitochondria and recruits Atg8, a key component of the autophagosome, to initiate mitophagy.

ii. **Phosphorylation of Atg32**

Phosphorylation of Atg32 by CK2 (casein kinase 2) enhances its interaction with Atg8, promoting mitophagy (Palikaras et al., 2018).

These molecular mechanisms ensure the selective elimination of damaged mitochondria, maintaining mitochondrial quality control and preventing the accumulation of dysfunctional mitochondria, which can contribute to various diseases (Zhang and Ney, 2009; Zong et al., 2024).

Figure 5. The diagram shows mitophagy's role in maintaining mitochondrial health and cellular function under physiological conditions, and its involvement in pathological conditions such as neurodegenerative diseases, cancer, metabolic disorders, Heart &Liver disorders and aging when dysregulated.

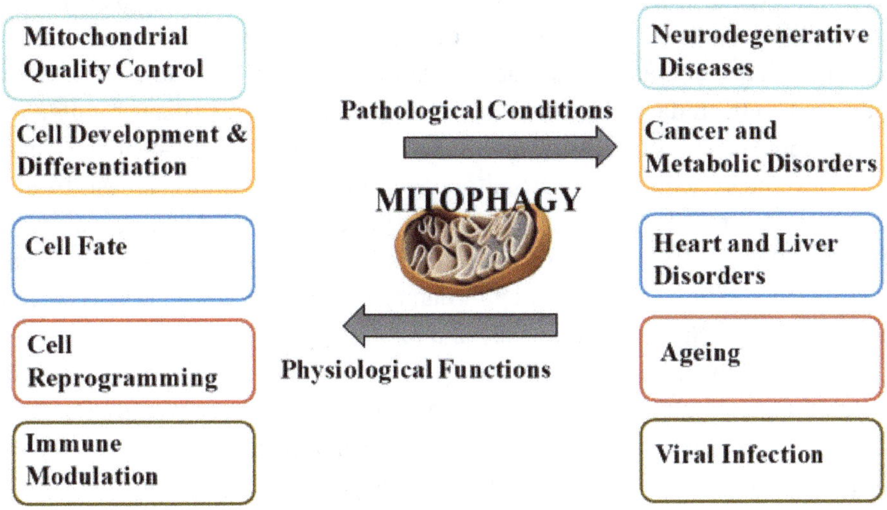

2.2.3. Relevance to Cancer

Why studying autophagy and mitophagy is crucial in cancer research. Autophagy and mitophagy are crucial cellular processes that have gained significant attention in recent years due to their multifaceted roles in cancer development and progression. These processes are essential for maintaining cellular homeostasis and quality control by degrading damaged organelles and proteins. In the context of cancer, understanding the mechanisms of autophagy and mitophagy is crucial for developing effective therapeutic strategies (Xu and Hu, 2022). Autophagy is a cellular process that involves the degradation of damaged organelles and proteins through the formation of autophagosomes, which then fuse with lysosomes to release the contents for recycling (Hippert et al., 2006; Settembre and Perera, 2024). This process is necessary for maintaining cellular homeostasis and quality control. In cancer, autophagy can have both tumor-suppressive and tumor-promoting effects, depending on the context (Li et al., 2020). For instance, autophagy can suppress cancer development by removing damaged organelles and proteins that can contribute to tumorigenesis (Pyo et al., 2012). However, under conditions of nutrient deprivation, autophagy can promote tumor growth and survival by providing energy and nutrients to the cells (Glick et al., 2010). Mitophagy, a form of autophagy, specifically targets damaged mitochondria for degradation (Guan et al., 2021). Mitochondria are critical for energy production and cellular metabolism, but they can also contribute to cancer development and progression by producing reactive oxygen species (ROS) and promoting cell survival (Bahar et al., 2022). Mitophagy plays an important role in maintaining mitochondrial homeostasis by amputating damaged mitochondria and preventing their accumulation, which can lead to increased ROS production and cell damage (Marinkovic and Novak, 2021). In cancer, mitophagy can have both tumor-suppressive and tumor-promoting effects, depending on the tumor type and stage. For instance, mitophagy can suppress tumorigenesis by eliminating damaged mitochondria that can contribute to cancer development further (Durcan and Fon, 2015). However, under conditions of chemotherapy, mitophagy can promote drug resistance by removing damaged mitochondria that can be targeted by chemotherapy. Studying autophagy and mitophagy is crucial in cancer research for several reasons. Firstly, understanding the mechanisms of these processes can provide insights into the development of effective therapeutic strategies for cancer treatment. For instance, modulating autophagy and mitophagy can be used to enhance the efficacy of chemotherapy and radiation therapy (Bahar et al., 2022). Secondly, studying these processes can provide insights into the molecular mechanisms of cancer development and progression, which can lead to the identification of new therapeutic targets. Finally, understanding the function of autophagy and mitophagy in cancer can provide insights into the development of novel diagnostic biomarkers for cancer (Pyo et al., 2012). In conclusion, studying autophagy and mitophagy is crucial in cancer research due to their multifaceted roles in cancer development and progression. These processes are vital for maintaining cellular homeostasis and quality control, and their dysregulation can contribute to cancer development and progression (Debnath et al., 2023). Understanding the mechanisms of autophagy and mitophagy can provide insights into the development of effective therapeutic strategies for cancer treatment and the identification of new therapeutic targets (Xu and Hu, 2022).

2.3. Cross-Talk Between Autophagy and Mitophagy

Autophagy and mitophagy are two closely intertwined cellular processes that play crucial roles in maintaining cellular homeostasis and preventing disease. The regulation of these processes involves a complex interplay of signaling pathways and molecular mechanisms, including the mTOR-AMPK axis and the Parkin-PINK1 pathway (Yu et al., 2018). Autophagy is a self-degradative process where cells recycle damaged or dysfunctional cellular components, such as proteins and organelles, to maintain cellular health (Chun and Kim, 2018). Mitophagy, a specific type of autophagy, is the process of selectively degrading damaged or dysfunctional mitochondria, which are essential for cellular energy production and maintenance (Lee et al., 2023).

Mitophagy is a critical component of the broader autophagy pathway, as it helps to remove damaged mitochondria that can contribute to cellular stress and disease (Gottlieb and Carreira, 2010). Mitophagy is essential for the selective removal of damaged or dysfunctional mitochondria, which can contribute to cellular stress and disease. The efficient removal of these harmful mitochondria through mitophagy is particularly important in long-lived, post-mitotic cells, such as cardiomyocytes and neurons, where the accumulation of defective mitochondria has been linked to the development of aging-related disorders (Zhang and Ney, 2009; Basak and Holzbaur, 2025).

Conversely, autophagy plays a crucial role in maintaining the quality and quantity of mitochondria by eliminating damaged or dysfunctional components, which can prevent the accumulation of defective mitochondria and the onset of mitophagy (Guan et al., 2021).

This interdependence is particularly evident in long-lived, post-mitotic cells, such as cardiomyocytes, neurons, and memory T cells, where the efficient removal of damaged mitochondria through mitophagy is essential for cellular homeostasis and function (Lee et al.,2023). The dysregulation of autophagy and mitophagy has been implicated in various diseases, including neurodegenerative disorders, cardiovascular diseases, and cancer. Understanding the intricate mechanisms underlying these processes and their roles in disease pathogenesis is crucial for the development of targeted therapeutic strategies (Zhang and Ney, 2009; Basak and Holzbaur, 2025).

As the field of autophagy and mitophagy research continues to evolve, the potential for therapeutic interventions targeting these processes holds promise for the treatment of a wide range of diseases. By modulating autophagy and mitophagy, researchers and clinicians may be able to harness the power of these fundamental cellular processes to improve human health and longevity (Gottlieb and Carreira, 2010).

2.3.1. Regulation of Autophagy and Mitophagy

The regulation of autophagy and mitophagy involves a complex interplay of molecular mechanisms and signaling pathways (fig. 6). The mammalian target of rapamycin (mTOR) and the 5′ adenosine monophosphate-activated protein kinase (AMPK) are key regulators of autophagy, with mTOR acting as a negative regulator while AMPK acting as a positive regulator (Sabatini, 2006). The activity of these kinases is influenced by various cellular signals, such as nutrient availability, energy status, and stress signals. Mitophagy, on the other hand, is regulated by a distinct set of molecular mechanisms, including the Parkin-PINK1 pathway (Zhang and Ney, 2009; Basak and Holzbaur, 2025). In this pathway, PINK1, a serine/threonine protein kinase, is recruited to damaged mitochondria, where it phosphorylates and activates the E3 ubiquitin ligase Parkin. Parkin then ubiquitinates mitochondrial proteins, marking them for degradation by autophagy (Lee et al., 2023).

2.3.1.1. Signaling Pathways and Molecular Mechanisms

The regulation of autophagy and mitophagy involves several signaling pathways and molecular mechanisms, including:

i. mTOR and AMPK Signaling

mTOR and AMPK are key regulators of autophagy, with mTOR acting as a negative regulator and AMPK acting as a positive regulator. The activity of these kinases is influenced by various cellular signals, such as nutrient availability, energy status, and stress signals (Shaw, 2009; Zamanian et al., 2024).

ii. Parkin-PINK1 Pathway

In this pathway, PINK1 is recruited to damaged mitochondria, where it phosphorylates and activates the E3 ubiquitin ligase Parkin. Parkin then ubiquitinates mitochondrial proteins, marking them for degradation by autophagy (Gehring, 2022).

iii. ULK1/ATG13/FIP200 Complex

This complex is essential for the formation of autophagosomes and is regulated by mTOR and AMPK (Shaw, 2009; Sankar et al., 2024).

BECN1 and BCL-2 Interaction

BECN1 (Beclin 1) interacts with BCL-2 to regulate autophagy, with BCL-2 inhibiting autophagy and BECN1 promoting it (Yu et al., 2018).

2.3.2. Mitochondrial Dynamics

Mitochondrial dynamics, including mitochondrial fusion and fission, play a significant role in regulating mitophagy. The balance between these processes can determine the fate of mitochondria, either leading to their degradation or preservation (Gottlieb and Carreira, 2010). These Signaling pathways and molecular mechanisms work in concert to fine-tune the regulation of autophagy and mitophagy, ensuring that these processes are responsive to various cellular cues and maintain cellular homeostasis (Bahar et al., 2022).

Figure 6. The figure illustrates the molecular pathways of autophagy and mitophagy. Autophagy is initiated by nutrient and energy deprivation via AMPK activation and mTOR1 inhibition, leading to phagophore formation and autophagosome development. Damaged mitochondria trigger mitophagy through Parkin-dependent or -independent mechanisms, especially under stress conditions like ROS and hypoxia. The autophagosome engulfs damaged mitochondria and fuses with lysosomes to form autolysosomes for degradation.

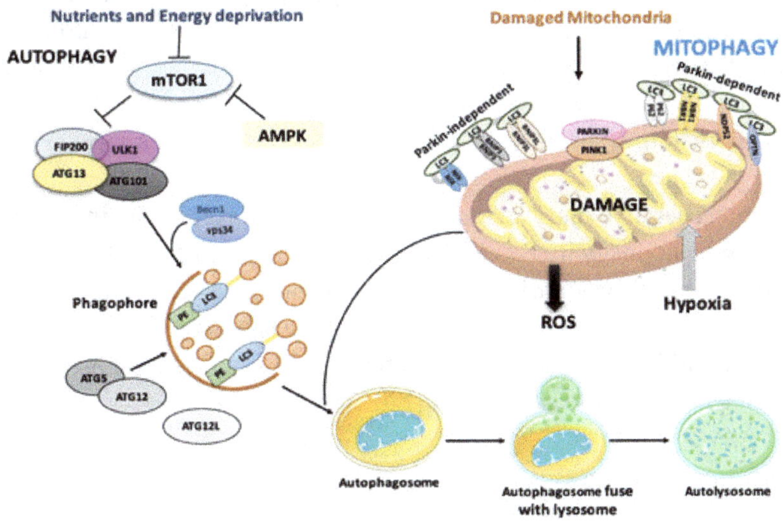

2.3.3. The Importance of Mitophagy

Mitophagy plays a vital role in maintaining mitochondrial integrity and cellular health. Damaged or dysfunctional mitochondria can cause the secretion of reactive oxygen species (ROS), cytochrome c, and other pro-apoptotic factors, which can lead to cellular damage and death (Gottlieb and Carreira, 2010). By selectively removing these harmful mitochondria, mitophagy helps to preserve the integrity of the remaining mitochondrial population and maintain cellular homeostasis.

Moreover, mitophagy is essential for the removal of mitochondria that are producing excessive ROS, thereby reducing the overall oxidative burden on the cell (Bahar et al., 2022). This link between mitophagy and the mitochondrial free radical theory of aging suggests that the efficient removal of damaged mitochondria through mitophagy may contribute to longevity, particularly in long-lived cells (Guan et al., 2021). Mitophagy is also crucial for cellular differentiation and development. For example, the maturation of reticulocytes into erythrocytes (red blood cells) involves the selective removal of mitochondria through mitophagy, a process that is essential for the formation of mature red blood cells. Similarly, mitophagy plays a role in the differentiation of T lymphocytes, highlighting its importance in various physiological processes (Gottlieb and Carreira, 2010).

2.3.4. Dysregulation of Autophagy and Mitophagy in Disease

The dysregulation of autophagy and mitophagy has been implicated in the pathogenesis of various diseases, including neurodegenerative disorders, cardiovascular diseases, and cancer.

i. Neurodegenerative Disorders

In neurodegenerative diseases, such as Parkinson's disease, the impairment of mitophagy and autophagy has been identified as a key contributor to the accumulation of damaged mitochondria and the subsequent neuronal death. The Parkin-PINK1 pathway, which is essential for mitophagy, has been extensively studied in the context of Parkinson's disease, as mutations in these genes have been linked to the development of the disease (Gehring, 2022).

ii. Cardiovascular Diseases

In the cardiovascular system, the impairment of autophagy and mitophagy has been associated with the development of aging-related disorders, such as heart failure and atherosclerosis. The gradual inhibition of autophagy in the aging heart, at least in part due to the accumulation of lipofuscin (a byproduct of lysosomal digestion), can lead to the accumulation of damaged mitochondria and the development of cardiac dysfunction. Therapeutic approaches aimed at enhancing autophagy and mitophagy have shown promise in mitigating these age-related cardiovascular diseases.

iii. Cancer

The role of autophagy and mitophagy in cancer is complex, as these processes can exhibit both tumor-suppressive and tumor-promoting effects, depending on the context. Autophagy can act as a tumor suppressor by removing damaged organelles and proteins, thereby preventing genomic instability and the accumulation of oncogenic mutations (Lee et al., 2023). On the other hand, autophagy and mitophagy can also support tumor growth by providing energy and nutrients to rapidly proliferating cancer cells, particularly in the tumor microenvironment (Xu and Hu, 2022).

In the tumor microenvironment, autophagy and mitophagy in cancer-associated fibroblasts (CAFs) can contribute to the metabolic symbiosis between cancer cells and their stromal counterparts. CAFs can engage in autophagy and mitophagy to generate and secrete various nutrients, such as amino acids and nucleotides, which can then be utilized by the neighbouring cancer cells to sustain their growth and proliferation (Guan et al, 2021).

Moreover, autophagy and mitophagy in immune cells within the tumor microenvironment can also influence the tumor's immune response. Autophagy in tumor-associated immune cells, such as T cells and macrophages, can modulate their cytokine secretion and function, potentially contributing to a tumor-promoting immune landscape (Lee et al., 2023).

2.3.5. Therapeutic Potential of Targeting Autophagy and Mitophagy

In the context of neurodegenerative disorders, enhancing mitophagy through the modulation of the Parkin-PINK1 pathway or other mitophagy-related mechanisms has been explored as a potential therapeutic approach. Similarly, in cardiovascular diseases, therapies aimed at increasing autophagy and mitophagy have shown promise in improving cardiac function and mitigating age-related cardiac dysfunction (Gehring, 2022).

In cancer, the dual roles of autophagy and mitophagy present both challenges and opportunities. While inhibiting autophagy in cancer cells can have a tumor-suppressive effect, targeting autophagy and mitophagy in the tumor microenvironment, particularly in CAFs and immune cells, may also hold therapeutic potential (Lee et al., 2023). Ongoing research is exploring the development of selective autophagy and mitophagy modulators that can be tailored to the specific context of the disease and the tumor microenvironment.

2.3.6. Autophagy: A Catabolic Pathway for Cellular Homeostasis

Autophagy is a highly conserved process that is active at basal levels in all cells. It is characterized by the formation of double-membrane vesicles called autophagosomes that deliver damaged organelles and extra proteins to lysosomes for recycling (Awan and Deng, 2014; Abdelkader and AboQuella, 2025). Autophagy is induced by various environmental and genetic factors, including nutrient starvation, oxidative stress, and genetic mutations (Chun and Kim, 2018).

Autophagy plays a crucial role in maintaining cellular homeostasis by recycling damaged organelles and aggregated or misfolded macromolecules. This process helps to maintain cellular health by removing damaged cellular components that can contribute to various diseases (Xu and Hu, 2022). Autophagy is important for maintaining cellular balance and is deeply connected with the pathogenesis of various diseases, including cancer, diabetes, neurodegenerative disorders, and infectious diseases (Awan and Deng, 2014; Abdelkader and AboQuella, 2025).

2.3.7. Mitophagy: A Specific Form of Autophagy for Mitochondrial Homeostasis

Mitophagy is a specific form of autophagy that targets damaged mitochondria for degradation. Mitochondria are critical organelles that generate energy for the cell through the process of cellular respiration. However, damaged mitochondria can accumulate and contribute to various diseases, including neurodegenerative diseases and cancer (Guan et al., 2021).

Mitophagy is essential for maintaining mitochondrial homeostasis by removing damaged mitochondria that can contribute to cellular stress and disease. Mitophagy is regulated by various Signaling pathways, including the PI3K/Akt and mTOR pathways, which play a crucial role in regulating mitochondrial dynamics and function (Palikaras et al., 2018; Zamanian et al., 2024).

2.3.8. Impact of Autophagy and Mitophagy on Diseases

Autophagy and mitophagy are two essential cellular processes that play a vital role in maintaining cellular homeostasis. Autophagy is a lysosomal degradation pathway that recycles damaged organelles and aggregated or misfolded macromolecules, while mitophagy specifically targets damaged mitochondria for degradation. Both processes are critical for maintaining cellular health and preventing the accumulation of damaged cellular components that can contribute to various diseases (Lee et al., 2023). They have a significant impact on various diseases, including cancer, diabetes, neurodegenerative disorders, and infectious diseases. These mechanisms are essential for maintaining cellular health and preventing the accumulation of damaged cellular components that can contribute to various diseases (Xu and Hu, 2022).

3. ROLE OF AUTOPHAGY IN CANCER METABOLIC REMODELING

Autophagy is an important physiological function that primarily shields organisms and cells against adverse conditions, such as low levels of adenosine triphosphate (ATP) or starvation. Cancer's hallmark, metabolic reprogramming, has recently developed a curiosity for cancer treatment (Chu et al., 2020).

3.1. Autophagy as a Double-Edged Sword in Cancer

Numerous internal and extrinsic stressors that impair development and homeostasis are encountered by cancer cells during the tumorigenic process. Even under stress, cancer cells exhibit the activation of unique pathways for growth and adaptability. One catabolic process that helps with intracellular material breakdown and metabolite recycling is autophagy. In situations of food deficiency, genotoxic stress, growth factor withdrawal, and hypoxia, this activity aids in meeting metabolic demands. Nevertheless, depending on the stage of tumor growth, autophagy has a contradictory effect on the formation of tumors. Autophagy is a tumor suppressor early in the carcinogenesis process by breaking down potentially carcinogenic chemicals. Nonetheless, in more advanced phases, autophagy helps tumor cells survive by reducing environmental stress. Because autophagy is connected to other unique cellular processes, it plays a variety of complex roles (Chavez-Dominguez et al., 2020).

3.1.1. Tumor Suppression vs. Tumor Promotion

i. Tumor Suppression:

Given that 40–75% of human breast, ovarian, and prostate malignancies have been shown to have allelic deletion of the key autophagy gene BECN1 (ATG6), autophagy was once believed to be a tumor suppression mechanism (Wang et al., 2024; Liang et al., 1999). The fact that BECN1 is located on chromosome 17q21, near the recognized tumor suppressor breast cancer 1, early onset (BRCA1), throws doubt on these studies. However, autophagy reduces DNA damage response, chronic inflammation, tissue damage, and genomic instability—all of which have been linked to the development of cancer (Mathew et al., 2014; Deretic et al., 2013; Karantza-Wadsworth et al., 2007; Mathew et al., 2009; Mathew et al., 2007; White, 2012). In mice, a mosaic loss of the ATG5 gene leads to ongoing liver injury, inflammation, and the formation of benign liver tumors that do not advance to cancer (Takamura et al., 2011). Chronic liver damage acts as a tumor promoter by causing hepatocyte death, activating Kupffer cells, and triggering cytokine production that enhances compensatory cell proliferation (White, 2012). This pattern is also observed in the pancreas, where chronic inflammation promotes benign tumor growth following ATG gene deletion (Zhou et al., 2024; Rosenfeldt et al., 2013). These findings imply that autophagy might inhibit the initiation of tumors in the liver and pancreas by maintaining protein and organelle quality control, which reduces tissue. Further understanding of the mechanisms behind tumor suppression by autophagy has been gained through additional genetically engineered mouse models. In the liver of mice, the deletion of an essential Atg gene leads to the buildup of the autophagy substrate p62, which plays a crucial role in promoting tumors. Notably, the suppression of this tumorigenesis occurs with compound p62 deficiency (Yang et al., 2014). p62 interacts with and inhibits Kelch-like ECH-associated protein 1, which is an inhibitor of Nuclear factor (erythroid-derived 2)-like 2 (NRF2), thus enhancing NRF2 activity. NRF2 is an oncogene, while KEAP1 is a tumor suppressor in humans. The antioxidant defense response is master-regulated by NRF2, a transcription factor that enhances the survival of cancer cells. The development and survival of cancer cells may thus be driven by the suppression of Kelch-like ECH-associated protein 1 by p62 accumulation in autophagy-defective tumors and the subsequent NRF2 activation. The temporary encouragement of tumor development in Atg7-deficient Loss of one allele of Becn1 accelerates the development of mammary tumors after pregnancy and when the oncogenic WNT1 pathway is activated in mammary tissue (Cicchini et al., 2014). Becn1 heterozygosity leads to the expansion of immature mammary epithelial stem or progenitor cells, which are thought to be the initial cells in WNT1-driven mammary tumorigenesis. Notably, Atg7 deletion in the mammary gland does not exhibit the same effect (Cicchini et al., 2014). This indicates that losing one allele of Becn1 increases the number of cells that can be transformed malignantly by WNT1 activation. BRAFV600E-driven lung cancers are caused by NRF2 induction (Strohecker and White, 2014). It is unknown if the loss of a Becn1 function that is autophagy-independent is the cause of this stem cell/progenitor expansion. It is significant to remember that Becn1 controls growth factor receptor signaling apart from its involvement in autophagy, which may promote the spread of cancer (Rohatgi et al., 2015). Additionally, distinct results might arise from suppression as opposed to total autophagy loss. It is also unknown if the above-described KEAP1/NRF2/p62 regulation is connected to this tumor promotion. Lastly, it is unknown if autophagy impairment occurs in people and if it uses these processes to induce cancer (White et al., 2015).

ii. Tumor promotion:

When a person is starved, autophagy is quickly elevated to a great degree, and the breakdown of intracellular components that results provides substrates to sustain metabolism in the lack of external nutrients. Although the precise autophagy substrates and metabolic pathways they support are unknown, one may anticipate that they would vary depending on the tissue under question and the conditions. Autophagy's role in promoting metabolic survival is also triggered in cancers. Certain cancer cell lines exhibit unusually high levels of autophagy even when nutrients are plentiful, indicating that oncogenic events induce intrinsic metabolic stress that requires autophagy for tumor cell survival (Yang et al., 2014; Degenhardt et al, 2006; Guo et al., 2011; Guo et al., 2013; Lazova et al., 2012; Lock et al., 2011; Ma et al., 2011; Yang et al., 2011). Recent studies show that Ras-driven pancreatic cancers enhance transcription programs for autophagy and lysosomal biogenesis by encouraging the nuclear localization of the master regulatory MiT/TFE family (Perera et al., 2015). Moreover, somatic mutation and other pathways in human tumors activate members of the MiT/TFE family (Ferguson, 2015), indicating the broader significance of the autophagy-lysosome system in driving tumor development. The functional significance of autophagy in tumor promotion may be demonstrated by reducing survival and tumorigenesis in cancer cell lines by either deleting or knocking down the expression of key autophagy genes. In hypoxic tumor areas, where autophagy is necessary for tumor cell survival, it is also increased (Degenhardt et al., 2006). Consequently, autophagy may be more necessary to support tumor growth and survival when cancer pathways are activated inside tumor cells and stress is present in the tumor microenvironment. (Aita et al., 1999).

3.2. Autophagy-Mediated Metabolic Adaptations

i. Nutrient recycling and energy production:

When faced with nutritional and energy shortages, cells must make prompt choices to manage the balance between nutrient and energy requirements, allocating the limited resources to sustain viability and essential functions while sacrificing non-essential cellular structures and activities. Autophagy, originating from the ancient Greek term for 'self-eating,' is a lysosomal breakdown pathway that has evolved across eukaryotes, from yeast to humans, to fulfill this role (He and Klionsky, 2009). The substrates that are suitable for autophagy are more versatile than those for another cellular degradation pathway, the ubiquitin-proteasomal pathway, which breaks down short-lived proteins and necessitates the unfolding of substrate proteins for proteasomes to feed on them. These substrates include long-lived proteins, non-protein structures, protein aggregates, and organelles that are either too big or too difficult to unfold for proteasomal degradation. Under normal circumstances, autophagy operates at a low baseline level. However, several stimuli, including hunger, endoplasmic reticulum stress, hypoxia, pathogen infection, and exercise, can increase autophagy activity (He and Klionsky, 2009; Kuma and Mizushima, 2010; Rocchi and He, 2017). Autophagy, not the ubiquitin-proteasomal system, is the primary mechanism necessary to sustain energy generation and cell survival under food deprivation (Weber et al., 2020).

Autophagy cargos ultimately arrive in the lysosomal lumen, where acid hydrolases break down the supplied lysosomal contents to produce sugars, amino acids, fatty acids, and nucleotides. These products are then recycled back into the cytoplasm and utilized again. Three forms of autophagy are distinguished: macroautophagy, microautophagy, and chaperone-mediated autophagy. These categories rely on the mechanistic variations in cargo translocation and delivery to lysosomes. Macroautophagy, also known as autophagy, is the process by which a phagophore—a developing autophagosomal membrane—becomes a typical double-membrane autophagosome. Autophagosomes are not involved in microautophagy; instead, they enclose and transfer cytosolic cargos to lysosomes for destruction. Rather, endosomal sorting complexes required for transport machinery are needed for microautophagy, which is the direct invasion of the lysosomal membrane followed by the disintegration of incorporated cargos. This process could be comparable to the emergence of endosomal multivesicular bodies (Schuck, 2020). During the period of stress, the three autophagy processes are crucial in controlling energy homeostasis and nutrient mobilization. The three forms of autophagy may break down a wide range of essential resources, including proteins, nucleic acids, carbs, and fats, into their components, such as amino acids, nucleotides, glucose, and fatty acid chains, for reuse and recycling purposes. These catabolic pathways interact with one another to supply substrates for biosynthetic processes, as well as supplying energy generation through glycolysis and mitochondria. Energy generation and expenditure are both regulated by autophagy. The Krebs cycle, glycolysis, and oxidative phosphorylation, which drive ATP synthase, are the three main biological processes that create the energy-storing molecule ATP. Three other activities also need energy expenditure: maintaining a baseline metabolic rate, engaging in vigorous physical activity, and producing heat (thermogenesis). To produce energy, fatty acid β-oxidation is a crucial mechanism that powers both the Krebs cycle and oxidative phosphorylation (He, 2022).

3.2.1. Impact on Glycolysis, Oxidative Phosphorylation (OXPHOS), and Fatty Acid Metabolism

i. Unveiling the impact on glycolysis:

Otto Warburg first laid out the variations in energy supply between healthy cells and cancerous cells in the early twentieth century. According to Dr. Warburg, cancer cells exhibit the "Warburg effect," which is an elevated level of glycolysis and lactate synthesis even in the presence of enough oxygen (Warburg, 1956; Seyfried et al., 2025). Metabolic reprogramming is frequently used by cancer cells to sustain their expansion, survival, multiplication, and metastasis. Autophagy is typically altered in cancer cells to satisfy the needs of metabolic alterations. Autophagy and metabolism have been the subject of much research in the last several years. The primary nutritional source that cells need to produce energy is glucose. A steady supply of glucose is necessary for the synthesis of ATP. Glycolysis is an essential biological activity for the metabolism of glucose and is inextricably linked to autophagy. Its capacity to control autophagy is one metabolic process that propels the growth of tumors. Glycolysis helps cancer cells survive by controlling the process of autophagy. Studies revealed that leukemia cell viability was supported by increased autophagy and oxidative phosphorylation, which is driven by reduced glycolysis (Kawaguchi et al., 2016). Glioma cells that were engineered to undergo autophagic cell death and glycolysis malfunction were less viable when exposed to RSL3. Furthermore, pyruvate supplementation stopped RSL3-induced cell death, suggesting that glioma cell autophagic cell death might be caused by glycolysis failure (Wang et al., 2019). According to Ji Hye Kim et al., the longevity of EGFR-mutant NSCLC depends on the EGFR mutation-mediated increase of glycolysis, which maintains EGFR stability. Because reduction of glucose-derived ATP synthesis may lead to ROS-mediated c-Jun N-terminal kinase (JNK) activation, which in turn may lead to autophagy-mediated EGFR degradation, glucose metabolism suppression might overcome T790 M-mediated resistance (Kim et al., 2018). Glycolysis modifies immunity against tumors and controls autophagy. Myeloid-derived suppressor cells (MDSCs) are a kind of heterogenetic myeloid cell that have been given the ability to suppress the immune system through the use of many effector chemicals, including inducible carbon oxide synthase (INOS), reactive oxygen species (ROS), and arginase1 (Arg1) (Mantovani, 2010; Thylur Puttalingaiah et al., 2024). The induction of AMP-activated protein kinase (AMPK)-unc-51-like kinase 1 (ULK1) signaling and autophagy establishment were hindered by high glycolytic rate in TNBC cells. This, in turn, reduced autophagy-mediated partial LAP reduction. Furthermore, LAP boosted the levels of granulocyte-colony stimulating factor (G-CSF) and granulocyte-macrophage colony stimulating factor (GM-CSF) to promote the proliferation of MDSCs and sustain tumor suppression of immunity (Li et al., 2018). Glycolysis controls autophagy and contributes significantly to cancer's susceptibility to chemotherapy. Hexokinase 2 (HK2), for example, increased autophagic activity and ERK1/2 activation in ovarian cancer cells, conferring resistance to cisplatin. The autophagy blocker 3-MA was used to block autophagy, which made resistant ovarian cancer cells more sensitive to cisplatin (Zhang et al., 2018). Because it can trigger pro-survival autophagy, 2-Deoxy-D-Glucose (2DG), an inhibitor of glycolysis, has a minimal therapeutic effect when used alone. A popular non-selective epinephrine receptor blocker, propranolol, has lately demonstrated anticancer effects. Propranolol + 2DG can efficiently trigger cell death, alter mitochondrial shape, prevent mitochondrial biological energy, exacerbate endoplasmic reticulum stress, and prevent tumor development in vivo, in addition to successfully inhibiting the proliferation of prostate cancer cells in vitro (Brohee et al., 2018). Human NSCLCs with EGFR activating mutations were resistant to tyrosine kinase inhibitors (TKIs) that target EGFR. Resistant cell lines have higher rates of glycolysis and greater uptake of glucose. Additionally, under glucose deprivation, drug-resistant cell lines exhibited active autophagy. Pairing autophagy inhibitors with glucose restriction may be able to overcome NSCLC resistance to EGFR-targeted treatment (Ye et al., 2017). Therefore, it is evident that targeting glycolysis and autophagy together is a successful cancer therapeutic strategy (Chu et al., 2020).

ii. **Unveiling the impact on fatty acid metabolism:**

Reduction of the autophagy protein ATG5 leads to a decline in hepatic fatty acid beta-oxidation triggered by thyroid hormones, implying that autophagy plays a favorable role in regulating fatty acid beta-oxidation in the liver (Sinha et al., 2012). Similarly, prolonged exposure to cold stress in brown adipose tissue stimulates both autophagy and fatty acid beta-oxidation, likely under central regulation by anorexigenic proopiomelanocortin neurons (Quan et al., 2012; Martinez-Lopez et al., 2016). Theoretically, mitochondrial ATP synthase should convert all autophagy-derived metabolites to acetyl-CoA and use them as fuel for aerobic respiration, but in practice, this does not happen. In addition to providing substrate metabolites for ATP synthesis and biosynthetic pathways, cold-stress-induced autophagy in brown adipose tissues also increases thermogenesis (Yau et al., 2021). Brown and beige adipose tissues, which are enriched with mitochondria, are responsible for thermogenesis. Protons enter the mitochondrial matrix through uncoupling protein 1, avoiding the ATP synthase. Thus, ATP synthesis, thermogenesis, and the availability of building blocks for biosynthetic pathways are the three consequences of metabolites obtained by autophagy. Autophagy has a complicated function in regulating energy use. White adipose tissue growth requires basal autophagy (Chang, 2023; Zhang et al., 2009), and activating autophagy increases the "whitening" of brown adipose tissue by breaking down mitochondria42. Disabling autophagy specifically in beige adipocytes through Atg5 or Atg12 knockout proves advantageous for maintaining beige fat and shields mice from obesity and insulin resistance induced by a high-fat diet (HFD) (Altshuler-Keylin et al., 2016). Moreover, while inhibiting liver-specific chaperone-mediated autophagy leads to hepatosteatosis in HFD-fed mice, this inhibition surprisingly boosts hepatic energy expenditure and promotes weight loss (Schneider et al., 2014). This effect could arise from the prevention of chaperone-mediated autophagy degradation of metabolic enzymes or compensatory increases in (macro)autophagy activity. Hence, autophagy activation can modify liver and adipose tissue, making them less thermogenic and requiring less energy expenditure; however, autophagy additionally has the potential to improve thermogenesis in mature brown adipose tissues in response to cold stress (Yau et al., 2021), most likely by supplying metabolites and substrates and enhancing mitochondrial quality control. Future quantitative analyses are required to simulate the circumstances in which autophagy can either regulate energy availability and demand, provide the best ATP production, or be energetically useless, preferably in individual cells or individual populations of homogeneous cells. Furthermore, it is unclear and needs further research how autophagy regulates activity-induced energy consumption vs resting energy consumption, also known as basal metabolic rate (Hawley et al., 2015).

4. ROLE OF MITOPHAGY IN CANCER METABOLIC REMODELLING

Mitophagy plays a crucial role in cancer metabolic remodeling by selectively removing damaged mitochondria, allowing cancer cells to adapt to stress and maintain their energy production. This process supports the metabolic shifts that enable tumor growth and survival in challenging environments.

4.1. Mitochondrial Dynamics in Cancer

Mitochondrial dynamics, which encompass the processes of mitochondrial biogenesis, fission, fusion, and quality control, are essential for cancer metabolism. To accommodate the higher energy requirements and biosynthetic requirements of rapidly dividing cells, these processes are frequently reprogrammed in cancer cells (Chen et al., 2023). In cancer, mitochondrial biogenesis, which involves the production of new mitochondria, is frequently stimulated, which facilitates the increased metabolic activity necessary for tumour growth. Furthermore, the maintenance of mitochondrial function and the adaptation to cellular duress are contingent upon the maintenance of the equilibrium between mitochondrial fission (division) and fusion (joining). This equilibrium is frequently disturbed in cancer, resulting in altered mitochondrial structure, distribution, and function, which can contribute to the progression of the tumour (Moindjie et al., 2021).

4.2. Mitochondrial Biogenesis, Dynamics, and Quality Control

Mitophagy and other mitochondrial quality control mechanisms are essential for the removal of damaged or dysfunctional mitochondria, thereby ensuring the mitochondrial network's health within the cell. Mitophagy selectively targets these defective mitochondria for degradation, thereby preventing the accumulation of toxic reactive oxygen species (ROS) and preserving cellular homeostasis (Wang et al., 2021). Mitophagy facilitates the metabolic adaptability of tumour cells in the context of cancer, enabling them to endure in the presence of stressors such as nutrient scarcity and hypoxia. Mitophagy also contributes to the metabolic shift known as the Warburg effect, in which cancer cells prioritise glycolysis over oxidative phosphorylation for energy production, by modulating the content and function of mitochondria (Seyfried et al., 2025). This change enables cancer cells to maintain their high metabolic demands and prevent oxidative stress, thereby promoting the growth and survival of the tumour (Deepak et al., 2024).

Mitophagy is essential for the metabolic remodelling observed in cancer, as it allows tumour cells to adapt to their microenvironment and resist apoptosis through these processes. The comprehension of mitophagy's function in these mitochondrial dynamics offers potential therapeutic strategies that could disrupt the metabolic flexibility of cancer cells by targeting mitochondrial quality control mechanisms (Ferro et al., 2020).

5. INTERACTION BETWEEN AUTOPHAGY, MITOPHAGY, AND CANCER THERAPIES

Autophagy and mitophagy are cellular processes that break down and recycle cellular components. These activities have important consequences in cancer treatments, including in chemotherapy and radiotherapy. Gaining a clear understanding of the functions they play in various therapies can offer valuable insights into the results of treatment and the causes of resistance, which may ultimately lead to the development of new and innovative therapeutic approaches (Xia et al., 2014).

5.1. Impact on Chemotherapy and Radiotherapy

Autophagy and mitophagy have both positive and negative effects in cancer treatment. One benefit is that they can enhance the survival of cancer cells by removing damaged organelles and proteins, which reduces cellular stress and prevents apoptosis (Frank et al., 2012). Conversely, an excessive amount of autophagy can result in autophagic cell death, particularly when the body is subjected to intense stress caused by therapies such as chemotherapy and radiotherapy (Yonekawa & Thorburn, 2013).

For instance, when exposed to chemotherapeutic treatments, cancer cells may increase autophagy as a defensive mechanism, enabling them to survive in conditions that would otherwise be deadly. The protective function can reduce the effectiveness of chemotherapy, resulting in treatment ineffectiveness. Autophagy can mitigate radiation-induced damage and decrease cell death, hence influencing treatment outcomes in radiotherapy (Wang et al., 2018).

5.2. Resistance Mechanisms: Drug Resistance Caused by Autophagy/Mitophagy

The involvement of autophagy and mitophagy in the emergence of drug resistance in cancer cells has been suggested. This resistance can arise via the targeted breakdown of apoptotic proteins, the preservation of mitochondrial function during periods of stress, or by supplying the necessary energy for cell survival. Mitophagy plays a crucial role in preserving the quality of mitochondria by eliminating damaged ones and replacing them. This process prevents cell death and enhances survival when the body is subjected to therapeutic stress (Deepak et al., 2024).

Overcoming the resistance caused by autophagy and mitophagy is a major obstacle in cancer treatment. An effective strategy involves employing autophagy inhibitors, which enhance the susceptibility of cancer cells to chemotherapy and radiotherapy by impeding the reutilization of cellular constituents and facilitating programmed cell death. The combination of these inhibitors with traditional treatments has demonstrated potential in preclinical animals. Moreover, the identification and manipulation of certain pathways, such as the PINK1/Parkin pathway, that are implicated in mitophagy, could potentially provide novel approaches to overcome resistance (Wang et al., 2023).

5.3. Innovative Therapeutic Methods: Inhibitors of Autophagy and Mitophagy

Research on inhibitors that target autophagy and mitophagy is a promising field of study. Chloroquine and hydroxychloroquine agents have been studied for their capacity to hinder autophagy by interrupting the fusion of autophagosomes with lysosomes (Chen et al., 2023). This action improves the effectiveness of chemotherapy and radiotherapy. Furthermore, researchers are also studying novel inhibitors that specifically target pathways involved in mitophagy. The objective is to hinder the survival strategies of cancer cells while leaving normal cells unaffected (Chen & Kuo, 2017). It is essential to identify biomarkers that can predict the autophagic or mitophagic response to therapy to design personalised treatment regimens. For example, the levels of autophagy-related genes or the activity of important mitophagy regulators could be used as biomarkers to help choose the most appropriate medication and forecast the results of treatment. Tailored strategies utilising these biomarkers have the potential to enhance treatment effectiveness and reduce the development of resistance (Miceli et al., 2023).

6. CASE STUDIES AND CLINICAL TRIALS

The aim of case studies and clinical trials focusing on autophagy and mitophagy in cancer has been to comprehend how these cellular functions can be altered to enhance treatment results. Strong evidence supporting the dual roles of autophagy and mitophagy in cancer has been produced by preclinical research employing a variety of cancer cell lines and animal models. These investigations have shown that these pathways can be used as therapeutic targets in addition to helping cancer cells survive stressful situations like chemotherapy and radiation (Pandey et al., 2021). For example, in vitro studies using human colorectal cancer cell lines have demonstrated that the combination of chemotherapeutic drugs like 5-fluorouracil (5-FU) and autophagy inhibitors like chloroquine promotes cancer cell death through the promotion of apoptosis. Autophagy suppression has the potential to improve the efficacy of chemotherapy, as demonstrated by the improved sensitivity of breast cancer cell lines treated with bafilomycin A1 and 3-methyladenine to doxorubicin and paclitaxel (Hareendran et al., 2022; Lauzier et al., 2019).

These findings have been further substantiated by animal studies, which have illustrated the influence of autophagy and mitophagy modulation on tumour growth and metastasis. For example, the knockout of autophagy-related gene 7 (ATG7) in genetically engineered murine models of colorectal cancer led to increased sensitivity to oxaliplatin, a chemotherapeutic drug, and reduced tumour growth (Scherr et al., 2020). Furthermore, xenograft models that utilise human cancer cells implanted in immunocompromised mice have demonstrated that the inhibition of mitophagy-specific pathways, including the PINK1/Parkin pathway, can suppress tumour growth and metastasis in melanoma and glioblastoma models. These results offer a compelling justification for the translation of preclinical research into clinical settings (Yang, 2021).

These preclinical insights have been expanded upon in clinical trials that target autophagy and mitophagy in cancer. These trials have concentrated on both completed and ongoing studies that are designed to validate these strategies in patients. The utilisation of autophagy inhibitors in conjunction with conventional therapies has been the subject of numerous completed trials. For instance, a Phase II trial investigated the efficacy of hydroxychloroquine in combination with gemcitabine and nab-paclitaxel in patients with advanced pancreatic cancer (Mohsen et al., 2022). Although the combination therapy was generally well-tolerated, the overall improvement in progression-free survival was relatively modest. This implies that additional refinement, such as patient selection based on specific biomarkers, may be required to attain superior outcomes. New combinations and inhibitors are being investigated in ongoing clinical trials to improve efficacy. This trial is assessing the safety and efficacy of DTP3, a novel selective autophagy inhibitor, in patients with relapsed or refractory multiple myeloma. In an additional trial, the combination of pembrolizumab, an immune checkpoint inhibitor, and chloroquine is being examined as a potential treatment for advanced non-small cell lung cancer (NSCLC) to circumvent resistance mechanisms (Sandomenico et al., 2020).

Although there have been significant advancements in the targeting of autophagy and mitophagy, there have also been setbacks. Certain trials, such as those that combine hydroxychloroquine with temozolomide in melanoma, have reported limited efficacy. This may be attributed to suboptimal dosing or insufficient inhibition of autophagy at clinically tolerable dosages (Kocak et al., 2021). Additionally, patients have encountered adverse effects, including gastrointestinal toxicity, which have resulted in the need for dose reductions or treatment discontinuation. Additionally, there is substantial heterogeneity in patient responses, with some patients demonstrating benefits and others not. This is likely a result of the varying modulation of autophagy across different cancer types and patient populations. (Qi & Cao, 2023)

In general, the lessons learnt from these studies comprise numerous critical points. Initially, it is imperative to implement a personalised medicine strategy, as the response to autophagy and mitophagy-targeted therapies is highly variable. The clinical utility of these therapies could be improved by the identification of biomarkers that predict patient response. Secondly, the use of combination strategies, such as the combination of autophagy inhibitors with conventional therapies or novel agents like immune checkpoint inhibitors, may enhance outcomes and provide a synergistic effect. Ultimately, the prudent management of adverse effects and the effective monitoring of autophagy and mitophagy activity are essential for the equilibrium of safety and efficacy in clinical trials.

7. CONCLUSIONS

The complex functions that autophagy and mitophagy play in the metabolic remodelling of cancer have been emphasised in this chapter. In the context of cancer, these processes, which are essential for sustaining cellular homeostasis, are both protective and exploitative. Autophagy facilitates the survival and proliferation of cancer cells by recycling cellular components and generating energy during metabolic duress. It has an impact on critical metabolic pathways, including glycolysis and oxidative phosphorylation, which are essential for the growth of tumours. In the same way, mitophagy is responsible for the regulation of reactive oxygen species (ROS) levels and the preservation of healthy mitochondria, which are essential for cancer cells to adapt to adverse conditions such as hypoxia and nutrient deprivation.

The dual nature of these processes poses both opportunities and challenges in the field of cancer therapy. Although they have the potential to exacerbate resistance to chemotherapy and radiotherapy, comprehending the underlying mechanisms has facilitated the development of novel therapeutic interventions. The potential to improve treatment efficacy and surmount drug resistance is present by targeting autophagy and mitophagy, either by inhibiting these processes or by modulating them in combination with existing therapies.

The chapter also emphasises the necessity of ongoing research in this discipline. There are still substantial voids in our comprehension of the regulation of autophagy and mitophagy in various cancer types and the interaction between these processes and other cellular pathways. The complexities of these pathways are poised to be further unravelled by emerging technologies, including advanced imaging and genetic tools, which will allow for more precise targeting in cancer treatment.

Ultimately, the incorporation of autophagy and mitophagy modulation into personalised medicine is a promising frontier in oncology. There is the potential to considerably enhance outcomes by customising therapies to the unique characteristics of individual patients' tumours. The critical role of autophagy and mitophagy in the future of cancer therapy will be underscored by the insights that will be obtained as research advances, which are expected to result in more effective and innovative strategies for combating cancer.

REFERENCES

Abdelkader, M., & AboQuella, N. M. (2025). Autophagy and Extracellular Nanovesicles: Communication and Their Therapeutic Application in Neurodegenerative Diseases. In Nanocarriers in Neurodegenerative Disorders (pp. 208-221). CRC Press.

Aita, V. M., Liang, X. H., Murty, V. V. V. S., Pincus, D. L., Yu, W., Cayanis, E., Kalachikov, S., Gilliam, T. C., & Levine, B. (1999). Cloning and genomic organization of beclin 1, a candidate tumor suppressor gene on chromosome 17q21. *Genomics*, *59*(1), 59–65. DOI: 10.1006/geno.1999.5851 PMID: 10395800

Altshuler-Keylin, S., Shinoda, K., Hasegawa, Y., Ikeda, K., Hong, H., Kang, Q., Yang, Y., Perera, R. M., Debnath, J., & Kajimura, S. (2016). Beige adipocyte maintenance is regulated by autophagy-induced mitochondrial clearance. *Cell Metabolism*, *24*(3), 402–419. DOI: 10.1016/j.cmet.2016.08.002 PMID: 27568548

Amaravadi, R. K., Kimmelman, A. C., & Debnath, J. (2019). Targeting autophagy in cancer: Recent advances and future directions. *Cancer Discovery*, *9*(9), 1167–1181. DOI: 10.1158/2159-8290.CD-19-0292 PMID: 31434711

Antico, O., Thompson, P. W., Hertz, N. T., Muqit, M. M., & Parton, L. E. (2025). Targeting mitophagy in neurodegenerative diseases. *Nature Reviews. Drug Discovery*, •••, 1–24. PMID: 39809929

Awan, M. U. F., & Deng, Y. (2014). Role of autophagy and its significance in cellular homeostasis. *Applied Microbiology and Biotechnology*, *98*(12), 5319–5328. DOI: 10.1007/s00253-014-5721-8 PMID: 24743981

Bahar, E., Han, S. Y., Kim, J. Y., & Yoon, H. (2022). Chemotherapy resistance: Role of mitochondrial and autophagic components. *Cancers (Basel)*, *14*(6), 1462. DOI: 10.3390/cancers14061462 PMID: 35326612

Barba, I., Carrillo-Bosch, L., & Seoane, J. (2024). Targeting the Warburg effect in cancer: Where do we stand? *International Journal of Molecular Sciences*, *25*(6), 3142. DOI: 10.3390/ijms25063142 PMID: 38542116

Basak, B., & Holzbaur, E. L. (2025). Mitophagy in Neurons: Mechanisms Regulating Mitochondrial Turnover and Neuronal Homeostasis. *Journal of Molecular Biology*, •••, 169161. DOI: 10.1016/j.jmb.2025.169161 PMID: 40268233

Brohee, L., Peulen, O., Nusgens, B., Castronovo, V., Thiry, M., Colige, A. C., & Deroanne, C. F. (2018). Propranolol sensitizes prostate cancer cells to glucose metabolism inhibition and prevents cancer progression. *Scientific Reports*, *8*(1), 7050. DOI: 10.1038/s41598-018-25340-9 PMID: 29728578

Bui, V., Liang, X., Ye, Y., Giang, W., Tian, F., Takahashi, Y., & Wang, H. G. (2025). Blocking autophagosome closure manifests the roles of mammalian Atg8-family proteins in phagophore formation and expansion during nutrient starvation. *Autophagy*, *21*(5), 1–16. DOI: 10.1080/15548627.2024.2443300 PMID: 39694607

Cao, W., Li, J., Yang, K., & Cao, D. (2021). An overview of autophagy: Mechanism, regulation and research progress. *Bulletin du Cancer*, *108*(3), 304–322. DOI: 10.1016/j.bulcan.2020.11.004 PMID: 33423775

Chang, J. S. (2023). Recent insights into the molecular mechanisms of simultaneous fatty acid oxidation and synthesis in brown adipocytes. *Frontiers in Endocrinology*, *14*, 1106544. DOI: 10.3389/fendo.2023.1106544 PMID: 36896177

Chavez-Dominguez, R., Perez-Medina, M., Lopez-Gonzalez, J. S., Galicia-Velasco, M., & Aguilar-Cazares, D. (2020). The double-edge sword of autophagy in cancer: From tumor suppression to pro-tumor activity. *Frontiers in Oncology*, *10*, 578418. DOI: 10.3389/fonc.2020.578418 PMID: 33117715

Chen, H. H., & Kuo, M. T. (2017). Improving radiotherapy in cancer treatment: Promises and challenges. *Oncotarget*, *8*(37), 62742–62758. DOI: 10.18632/oncotarget.18409 PMID: 28977985

Chen, J., Huang, Z., Chen, Y., Tian, H., Chai, P., Shen, Y., Yao, Y., Xu, S., Ge, S., & Jia, R. (2025). Lactate and lactylation in cancer. *Signal Transduction and Targeted Therapy*, *10*(1), 38. DOI: 10.1038/s41392-024-02082-x PMID: 39934144

Chen, J. L., Wu, X., Yin, D., Jia, X. H., Chen, X., Gu, Z. Y., & Zhu, X. M. (2023). Autophagy inhibitors for cancer therapy: Small molecules and nanomedicines. *Pharmacology & Therapeutics*, *249*, 108485. DOI: 10.1016/j.pharmthera.2023.108485 PMID: 37406740

Chen, W., Zhao, H., & Li, Y. (2023). Mitochondrial dynamics in health and disease: Mechanisms and potential targets. *Signal Transduction and Targeted Therapy*, *8*(1), 333. Advance online publication. DOI: 10.1038/s41392-023-01547-9 PMID: 37669960

Chu, Y., Chang, Y., Lu, W., Sheng, X., Wang, S., Xu, H., & Ma, J. (2020). Regulation of autophagy by glycolysis in cancer. *Cancer Management and Research*, *12*, 13259–13271. DOI: 10.2147/CMAR.S279672 PMID: 33380833

Chun, Y., & Kim, J. (2018). Autophagy: An essential degradation program for cellular homeostasis and life. *Cells*, *7*(12), 278. DOI: 10.3390/cells7120278 PMID: 30572663

Cicchini, M., Chakrabarti, R., Kongara, S., Price, S., Nahar, R., Lozy, F., Zhong, H., Vazquez, A., Kang, Y., & Karantza, V. (2014). Autophagy regulator BECN1 suppresses mammary tumorigenesis driven by WNT1 activation and following parity. *Autophagy*, *10*(11), 2036–2052. DOI: 10.4161/auto.34398 PMID: 25483966

Cruzat, V., Macedo Rogero, M., Noel Keane, K., Curi, R., & Newsholme, P. (2018). Glutamine: Metabolism and immune function, supplementation and clinical translation. *Nutrients*, *10*(11), 1564. DOI: 10.3390/nu10111564 PMID: 30360490

DeBerardinis, R. J., & Chandel, N. S. (2016). Fundamentals of cancer metabolism. *Science Advances*, *2*(5), e1600200. DOI: 10.1126/sciadv.1600200 PMID: 27386546

Debnath, J., Gammoh, N., & Ryan, K. M. (2023). Autophagy and autophagy-related pathways in cancer. *Nature Reviews. Molecular Cell Biology*, *24*(8), 560–575. DOI: 10.1038/s41580-023-00585-z PMID: 36864290

Deepak, K., Roy, P. K., Das, C. K., Mukherjee, B., & Mandal, M. (2024). Mitophagy at the crossroads of cancer development: Exploring the role of mitophagy in tumor progression and therapy resistance. *Biochimica Et Biophysica Acta (BBA) -. Biochimica et Biophysica Acta. Molecular Cell Research*, *1871*(6), 119752. DOI: 10.1016/j.bbamcr.2024.119752 PMID: 38776987

Degenhardt, K., Mathew, R., Beaudoin, B., Bray, K., Anderson, D., Chen, G., Mukherjee, C., Shi, Y., Gélinas, C., Fan, Y., Nelson, D. A., Jin, S., & White, E. (2006). Autophagy promotes tumor cell survival and restricts necrosis, inflammation, and tumorigenesis. *Cancer Cell*, *10*(1), 51–64. DOI: 10.1016/j.ccr.2006.06.001 PMID: 16843265

Deretic, V., Saitoh, T., & Akira, S. (2013). Autophagy in infection, inflammation and immunity. *Nature Reviews. Immunology*, *13*(10), 722–737. DOI: 10.1038/nri3532 PMID: 24064518

Durcan, T. M., & Fon, E. A. (2015). The three 'P's of mitophagy: PARKIN, PINK1, and post-translational modifications. *Genes & Development*, *29*(10), 989–999. DOI: 10.1101/gad.262758.115 PMID: 25995186

Ferguson, S. M. (2015). Beyond indigestion: Emerging roles for lysosome-based signaling in human disease. *Current Opinion in Cell Biology*, *35*, 59–68. DOI: 10.1016/j.ceb.2015.04.014 PMID: 25950843

Ferro, F., Servais, S., Besson, P., Roger, S., Dumas, J. F., & Brisson, L. (2020). Autophagy and mitophagy in cancer metabolic remodelling. *Seminars in Cell & Developmental Biology*, *98*, 129–138. DOI: 10.1016/j.semcdb.2019.05.029 PMID: 31154012

Geisler, S., Holmström, K. M., Skujat, D., Fiesel, F. C., Rothfuss, O. C., Kahle, P. J., & Springer, W. (2010). PINK1/Parkin-mediated mitophagy is dependent on VDAC1 and p62/SQSTM1. *Nature Cell Biology*, *12*(2), 119–131. DOI: 10.1038/ncb2012 PMID: 20098416

Glick, D., Barth, S., & Macleod, K. F. (2010). Autophagy: Cellular and molecular mechanisms. *The Journal of Pathology*, *221*(1), 3–12. DOI: 10.1002/path.2697 PMID: 20225336

Gottlieb, R. A., & Carreira, R. S. (2010). Autophagy in health and disease. 5. Mitophagy as a way of life. *American Journal of Physiology. Cell Physiology*, *299*(2), C203–C210. DOI: 10.1152/ajpcell.00097.2010 PMID: 20357180

Guan, Y., Wang, Y., Li, B., Shen, K., Li, Q., Ni, Y., & Huang, L. (2021). Mitophagy in carcinogenesis, drug resistance and anticancer therapeutics. *Cancer Cell International*, *21*(1), 1–9. DOI: 10.1186/s12935-021-02065-w PMID: 34225732

Guo, J. Y., Chen, H. Y., Mathew, R., Fan, J., Strohecker, A. M., Karsli-Uzunbas, G., Kamphorst, J. J., Chen, G., Lemons, J. M. S., Karantza, V., Coller, H. A., DiPaola, R. S., Gelinas, C., Rabinowitz, J. D., & White, E. (2011). Activated Ras requires autophagy to maintain oxidative metabolism and tumorigenesis. *Genes & Development*, *25*(5), 460–470. DOI: 10.1101/gad.2016311 PMID: 21317241

Guo, J. Y., Karsli-Uzunbas, G., Mathew, R., Aisner, S. C., Kamphorst, J. J., Strohecker, A. M., Chen, G., Price, S., Lu, W., Teng, X., Snyder, E., Santanam, U., DiPaola, R. S., Jacks, T., Rabinowitz, J. D., & White, E. (2013). Autophagy suppresses progression of K-ras-induced lung tumors to oncocytomas and maintains lipid homeostasis. *Genes & Development*, *27*(13), 1447–1461. DOI: 10.1101/gad.219642.113 PMID: 23824538

Halama, A., & Suhre, K. (2022). Advancing cancer treatment by targeting glutamine metabolism—A roadmap. *Cancers (Basel)*, *14*(3), 553. DOI: 10.3390/cancers14030553 PMID: 35158820

Hareendran, S., Yang, X., Sharma, V. K., & Loh, Y. P. (2022). Carboxypeptidase E and its splice variants: Key regulators of growth and metastasis in multiple cancer types. *Cancer Letters*, *548*, 215882. DOI: 10.1016/j.canlet.2022.215882 PMID: 35988818

Hawley, J. A., Maughan, R. J., & Hargreaves, M. (2015). Exercise metabolism: Historical perspective. *Cell Metabolism*, *22*(1), 12–17. DOI: 10.1016/j.cmet.2015.06.016 PMID: 26154050

He, C. (2022). Balancing nutrient and energy demand and supply via autophagy. *Current Biology, 32*(12), R684–R696. DOI: 10.1016/j.cub.2022.04.071 PMID: 35728554

He, C., & Klionsky, D. J. (2009). Regulation mechanisms and signaling pathways of autophagy. *Annual review of genetics, 43*, 67-93.8

Hippert, M. M., O'Toole, P. S., & Thorburn, A. (2006). Autophagy in cancer: Good, bad, or both? *Cancer Research, 66*(19), 9349–9351. DOI: 10.1158/0008-5472. CAN-06-1597 PMID: 17018585

Jacobo-Herrera, N., & Ozsvari, B. (2023). Reviews in cancer metabolism. *Frontiers in Oncology, 13*, 1216. DOI: 10.3389/fonc.2023.1167484 PMID: 37056333

Jang, M., Kim, S. S., & Lee, J. (2013). Cancer cell metabolism: Implications for therapeutic targets. *Experimental & Molecular Medicine, 45*(10), e45–e45. DOI: 10.1038/emm.2013.85 PMID: 24091747

Karantza-Wadsworth, V., Patel, S., Kravchuk, O., Chen, G., Mathew, R., Jin, S., & White, E. (2007). Autophagy mitigates metabolic stress and genome damage in mammary tumorigenesis. *Genes & Development, 21*(13), 1621–1635. DOI: 10.1101/ gad.1565707 PMID: 17606641

Kawaguchi, M., Aoki, S., Hirao, T., Morita, M., & Ito, K. (2016). Autophagy is an important metabolic pathway to determine leukemia cell survival following suppression of the glycolytic pathway. *Biochemical and Biophysical Research Communications, 474*(1), 188–192. DOI: 10.1016/j.bbrc.2016.04.098 PMID: 27107693

Kim, J. H., Nam, B., Choi, Y. J., Kim, S. Y., Lee, J. E., Sung, K. J., Kim, W. S., Choi, C.-M., Chang, E.-J., Koh, J. S., Song, J. S., Yoon, S., Lee, J. C., Rho, J. K., & Son, J. (2018). Enhanced glycolysis supports cell survival in EGFR-mutant lung adenocarcinoma by inhibiting autophagy-mediated EGFR degradation. *Cancer Research, 78*(16), 4482–4496. DOI: 10.1158/0008-5472.CAN-18-0117 PMID: 29945964

Kocak, M., Erdi, S. E., Jorba, G., Maestro, I., Farrés, J., Kirkin, V., Martinez, A., & Pless, O. (2021). Targeting autophagy in disease: Established and new strategies. *Autophagy, 18*(3), 473–495. DOI: 10.1080/15548627.2021.1936359 PMID: 34241570

Kondapalli, C., Kazlauskaite, A., Zhang, N., Woodroof, H. I., Campbell, D. G., Gourlay, R., Burchell, L., Walden, H., Macartney, T. J., Deak, M., Knebel, A., Alessi, D. R., & Muqit, M. M. K. (2012). PINK1 is activated by mitochondrial membrane potential depolarization and stimulates Parkin E3 ligase activity by phosphorylating Serine 65. *Open Biology, 2*(5), 120080. DOI: 10.1098/rsob.120080 PMID: 22724072

Kong, L., Li, S., Fu, Y., Cai, Q., Du, X., Liang, J., & Ma, T. (2025). Mitophagy in relation to chronic inflammation/ROS in aging. *Molecular and Cellular Biochemistry*, *480*(2), 721–731. DOI: 10.1007/s11010-024-05042-9 PMID: 38834837

Kuma, A., & Mizushima, N. (2010, September). Physiological role of autophagy as an intracellular recycling system: With an emphasis on nutrient metabolism. []). Academic Press.]. *Seminars in Cell & Developmental Biology*, *21*(7), 683–690. DOI: 10.1016/j.semcdb.2010.03.002 PMID: 20223289

Kundu, M., Lindsten, T., Yang, C. Y., Wu, J., Zhao, F., Zhang, J., Selak, M. A., Ney, P. A., & Thompson, C. B. (2008). Ulk1 plays a critical role in the autophagic clearance of mitochondria and ribosomes during reticulocyte maturation. *Blood*, *112*(4), 1493–1502. DOI: 10.1182/blood-2008-02-137398 PMID: 18539900

Lauzier, A., Normandeau-Guimond, J., Vaillancourt-Lavigueur, V., Boivin, V., Charbonneau, M., Rivard, N., Scott, M. S., Dubois, C. M., & Jean, S. (2019). Colorectal cancer cells respond differentially to autophagy inhibition in vivo. *Scientific Reports*, *9*(1), 11316. Advance online publication. DOI: 10.1038/s41598-019-47659-7 PMID: 31383875

Lazova, R., Camp, R. L., Klump, V., Siddiqui, S. F., Amaravadi, R. K., & Pawelek, J. M. (2012). Punctate LC3B expression is a common feature of solid tumors and associated with proliferation, metastasis, and poor outcome. *Clinical Cancer Research*, *18*(2), 370–379. DOI: 10.1158/1078-0432.CCR-11-1282 PMID: 22080440

Lee, S., Son, J. Y., Lee, J., & Cheong, H. (2023). Unraveling the Intricacies of Autophagy and Mitophagy: Implications in Cancer Biology. *Cells*, *12*(23), 2742. DOI: 10.3390/cells12232742 PMID: 38067169

Li, W., Tanikawa, T., Kryczek, I., Xia, H., Li, G., Wu, K. E., Wei, S., Zhao, L., Vatan, L., Wen, B., Shu, P., Sun, D., Kleer, C., Wicha, M., Sabel, M., Tao, K., Wang, G., & Zou, W. (2018). Aerobic glycolysis controls myeloid-derived suppressor cells and tumor immunity via a specific CEBPB isoform in triple-negative breast cancer. *Cell Metabolism*, *28*(1), 87–103. DOI: 10.1016/j.cmet.2018.04.022 PMID: 29805099

Li, X., He, S., & Ma, B. (2020). Autophagy and autophagy-related proteins in cancer. *Molecular Cancer*, *19*(1), 12. DOI: 10.1186/s12943-020-1138-4 PMID: 31969156

Li, Y., Zheng, W., Lu, Y., Zheng, Y., Pan, L., Wu, X., Yuan, Y., Shen, Z., Ma, S., Zhang, X., Wu, J., Chen, Z., & Zhang, X. (2021). BNIP3L/NIX-mediated mitophagy: Molecular mechanisms and implications for human disease. *Cell Death & Disease*, *13*(1), 14. DOI: 10.1038/s41419-021-04469-y PMID: 34930907

Liang, C., Feng, P., Ku, B., Dotan, I., Canaani, D., Oh, B. H., & Jung, J. U. (2006). Autophagic and tumour suppressor activity of a novel Beclin1-binding protein UVRAG. *Nature Cell Biology, 8*(7), 688–698. DOI: 10.1038/ncb1426 PMID: 16799551

Liang, H., Ma, Z., Zhong, W., Liu, J., Sugimoto, K., & Chen, H. (2024). Regulation of mitophagy and mitochondrial function: Natural compounds as potential therapeutic strategies for Parkinson's disease. *Phytotherapy Research, 38*(4), 1838–1862. DOI: 10.1002/ptr.8156 PMID: 38356178

Liang, X. H., Jackson, S., Seaman, M., Brown, K., Kempkes, B., Hibshoosh, H., & Levine, B. (1999). Induction of autophagy and inhibition of tumorigenesis by beclin 1. *Nature, 402*(6762), 672–676. DOI: 10.1038/45257 PMID: 10604474

Liu, J., Ma, H., Wu, Z., Ji, Y., & Liang, Y. (2024). The Knowns and Unknowns of Membrane Features and Changes During Autophagosome–Lysosome/Vacuole Fusion. *International Journal of Molecular Sciences, 25*(20), 11160. DOI: 10.3390/ijms252011160 PMID: 39456939

Lock, R., Roy, S., Kenific, C. M., Su, J. S., Salas, E., Ronen, S. M., & Debnath, J. (2011). Autophagy facilitates glycolysis during Ras-mediated oncogenic transformation. *Molecular Biology of the Cell, 22*(2), 165–178. DOI: 10.1091/mbc.e10-06-0500 PMID: 21119005

Ma, X. H., Piao, S., Wang, D., Mcafee, Q. W., Nathanson, K. L., Lum, J. J., Li, L. Z., & Amaravadi, R. K. (2011). Measurements of tumor cell autophagy predict invasiveness, resistance to chemotherapy, and survival in melanoma. *Clinical Cancer Research, 17*(10), 3478–3489. DOI: 10.1158/1078-0432.CCR-10-2372 PMID: 21325076

Mantovani, A. (2010). The growing diversity and spectrum of action of myeloid-derived suppressor cells. *European Journal of Immunology, 40*(12), 3317–3320. DOI: 10.1002/eji.201041170 PMID: 21110315

Marinković, M., & Novak, I. (2021). A brief overview of BNIP3L/NIX receptor-mediated mitophagy. *FEBS Open Bio, 11*(12), 3230–3236. DOI: 10.1002/2211-5463.13307 PMID: 34597467

Martinez-Lopez, N., Garcia-Macia, M., Sahu, S., Athonvarangkul, D., Liebling, E., Merlo, P., Cecconi, F., Schwartz, G. J., & Singh, R. (2016). Autophagy in the CNS and periphery coordinate lipophagy and lipolysis in the brown adipose tissue and liver. *Cell Metabolism, 23*(1), 113–127. DOI: 10.1016/j.cmet.2015.10.008 PMID: 26698918

Martínez-Reyes, I., & Chandel, N. S. (2021). Cancer metabolism: Looking forward. *Nature Reviews. Cancer*, *21*(10), 669–680. DOI: 10.1038/s41568-021-00378-6 PMID: 34272515

Mathew, R., Karp, C. M., Beaudoin, B., Vuong, N., Chen, G., Chen, H. Y., Bray, K., Reddy, A., Bhanot, G., Gelinas, C., DiPaola, R. S., Karantza-Wadsworth, V., & White, E. (2009). Autophagy suppresses tumorigenesis through elimination of p62. *Cell*, *137*(6), 1062–1075. DOI: 10.1016/j.cell.2009.03.048 PMID: 19524509

Mathew, R., Khor, S., Hackett, S. R., Rabinowitz, J. D., Perlman, D. H., & White, E. (2014). Functional role of autophagy-mediated proteome remodeling in cell survival signaling and innate immunity. *Molecular Cell*, *55*(6), 916–930. DOI: 10.1016/j.molcel.2014.07.019 PMID: 25175026

Mathew, R., Kongara, S., Beaudoin, B., Karp, C. M., Bray, K., Degenhardt, K., Chen, G., Jin, S., & White, E. (2007). Autophagy suppresses tumor progression by limiting chromosomal instability. *Genes & Development*, *21*(11), 1367–1381. DOI: 10.1101/gad.1545107 PMID: 17510285

McWilliams, T. G., & Muqit, M. M. (2017). PINK1 and Parkin: Emerging themes in mitochondrial homeostasis. *Current Opinion in Cell Biology*, *45*, 83–91. DOI: 10.1016/j.ceb.2017.03.013 PMID: 28437683

Miceli, C., Leri, M., Stefani, M., & Bucciantini, M. (2023). Autophagy-related proteins: Potential diagnostic and prognostic biomarkers of aging-related diseases. *Ageing Research Reviews*, *89*, 101967. DOI: 10.1016/j.arr.2023.101967 PMID: 37270146

Mishra, T., Singh, S., & Singh, T. G. (2024). Therapeutic Implications and Regulations of Protein Post-translational Modifications in Parkinsons Disease. *Cellular and Molecular Neurobiology*, *44*(1), 53. DOI: 10.1007/s10571-024-01471-8 PMID: 38960968

Mizushima, N., & Levine, B. (2020). Autophagy in human diseases. *The New England Journal of Medicine*, *383*(16), 1564–1576. DOI: 10.1056/NEJMra2022774 PMID: 33053285

Mohsen, S., Sobash, P. T., Algwaiz, G. F., Nasef, N., Al-Zeidaneen, S. A., & Karim, N. A. (2022). Autophagy Agents in Clinical Trials for Cancer Therapy: A Brief Review. *Current Oncology (Toronto, Ont.)*, *29*(3), 1695–1708. DOI: 10.3390/curroncol29030141 PMID: 35323341

Moindjie, H., Rodrigues-Ferreira, S., & Nahmias, C. (2021). Mitochondrial Metabolism in Carcinogenesis and Cancer Therapy. *Cancers (Basel)*, *13*(13), 3311. DOI: 10.3390/cancers13133311 PMID: 34282749

Nakatogawa, H., Suzuki, K., Kamada, Y., & Ohsumi, Y. (2009). Dynamics and diversity in autophagy mechanisms: Lessons from yeast. *Nature Reviews. Molecular Cell Biology*, *10*(7), 458–467. DOI: 10.1038/nrm2708 PMID: 19491929

Narendra, D. P., & Youle, R. J. (2024). The role of PINK1–Parkin in mitochondrial quality control. *Nature Cell Biology*, *26*(10), 1639–1651. DOI: 10.1038/s41556-024-01513-9 PMID: 39358449

Ney, P. A. (1853). 2015. Mitochondrial autophagy: Origins, significance, and role of BNIP3 and NIX. *Biochimica et Biophysica Acta (BBA)-. Molecular Cell Research*, (10), 2775–2783.

Niemi, N. M., & Friedman, J. R. (2024). Coordinating BNIP3/NIX-mediated mitophagy in space and time. *Biochemical Society Transactions*, *52*(5), 1969–1979. DOI: 10.1042/BST20221364 PMID: 39377319

Ohsumi, Y. (2014). Historical landmarks of autophagy research. *Cell Research*, *24*(1), 9–23. DOI: 10.1038/cr.2013.169 PMID: 24366340

Ortega, M. A., Fraile-Martinez, O., de Leon-Oliva, D., Boaru, D. L., Lopez-Gonzalez, L., García-Montero, C., Alvarez-Mon, M. A., Guijarro, L. G., Torres-Carranza, D., Saez, M. A., Diaz-Pedrero, R., Albillos, A., & Alvarez-Mon, M. (2024). Autophagy in its (proper) context: Molecular basis, biological relevance, pharmacological modulation, and lifestyle medicine. *International Journal of Biological Sciences*, *20*(7), 2532–2554. DOI: 10.7150/ijbs.95122 PMID: 38725847

Palikaras, K., Lionaki, E., & Tavernarakis, N. (2018). Mechanisms of mitophagy in cellular homeostasis, physiology and pathology. *Nature Cell Biology*, *20*(9), 1013–1022. DOI: 10.1038/s41556-018-0176-2 PMID: 30154567

Palma, F. R., Gantner, B. N., Sakiyama, M. J., Kayzuka, C., Shukla, S., Lacchini, R., Cunniff, B., & Bonini, M. G. (2024). ROS production by mitochondria: Function or dysfunction? *Oncogene*, *43*(5), 295–303. DOI: 10.1038/s41388-023-02907-z PMID: 38081963

Pandey, A., Yadav, P., & Shukla, S. (2021). Unfolding the role of autophagy in the cancer metabolism. *Biochemistry and Biophysics Reports*, *28*, 101158. DOI: 10.1016/j.bbrep.2021.101158 PMID: 34754952

Perera, R. M., Stoykova, S., Nicolay, B. N., Ross, K. N., Fitamant, J., Boukhali, M., Lengrand, J., Deshpande, V., Selig, M. K., Ferrone, C. R., Settleman, J., Stephanopoulos, G., Dyson, N. J., Zoncu, R., Ramaswamy, S., Haas, W., & Bardeesy, N. (2015). Transcriptional control of autophagy–lysosome function drives pancreatic cancer metabolism. *Nature*, *524*(7565), 361–365. DOI: 10.1038/nature14587 PMID: 26168401

Pyo, J. O., Nah, J., & Jung, Y. K. (2012). Molecules and their functions in autophagy. *Experimental & Molecular Medicine*, *44*(2), 73–80. DOI: 10.3858/emm.2012.44.2.029 PMID: 22257882

Qi, T., & Cao, Y. (2023). Dissecting sources of variability in patient response to targeted therapy: anti-HER2 therapies as a case study. *European Journal of Pharmaceutical Sciences*, *186*, 106467. DOI: 10.1016/j.ejps.2023.106467 PMID: 37196833

Quan, W., Kim, H. K., Moon, E. Y., Kim, S. S., Choi, C. S., Komatsu, M., Jeong, Y. T., Lee, M.-K., Kim, K.-W., Kim, M.-S., & Lee, M. S. (2012). Role of hypothalamic proopiomelanocortin neuron autophagy in the control of appetite and leptin response. *Endocrinology*, *153*(4), 1817–1826. DOI: 10.1210/en.2011-1882 PMID: 22334718

Rocchi, A., & He, C. (2017). Regulation of exercise-induced autophagy in skeletal muscle. *Current Pathobiology Reports*, *5*(2), 177–186. DOI: 10.1007/s40139-017-0135-9 PMID: 29057166

Rohatgi, R. A., Janusis, J., Leonard, D., Bellvé, K. D., Fogarty, K. E., Baehrecke, E. H., Corvera, S., & Shaw, L. M. (2015). Beclin 1 regulates growth factor receptor signaling in breast cancer. *Oncogene*, *34*(42), 5352–5362. DOI: 10.1038/onc.2014.454 PMID: 25639875

Rosenfeldt, M. T., O'Prey, J., Morton, J. P., Nixon, C., MacKay, G., Mrowinska, A., Au, A., Rai, T. S., Zheng, L., Ridgway, R., Adams, P. D., Anderson, K. I., Gottlieb, E., Sansom, O. J., & Ryan, K. M. (2013). p53 status determines the role of autophagy in pancreatic tumour development. *Nature*, *504*(7479), 296–300. DOI: 10.1038/nature12865 PMID: 24305049

Sabatini, D. M. (2006). mTOR and cancer: Insights into a complex relationship. *Nature Reviews. Cancer*, *6*(9), 729–734. DOI: 10.1038/nrc1974 PMID: 16915295

Sandomenico, A., Di Rienzo, L., Calvanese, L., Iaccarino, E., D'Auria, G., Falcigno, L., Chambery, A., Russo, R., Franzoso, G., Tornatore, L., D'Abramo, M., Ruvo, M., Milanetti, E., & Raimondo, D. (2020). Insights into the Interaction Mechanism of DTP3 with MKK7 by Using STD-NMR and Computational Approaches. *Biomedicines*, *9*(1), 20. DOI: 10.3390/biomedicines9010020 PMID: 33396582

Sankar, D. S., Kaeser-Pebernard, S., Vionnet, C., Favre, S., de Oliveira Marchioro, L., Pillet, B., Zhou, J., Stumpe, M., Kovacs, W. J., Kressler, D., Antonioli, M., Fimia, G. M., & Dengjel, J. (2024). The ULK1 effector BAG2 regulates autophagy initiation by modulating AMBRA1 localization. *Cell Reports*, *43*(9), 114689. DOI: 10.1016/j.celrep.2024.114689 PMID: 39207901

Sauve Brohée, V., Sung, G., MacDougall, E. J., Kozlov, G., Saran, A., Fakih, R., Fon, E. A., & Gehring, K. (2022). Structural basis for feedforward control in the PINK1/Parkin pathway. *The EMBO Journal*, *41*(12), e109460. DOI: 10.15252/embj.2021109460 PMID: 35491809

Scherr, A. L., Jassowicz, A., Pató, A., Elssner, C., Ismail, L., Schmitt, N., Hoffmeister, P., Neukirch, L., Gdynia, G., Goeppert, B., Schulze-Bergkamen, H., Jäger, D., & Köhler, B. C. (2020). Knockdown of Atg7 Induces Nuclear-LC3 Dependent Apoptosis and Augments Chemotherapy in Colorectal Cancer Cells. *International Journal of Molecular Sciences*, *21*(3), 1099. DOI: 10.3390/ijms21031099 PMID: 32046105

Schneider, J. L., Suh, Y., & Cuervo, A. M. (2014). Deficient chaperone-mediated autophagy in liver leads to metabolic dysregulation. *Cell Metabolism*, *20*(3), 417–432. DOI: 10.1016/j.cmet.2014.06.009 PMID: 25043815

Schuck, S. (2020). Microautophagy–distinct molecular mechanisms handle cargoes of many sizes. *Journal of Cell Science*, *133*(17), jcs246322. DOI: 10.1242/jcs.246322 PMID: 32907930

Settembre, C., & Perera, R. M. (2024). Lysosomes as coordinators of cellular catabolism, metabolic signalling and organ physiology. *Nature Reviews. Molecular Cell Biology*, *25*(3), 223–245. DOI: 10.1038/s41580-023-00676-x PMID: 38001393

Seyfried, T. N., Lee, D. C., Duraj, T., Ta, N. L., Mukherjee, P., Kiebish, M., Arismendi-Morillo, G., & Chinopoulos, C. (2025). The Warburg hypothesis and the emergence of the mitochondrial metabolic theory of cancer. *Journal of Bioenergetics and Biomembranes*, •••, 1–27. DOI: 10.1007/s10863-025-10059-w PMID: 40199815

Shang, J. N., Yu, C. G., Li, R., Xi, Y., Jian, Y. J., Xu, N., & Chen, S. (2024). The nonautophagic functions of autophagy-related proteins. *Autophagy*, *20*(4), 720–734. DOI: 10.1080/15548627.2023.2254664 PMID: 37682088

Shaw, R. J. (2009). LKB1 and AMP-activated protein kinase control of mTOR Signaling and growth. *Acta Physiologica (Oxford, England)*, *196*(1), 65–80. DOI: 10.1111/j.1748-1716.2009.01972.x PMID: 19245654

Sinha, R. A., You, S. H., Zhou, J., Siddique, M. M., Bay, B. H., Zhu, X., Privalsky, M. L., Cheng, S.-Y., Stevens, R. D., Summers, S. A., Newgard, C. B., Lazar, M. A., & Yen, P. M. (2012). Thyroid hormone stimulates hepatic lipid catabolism via activation of autophagy. *The Journal of Clinical Investigation*, *122*(7), 2428–2438. DOI: 10.1172/JCI60580 PMID: 22684107

Strohecker, A. M., & White, E. (2014). Targeting mitochondrial metabolism by inhibiting autophagy in BRAF-driven cancers. *Cancer Discovery*, *4*(7), 766–772. DOI: 10.1158/2159-8290.CD-14-0196 PMID: 24860158

Takamura, A., Komatsu, M., Hara, T., Sakamoto, A., Kishi, C., Waguri, S., Eishi, Y., Hino, O., Tanaka, K., & Mizushima, N. (2011). Autophagy-deficient mice develop multiple liver tumors. *Genes & Development*, *25*(8), 795–800. DOI: 10.1101/gad.2016211 PMID: 21498569

Thylur Puttalingaiah, R., Dean, M. J., Zheng, L., Philbrook, P., Wyczechowska, D., Kayes, T., Del Valle, L., Danos, D., & Sanchez-Pino, M. D. (2024). Excess Potassium Promotes Autophagy to Maintain the Immunosuppressive Capacity of Myeloid-Derived Suppressor Cells Independent of Arginase 1. *Cells*, *13*(20), 1736. DOI: 10.3390/cells13201736 PMID: 39451254

Vander Heiden, M.G., Cantley, L.C. and Thompson, C.B., 2009. Understanding the Warburg effect: the metabolic requirements of cell proliferation. *science, 324*(5930), pp.1029-1033.

Voronina, M. V., Frolova, A. S., Kolesova, E. P., Kuldyushev, N. A., Parodi, A., & Zamyatnin, A. A.Jr. (2024). The Intricate Balance between Life and Death: ROS, cathepsins, and their interplay in cell death and autophagy. *International Journal of Molecular Sciences*, *25*(7), 4087. DOI: 10.3390/ijms25074087 PMID: 38612897

Wang, J. Z., Paulus, P., Niu, Y., Zhu, L., Morisseau, C., Rawling, T., Murray, M., Hammock, B. D., & Zhou, F. (2024). The Role of Autophagy in Human Uveal Melanoma and the Development of Potential Disease Biomarkers and Novel Therapeutic Paradigms. *Biomedicines*, *12*(2), 462. DOI: 10.3390/biomedicines12020462 PMID: 38398064

Wang, S., Long, H., Hou, L., Feng, B., Ma, Z., Wu, Y., Zeng, Y., Cai, J., Zhang, D. W., & Zhao, G. (2023). The mitophagy pathway and its implications in human diseases. *Signal Transduction and Targeted Therapy*, *8*(1), 304. Advance online publication. DOI: 10.1038/s41392-023-01503-7 PMID: 37582956

Wang, X., Lu, S., He, C., Wang, C., Wang, L., Piao, M., Chi, G., Luo, Y., & Ge, P. (2019). RSL3 induced autophagic death in glioma cells via causing glycolysis dysfunction. *Biochemical and Biophysical Research Communications*, *518*(3), 590–597. DOI: 10.1016/j.bbrc.2019.08.096 PMID: 31445705

Wang, X. L., Feng, S. T., Wang, Z. Z., Chen, N. H., & Zhang, Y. (2021). Role of mitophagy in mitochondrial quality control: Mechanisms and potential implications for neurodegenerative diseases. *Pharmacological Research*, *165*, 105433. DOI: 10.1016/j.phrs.2021.105433 PMID: 33454337

Warburg, O. (1956). On the origin of cancer cells. *Science*, *123*(3191), 309–314. DOI: 10.1126/science.123.3191.309 PMID: 13298683

Weber, C. A., Sekar, K., Tang, J. H., Warmer, P., Sauer, U., & Weis, K. (2020). β-Oxidation and autophagy are critical energy providers during acute glucose depletion in S accharomyces cerevisiae. *Proceedings of the National Academy of Sciences of the United States of America*, *117*(22), 12239–12248. DOI: 10.1073/pnas.1913370117 PMID: 32430326

Wei, Z., Liu, X., Cheng, C., Yu, W., & Yi, P. (2021). Metabolism of amino acids in cancer. *Frontiers in Cell and Developmental Biology*, *8*, 603837. DOI: 10.3389/fcell.2020.603837 PMID: 33511116

White, E. (2012). Deconvoluting the context-dependent role for autophagy in cancer. *Nature Reviews. Cancer*, *12*(6), 401–410. DOI: 10.1038/nrc3262 PMID: 22534666

White, E., Mehnert, J. M., & Chan, C. S. (2015). Autophagy, metabolism, and cancer. *Clinical Cancer Research*, *21*(22), 5037–5046. DOI: 10.1158/1078-0432.CCR-15-0490 PMID: 26567363

Xu, H. M., & Hu, F. (2022). The role of autophagy and mitophagy in cancers. *Archives of Physiology and Biochemistry*, *128*(2), 281–289. DOI: 10.1080/13813455.2019.1675714 PMID: 31596150

Yamashita, S. I., Arai, R., Hada, H., Padman, B. S., Lazarou, M., Chan, D. C., Kanki, T., & Waguri, S. (2025). The mitophagy receptors BNIP3 and NIX mediate tight attachment and expansion of the isolation membrane to mitochondria. *The Journal of Cell Biology*, *224*(7), e202408166. DOI: 10.1083/jcb.202408166 PMID: 40358358

Yang, A., Rajeshkumar, N. V., Wang, X., Yabuuchi, S., Alexander, B. M., Chu, G. C., Von Hoff, D. D., Maitra, A., & Kimmelman, A. C. (2014). Autophagy is critical for pancreatic tumor growth and progression in tumors with p53 alterations. *Cancer Discovery*, *4*(8), 905–913. DOI: 10.1158/2159-8290.CD-14-0362 PMID: 24875860

Yang, J., Shay, C., Saba, N. F., & Teng, Y. (2024). Cancer metabolism and carcinogenesis. *Experimental Hematology & Oncology*, *13*(1), 10. DOI: 10.1186/s40164-024-00482-x PMID: 38287402

Yang, J., Shay, C., Saba, N. F., & Teng, Y. (2024). Cancer metabolism and carcinogenesis. *Experimental Hematology & Oncology*, *13*(1), 10. DOI: 10.1186/s40164-024-00482-x PMID: 38287402

Yang, Q. E. (2021). Human cancer xenografts in immunocompromised mice provide an advanced genuine tumor model for research and drug development-A revisit of murine models for human cancers. *Biochimica Et Biophysica Acta (BBA) -. Biochimica et Biophysica Acta. G, General Subjects*, *1865*(8), 129929. DOI: 10.1016/j.bbagen.2021.129929 PMID: 33991617

Yang, S., Wang, X., Contino, G., Liesa, M., Sahin, E., Ying, H., Bause, A., Li, Y., Stommel, J. M., Dell'Antonio, G., Mautner, J., Tonon, G., Haigis, M., Shirihai, O. S., Doglioni, C., Bardeesy, N., & Kimmelman, A. C. (2011). Pancreatic cancers require autophagy for tumor growth. *Genes & Development*, *25*(7), 717–729. DOI: 10.1101/gad.2016111 PMID: 21406549

Yau, W. W., Wong, K. A., Zhou, J., Thimmukonda, N. K., Wu, Y., Bay, B. H., Singh, B. K., & Yen, P. M. (2021). Chronic cold exposure induces autophagy to promote fatty acid oxidation, mitochondrial turnover, and thermogenesis in brown adipose tissue. *iScience*, *24*(5), 102434. DOI: 10.1016/j.isci.2021.102434 PMID: 34027318

Ye, M., Wang, S., Wan, T., Jiang, R., Qiu, Y., Pei, L., Pang, N., Huang, Y., Huang, Y., Zhang, Z., & Yang, L. (2017). Combined inhibitions of glycolysis and AKT/autophagy can overcome resistance to EGFR-targeted therapy of lung cancer. *Journal of Cancer*, *8*(18), 3774–3784. DOI: 10.7150/jca.21035 PMID: 29151965

Yu, L., Chen, Y., & Tooze, S. A. (2018). Autophagy pathway: Cellular and molecular mechanisms. *Autophagy*, *14*(2), 207–215. DOI: 10.1080/15548627.2017.1378838 PMID: 28933638

Zamanian, M. Y., Golmohammadi, M., Yumashev, A., Hjazi, A., Toama, M. A., AbdRabou, M. A., Gehlot, A., Alwaily, E. R., Shirsalimi, N., Yadav, P. K., & Moriasi, G. (2024). Effects of metformin on cancers in experimental and clinical studies: Focusing on autophagy and AMPK/mTOR signaling pathways. *Cell Biochemistry and Function*, *42*(4), e4071. DOI: 10.1002/cbf.4071 PMID: 38863255

Zhang, J., & Ney, P. A. (2009). Role of BNIP3 and NIX in cell death, autophagy, and mitophagy. *Cell Death and Differentiation*, *16*(7), 939–946. DOI: 10.1038/cdd.2009.16 PMID: 19229244

Zhang, X. Y., Zhang, M., Cong, Q., Zhang, M. X., Zhang, M. Y., Lu, Y. Y., & Xu, C. J. (2018). Hexokinase 2 confers resistance to cisplatin in ovarian cancer cells by enhancing cisplatin-induced autophagy. *The International Journal of Biochemistry & Cell Biology*, *95*, 9–16. DOI: 10.1016/j.biocel.2017.12.010 PMID: 29247711

Zhang, Y., Goldman, S., Baerga, R., Zhao, Y., Komatsu, M., & Jin, S. (2009). Adipose-specific deletion of autophagy-related gene 7 (atg7) in mice reveals a role in adipogenesis. *Proceedings of the National Academy of Sciences of the United States of America*, *106*(47), 19860–19865. DOI: 10.1073/pnas.0906048106 PMID: 19910529

Zhou, Y., Tao, L., Qiu, J., Xu, J., Yang, X., Zhang, Y., Tian, X., Guan, X., Cen, X., & Zhao, Y. (2024). Tumor biomarkers for diagnosis, prognosis and targeted therapy. *Signal Transduction and Targeted Therapy*, *9*(1), 132. DOI: 10.1038/s41392-024-01823-2 PMID: 38763973

Zong, Y., Li, H., Liao, P., Chen, L., Pan, Y., Zheng, Y., Zhang, C., Liu, D., Zheng, M., & Gao, J. (2024). Mitochondrial dysfunction: Mechanisms and advances in therapy. *Signal Transduction and Targeted Therapy*, *9*(1), 124. DOI: 10.1038/s41392-024-01839-8 PMID: 38744846

Chapter 3
How to Target Mitophagy and Link-Related Pathways in Anticancer Therapy

K. R. Padma
https://orcid.org/0000-0002-6783-3248
Sri Padmavati Mahila Visva Vidyalayam (Women's) University, India

K. R. Don
Sree Balaji Dental College and Hospital, India

ABSTRACT

Mitophagy the deliberate breakdown of mitochondria by the autophagic pathway is a crucial component of cell-level mitochondrial quality control. Mitophagy, the act of eliminating damaged or malfunctioning mitochondria, is a crucial part of normal cellular physiology and tissue creation. Shared pathways governing mitophagy, cancer, and cell death could be triggered by a solitary upstream signal convening at the mitochondria. We also discuss the pivotal roles that these processes perform in the cancer microenvironment. Recent studies have contributed to the development of anticancer treatments that either promote or inhibit autophagy, shedding light on the role autophagy and related mechanisms play in the initiation and spread of cancer. In this review paper, we have looked at and investigated the different roles that autophagy and related systems play in the development, maintenance, and expansion of malignancies.

DOI: 10.4018/979-8-3693-3836-0.ch003

INTRODUCTION

One of the significant homeostatic pathways that enhance breakdown and recycling of cellular content is the macroautophagy or autophagy (Klionsky et al., 2021). In diseases, the benefits of autophagy induction were becoming one of the leading areas that helped the cure of such issues as removal of protein aggregates that cause or cause neurodegeneration, for example. However, one might say that autophagy has a more complex role in cancer, which depends on the biology and stage of a tumor as well as surrounding microenvironment. The process of autophagy includes the formation of a double-membrane vesicle called an autophagosome that encloses the cellular cargo and meets with lysosomes and breaks down by lysosomal hydrolases2. This process is regulated by a panel of autophagy – related (ATG) gene products (Fig. 1).

Figure 1. A schematic illustration of autophagy. ULK1 complex is activated, and several ATG proteins are participating where PAS is the place where they are localized. The series of events involved during phagophore formation include: recruitment of lipids and ATG proteins, elongation that includes wrapping and engulfment of cytoplasm and organelles and maturation, completion and transport of autophagosome. The docking, fusing, and fusion process of autophagosome-lysosome. Degradation takes place in the autolysosome with regards to the cargo. ULK1, ATG13, FIP200 and ATG101 make up for ULK1 kinase core complex. Beclin1, VPS34, VPS15 and ATG14L form the complex I of class III PI3K. All three namely, ATG9A, ATG2 and WIPI1/2 are the subunits of the ATG9A/Atg2- WIPI1/2 trafficking system. ATG12-conjugation system has the following components: ATG12, ATG7, ATG10, ATG5 and ATG16L. ProLC3, ATG4, LC3-I, ATG7, ATG3 and LC3-II (LC3-I/PE) all make up the LC3-conjugation system.

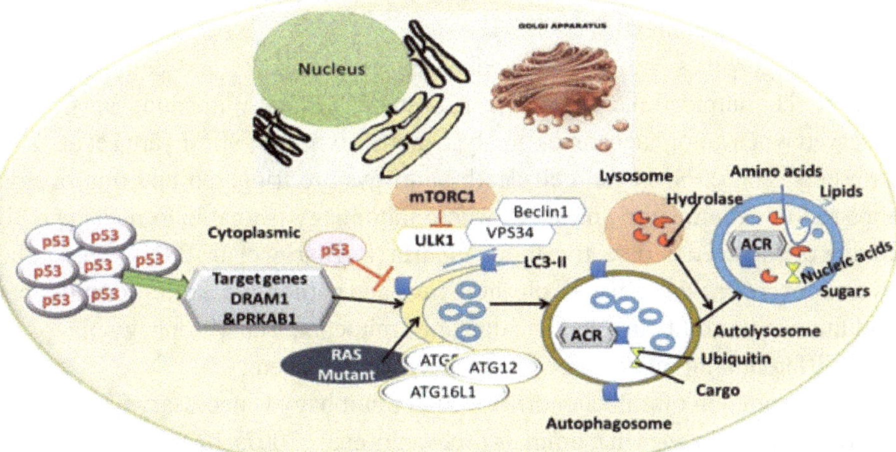

Autophagy begins with the formation of a phagophore, a double membrane originating from the endoplasmic reticulum and other sources. This process is regulated by ULK1 kinase and the class III PI3K complex, including beclin-1 and VPS34, which produce phosphatidylinositol-3-phosphate essential for autophagosome membrane expansion. The ATG8 family proteins conjugate to phosphatidylethanolamine through the ATG5-ATG12-ATG16L1 complex, converting LC3 into its lipidated form, LC3-II, which remains on the phagophore membrane to assist autophagosome formation (Mathiassen et al., 2017; Lee et al., 2012).

Lipidated ATG8 proteins facilitate selective autophagy by binding to autophagy cargo receptors (ACRs) that recognize ubiquitinated cargo. Once fully formed, the autophagosome fuses with lysosomes, where cargo is degraded by lysosomal enzymes into amino acids, lipids, or carbohydrates for cellular reuse. This degradation prevents accumulation of unfolded proteins, damaged organelles, and excessive reactive oxygen species (ROS), which could otherwise lead to inflammation, cellular dysfunction, or malignant transformation. Autophagy thus maintains cellular homeostasis and prevents disease progression.

Autophagy can suppress tumors by degrading elements like the cargo receptor p62, which is linked to cancer development. Key regulators such as tumor suppressor p53 and oncogenic RAS influence autophagy and tumor progression. Nutrient-sensing mechanistic target of rapamycin complex 1 (mTORC1) represses autophagy, while AMP-activated protein kinase (AMPK) activates it under energy stress. Basal p53 inhibits autophagy, but stress-induced p53 promotes it by activating genes like damage-regulated autophagy modulator 1(DRAM1) and AMPK through its subunit PRKAB1 (protein kinase AMP-activated non-catalytic subunit beta 1). Mutant RAS has a complex role, both stimulating and potentially suppressing autophagy depending on the context.

Autophagosomes are where depolarized mitochondria and cellular proteins are kept. The intracellular environment is stabilized and mitochondrial fitness is preserved when autophagosomes and lysosomes combine (Matsuyama et al., 2000; Lemasters, 2005). However, cell death pathways are triggered and mitophagy is repressed in extreme circumstances where mitophagy is unable to manage a high number of damaged or defective mitochondria (Pagliarini et al., 2012). Researchers have discovered a wide range of physiological and pathological roles for mitophagy in addition to its ability to eliminate damaged mitochondria. Mitophagy plays a role in the differentiating of erythrocytes and cell development.

The elimination of mitochondria through mitophagy is necessary for the differentiating of erythrocytes in mammals (Schweers et al., 2007). In animals lacking the mitophagy-related gene BCL2/adenovirus E1B 19 kDa protein-interacting protein 3-like (BNIP3L), erythrocytes accumulate mitochondria, leading to anemia (Sandoval et al., 2008). To encourage the shift of beige to white adipocytes, mitophagy removes extra mitochondria from adipocytes (Lu et al., 2018). Dysregulation of mitophagy is not surprising because it has a function in human disorders because it maintains mitochondrial homeostasis. Patients with Parkinson's disease have brain tissue that has an excess of defective mitochondria and has been shown to have PTEN-induced putative kinase 1 (PINK1) mutation (Nah et al., 2015). PINK1 is then demonstrated to be a gene associated to mitophagy (Valente et al., 2004). Furthermore, patients with Alzheimer's disease exhibit a similar phenomenon, suggesting that mitophagy protects against neurodegenerative illnesses (Manczak et al., 2018). malignancies arise from complex pathophysiological processes; the impact of mitophagy on malignancies will be covered in a later section. We provide a succinct overview of the primary processes governing mitophagy control in this study. We also clarified the functions of mitophagy in drug resistance, anticancer therapies, and carcinogenesis.

MITOPHAGY AND ITS COMMON FUNCTIONS

The process of mitophagy is a type of selective autophagy in which the autophagolysosome exclusively targets mitochondria for breakdown (Springer & Macleod 2016; Bernardini, 2017). For this reason, the mitophagy process depends on in addition to the general autophagy mechanism, it is dependent on an expanding array of regulatory molecules and "mitophagy adaptors" that choose which mitochondria will undergo autophagic turnover (see Table 1). Although mitophagy can be synthetically generated by respiratory chain inhibitors and uncoupling agents that depolarize mitochondria, including carbonyl cyanide 3-chlorophenylhydrazone (CCCP) (Al Rawi et al., 2011; Sato, 2011), it is also a natural response to important physiological stresses like hypoxia and nutritional restriction.

Furthermore, removal of mitochondria during red blood cell synthesis (Rojansky et al., 2016), muscle differentiation, and elimination of paternal mitochondria from the fertilized egg (Schweers et al., 2007) are all examples of the planned components of developmental and differentiation processes that include mitophagy. Mitophagy is essential for preserving the integrity of the mitochondria and the cell because it facilitates the removal of old, defective, and/or supernumerary mitochondria. On the other hand, aberrant macrophagy may result in the breakdown of tissue homeostasis and the emergence of illnesses, such as cancer (Sin et al., 2016). Many mitophagy modulators, such as PARK2, BNIP3, BNIP3L, FANCC, and p62/SQSTM1, have been demonstrated to be dysregulated in human malignancies; further modulators are probably going to surface as this field of study develops. The problem in research involves figuring out what selective advantage the tumor gains from mitophagy dysregulation and whether mitophagy encourages or inhibits growth.

Table 1. Regulators and functions of mitophagy in association with cancer/disease

Protein/gene	Functions associated with the process of mitophagy	Links to cancer/disease	Reference
PARK8/LRRK2	An innovative PD predisposition gene that codes for a protein that interacts with Miro to encourage its breakdown, obstructs mitophagy, and prevents mitochondria from being sequestered. Specific kinase activity of LRRK2 is shown for Rab GTPases (Rab1b, Rab8a, and Rab10) involved in cellular trafficking; mutant LRRK2 (G2019S) exhibits enhanced kinase activity for these substrates.	mutated in Parkinson's disease (e.g., G2019S)	(Hsieh et al., 2016)
PARK6/PINK1	Phosphorylates Parkin and ubiquitin chains on the IMM via voltage-dependent import and degradation of serine/threonine kinase, which is stabilized at the OMM by modified $\Delta\Psi mt$. S65 to suppress its auto-inhibitory function, which causes Parkin to recruit and activate at the OMM.	Parkinson's disease and PARK6 loss are related.	(Heo et al., 2015)
TAZ/tafazzin	Cardiolipin-remodeling phospholipid trans-acylase; absence of TAZ prevents mitophagy because LC3 is unable to identify CL; low TAZ causes less acylation of CL and its removal from mitochondria.	Barth syndrome mutation	(Hsu et al., 2015)
Caspase-1	Proto-typical caspase that is important for cytokine processing and is part of the NLRP3 inflammasome. It is attracted to the OMM and is activated by oxidized mtDNA and changed $\Delta\Psi mt$ ROS in a positive feedback loop. It also cleaves Parkin. Inflammasome activity is reduced by mitophagy.	Breast and stomach malignancies, as well as fibrosarcoma, are encouraged by IL-1 signaling and inflammatory proteins.	(Nakahira et al., 2011; Shimada et al., 2012)
OPTN/ Optineurin	OPTN is an adapter for autophagic cargo that has the ability to bind ubiquitin and LC3 at the same time at the OMM. becomes attracted to depolarized mitochondria in a way that is reliant on Parkin	ALS-related mutation. in cell lines of lung cancer downregulated. Poor prognosis in lung cancer patients is correlated with low expression.	(Wong & Holzbaur, 2014)
FUNDC1	Hypoxia-induced OMM protein interacts directly with LC3, which is controlled by ULK1, SRC, CK2, and PGAM5. Through interactions with calnexin, OMM protein accumulates at ER-mito contact sites and is necessary for Drp1 and LC3 recruitment during hypoxia-induced mitophagy.	Unknown. Platelet maturation abnormalities are present in knockout mice.	(Liu et al., 2012; Wu et al., 2014)

continued on following page

Table 1. Continued

Protein/gene	Functions associated with the process of mitophagy	Links to cancer/disease	Reference
FANC-C	A portion of the DNA repair pathway for Fanconi Anemia (FA); found in a screen for genes that rescue selective autophagy; interacts with Parkin, which is necessary for mitophagy and localizes to mitochondria; FANCC has a distinct genetic function apart from its role in DNA repair. FANCA, FANCD1 (BRCA2), FANCD2, FANCF, FANCL, and FANCS (BRCA1) are additional FA genes that have also been linked to mitophagy.	Other FANC genes include BRCA2 and BRCA1, which are lost in hereditary ovarian and breast cancer, and are inactivated in Fanconi Anemia.	(Sumpter et al., 2016)
Cardiolipin (CL)	Stress causes CL to relocalize to OMM; LC3 binds to CL and is necessary for LC3-mediated mitophagy; IMM phospholipid is involved in attaching proteins to cristae, including ETC components.	Not known	(Chu et al., 2013)

Mitophagy is Facilitated by Parkin Recruitment to Depolarized Mitochondria

When human Parkinson's disease (PD) was first linked to mutations in the PARK2 (Parkin) and PARK6 (PINK1) gene products, it was later demonstrated that these gene products worked together to increase mitophagy, suggesting that defective mitochondria were a possible cause of PD (Youle & Narendra, 2011). In human chromosome 6q25–q26, PARK2 (Parkin) aligns to a common fragile site that is frequently deleted in malignancies of the ovary, breast, bladder, lung, and other tissues (Cesari et al., 2003; Gong et al., 2014). In a nutshell when mitochondrial depolarization occurs, PINKB1 builds up at the outer mitochondrial membrane (OMM). As a ubiquitin kinase at the OMM, PINK1 phosphorylates Parkin on S65 in its ubiquitin-like domain, encouraging more active Parkin to be localized to the OMM. Parkin binds ubiquitin chains to important mitochondrial substrates, including as mitofusins, Vdac1, Miro, and other OMM proteins. Pink1 then phosphorylates these ubiquitin chains, amplifying the signal for mitophagy (Fig. 1A). The recruitment of mitophagy cargo adaptors, such as p62/Sqstml, OPTN, and NDP52, which bind to the phospho-ubiquitin chains produced by PINK1/Parkin, requires both PINK1 and Parkin.

Upon being ubiquitinated by Parkin, certain substrates (like ubiquitinated Vdac1) establish a docking location for the LC3 interacting proteins p62/SQSTM1 and NBR-1 (Lee et al., 2010;-Geisler et al., 2010). This enables the selective destruction of mitochondria by Parkin at the autophagosome (Figure 1). The anti-apoptotic proteins Bcl-XL, Mcl-1, and Bcl-W, but not Bcl-2 itself, hinder Parkin's recruitment to depolarized membranes in a way that is not dependent on Beclin. Bcl-XL, Mcl-1, and Bcl-W inhibited mitophagy by directly interacting with Parkin, which blocked Parkin's association with PINK1 and, consequently, prevented the ubiquitination of mitochondrial targets by Parkin. On the other hand, the noncanonical BH3 proteins BNIP3, Nix, or Beclin1 did not increase Parkin translocation to mitochondria, whereas the pro-apoptotic BH3 proteins Puma, Noxa, Bim, and Bad did (Novak, 2012). This may have happened via limiting Parkin's interaction with the previously described Bcl-2-related molecules.

The Key Aspects of Mitochondrial Behaviour in Cancer

The origin, spread, invasion, and metastasis of cancer are all significantly influenced by mitochondria. Cancer and the destiny of mitochondria have a strong link (Wallace, 2012). Cancer cells often experience a fast metabolic reprogramming that limits the tricarboxylic acid cycle (TCA) and mitochondrial oxidative phosphorylation (OXPHOS) due to numerous mutations in critical enzymes (Van et al., 2015). This makes it possible for cancer cells to switch their energy metabolism from ATP synthesis via glycolysis; however, changed metabolism is not the only way that mitochondrial malfunction and cancer are related (Warburg, 1956). There is mounting evidence that mitochondrial malfunction plays a role in the development of cancer, with the exact relationship varying depending on the kind of cancer. Decreased mitochondrial efficiency leads to the build-up of damaged mitochondria, which intensifies oxidative damage, including reactive oxygen species (ROS)-induced DNA alterations, and upsets the redox equilibrium. Genetic instability causes an increase in free radical generation, which in turn contributes to the growth of tumors (Kryston et al., 2011). Furthermore, cancer cells modify their metabolism to lower the regulation of reactive oxygen species (ROS) produced by malfunctioning mitochondria. Therefore, changes in cancer cell metabolism are strongly linked to mitophagy, a process that selectively degrades damaged mitochondria and further impacts the course of cancer.

The relationship between cancer and mitophagy is still intricate and varied. One way in which mitophagy is important is that it keeps damaged mitochondria from building up and causing tumors. Conversely, aberrant mitophagy is linked to drug resistance, cancer cell survival, and avoidance of cell death; yet the majority of research has not directly demonstrated mitophagy during tumor development. In order to determine the precise elements that contribute to general mitophagy deficits or their repercussions, these processes need to be investigated further (Table 2).

Table 2. Cancer's mitophagy's molecular effects

Gene of target	Effect	Type	Reference
PINK1	The elevated level of PINK1 expression promotes proliferation throughout the course of NSCLC in addition to chemoresistance.	(Oncogene) lung cancer	(Zhang et al., 2017; Lu et al., 2020)
MFN2	In a pancreatic ductal adenocarcinoma (PDAC) model, the oral medication leflunomide, which is used to treat arthritis, increases Mfn2 expression twofold. This results in a 50% increase in the average survival rate of tumor-bearing mice when compared to the vehicle group.	(Tumor suppressor) Pancreatic cancer	(Yu et al., 2019)
AMBRA1	Ambra1 deficiency increases the development of melanocytic nevi and speeds up the evolution of melanoma, ultimately increasing the risk of metastasis.	(Oncogene) Melanoma	(Di Leo et al., 2021)
Parkin	Adenomatous polyposis coli (APC) deficiency in human colon cancer is substantially linked to a deficiency in PARK2 expression.	(Tumor suppressor) Colorectal cancer	(Poulogiannis et al., 2010)
BNIP3	The methylation of the hypoxia-responsive element (HRE) site was linked to the suppression of BNIP3 production, and this in turn prevented HIF-1 from attaching to the BNIP3 promoter.	(Tumor suppressor) Pancreatic cancer	(Li et al., 2017)
DRP1	Drp1 is essential for both the oxidative metabolism and the carcinogenic process in a pancreatic cancer tumor model that is triggered by KRas. The survival rate for pancreatic cancer is increased by inhibiting Drp1.	(Oncogene) Pancreatic cancer	(Nagdas et al., 2019)
NIX	In a mouse model of PDAC (pancreatic ductal adenocarcinoma), NIX knockdown dramatically slows the advancement of pancreatic cancer and increases survival rates.	(Oncogene) Pancreatic cancer	(Humpton et al., 2019)
PGAM5	A poor prognostic characteristic in HCC is linked to elevated PGAM5 expression. In HCC cells, PGAM5 knockdown increased chemosensitivity and decreased cell survival.	(Oncogene) Hepatocellular carcinoma	(Cheng et al., 2018)

Mitophagy Encourages the Growth of Tumors

According to Levy et al. (2017), autophagy has a multifaceted function in tumor biology that varies depending on the kind, stage, and setting of the tumor. Since autophagy reduces inflammation and genomic instability, it generally helps prevent the start of cancer. On the other hand, in tumors that have already grown, cancer cells might use autophagy to meet their metabolic needs and strengthen their resistance to cell death, which would promote their growth and invasiveness. Similarly, one of the hallmarks of cancer is defective mitophagy. The majority of mitophagy regulators or receptors are implicated in cancer; however, the kind of tumor and

TME (Table 3), as is explained below, appear to have a significant influence on whether these regulators or receptors function as tumor promoters or suppressors (Panigrahi et al., 2019; Praharaj et al., 2019; Ferro et al., 2020).

Table 3. Regulations of mitophagy in the progression of tumors

Regulators of Mitophagy	Type of Tumor	Functions related to cancer	Mechanism	Reference
BNIP3	Gastric cancer	Tumor Suppressor	Induces cell death due to hypoxia	(Murai et al., 2005)
PRKN	Colon cancer	Tumor Suppressor	Inhibits the proliferation of cells	(Yin et al., 2018)
PINK1	Pancreatic ductal adenocarcinoma	Tumor Suppressor	Reduces inflammation and immune response against tumors	(Li et al., 2018)
FUNDC1	Hepatocellular carcinoma	Tumor Suppressor	Reduces inflammation	(Li et al., 2019a)
PHB2	Non-small cell lung carcinoma	Tumor Promoter	Stimulates migration and multiplication of cells	(Zhang et al., 2020)
Ceramide	Head and neck squamous cell carcinoma, acute myeloid leukemia cells	Tumor Suppressor	Promotes cellular apoptosis	(Dany et al., 2016)
BNIP3	Breast tumor	Tumor Suppressor	Prevents angiogenesis and glycolysis	(Chourasia et al., 2015)
FUNDC1	Laryngeal cancer	Tumor Promoter	Encourages the survival and multiplication of cells	(Hui et al., 2019)

Anticancer Therapy: Mitophagy as a Target

Mitophagy is involved in many different aspects of cancer development and progression. The characteristics and subtypes of cancer cells determine whether it acts as a tumor suppressor or promoter (Fei, 2004; Kulikov et al., 2017). To preserve the balance between the amount and quality of mitochondria, mitophagy can eliminate damaged or defective mitochondria. Functional mitochondria reduce ROS production and their ability to initiate tumors after mitophagy (Waris & Ahsan, 2006). However, once the malignancies have progressed, mitophagy can serve as a cytoprotective strategy to direct the tumor's growth in order to prevent chemotherapy-induced apoptosis (Yan et al., 2017; Im et al., 2016). Carcinogenesis is prevented and the build-up of damaged mitochondria is inhibited by functional mitophagy. According to a study on liver cancer in mice, thyroid hormone T3 inhibits the growth of new cancer cells by turning on the PINK1/Parkin pathway (Chi et al., 2017).

Various chemotherapeutic agents cause mitochondrial malfunction, release harmful compounds including ROS, and disrupt regular metabolic processes (Carew et al., 2003; Li et al., 2003; Lu et al., 2007). An adaptation mechanism to chemotherapy drug treatment is mitophagy, a cytoprotective mechanism. As such, mitochondrial targeting is seen to be a promising anticancer treatment. The platinum-based substance cisplatin is commonly utilized and has anticancer properties against a variety of malignancies. Cisplatin resistance in cancers gradually develops. Thus, it is extremely difficult to avoid medication resistance (Liu et al., 2020). The cisplatin resistance of the non-small cell lung cancer cell line A549 is partly attributed to caveolin-1 (Cav-1)/Parkin-mediated mitophagy. Due to the decreased Rho-associated coiled-coil-containing protein kinase 1 (ROCK1), the cav-1-knockdown A549 cells look more susceptible to cisplatin, which in turn inhibits Parkin-mediated mitophagy (Li et al., 2019).

Through the triggering of mitochondrial apoptosis, a novel betulinic acid (BA) derivative called B5G1 exhibits strong anticancer action against multidrug-resistant cancer cells. On the other hand, B5G1 can cause mitophagy by upregulating PINK1 and then recruiting Parkin. Drug-resistant cancer cells become sensitive to B5G1 when mitophagy is inhibited by mitochondrial division inhibitor 1 (mdivi-1) or bafilomycin (Yao et al., 2019). The DNA-damaging drug doxorubicin significantly reduces cell viability by causing cell death and mitochondrial malfunction. But in colorectal cancer, BNIP3L-mediated mitophagy eliminates damaged mitochondria to lessen oxidative stress and promote cell survival.

While mitophagy helps cells adapt to stress, too much mitochondrial clearance can cause a cell to die. Thus, in the therapy of cancer, mitophagy inducers and inhibitors might be just as beneficial. Downregulating cancer cells' drug resistance is mostly dependent on the inhibition of mitophagy (Yao et al., 2019). Drug resistance to cisplatin inhibits the effectiveness of chemotherapy in cervical cancer. Renowned for its ability to minimize hypoxia-ischemia damage and enhance sleep, melatonin (N-acetyl-5-methoxytryptamine) is an endogenous indoleamine and antioxidant. Along with blocking mitophagy, it can help regulate the growth of tumors. Mechanistically, melatonin worsens cervical cancer cell apoptosis and suppresses mitophagy via downregulating c-Jun N-terminal kinase (JNK) and subsequently Parkin (MacKeigan, 2005). Chemotherapeutic medications like cisplatin are not very effective at curing liver cancer.

A lack of functioning mitochondria may cause enhanced mitophagy and consequent cell death. For therapeutic intervention in other malignancies, enhanced mitophagy can potentially offer a promising approach. By downregulating the expression of COX-2, an oral antifungal medication called ketoconazole induces PINK1/Parkin-mediated mitophagy and stimulates hepatic carcinoma cells to undergo apoptosis (Chen et al., 2018). Furthermore, via PINK1/Parkin-mediated mitophagy, sorafenib promotes the death of liver cancer cells. It attracts Parkin to malfunctioning mitochondria to start mitophagy and stabilizes PINK1 on the outer membrane of mitochondria (Chen et al., 2019). Two mitochondria-targeting medications, Mito-CP and Mito-Metformin, limit the growth of colorectal cancer cells by inhibiting mitophagy, releasing ULK1 from mTOR-mediated regulation, and lowering mitochondrial membrane potential (Zhang et al., 2017; Boyle et al., 2018).

CONCLUSIONS AND FUTURE DIRECTIONS

Deleting damaged mitochondria using mitophagy is a significant and complex role in cancer science. While cellular homeostasis can help prevent tumors, under stress it can increase tumor survival. Links between mitophagy and CSC self-renewal, the control of key cancer signals, and tumor growth are still not fully understood. Researchers are still trying to understand how modulating mitophagy could boost therapies that rely on checkpoint inhibitors or oncolytic virus therapy. Exploring how hypoxia, nutrient shortage, and ROS affect it is important as well. More knowledge about how mitophagy responds to oncometabolites might help find new approaches for treatment. By identifying specific receptors, we now better understand the part autophagy plays in tumors. It is important to find biomarkers that can track mitophagy and learn its functions in both normal and cancer cells. By studying these insights, researchers may develop better, more targeting treatments for cancer.

Although the proteins that regulate mitophagy are known, there are still important questions. With basal mitophagy, the cells discard malfunctioning mitochondria, which helps the cells survive when the stress is not too strong. But if the damage to mitochondria is too serious, the process of mitophagy is suppressed, which leads to cell death. The role of mitophagy in cancer is two-sided: it can lead to survival or to suppression. By stopping mitophagy, this treatment could disrupt tumor cell adaptation and cause their death.

ACKNOWLEDGMENTS

Dr.K.R. Padma and Dr.K.R.Don solely drafted the paper. All the authors are thankful to the Department of Biotechnology Sri Padmavati Mahila Visvavidyalayam (Women's) University, Tirupati-India. and the Department of Oral Pathology and Microbiology, Sri Balaji Dental College and Hospital, Bharath Institute of Higher Education and Research (BIHER) Bharath University, Chennai, Tamil Nadu.

Competing Interests:

The authors declare that they have no competing interests.

Consent for Publication:

Not applicable.

REFERENCES

Al Rawi, S., Louvet-Vallée, S., Djeddi, A., Sachse, M., Culetto, E., Hajjar, C., Boyd, L., Legouis, R., & Galy, V. (2011). Postfertilization autophagy of sperm organelles prevents paternal mitochondrial DNA transmission. *Science*, *334*(6059), 1144–1147. DOI: 10.1126/science.1211878 PMID: 22033522

Bernardini, J. P., Lazarou, M., & Dewson, G. (2017). Parkin and mitophagy in cancer. *Oncogene*, *36*(10), 1315–1327. DOI: 10.1038/onc.2016.302 PMID: 27593930

Boyle, K., Van Wickle, J., Hill, R., Marchitti, S. A., Kresty, L., & Dorr, R. T. (2018). Mitochondria-targeted drugs stimulate mitophagy and abrogate colon cancer cell proliferation. *The Journal of Biological Chemistry*, *293*(38), 14891–14904. DOI: 10.1074/jbc.RA117.001469 PMID: 30087121

Carew, J. A., Zhou, Y., Albitar, M., Keating, M. J., & Huang, P. (2003). Mitochondrial DNA mutations in primary leukemia cells after chemotherapy: Clinical significance and therapeutic implications. *Leukemia*, *17*(8), 1437–1447. DOI: 10.1038/sj.leu.2403043 PMID: 12886229

Cesari, R., Martin, E. S., Calin, G. A., Pentimalli, F., Bichi, R., McAdams, H., & Croce, C. M. (2003). Parkin, a gene implicated in autosomal recessive juvenile parkinsonism, is a candidate tumor suppressor gene on chromosome 6q25–q27. *Proceedings of the National Academy of Sciences of the United States of America*, *100*(10), 5956–5961.

Chen, L., Liu, L., Li, Y., Li, Y., Duan, Q., Liang, Y., Ma, B., & Yuan, Y. (2018). Melatonin increases human cervical cancer HeLa cells apoptosis induced by cisplatin via inhibition of JNK/Parkin/mitophagy axis. *In Vitro Cellular & Developmental Biology. Animal*, *54*(1), 1–10. DOI: 10.1007/s11626-017-0200-z PMID: 29071589

Chen, Y., Chen, H. N., Wang, K., Chen, Y., Wang, Y., Zhu, X., Li, P., Zhang, H., Liu, Z., & Yu, J. (2019). Ketoconazole exacerbates mitophagy to induce apoptosis by downregulating cyclooxygenase-2 in hepatocellular carcinoma. *Journal of Hepatology*, *70*(1), 66–77. DOI: 10.1016/j.jhep.2018.09.022 PMID: 30287340

Cheng, J., Qian, D., Ding, X., Song, T., Cai, M., Dan, X., Wang, Y., Zhao, J., Liu, Z., Wu, Z., Zhang, X., & Wang, X. (2018). High PGAM5 expression induces chemoresistance by enhancing Bcl-xL-mediated anti-apoptotic signaling and predicts poor prognosis in hepatocellular carcinoma patients. *Cell Death & Disease*, *9*(10), 991. DOI: 10.1038/s41419-018-1017-8 PMID: 30250224

Chi, H., Chen, S., Lin, S., Wang, X., Zhang, Q., Liu, Y., Wang, T., Zhang, Y., & Wang, Q. (2017). Thyroid hormone protects hepatocytes from HBx-induced carcinogenesis by enhancing mitochondrial turnover. *Oncogene*, *36*(37), 5274–5284. DOI: 10.1038/onc.2017.136 PMID: 28504722

Chourasia, A. H., Tracy, K., Frankenberger, C., Boland, M. L., Sharifi, M. N., Drake, L. E., Sachleben, J. R., & Macleod, K. F. (2015). Mitophagy defects arising from BNip3 loss promote mammary tumor progression to metastasis. *EMBO Reports*, *16*(9), 1145–1163. DOI: 10.15252/embr.201540759 PMID: 26232272

Chu, C. T., Ji, J., Dagda, R. K., Jiang, J., Tyurina, Y. Y., Kapralov, A. A., Tyurin, V. A., Yanamala, N., Shrivastava, I. H., Mohammadyani, D., Wang, K., Zhu, J., Klein-Seetharaman, J., Balasubramanian, R., Amoscato, A. A., Borisenko, G. G., Huang, Z., Gusdon, A. M., Cheikhi, A., & Kagan, V. E. (2013). Cardiolipin externalization to the outer mitochondrial membrane acts as an elimination signal for mitophagy in neuronal cells. *Nature Cell Biology*, *15*(10), 1197–1205. DOI: 10.1038/ncb2837 PMID: 24036476

Dany, M., Gencer, S., Nganga, R., Thomas, R. J., Oleinik, N., Baron, K. D., Szulc, Z. M., Ruvolo, P. P., Kornblau, S. M., & Ogretmen, B. (2016). Targeting FLT3-ITD signaling mediates ceramide-dependent mitophagy and attenuates drug resistance in AML. *Blood*, *128*(15), 1944–1958. DOI: 10.1182/blood-2016-04-708750 PMID: 27540013

Di Leo, L., Bodemeyer, V., Bosisio, F. M., Claps, G., Carretta, M., Rizza, S., Faienza, F., Frias, A., Khan, S., Bordi, M., Pacheco, M. P., Di Martino, J., Bravo-Cordero, J. J., Daniel, C. J., Sears, R. C., Donia, M., Madsen, D. H., Guldberg, P., Filomeni, G., & Cecconi, F. (2021). Loss of Ambra1 promotes melanoma growth and invasion. *Nature Communications*, *12*(1), 2550. Advance online publication. DOI: 10.1038/s41467-021-22772-2 PMID: 33953176

Fei, P., Wang, W., Kim, S., Wang, S., Burns, T. F., Sax, J. K., Buzzai, M., Dicker, D. T., McKenna, W. G., Bernhard, E. J., & El-Deiry, W. S. (2004). Bnip3L is induced by p53 under hypoxia, and its knockdown promotes tumor growth. *Cancer Cell*, *6*(6), 597–609. DOI: 10.1016/j.ccr.2004.10.012 PMID: 15607964

Ferro, F., Servais, S., Besson, P., Roger, S., Dumas, J. F., & Brisson, L. (2020). Autophagy and mitophagy in cancer metabolic remodelling. *Seminars in Cell & Developmental Biology*, *98*, 129–138. DOI: 10.1016/j.semcdb.2019.05.029 PMID: 31154012

Geisler, S., Holmström, K. M., Skujat, D., Fiesel, F. C., Rothfuss, O. C., Kahle, P. J., & Springer, W. (2010). PINK1/Parkin-mediated mitophagy is dependent on VDAC1 and p62/SQSTM1. *Nature Cell Biology*, *12*(2), 119–131. DOI: 10.1038/ncb2012 PMID: 20098416

Gong, Y., Zack, T. I., Morris, L. G. T., Lin, K. H., Hukkelhoven, E., Raheja, R., Mendenhall, E. M., Deng, Y., Diala, I., & Ni, M.. (2014). Pan-cancer genetic analysis identifies PARK2 as a master regulator of G1/S cyclins. *Nature Genetics*, *46*(6), 588–594. DOI: 10.1038/ng.2981 PMID: 24793136

Heo, J. M., Ordureau, A., Paulo, J. A., Rinehart, J., & Harper, J. W. (2015). The PINK1-PARKIN mitochondrial ubiquitylation pathway drives a program of OPTN/NDP52 recruitment and TBK1 activation to promote mitophagy. *Molecular Cell*, *60*(1), 7–20. DOI: 10.1016/j.molcel.2015.08.016 PMID: 26365381

Hsieh, C. H., Shaltouki, A., & Gonzalez, A. E.. (2016). Functional impairment in Miro degradation and mitophagy is a shared feature in familial and sporadic Parkinson's disease. *Cell Stem Cell*, *19*(6), 709–724. DOI: 10.1016/j.stem.2016.08.002 PMID: 27618216

Hsu, P., Liu, X., Zhang, J., Hong-Gang, W., Ji-Ming, Ye., & Yuguang, S. (2015). Cardiolipin remodeling by TAZ/tafazzin is selectively required for the initiation of mitophagy. *Autophagy*, *11*(4), 643–652. DOI: 10.1080/15548627.2015.1023984 PMID: 25919711

Hui, L., Wu, H., Wang, T., Yang, N., Guo, X., & Jang, X. (2019). Hydrogen peroxide-induced mitophagy contributes to laryngeal cancer cells survival via the upregulation of FUNDC1. *Clinical & Translational Oncology*, *21*(5), 596–606. DOI: 10.1007/s12094-018-1958-5 PMID: 30284230

Humpton, T. J., Alagesan, B., DeNicola, G. M., Lu, D., Yordanov, G. N., Leonhardt, C. S., Yao, M. A., Alagesan, P., Zaatari, M. N., Park, Y., & Aghajan, M.. (2019). Oncogenic KRAS induces NIX-mediated mitophagy to promote pancreatic cancer. *Cancer Discovery*, *9*(9), 1268–1287. DOI: 10.1158/2159-8290.CD-18-1409 PMID: 31263025

Im, E., Yoo, L., Hyun, M. S., Lee, J., Lee, S., Park, J. H., & Lee, H. S. (2016). Covalent ISG15 conjugation positively regulates the ubiquitin E3 ligase activity of parkin. *Open Biology*, *6*(8), 160193. DOI: 10.1098/rsob.160193 PMID: 27534820

Klionsky, D. J., Abdel-Aziz, A. K., Abdelfatah, S., & Abdellatif, M. (2021). Autophagy in major human diseases. *The EMBO Journal*, *40*(19), e108863. DOI: 10.15252/embj.2021108863 PMID: 34459017

Kryston, T. B., Georgiev, A. B., Pissis, P., & Georgakilas, A. G. (2011). Role of oxidative stress and DNA damage in human carcinogenesis. *Mutation Research*, *711*(1-2), 193–201. DOI: 10.1016/j.mrfmmm.2010.12.016 PMID: 21216256

Kulikov, A., Luchkina, E., Gogvadze, V., & Zhivotovsky, B. (2017). Mitophagy: Link to cancer development and therapy. *Biochemical and Biophysical Research Communications*, *482*(3), 432–439. DOI: 10.1016/j.bbrc.2016.10.088 PMID: 28212727

Lee, I. H., Kawai, Y., Fergusson, M. M., Rovira, I. I., Bishop, A. J. R., Motoyama, N., Cao, L., & Finkel, T. (2012). Atg7 modulates p53 activity to regulate cell cycle and survival during metabolic stress. *Science*, *336*(6078), 225–228. DOI: 10.1126/science.1218395 PMID: 22499945

Lee, J. Y., Nagano, Y., Taylor, J. P., Lim, K. L., & Yao, T. P. (2010). Disease-causing mutations in parkin impair mitochondrial ubiquitination, aggregation, and HDAC6-dependent mitophagy. *The Journal of Cell Biology*, *189*(4), 671–679. DOI: 10.1083/jcb.201001039 PMID: 20457763

Lemasters, J. J. (2005). Selective mitochondrial autophagy, or mitophagy, as a targeted defense against oxidative stress, mitochondrial dysfunction, and aging. *Rejuvenation Research*, *8*(1), 3–5. DOI: 10.1089/rej.2005.8.3 PMID: 15798367

Levy, J. M. M., Towers, C. G., & Thorburn, A. (2017). Targeting autophagy in cancer. *Nature Reviews. Cancer*, *17*(9), 528–542. DOI: 10.1038/nrc.2017.53 PMID: 28751651

Li, C., Zhang, Y., Cheng, X., Yuan, H., Zhu, S., Liu, J., Wen, Q., Wang, X., Zhang, Y., & Kang, R. (2018). PINK1 and PARK2 suppress pancreatic tumorigenesis through control of mitochondrial iron-mediated immunometabolism. *Developmental Cell, 46*(4), 441–455. DOI: 10.1016/j.devcel.2018.07.012 PMID: 30100261

Li, N., Ragheb, K., Lawler, G., Sturgis, J., Rajwa, B., Melendez, J. A., & Robinson, J. P. (2003). Mitochondrial complex I inhibitor rotenone induces apoptosis through enhancing mitochondrial reactive oxygen species production. *The Journal of Biological Chemistry, 278*(10), 8516–8525. DOI: 10.1074/jbc.M210432200 PMID: 12496265

Li, Y., Zhang, X., Yang, J., Zhang, Y., Zhu, D., Zhang, L., Zhu, Y., Li, D., & Zhou, J. (2017). Methylation of BNIP3 in pancreatic cancer inhibits the induction of mitochondrial-mediated tumor cell apoptosis. *Oncotarget, 8*(38), 63208–63222. DOI: 10.18632/oncotarget.18736 PMID: 28968982

Li, Z., Wang, Y., Wu, L., Wang, C., Wang, P., Ma, Q., & Zhang, L. (2019). Apurinic endonuclease 1 promotes the cisplatin resistance of lung cancer cells by inducing Parkin-mediated mitophagy. *Oncology Reports, 42*(6), 2245–2254. DOI: 10.3892/or.2019.7345 PMID: 31578585

Li, W., Li, Y., Siraj, S., Jin, H., Fan, Y., Yang, X., & Chen, Q. (2019). FUN14 Domain-containing 1–mediated mitophagy suppresses hepatocarcinogenesis by inhibition of inflammasome activation in mice. *Hepatology (Baltimore, Md.), 69*(2), 604–621.

Liu, L., Feng, D., Chen, G., Chen, M., Zheng, Q., Song, P., Ma, Q., Zhu, C., Wang, R., Qi, W., Huang, L., Xue, P., Li, B., Wang, X., Jin, H., Wang, J., Yang, F., Liu, Y., & Chen, Q. (2012). Mitochondrial outer-membrane protein FUNDC1 mediates hypoxia-induced mitophagy in mammalian cells. *Nature Cell Biology, 14*(2), 177–185. DOI: 10.1038/ncb2422 PMID: 22267086

Liu, Y., Fu, Y., Hu, X., Wang, Y., Zhou, Y., Zhang, L., & Wang, L. (2020). Caveolin-1 knockdown increases the therapeutic sensitivity of lung cancer to cisplatin-induced apoptosis by repressing Parkin-related mitophagy and activating the ROCK1 pathway. *Journal of Cellular Physiology, 235*(2), 1197–1208. DOI: 10.1002/jcp.29033 PMID: 31270811

Lu, J., Chew, E. L., & Holmgren, A. (2007). Targeting thioredoxin reductase is a basis for cancer therapy by arsenic trioxide. *Proceedings of the National Academy of Sciences of the United States of America, 104*(30), 12288–12293. DOI: 10.1073/pnas.0701549104 PMID: 17640917

Lu, X., Altshuler-Keylin, S., Wang, Q., Chen, Y. C., Sponton, C. H., & Kajimura, S. (2018). Mitophagy controls beige adipocyte maintenance through a Parkin-dependent and UCP1-independent mechanism. *Science Signaling*, *11*(527), eaap8526. Advance online publication. DOI: 10.1126/scisignal.aap8526 PMID: 29692364

Lu, X., Liu, Q., Zhang, J., Zhou, D., Yang, G., Li, M., Qiu, Y., Chen, Q., Zheng, H., & Dai, J. (2020). PINK1 overexpression promotes cell migration and proliferation via regulation of autophagy and predicts a poor prognosis in lung cancer cases. *Cancer Management and Research*, *12*, 7703–7714. DOI: 10.2147/CMAR.S262466 PMID: 32904694

MacKeigan, J. P., Murphy, L. O., & Blenis, J. (2005). Sensitized RNAi screen of human kinases and phosphatases identifies new regulators of apoptosis and chemoresistance. *Nature Cell Biology*, *7*(6), 591–600. DOI: 10.1038/ncb1258 PMID: 15864305

Manczak, M., Kandimalla, R., Yin, X., & Reddy, P. H. (2018). Hippocampal mutant APP and amyloid beta-induced cognitive decline, dendritic spine loss, defective autophagy, mitophagy and mitochondrial abnormalities in a mouse model of Alzheimer's disease. *Human Molecular Genetics*, *27*(8), 1332–1342. DOI: 10.1093/hmg/ddy042 PMID: 29408999

Mathiassen, S. G., De Zio, D., & Cecconi, F. (2017). Autophagy and the cell cycle: A complex landscape. *Frontiers in Oncology*, *7*, 51. Advance online publication. DOI: 10.3389/fonc.2017.00051 PMID: 28409123

Matsuyama, S., Llopis, J., Deveraux, Q. L., Tsien, R. Y., & Reed, J. C. (2000). Changes in intramitochondrial and cytosolic pH: Early events that modulate caspase activation during apoptosis. *Nature Cell Biology*, *2*(6), 318–325. DOI: 10.1038/35014006 PMID: 10854321

Murai, M., Toyota, M., Suzuki, H., Satoh, A., Sasaki, Y., Akino, K., Kikuchi, T., Mita, H., Tanaka, N., Itoh, F., & Tokino, T. (2005). Aberrant methylation and silencing of the BNIP3 gene in colorectal and gastric cancer. *Clinical Cancer Research*, *11*(3), 1021–1027. DOI: 10.1158/1078-0432.1021.11.3 PMID: 15709167

Nagdas, S. K., Daniel, F., Nascimento, A. L., Hussain, S. S., Trainor, R. E., Pollock, S. R., Adair, S. J., Michaels, A. D., Sesaki, H. S., & Elizabeth, B.. (2019). Drp1 promotes KRas-driven metabolic changes to drive pancreatic tumor growth. *Cell Reports*, *28*(7), 1845–1859.e5. DOI: 10.1016/j.celrep.2019.07.031 PMID: 31412251

Nah, J., Yuan, J., & Jung, Y. K. (2015). Autophagy in neurodegenerative diseases: From mechanism to therapeutic approach. *Molecules and Cells*, *38*(5), 381–389. DOI: 10.14348/molcells.2015.0034 PMID: 25896254

Nakahira, K., Haspel, J. A., Rathinam, V. A. K., Lee, S. J., Dolinay, T., Lam, H. C., Englert, J. A., Rabinovitch, M., Cernadas, M., Kim, H. P., Fitzgerald, K. A., Ryter, S. W., & Choi, A. M. K. (2011). Autophagy proteins regulate innate immune responses by inhibiting the release of mitochondrial DNA mediated by the NALP3 inflammasome. *Nature Immunology*, *12*(3), 222–230. DOI: 10.1038/ni.1980 PMID: 21151103

Novak, I. (2012). Mitophagy: A complex mechanism of mitochondrial removal. *Antioxidants & Redox Signaling*, *17*(5), 794–802. DOI: 10.1089/ars.2011.4407 PMID: 22077334

Pagliarini, V., Wirawan, E., Romagnoli, A., Ciccosanti, F., Lisi, S., Lippens, S., Cecconi, F., Fimia, G. M., Vandenabeele, P., & Piacentini, M. (2012). Proteolysis of Ambra1 during apoptosis has a role in the inhibition of the autophagic pro-survival response. *Cell Death and Differentiation*, *19*(9), 1495–1504. DOI: 10.1038/cdd.2012.27 PMID: 22441670

Panigrahi, D. P., Praharaj, P. P., Bhol, S., Mahapatra, K. K., Patra, S., Behera, B. P., Mishra, S. R., & Bhutia, S. K. (2019). The emerging, multifaceted role of mitophagy in cancer and cancer therapeutics. *Seminars in Cancer Biology*, *66*, 45–58. DOI: 10.1016/j.semcancer.2019.07.015 PMID: 31351198

Poulogiannis, G., McIntyre, R. E., Dimitriadi, M., Apps, J. R., Wilson, C. H., Ichimura, K., Luo, F., Cantley, L. C., Wyllie, A. H., Adams, D. J., & Malliri, A. (2010). PARK2 deletions occur frequently in sporadic colorectal cancer and accelerate adenoma development in Apc mutant mice. *Proceedings of the National Academy of Sciences of the United States of America*, *107*(34), 15145–15150. DOI: 10.1073/pnas.1009941107 PMID: 20696900

Praharaj, P. P., Naik, P. P., Panigrahi, D. P., Bhol, C. S., Mahapatra, K. K., Patra, S., Mishra, S. R., Behera, B. P., & Bhutia, S. K. (2019). Intricate role of mitochondrial lipid in mitophagy and mitochondrial apoptosis: Its implication in cancer therapeutics. *Cellular and Molecular Life Sciences : CMLS*, *76*(9), 1641–1652. DOI: 10.1007/s00018-018-2990-x PMID: 30539200

Rojansky, R., Cha, M. Y., & Chan, D. C. (2016). Elimination of paternal mitochondria in mouse embryos occurs through autophagic degradation dependent on PARKIN and MUL1. *eLife*, *5*, e17896. DOI: 10.7554/eLife.17896 PMID: 27852436

Sandoval, H., Thiagarajan, P., Dasgupta, S. K., Schumacher, A., Prchal, J. T., Chen, M., & Wang, J. (2008). Essential role for Nix in autophagic maturation of erythroid cells. *Nature*, *454*(7201), 232–235. DOI: 10.1038/nature07006 PMID: 18454133

Sato, M., & Sato, K. (2011). Degradation of paternal mitochondria by fertilization-triggered autophagy in C. elegans embryos. *Science*, *334*(6059), 1141–1144. DOI: 10.1126/science.1210333 PMID: 21998252

Schweers, R. L., Zhang, J., Randall, M. S., Loyd, M. R., Li, W., Dorsey, F. C., Kundu, M., Opferman, J. T., Cleveland, J. L., Miller, J. L., & Ney, P. A. (2007). NIX is required for programmed mitochondrial clearance during reticulocyte maturation. *Proceedings of the National Academy of Sciences of the United States of America*, *104*(49), 19500–19505. DOI: 10.1073/pnas.0708818104 PMID: 18048346

Shimada, K., Crother, T. R., Karlin, J., Dagvadorj, J., Chiba, N., Chen, S. Y., Ramanujan, V. K., Wolf, A. J., Vergnes, L., Ojcius, D. M., Rentsendorj, A., Vargas, M., Guerrero, C., Wang, Y., Fitzgerald, K. A., Underhill, D. M., Town, T., & Arditi, M. (2012). Oxidized mitochondrial DNA activates the NLRP3 inflammasome during apoptosis. *Immunity*, *36*(3), 401–414. DOI: 10.1016/j.immuni.2012.01.009 PMID: 22342844

Sin, J. S., Andres, A. M., Taylor, D. J., Weston, T., Hiraumi, Y., Stotland, A., Kim, B. J., Huang, C., Doran, K. S., & Gottlieb, R. A. (2016). Mitophagy is required for mitochondrial biogenesis and myogenic differentiation of C2C12 myoblasts. *Autophagy*, *12*(2), 369–380. DOI: 10.1080/15548627.2015.1115172 PMID: 26566717

Springer, M. Z., & Macleod, K. F. (2016). Mitophagy: Mechanisms and role in human disease. *The Journal of Pathology*, *240*(3), 253–255. DOI: 10.1002/path.4774 PMID: 27453450

Sumpter, R. J., Sirasanagandla, S., Fernández, A. F., Wei, Y., Dong, X., Franco, L., Zou, Z., Marchal, C., Lee, M. Y., Clapp, D. W., & Levine, B. (2016). Fanconi anemia proteins function in mitophagy and immunity. *Cell*, *165*(4), 867–881. DOI: 10.1016/j.cell.2016.04.006 PMID: 27133164

Valente, E. M., Abou-Sleiman, P. M., Caputo, V., Muqit, M. M. K., Harvey, K., Gispert, S., Ali, Z., Del Turco, D., Bentivoglio, A. R., Healy, D. G., Albanese, A., Nussbaum, R., González-Maldonado, R., Deller, T., Salvi, S., Cortelli, P., Gilks, W. P., Latchman, D. S., Harvey, R. J., & Wood, N. W. (2004). Hereditary early-onset Parkinson's disease caused by mutations in PINK1. *Science*, *304*(5674), 1158–1160. DOI: 10.1126/science.1096284 PMID: 15087508

Van, G., Marjolein, W., Voets, A. M., Starmans, M. H., de Coo, I. F., Yadak, R., Hoffmann, R. F., Boutros, P. C., Smeets, H. J., Dubois, L., & Lambin, P. (2015). How do changes in the mtDNA and mitochondrial dysfunction influence cancer and cancer therapy? Challenges, opportunities and models. *Mutation Research/ Reviews in Mutation Research*, *764*, 16–30. DOI: 10.1016/j.mrrev.2015.01.001 PMID: 26041263

Wallace, D. C. (2012). Mitochondria and cancer. *Nature Reviews. Cancer*, *12*(10), 685–698. DOI: 10.1038/nrc3365 PMID: 23001348

Warburg, O. (1956). On the origin of cancer cells. *Science*, *123*(3191), 309–314. DOI: 10.1126/science.123.3191.309 PMID: 13298683

Waris, G., & Ahsan, H. (2006). Reactive oxygen species: Role in the development of cancer and various chronic conditions. *Journal of Carcinogenesis*, *5*(1), 14. Advance online publication. DOI: 10.1186/1477-3163-5-14 PMID: 16689993

Wong, Y. C., & Holzbaur, E. L. F. (2014). Optineurin is an autophagy receptor for damaged mitochondria in parkin-mediated mitophagy that is disrupted by an ALS-linked mutation. *Proceedings of the National Academy of Sciences of the United States of America*, *111*(42), E4439–E4448. DOI: 10.1073/pnas.1405752111 PMID: 25294927

Wu, W. K. K., Tian, Y., Zhan, W., Li, X., He, J., Li, S., Wang, J., Zhang, J., Chan, M. T. Y., Yu, J., Sung, J. J. Y., Hu, Z. Q., & Pan, W. (2014). ULK1 translocates to mitochondria and phosphorylates FUNDC1 to regulate mitophagy. *EMBO Reports*, *15*(5), 566–575. DOI: 10.1002/embr.201438501 PMID: 24671035

Yan, C., Luo, L., Guo, C., Wang, H., & Jin, J. (2017). Doxorubicin-induced mitophagy contributes to drug resistance in cancer stem cells from HCT8 human colorectal cancer cells. *Cancer Letters*, *388*, 34–42. DOI: 10.1016/j.canlet.2016.11.018 PMID: 27913197

Yao, N., Wang, C., Hu, N., Yao, M., Li, H., Zhang, L., He, C., Wang, H., & Zhou, Q. (2019). Inhibition of PINK1/Parkin-dependent mitophagy sensitizes multidrug-resistant cancer cells to B5G1, a new betulinic acid analog. *Cell Death & Disease*, *10*(3), 232. Advance online publication. DOI: 10.1038/s41419-019-1470-z PMID: 30850585

Yin, J., Guo, J., Zhang, Q., Cui, L., Zhang, L., Zhang, T., Wang, C., Liu, Y., & Wang, H. (2018). Doxorubicin-induced mitophagy and mitochondrial damage is associated with dysregulation of the PINK1/parkin pathway. *Toxicology In Vitro*, *51*, 1–10. DOI: 10.1016/j.tiv.2018.05.001 PMID: 29729358

Youle, R. J., & Narendra, D. P. (2011). Mechanisms of mitophagy. *Nature Reviews. Molecular Cell Biology*, *12*(1), 9–14. DOI: 10.1038/nrm3028 PMID: 21179058

Yu, M., Nguyen, N. D., Huang, Y., Lin, D., Fujimoto, T. N., Molkentine, J. M., Deorukhkar, A., Kang, Y., San Lucas, F. A., Fernandes, C. J., & Jimenez, C. R.. (2019). Mitochondrial fusion exploits a therapeutic vulnerability of pancreatic cancer. *JCI Insight*, *5*(16), e126915. DOI: 10.1172/jci.insight.126915 PMID: 31335325

Zhang, C., Liu, Z., Bunker, E., Ramamoorthy, S., Rodrigues, L. O., Djaballah, H., & Pfeiffer, S. (2017). Sorafenib targets the mitochondrial electron transport chain complexes and ATP synthase to activate the PINK1–Parkin pathway and modulate cellular drug response. *The Journal of Biological Chemistry*, *292*(36), 15105–15120. DOI: 10.1074/jbc.M117.783175 PMID: 28673964

Zhang, H., Yin, C., Liu, X., Bai, X., Wang, L., Xu, H., Li, F., Zhang, J., & Zhao, Q. (2020). Prohibitin 2/PHB2 in parkin-mediated mitophagy: A potential therapeutic target for non-small cell lung carcinoma. *Medical Science Monitor*, *26*, e923227. DOI: 10.12659/MSM.923227 PMID: 32320388

Zhang, R., Gu, J., Chen, J., Ni, J., Hung, J., Wang, Z., Zhang, X., Feng, J., & Ji, L. (2017). High expression of PINK1 promotes proliferation and chemoresistance of NSCLC. *Oncology Reports*, *37*(4), 2137–2146. DOI: 10.3892/or.2017.5486 PMID: 28259921

Chapter 4

Mitophagy Regulation and Molecular Mechanistic Treatment for Neuroblastoma

R. Prakash
B.S. Abdur Rahman Crescent Institute of Science and Technology, India

E. A. K. Nivethaa
B.S. Abdur Rahman Crescent Institute of Science and Technology, India

J. Sivasankari
B.S. Abdur Rahman Crescent Institute of Science and Technology, India

ABSTRACT

The second most frequent extracranial malignant tumour in children and the most common solid tumour in infants is neuroblastoma, a cancer of the sympathetic nervous system. Patients' survival rates gradually increase as a result of the most recent developments in neuroblastoma treatment being gradually included into clinical trials and clinical practice guidelines. The capacity to develop treatments for certain molecular targets in neuroblastoma is critical as technologies develop. ALK inhibitors and anti-GD2 treatments are currently the most prominent targeted medicines available for high-risk neuroblastoma; they have both established themselves as cornerstones of treatment in both the upfront and relapsed contexts. Additional molecular targeted therapeutic development has proven difficult and has had mixed results. The identification of possible therapeutic targets keeps up with the rapid advancement of technologies in molecular profiling and diagnostics. Here, in the era of precision medicine, we address the present state of clinical

DOI: 10.4018/979-8-3693-3836-0.ch004

neuroblastoma therapy.

INTRODUCTION TO NEUROBLASTOMA

Neuroblastoma (NBL) is the most common extracranial paediatric tumour. It usually starts in the nerve tissue of the adrenal gland or in sympathetic nerve. In the rear of the upper abdomen, two adrenal glands are located, one on top of each kidney. The adrenal glands produce vital hormones that regulate heart rate, blood pressure, blood sugar, and the body's response to stress. Apart from this the neuroblastoma can also originate in the sympathetic ganglia in the pelvis, chest, or neck, close to the spine (Colon, 2011; Maris, 2010).Most cases of neuroblastoma start in infancy, between the first month of birth and age five, a diagnosis is often made. When the tumour starts to develop and exhibit symptoms, it is discovered. It can occasionally develop prenatally and be discovered during a baby ultrasound. Most of the time, cancer has spread (metastasized) by the time it is diagnosed. In babies and children, neuroblastoma most commonly spreads to the skin, liver, bone marrow, lymph nodes, and bones.

Neuroblastoma develops from neuroblasts, which are immature nerve cells in the foetus that are expected to grow into functional nerve cells. In neuroblastoma, neuroblasts fail to develop normally and begin to grow in an uncontrolled manner, resulting in a tumour. The actual source of this problem is unknown, however it is thought to be genetic abnormalities. Changes in the way neuroblast cells behave, particularly in their growth and division into new cells, are the cause of neuroblastoma. The majority of neuroblastoma cases are sporadic, which means that the disease arises randomly without any familial history. However, a small proportion of the cases are hereditary, caused by inherited genetic abnormalities. The most prevalent mutations associated with familial neuroblastoma are in the ALK and PHOX2B genes (Maris, 2010; Park, 2013). These genes have a role in nerve cell formation and function. Some genetic markers are linked to more aggressive forms of neuroblastoma, these include: MYCN amplification which is a strong predictor of poor prognosis, linked to high-risk disease and found in 20–25% of cases; chromosome 1p and 11q Deletions and DNA Ploidy(Cohn, 2009; Matthay, 2016).

The location of the tumor and whether it has migrated to other regions of the body determine the symptoms of neuroblastoma. Typical symptoms include an abdominal lump or mass, frequently indicating adrenal gland or abdomen malignancy, discomfort in the back, belly, chest, or limbs, depending on where the tumor is located, swelling that obstructs breathing or swallowing if the tumor is located in the neck, Horner's syndrome, which is characterized by drooping of one eyelid (ptosis), constricted pupil (miosis), and absence of perspiration on one side of the face, can be brought on by tumors in the neck, an inexplicable fever is a typical sign, loss of appetite or weight loss brought on by the tumor's metabolic needs, bone Pain in cases where malignancy has progressed to the bone marrow, metastasis to the skin can result in bluish nodules called blueberry muffin spots in infants, periorbital ecchymosis and elevated blood pressure, particularly in cases when the tumor affects the adrenal glands(Maris, 2010).

According to the severity of the disease, neuroblastoma is categorized into four stages: Stage 1 is a localized tumor that can be surgically removed either with or without microscopic residual disease; representative ipsilateral lymph nodes are tumor-negative (albeit nodes that were removed along with the main tumor may have tested positive); Stage 2A: One-sided tumor with partial gross excision; ipsilateral non-adherent lymph nodes are representative and tumor-negative; Stage 2B: tumor with or without total gross excision, and tumor-positive ipsilateral non-adherent lymph nodes; Stage 3 is an unresectable tumor that has crossed the midline or is in lymph nodes on both sides of the body; Stage 4 is a tumor that has spread to distant lymph nodes, bone marrow, bone, liver, skin, or other organs; and Stage 4S is a special category for infants under one year old, where the cancer is widespread but occasionally regresses on its own(Cohn et al., 2009).

NBL is associated with a wide range of risk factors, many of which do not cause cancer directly. Rather, they raise the possibility of DNA damage in cells, which can result in neuroblastoma. Maternal anaemia, newborn hemolytic illness, a poor 1-minute Apgar score, and neonatal respiratory distress were shown to be risk factors for instances of neuroblastoma detected before the age of one year in this population-based linked-registry study conducted in Sweden. Larger, more comprehensive investigations should be conducted on the often more aggressive and treatment-resistant cases of neuroblastoma found after one year of life, as these illnesses were not linked to these perinatal problems(Bluhm, 2008).

ORIGIN OF NEUROBLASTOMA

Neural crest cells are present solely in mammals. The neural crest originates from the embryonic ectoderm and grows from the neural tube following closure (Simões-Costa, 2013)). Neural crest cells differentiate into various cell types during the epithelial-to-mesenchymal transition (EMT). This process causes cells to lose polarity and adhesion, allowing them to migrate from the neural tube and form diverse anatomical structures. Cells migrate along stereotyped paths to remote parts of the embryo and differentiate into various cell types, such as melanocytes, craniofacial cartilage cells, smooth muscle cells, peripheral neurons, and glial cells (Bronner, 2016). Epigenetic and transcriptional processes regulate neural crest cell delamination, migration, and differentiation. These programs involve histone modification, DNA methylation, and the production of bone morphogenetic proteins and transcription factors (Simões-Costa, 2015). Neural crest cells are classified into five functional types: vagal, sacral, cranial, cardiac, and trunk. Neural crest cells rapidly convert from multipotent progenitors to differentiated cell types, including neurons and glia.

The peripheral nervous system communicates with melanocytes, cartilage, and bone cells in the craniofacial skeleton. Initially, neural crest cells were thought to lose their multipotency and plasticity after migration. Research has shown that certain subpopulations with great flexibility and the potential to form spheres in vitro can be found in diverse tissues during late embryonic and postnatal stages, as well as in adults. Adult neural crest progenitor cells can be found in various organs, such as the epidermis, dorsal root ganglia, adrenal medulla, bone marrow, and others. Research indicates that adult neural crest-derived cells have stem cell characteristics. Numerous studies show that neural crest stem cell populations exhibit transcriptional patterns similar to embryonic stem cells and neural crest progenitor cells (Simões-Costa Bronner, 2015). The presence of neural crest progenitor cells in adult tissues may contribute to the development of neural crest-derived malignancies.

The neural crest's multipotent progenitor cells can cause various cancers in adulthood. Neural crest progenitor cells can be found in various locations throughout the body, leading to a broad range of malignancies developing from them. Melanoma, neuroblastoma, paraganglioma, pheochromocytoma, schwannoma, esthesioneuroblastoma, malignant peripheral nerve sheath tumors, granular cell tumors, neurofibroma, perineurioma, neurothekeoma, nerve sheath myxoma, and medullary thyroid cancer are among the most common cancers in adults and children (Zage, 2017). Researchers propose that neural crest cancers may be more likely to develop metastatic illness due to their ability to self-renew and migrate (Bailey, 2012; Gupta, 2005). Gene expression patterns and processes in neural crest and tumor cells share significant similarities. Both neural crest and tumor cells exhibit similar EMT processes, expressing matrix metalloproteinases (MMPs) and disintegrin and metalloproteinases (ADAMs) that aid in cell invasion and migration (Theveneau, 2012). These parallels suggest that the genetic changes driving cancer may be largely attributable to reactivation of factors. Signals necessary for neural crest cell migration and delamination are often inhibited post-embryogenesis.

While the biochemical features of NB formation and progression have been extensively investigated, little is known about the early phases of its pathogenesis. Additionally, the cells that cause this tumor have yet to be identified. Previously, it was thought that NB originated from sympathetic nervous system cells, namely sympathoadrenal progenitor cells that differentiate into sympathetic ganglion cells and adrenal chromaffin cells (Matthay et al., 2016). The sympathoadrenal lineage is formed when neural crest cells migrate along the ventral route and collect on the dorsal aorta (Anderson, 1993). These cells originate in the dorsal aorta and move to the developing adrenal glands to form chromaffin cells or sympathetic ganglia. As cells differentiate into sympathetic ganglia, they increase neuronal markers, while chromaffin cells increase adrenal gland proteins (Ernsberger, 2005; Howard, 2000). BMPs determine whether neural crest cells develop into catecholaminergic/adrenal chromaffin cells or sympathetic neurons (Reissmann, 1996; Schneider, 1999). Nerve growth factor (NGF) binding to the cell-surface receptor TrkA is necessary for the survival of differentiated cells. Excess sympathoadrenal cells undergo apoptosis at the end of differentiation due to NGF deprivation. Neuroblastoma is distinguished by the existence of sympathoadrenal neuroblasts, which can survive in the absence of NGF (Yuan, 2000). An experimental finding supports the theory that neuroblastoma originates from sympathoadrenal progenitor cells in the neural crest. Neuroblastoma tumors typically occur in areas where sympathoadrenal progenitor cells of the neural crest are located, such as the adrenal cortex, paraspinal ganglia, or abdominal cavity near the aorta in the kidney region (Brodeur, 2003; Maris, 2010).

Neuroblastoma is believed to originate from sympathoadrenal progenitor cells in the neural crest, as evidenced by the following facts:

- In situ neuroblastomas, which occur in the adrenal glands of 1 in 200 neonates and typically resolve on their own, have histological similarities to residual sympathogonia configurations (Beckwith, 1963).
- MYCN transgenic mice form neuroblastomas of their own accord (Weiss, 1997).
- Neuroblastoma cell lines can travel along neural crest pathways and invade neural crest-specific tissues (Bailey, 2014).
- Neuroblastoma gene expression patterns are comparable to those found in neural crest progenitor cells (De Preter, 2006).

Epidemiology

With neuroblastoma accounting for 8%–10% of all paediatric tumours, it is the most prevalent extracranial solid tumour in both babies and children. In children, it is responsible for around 15% of all cancer-related fatalities. Nearly 500 new cases of neuroblastoma are recorded each year, with an incidence of 10.2 cases per million children under the age of 15 years(Ward, 2014). Despite the fact that 90% of cases are identified before the age of five, 30% do so in the first year. 22 months is the median age upon diagnosis. Although results are significantly worse in this age range, it seldom manifests in adolescence and maturity(Cohn et al., 2009).

Neuroblastoma incidence varies slightly by area, with greater rates recorded in developed nations including the United States, Canada, and Western Europe. In contrast, the incidence seems to be lower in African and Asian countries (Stiller, 1992).

Autosomal dominant inheritance patterns have been seen in 1-2% of diagnosis. Patients in such pedigrees are usually diagnosed at a younger age (median age of 9 months) than those with sporadic illness, and they are more likely to have numerous primary malignancies. Neuroblastoma has also been associated with other congenital diseases, including Hirschsprung's disease, congenital hypoventilation disorder, and neurofibromatosis type 1. Because neuroblastoma and neurofibromatosis are both neural crest cell illnesses, the co-occurrence of the two was initially investigated. However, this might be chance rather than a real link.Over the past 30 years, neuroblastoma patient outcomes have significantly improved, with 5-year survival rates increasing from 52% to 74%. With up to 92% survival rates in the low-risk category, the increase is probably a byproduct of better cure rates. Relapse is thought to occur in 50–60% of patients in the high-risk category; hence, their death rate has only slightly decreased. According to research conducted by the International Neuroblastoma Risk Group, 73% of patients who relapsed were 18 months of age or older, with a median duration to relapse of 13.2 months. Combined, even with more rigorous therapy, their overall survival chances are still extremely low (about 20% after 5 years)(Colon Chung, 2011; J. E. Heck, 2009; Julia E. Heck, 2009).

Epigenetic Regulation

Over a decade ago, epigenetic changes impacting gene expression in neuroblastoma were first documented. Recent investigations have linked abnormalities in gene DNA methylation or histone modification to clinical outcomes (Olsson, 2016). Alaminos et al. used methylation-specific PCR to analyze promoter hypermethylation in 45 genes in 10 neuroblastoma cell lines and 10 genes in 118 primary neuroblastomas. They found distinct patterns in CpG island hypermethylation for MYCN-amplified versus nonamplified tumors(Alaminos, 2004). Researchers found that HOXA9 promoter hypermethylation was associated with higher mortality rates in elderly individuals compared to babies and tumors without MYCN amplification. Hypermethylation of TMS1 (proapoptotic gene) and CCND2 (cell cycle-related gene) was linked to advanced-stage cancers. Stage 4S tumors showed distinct hypermethylation or hypomethylation of particular chromosomal locations compared to other stages. They included transcription factors, genes related to neural crest formation, and genes involved in sympathetic neural differentiation. E2F1 binds to the hypermethylated TERT promoter in stage 4S cancers, unlike stage 4 tumors. Stage 4S neuroblastoma has lower TERT expression relative to stage 4 tumors, suggesting that TERT DNA methylation affects telomerase activity. Infinium Human 450 K Bead Chips have been used to conduct genome-wide methylation research, leading to more comprehensive investigations. Henrich et al. used an integrative strategy to assess the global methylation patterns, transcriptomes, and copy number aberrations of 105 neuroblastoma patients. This was supplemented by primary tumor- and cell line-derived global histone modification analysis and epigenetic medication therapy in vitro (Henrich, 2016). The study found unique DNA methylation patterns that correspond with survival and clinical/biological factors, such as MYCN amplification and copy number alterations. Gomez et al. found similar findings using the same strategy on 35 primary neuroblastomas (Gómez, 2015). Non-CpG methylation was linked to cancers with favorable clinicopathological characteristics.

Genetic Risk Factors

Genome-wide association studies (GWAS) have revealed that neuroblastoma is a complicated genetic disorder influenced by common polymorphism alleles. There are 12 extremely significant polymorphism variants that can affect neuroblastoma development (Bosse, 2016). Multiple perturbations can work together to induce malignant transformation during neurodevelopment, even if each has a little impact on illness start. GWAS has revealed several genes related with neuroblastoma susceptibility, including CASC15, BRCA1-associated RING domain protein 1 (BARD1), LMO1, DUSP12, DDX4, IL31RA, HSD17B12, HACE1, LIN28B, LINC00340, LOC729177 (FLJ44180) and NEFL. These genes have oncogenic or tumor-suppressive actions linked to the disease (Decock, 2011; Fetahu, 2021). The identification of susceptibility loci highlights the importance of evaluating GWAS data for understanding the biology of neuroblastoma genesis. However, unlike retinoblastoma, familial neuroblastoma is extremely rare (1%-2% of cases) (Ritenour, 2018). Familial neuroblastoma is often inherited through an autosomal dominant pattern with imperfect penetrance. Clinical behaviour varies significantly across pedigrees, including age at diagnosis, histology, and aggression. Although familial neuroblastoma is rare, pedigrees offer a unique chance to identify genetic causes. PHOX2B, a gene that promotes cell cycle exit and neuronal differentiation, was discovered as the first predisposition gene in neuroblastoma. This gene is crucial for the formation of neural crest-derived autonomic neurons. PHOX2B mutations affect less than 10% of hereditary neuroblastoma cases, but somatic mutations are uncommon in spontaneous cases (Raabe, 2008). PHOX2B mutations are typically seen in neural crest-derived illnesses, including congenital central hypoventilation syndrome and Hirschsprung's disease. Families with nonpolyalanine repeat expansion mutations have the highest risk of developing neuroblastoma, Hirschsprung's illness, and hypoventilation syndrome. These findings show that disruptions in the PHOX2B-regulated differentiation pathway may be a prevalent hereditary component behind neural crest disorders. The ALK locus is linked to a frequent lesion in familial neuroblastoma. ALK mutations are seen in 80% of neuroblastoma families and in rare cases in spontaneous neuroblastoma tumor cells (Chen, 2008; Mossé, 2008). Mutations in the tyrosine kinase domain cause constitutive phosphorylation, suggesting that ALK mutations in neuroblastoma may be cancer-causing. Midkine and pleiotrophin are naturally occurring ALK ligands (Stoica, 2002). ALK is highly expressed in the developing sympathoadrenal progenitor of the neural crest. It regulates the balance between proliferation and differentiation via many signalling pathways, including MAPK and RAS-related protein 1. Mutations in ALK are responsible for the first familial pediatric cancer caused by an oncogene.

Pathogenesis

The pathogenesis of neuroblastoma involves a complex interplay of genetic, developmental, and environmental factors that contribute to the initiation and progression of the disease(Park, 2008). While the exact cause of neuroblastoma is not fully understood, several key factors play a role in its development:

Genetic and molecular factors: Neuroblastoma is frequently caused by genetic mutations that occur early in foetal development. These mutations can impact genes that control cell development, differentiation, and apoptosis (programmed cell death). One of the most frequently mutated genes in neuroblastoma is the ALK gene (Anaplastic Lymphoma Kinase), which is shown to be changed in a minority of patients. Mutations in the ALK (anaplastic lymphoma kinase) gene are seen in both familial and spontaneous neuroblastoma cases. ALK is a receptor tyrosine kinase that regulates cell growth and survival. Mutations that activate ALK cause constitutive signalling, which enhances neuroblast survival and proliferation, hence leading to tumor growth. ALK mutations are seen in 8-10% of spontaneous neuroblastomas and are a leading source of familial neuroblastoma.Other genetic modifications commonly found in neuroblastoma tumours include MYCN amplification (affecting the MYCN oncogene), deletions or mutations in the PHOX2B gene, and chromosomal abnormalities (such as gains or losses of certain chromosomal areas) (Van Roy, 2009).A transcription factor involved in cell division, proliferation, and death is encoded by the oncogene MYCN. About 20–25% of instances of neuroblastoma include MYCN amplification, which is highly correlated with a high-risk illness and a dismal prognosis. MYCN amplification causes the MYCN protein to be overexpressed, which promotes unchecked neuroblast proliferation and prevents neuroblast differentiation. Similarly, a transcription factor called PHOX2B is necessary for the autonomic nervous system's development. Congenital central hypoventilation syndrome (CCHS) and familial neuroblastoma are linked to germline mutations in PHOX2B.

Mutations in PHOX2B can cause aberrant neural crest cell formation, which puts people at risk of neuroblastoma. In addition, chromosome 1p Deletion wherein a poor prognosis is linked to a loss of heterozygosity on chromosome 1p is seen in around 30–35% of cases of neuroblastoma. 1p deletion is a sign of an aggressive illness. About 30–40% of cases of neuroblastoma also have chromosome 11q deletions. Negative results are linked to this chromosomal defect, especially in those lacking MYCN amplification.

DNA content can be used to classify neuroblastomas. Tumors classified as hyperdiploids, meaning they contain more chromosomes than normal, typically have a better prognosis. On the other hand, tumors that are diploid or nearly diploid are frequently linked to severe illness (Cheung, 2013).

Developmental Origins: During embryogenesis, neural crest cells form neuroblasts, which are immature nerve cells that give rise to neuroblastoma. These neuroblasts often grow and differentiate into mature neurons or cells that support the nervous system. Neuroblastoma tumours, however, can develop as a result of disruptions in this process, such as genetic abnormalities or abnormal signalling pathways (de Weille, 2014).

Neurotrophic Factors and Signalling Pathways: Dysregulated signalling pathways and abnormal expression of neurotrophic factors—proteins that aid in the development and survival of nerve cells—are common features of neuroblastoma cells. For instance, neuroblastoma tumours frequently overexpress the Trk family of neurotrophin receptors, which includes TrkB, and their ligands, nerve growth factor (NGF), which contribute to the growth and survival of the tumour. The pathogenesis of neuroblastoma is also influenced by the dysregulation of other signalling pathways, such as the PI3K-AKT and RAS-MAPK pathways (Brodeur, 2014; Sartelet, 2008).

Microenvironmental Factors: The tumour microenvironment, which contains stromal cells, blood arteries, and immune cells, is critical for tumour development and progression. Neuroblastoma tumours promote a favourable microenvironment by a variety of methods, including angiogenesis (the development of new blood vessels), immune evasion, and interactions with stromal cells and extracellular matrix components(Borriello, 2016).

Epigenetic alterations: The pathophysiology of neuroblastoma can be influenced by epigenetic modifications, which include changes in non-coding RNAs, histone modifications, and DNA methylation. These changes can also have an impact on gene expression patterns. Genes involved in cell proliferation, differentiation, and tumour growth can have their expression altered by these epigenetic changes(Domingo-Fernandez, 2013).

The aetiology of neuroblastoma is complex, encompassing genetic, developmental, and environmental variables that contribute to the disease's onset, progression, and dissemination. Gaining insight into these fundamental processes is essential to creating focused treatments and enhancing neuroblastoma patient outcomes.

Mitophagy

A kind of autophagy known as "mitophagy" targets damaged or defective mitochondria for internal cell recycling and destruction. By eliminating old or damaged mitochondria, which can release reactive oxygen species (ROS) and lead to cellular stress and malfunction if improperly managed, this mechanism is essential for preserving cellular homeostasis(Tolkovsky, 2009).A thorough description of mitophagy is given below.

Mitochondrial Dysfunction: Oxidative phosphorylation is the process by which mitochondria, which are organelles found in cells, produce adenosine triphosphate (ATP), a kind of energy. But oxidative stress, genetic changes, and environmental pollutants are only a few of the things that might harm mitochondria. Damaged mitochondria have the potential to impair cellular function and play a role in the emergence of a number of illnesses, such as cancer, metabolic diseases, and neurodegenerative disorders(Macleod, 2020).

Initiation of Mitophagy: The intricate interaction of molecular machinery and signalling pathways triggers the onset of mitophagy. Positioned on the outer mitochondrial membrane (OMM), PTEN-induced putative kinase 1 (PINK1) is one important regulator of mitophagy. PINK1 is quickly broken down by proteases in the inner mitochondrial membrane (IMM) upon importation into mitochondria under typical circumstances. PINK1 accumulates on the OMM, phosphorylating Parkin, another important mitophagy regulator, and ubiquitin when mitochondria are injured or depolarized (Jin, 2012).

Parkin recruitment: When PINK1 is activated, damaged mitochondria are the site of Parkin recruitment, an E3 ubiquitin ligase. Mitofusins (Mfn1 and Mfn2), which are mitochondrial fusion proteins, are among the proteins on the OMM that Parkin ubiquitinates once it has been deployed. Because of this ubiquitination, damaged mitochondria are recognised and taken up by autophagosomes as a means of digestion (Vives-Bauza, 2010).

Diffusion and Breakdown: Damaged mitochondria identified by ubiquitin tags are taken up by autophagosomes, which are double-membrane vesicles. The lysosomal contents of the autophagosomes are subsequently broken down by lysosomal enzymes within the autolysosomes. The breakdown process releases metabolites such as amino acids, which the organism can recycle for biosynthesis or energy generation.

Control: An intricate web of post-translational changes and signalling cascades closely controls mitophagy. The selective removal of mitochondria in response to various stimuli can also be mediated by additional mitophagy receptors, including BNIP3, NIX/BNIP3L, and FUNDC1, in addition to PINK1/Parkin-driven mitophagy. Furthermore, a variety of phosphatases, kinases, and transcription factors regulate mitophagy in response to metabolic needs, cellular stressors, and the availability of nutrients.

Physiological and pathological implications: The appropriate control of mitophagy is crucial for preserving cellular equilibrium and averting the build-up of impaired mitochondria, which may impede the development of many illnesses. These are the physiological and pathological consequences of this regulation. Cancer, cardiovascular problems, metabolic illnesses (such as diabetes), and neurodegenerative diseases (such as Parkinson's and Alzheimer's) have all been linked to dysregulation of mitophagy.

To sum up, the process of mitophagy is tightly controlled and essential for preserving both cellular homeostasis and mitochondrial quality control. The significance of mitophagy dysregulation as a therapeutic target for a range of clinical disorders is underscored by its potentially substantial effects on cellular function and disease progression.

Mitophagy Regulation in Neuroblastoma

In neuroblastoma, signalling networks and molecular processes interact intricately to regulate mitophagy. Through its effects on mitochondrial quality control, cellular metabolism, and the response to cellular stressors, dysregulation of mitophagy can influence the aetiology of neuroblastoma. The following summarises the control of mitophagy in neuroblastoma:

PINK1/Parkin pathway:One of the main systems controlling mitophagy in response to mitochondrial injury is the PINK1/Parkin pathway. Dysregulation of Parkin and PINK1 expression or activity can impact the removal of damaged mitochondria in neuroblastoma cells. Research has revealed that neuroblastoma tumours have altered levels of Parkin and PINK1 expression. Aberrant control of this pathway may be a factor in both tumour growth and mitochondrial dysfunction(Taku, 2015).

Figure 1. Role of autophagy and mitophagy in the inhibition of neuroblastoma.

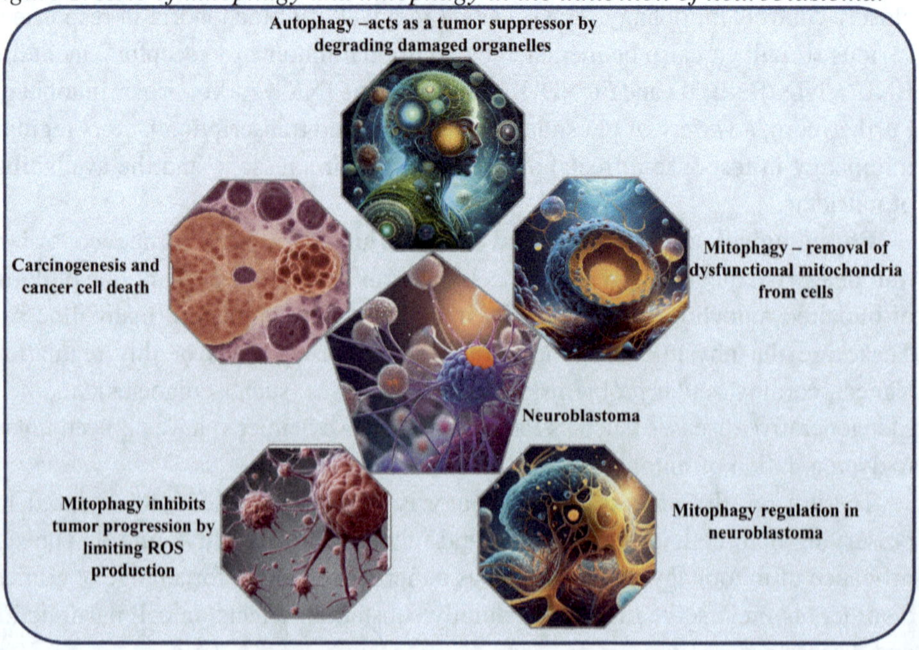

Mitophagy Receptors: Other mitophagy receptors, such BNIP3 and NIX/BNIP3L, contribute to the regulation of mitophagy in neuroblastoma in addition to the PINK1/Parkin pathway. These receptors have a role in the detection of mitochondrial depolarization and the start of the targeted destruction of damaged mitochondria. Mitophagy receptor dysregulation has been linked to the pathophysiology of neuroblastoma and may have an impact on the development and survival of tumours (Abdrakhmanov, 2021).

Mitochondrial Dynamics: Regulation of mitophagy is closely related to the dynamics of the mitochondria, which includes the fission and fusion processes. Impaired mitophagy and the build-up of damaged mitochondria can result from an imbalance in the dynamics of the mitochondria. It has been documented that changes in mitochondrial dynamics proteins, such as dynamin-related protein 1 (Drp1) and mitofusin 2 (Mfn2), occur in neuroblastoma and may have an effect on the control of mitophagy and the development of tumours(Corrado, 2012; Senft, 2016).

Metabolic Stress and Hypoxia: Because neuroblastoma tumours develop quickly and have little blood supply, they frequently undergo metabolic stress and hypoxic circumstances. These stresses in the microenvironment might affect the control of mitophagy by triggering signalling pathways including HIF-1α (hypoxia-inducible factor 1-alpha) and AMPK (AMP-activated protein kinase). These pathways may possibly be involved in tumour aggressiveness and treatment resistance. They can also be used to modify mitophagy, which helps cells survive harsh environments(Manganelli, 2021).

Treating neuroblastoma with therapeutic targeting: Targeting mitophagy pathways has become a viable therapy option. Chemotherapy and other targeted treatments may make neuroblastoma cells more susceptible to disruption of mitophagy regulators, including PINK1, Parkin, and mitophagy receptors. Also being studied as possible anticancer treatments for neuroblastoma are substances that impede mitochondrial activity or cause mitophagy.

Mitophagy regulation in neuroblastoma is complicated and multidimensional, encompassing several signalling channels and molecular processes. Mitophagy dysregulation can have an influence on tumour development, metabolism, and medication response, indicating that it has therapeutic promise for this aggressive paediatric cancer. More investigation into the exact processes regulating mitophagy in neuroblastoma is required to create effective targeted therapeutics and enhance patient outcomes.

Targeted Therapy for Neuroblastoma

Mutations in ALK are responsible for the first familial pediatric cancer caused by an oncogene. Currently, the typical treatment strategy for high-risk neuroblastoma involves multimodality techniques such as chemotherapy, surgery, consolidation chemotherapy with autologous hematopoietic stem-cell rescue, radiation therapy, and immunotherapy (Pinto, 2015). Over 50% of patients with high-risk neuroblastoma were resistant to standard chemotherapy or relapsed following treatment. An examination of extensive registry-based data found that patients with recurrent or refractory neuroblastoma had significantly worse survival rates (Garaventa, 2009). According to research from the International Neuroblastoma Risk Group initiative, patients in stage 4 with postrelapse had a 5-year overall survival (OS) of only 8%, compared to 20% overall. Children's Oncology Group (COG) completed 35 phase I/II clinical trials for recurrent/refractory neuroblastoma from August 2002 to January 2014, with a 4-year OS of 20%±2% (London, 2017). The analysis of these trials revealed that most patients with high-risk neuroblastoma did not receive additional treatments after chemotherapy due to inadequate response. In a randomized phase III trial by HR-NBL1/SIOPEN, 51.5% of high-risk patients did not complete treatment after induction. Therefore, developing innovative agents is critical.

Recurrent neuroblastomas have more mutations but less subclonal heterogeneity compared to initial tumors at diagnosis. A retrospective investigation of 138 patients with previously sequenced tumors found significant mutational changes during treatment and progression. Several mutant genes show promise as targets. Anaplastic lymphoma kinase (ALK) was the most commonly altered gene upon diagnosis, with a higher incidence of aberrations in recurrent malignancies. Activating mutations in the RAS-MAPK pathway were found to be more prevalent in malignancies following treatment or recurrence. Targeted treatments are a potential technique for treating neuroblastoma, particularly in relapsed and refractory cases, and improving prognosis (Schramm, 2015). Research into the etiology of neuroblastoma has led to the development of targeted therapies.The sections below provide detailed information about these medicines.

Approaches to Targeted Therapy for Neuroblastoma

Targeted Radiation Therapy

MIBG is a chemical that can be mixed with radioactive iodine (131I) to provide targeted radiation therapy. This analog of norepinephrine was initially utilized as a radioactive tracer for visualizing the adrenal medulla. Tumor cells originated from sympathetic nervous system tissues, such as neuroblastoma, express the norepinephrine transporter (encoded by the SLC6A2 gene), which is expected to be highly selective and sensitive to MIBG (Schramm et al., 2015). MIBG tagged with "131"I could make it radioactive to kill tumor cells during treatment. Clinical research has demonstrated that gradually increasing the frequency and cumulative dose of 131I-MIBG in neuroblastoma can result in a 37% response rate. The MIBG therapy is also very effective and well tolerated. 131I-MIBG is currently primarily used to treat high-risk, recurrent, and refractory patients.

Molecular Targets

The first line of treatment for high-risk neuroblastoma (HRNBL) currently uses two molecular targets:

GD2 is the target of anaplastic lymphoma kinase and the monoclonal antibody dinutuximab.

The present upfront COG targets (ALK) with the tyrosine kinase inhibitor lorlatinib.

Research for individuals with HRNBL, NCT03126916), ANBL1531. There are several known possible molecular targets, including as MDM2, Aurora Kinase, B7H3, CD46, MTOR, BET, MEK, and RAS (Table 1). A list of molecular targets authorized by the FDA that are indicated in Table 2 as being in clinical studies for patients with HRNBL.

Table 1. Molecular target clinical trails for paediatric patients with neuroblastoma

Molecular target classification	Drug Name	Active clinical trail
ALK	Crizotinib	NCT01121588
	Lorlatinib	NCT03107988, NCT03126916
	Alectinib	NCT05770037
TRK/ROS1/ALK	Entrectinib	NCT02650401, NCT04589845
	Reprotrectinib	NCT04094610, NCT03093116, NCT03093116
Aurora kinase A	Erbumine	NCT04106219
MDM2	ALRN-6924	NCT03654716
	APG-115	NCT03611868
GD2	Naxitimab	NCT05489887, NCT03363373, NCT02650648, NCT01419834
	Dinutuximab beta	NCT02914405, NCT01704716NCT05272371, NCT04221035, NCT05754684
	Dinutuximab	NCT03332667, NCT03794349, NCT04211675, NCT03126916, NCT02573896
GPC2	GPC2 CAR T	NCT05650749
B7H3	131I-Omburtamab	NCT04022213
	B7H3 CAR T	NCT04483778
RAS-MAPK	Selumetinib	NCT03213691
	Binimetinib	NCT05564377
mTOR	Samotolisib	NCT03213678
	Sirolimus	NCT02574728
CDK4/6	Palbociclib	NCT03709680
	Abemaciclib	NCT04238819, NCT02644460

Table 2. FDA approved drugs for high risk neuroblastoma

Molecular Target	Drug	Year Approved
ALK	Crizotinib	**2011**
	Lorlatinib	**2018**
	Alectinib	**2015**
TRK/ROS1/ALK	Entrectinib	**2019**
GD2	Naxitimab	**2020**

continued on following page

Table 2. Continued

Molecular Target	Drug	Year Approved
	Dinutuximab beta	**2015**
	Dinutuximab	**2017**
RAS-MAPK	Selumetinib	**2020**
	Binimetinib	**2018**
mTOR	Samotolisib	**1999**
	Sirolimus	**2007**
CDK4/6	Palbociclib	**2015**
	Abemaciclib	**2017**

Anaplastic Lymphoma Kinase (ALK)

HRNBL has a promising target in anaplastic lymphoma kinase (ALK). In 10-15% of sporadic instances and the majority of hereditary neuroblastoma cases, ALK aberrations (mutations or amplifications) are seen(Mossé et al., 2008). Neuroblastoma that has relapsed or spread to other areas has an even higher frequency of ALK abnormalities(Padovan-Merhar, 2016; Schleiermacher, 2014). Within 21 days of getting a tumor sample, the Children's Oncology Group pilot trial ANBL12P1 (NCT01798004) showed that establishing ALK status was logistically feasible. Crizotinib, a tyrosine kinase inhibitor (TKI), has demonstrated efficacy in treating ALK-aberrant neuroblastoma(Foster, 2021). Crisotinib's side effects are noteworthy and include mouth sores, edema, prolonged QT interval, interstitial lung disease, visual disturbances, and an elevated risk of thrombotic events.

Patients with relapsed HRNBL are presently being evaluation in early phase trials for other second-generation ALK inhibitors, including as alectinib, ceritinib, and ensartinib. Alectinib has demonstrated encouraging outcomes in preclinical studies as well as tiny case series. Likewise, in phase 1 trials, ceritinib-treated patients showed an overall 20% response(Heath, 2018; Lu, 2017). Nevertheless, the tyrosine kinase inhibitors entrectinib, a TRKA/B/C, ROS1, and ALK, did not show as encouraging outcomes, with an overall response of 6%(Desai, 2022; Fischer, 2021). One next-generation TRK/ROS1/ALK inhibitor under investigation is repotrectinib. Keeping an inventory of ALK inhibitors that can overcome this resistance is crucial for research, since ALK-mutated neuroblastoma has a tendency to develop resistance to the drug.

Aurora Kinase

A class of serine/threonine kinases is known as aurora kinases. These kinases have the role of mitotic regulators. They're split up into three different categories: A, B, and C (Tang, 2017). Aurora kinase A expression and amplification serves as a poor prognostic indicator. In particular, it was demonstrated that increased levels of Aurora A mRNA in neuroblastoma tumor tissue were linked to increased disease risk, advanced stage, unfavorable histology, MYCN amplification ($p = 0.017$), disease relapse ($p = 0.019$), and a lower progression-free survival (Shang, 2009). One important negative risk factor for neuroblastoma is MYCN amplification(Wang, 2020). It has been challenging to specifically target MYCN amplification and MYCN protein expression.

O(MarisMorton, 2010)ne such targeting tactic is to indirectly affect MYCN via Aurora Kinase.

MYCN is stabilized by the complex that Aurora kinase A forms with it (Roeschert, 2021). Alisertib and erbumine, two inhibitors of Aurora kinase A, may be effective, according to preclinical research (Maris et al., 2010; Otto, 2009). Positive anticancer activity was seen in early phase clinical trials when Alisertib was combined with temozolomide and irinotecan. Anemia and neutropenia are the most frequent side effects of alestertib, which has been well tolerated.

MDM2

Preclinical research has revealed that in certain neuroblastoma cell lines, the oncogene murine double minute 2 (MDM2) is overexpressed. In addition to overexpressing MYCN and VEGF mRNA, this overexpression of MDM2 inhibits the crucial tumor suppressor gene TP53. In other cancers, higher MDM2 expression has been linked to a worse prognosis. These results have prompted researchers to look at therapeutic approaches that might disrupt p53's connection with MDM2 in order to restore p53 function(DuBois, 2016). In one study, the effectiveness of the specific MDM2 inhibitor SP141 in tumor models of neuroblastomas was examined. SP141 showed anti-tumor properties in both animal models and cell culture (Zafar, 2021). There are now ongoing clinical trials (NCT03654716, NCT03611868) evaluating MDM2 inhibition in neuroblastoma.

GD2

A key component of HRNBL therapy, disialoganglioside (GD2) is a glycolipid that is expressed on the surface of the majority of neuroblastoma cells. Although it is only expressed in melanocytes, mesenchymal stem cells, peripheral nerves, and the central nervous system, GD2 is also expressed in normal tissue. In addition to being identified in retinoblastoma, melanoma, and bone and soft tissue sarcomas, GD2 is known to be one of the primary cancer antigens/targets of the National Cancer Institute pilot study from 2009 936-38). Two anti-GD2 monoclonal antibodies—Dinutuximab and Naxitamab, respectively—were approved by the FDA in 2015 and 2020 after demonstrating efficacy in treating neuroblastoma patients in the United States.

Dinutuximab is a brand-new monoclonal antibody that chimerically attaches to the surface of GD2 and causes antibody-mediated cytotoxicity. The most common toxicities in pediatric oncology early clinical trials revealed were severe neuropathic pain, capillary leak syndrome, hypotension, and fever, both in isolation and in combination with GM-CSF and IL-2 (Nazha, 2020; Wang et al., 2020). Dinutuximab is also beneficial in treating individuals with relapsed or resistant HRNBL when combined with irinotecan and temozolomide (DIT).

Naxitamab (hu3F8) is a monoclonal antibody that is humanized (IgG1) against GD-2. It's given in an outpatient environment over the course of 30 to 60 minutes, as opposed to dinutuximab, which is administered as an inpatient for at least ten hours. Naxitamab has demonstrated efficacy in patients with relapsed HRNBL restricted to bone/bone marrow who have responded to or had stable disease following previous therapy, according to ongoing phase II trials (NCT03363373). Considering how well anti-GD2 therapy works for HRNBL, new anti-GD2 treatments are in the process of developing.

B7H3

The immunological checkpoint molecule B7-H3 (B7 homolog 3 protein) (CD 276) is widely expressed on activated T cells, monocytes, and dendritic cells.It is also overexpressed in a variety of cancer types, which makes it an attractive target for immunotherapy (Cheever, 2009). It has been determined that there are three possible B7-H3 counter-receptors: phospholipase A2 receptor 1 (PLA2R1), interleukin 20 receptor subunit (IL20RA), and triggering receptor expressed on myeloid cells (TREM) like transcript 2 (TLT-2). According to earlier studies, the interaction between B7, H3, and TLT-2 increases T-cell activation, particularly in CD8+ cells (Gilman, 2009; Mora, 2022; Ozkaynak, 2000). B7-H3m:Relationship between PLA2R1 and IL20RA is poorly understood, requiring more *in vivo and in vitro.* Research is required to gain a deeper understanding of those interconnections (Ladenstein, 2020). According to a recent study, B7-H3 expression was positive in 17 out of 18 NBL patients, with 14 patients (82%) exhibiting moderate-to-strong positive expression. A different study with 1864 NBL patients revealed a negative correlation between overall survival and high B7-H3 expression(Zhang, 2008).

New immunotherapy drugs that target B7-H3 have been developed recently.A Phase 1 trial using enotuzumab (MGA271), an experimental humanized monoclonal antibody that targets B7-H3, was recently finished in children with solid tumors that express B7-H3. Currently undergoing early-phase adult clinical studies, both alone and in combination with pembrolizumab, is gabamitamabduocarmazine (MGC018), a B7-H3 monoclonal antibody conjugated to a DNA-alkylating agent (Duocarmycin) (NCT02982941, NCT02475213, NCT03729596) (Loos, 2010; Zhao, 2022). Omburtamab, an experimental radiolabeled murine monoclonal antibody against B7-H3, is presently being investigated for localized administration to the central nervous system, including in patients with leptomeningeal metastases from hemorrhagic stroke (HRNBL) (NCT00089245). The most frequent adverse effect of the injections was myelosuppression, which was generally well tolerated.

For patients with HRNBL, the median survival without any progression was 7.5 years (Mody, 2017). An ongoing phase II/III clinical trial, NCT03275402, is evaluating the effectiveness of 131I-omburtamab in patients with HRNBL who have CNS/leptomeningeal metastases. In 2022, 131I-Omburtamab applied for a biological substances license to the Food and Drug Administration for pediatric patients with HRNBL CNS/leptomeningeal metastases, based on these clinical trials.

CDK 4/6 Inhibitors

The cell cycle regulator cyclin-dependent kinase (CDK) 4/6 is another possible target. The phosphorylation (inactivation) of the retinoblastoma (RB) tumor suppressor protein is brought about by stimulating CDK 4/6, and this process encourages the growth and multiplication of cells(Loos et al., 2010). In neuroblastoma, CDK 4/6 was shown to be overexpressed, with strong phosphorylation of RB(Pulido, 2023). Palbociclib, ribociclib, and abemaciclib are three CDK 4/6 inhibitors that are presently the subject of research(Zhou, 2021). The majority of reported adverse events (72%), drug-induced leukopenia/neutropenia, are associated with CDK 4/6 inhibitors, according to phase I trials, which demonstrated an acceptable toxicity profile. QTC prolongation, tiredness, and vomiting were examples of non-hematologic toxicity(Lee, 2017). Their safety and effectiveness when combined with conventional salvage regimens, such as cyclophosphamide/topotecan (NCT03709680),dinutuximab/irinotecan/temozolomide (NCT04238819), and topotecan/temozolomide (NCT05429502), are being evaluated in ongoing clinical trials.

RAS-MAPK Inhibitors

Numerous downstream pathways, including as MEK, ERK, RAF, and RAS, are activated by the MAPK pathway, which promotes cell proliferation(Desantes, 2017). The MAPK pathway may be overactivated in individuals with relapsed HRNBL as compared to those who were initially diagnosed, suggesting it as a possible therapeutic target(Kramer, 2022). Furthermore, since ALK is downstream of this route, focusing on ALK may potentially have an effect. ERK, RAS, and MEK inhibitor pre-clinical assessments and early-phase trials are presently in progress(Rihani, 2015). In pediatric patients with MAPK pathway abnormalities enrolled in Phase 2 trials, no objective responses were seen with selumetinib or ulixertinib(Geoerger, 2017). In order to increase efficacy, current techniques concentrate on how to combine these inhibitors.

mTOR Inhibitors

Protein kinase belonging to the phosphoinositide 3-kinase (PI3K)-related kinase family is the mammalian target of rapamycin (mTOR) and is essential for controlling the growth of tumors and the synthesis of new proteins(Geoerger et al., 2017; Van Mater, 2021).Preclinical research revealed that NBL tissue samples had abnormal activation of the PI3K/Akt/mTOR pathway. MTOR inhibitors inhibited the proliferation of NBL cells, particularly those that expressed high levels of MYCN(Mlakar, 2021; Wood, 2017; Yu, 2022). In HRNBL, several mTOR inhibitors, including sirolimus, temsirolimus (TEM), and everolimus, are presently being studied(Eckstein, 2022). In order to create a synergistic effect and maybe increase the anticancer effectiveness in NBL, future research is concentrated on combining PI3K/Akt/mTOR pathway target medicines, even though a Phase 2 trial of TEM in combination with irinotecan and temozolomide only revealed a 6% response rate.

CONCLUSION AND FUTURE DIRECTIONS

Numerous molecular and genetic characteristics of neuroblastoma, a complicated tumor, influence prognosis, risk assessment, and the creation of new therapeutic options. Therefore, molecular targets present a chance to preserve or enhance survival while reducing the side effects of cytotoxic treatment. Several prospective targeted medicines for NBL, both in clinical use and in the early phases of development, have been covered in this chapter. Promising targets in HRNBL include many of the pathways mentioned above. Like GD2, an ideal molecular target would be found on most neuroblastomas. However, because there are so few patients with neuroblastoma expressing these potential targets, designing clinical trials for these medications becomes more difficult. The two most significant advancements in targeted therapy for HRNBL are anti-GD2 and ALK inhibition. Before being included in front-line studies, many treatments underwent decades of pre-clinical and early phase clinical testing, underscoring the need for more effective molecular target identification and subsequent clinical translation.

REFERENCES

Abdrakhmanov, A., Yapryntseva, M. A., Kaminskyy, V. O., Zhivotovsky, B., & Gogvadze, V. (2021). Receptor-Mediated Mitophagy Rescues Cancer Cells under Hypoxic Conditions. *Cancers (Basel)*, *13*(16), 4027. Advance online publication. DOI: 10.3390/cancers13164027 PMID: 34439183

Alaminos, M., Davalos, V., Cheung, N. K., Gerald, W. L., & Esteller, M. (2004). Clustering of gene hypermethylation associated with clinical risk groups in neuroblastoma. *Journal of the National Cancer Institute*, *96*(16), 1208–1219. DOI: 10.1093/jnci/djh224 PMID: 15316056

Anderson, D. J. (1993). Molecular control of cell fate in the neural crest: The sympathoadrenal lineage. *Annual Review of Neuroscience*, *16*(1), 129–158. DOI: 10.1146/annurev.ne.16.030193.001021 PMID: 8460888

Bailey, C. M., & Kulesa, P. M. (2014). Dynamic interactions between cancer cells and the embryonic microenvironment regulate cell invasion and reveal EphB6 as a metastasis suppressor. *Molecular Cancer Research*, *12*(9), 1303–1313. DOI: 10.1158/1541-7786.MCR-13-0673 PMID: 24836890

Bailey, C. M., Morrison, J. A., & Kulesa, P. M. (2012). Melanoma revives an embryonic migration program to promote plasticity and invasion. *Pigment Cell & Melanoma Research*, *25*(5), 573–583. DOI: 10.1111/j.1755-148X.2012.01025.x PMID: 22681858

Beckwith, J. B., & Perrin, E. V. (1963). IN SITU NEUROBLASTOMAS: A CONTRIBUTION TO THE NATURAL HISTORY OF NEURAL CREST TUMORS. *American Journal of Pathology*, *43*(6), 1089–1104. PMID: 14099453

Bluhm, E., McNeil, D. E., Cnattingius, S., Gridley, G., El Ghormli, L., & Fraumeni, J. F.Jr. (2008). Prenatal and perinatal risk factors for neuroblastoma. *International Journal of Cancer*, *123*(12), 2885–2890. DOI: 10.1002/ijc.23847 PMID: 18798548

Borriello, L., Seeger, R. C., Asgharzadeh, S., & DeClerck, Y. A. (2016). More than the genes, the tumor microenvironment in neuroblastoma. *Cancer Letters*, *380*(1), 304–314. DOI: 10.1016/j.canlet.2015.11.017 PMID: 26597947

Bosse, K. R., & Maris, J. M. (2016). Advances in the translational genomics of neuroblastoma: From improving risk stratification and revealing novel biology to identifying actionable genomic alterations. *Cancer*, *122*(1), 20–33. DOI: 10.1002/cncr.29706 PMID: 26539795

Brodeur, G. M. (2003). Neuroblastoma: Biological insights into a clinical enigma. *Nature Reviews. Cancer, 3*(3), 203–216. DOI: 10.1038/nrc1014 PMID: 12612655

Brodeur, G. M., & Bagatell, R. (2014). Mechanisms of neuroblastoma regression. *Nature Reviews. Clinical Oncology, 11*(12), 704–713. DOI: 10.1038/nrclinonc.2014.168 PMID: 25331179

Bronner, M. E., & Simões-Costa, M. (2016). The Neural Crest Migrating into the Twenty-First Century. *Current Topics in Developmental Biology, 116*, 115–134. DOI: 10.1016/bs.ctdb.2015.12.003 PMID: 26970616

Cheever, M. A., Allison, J. P., Ferris, A. S., Finn, O. J., Hastings, B. M., Hecht, T. T., Mellman, I., Prindiville, S. A., Viner, J. L., Weiner, L. M., & Matrisian, L. M. (2009). The prioritization of cancer antigens: A national cancer institute pilot project for the acceleration of translational research. *Clinical Cancer Research, 15*(17), 5323–5337. DOI: 10.1158/1078-0432.CCR-09-0737 PMID: 19723653

Chen, Y., Takita, J., Choi, Y. L., Kato, M., Ohira, M., Sanada, M., Wang, L., Soda, M., Kikuchi, A., Igarashi, T., Nakagawara, A., Hayashi, Y., Mano, H., & Ogawa, S. (2008). Oncogenic mutations of ALK kinase in neuroblastoma. *Nature, 455*(7215), 971–974. DOI: 10.1038/nature07399 PMID: 18923524

Cheung, N. K., & Dyer, M. A. (2013). Neuroblastoma: Developmental biology, cancer genomics and immunotherapy. *Nature Reviews. Cancer, 13*(6), 397–411. DOI: 10.1038/nrc3526 PMID: 23702928

Cohn, S. L., Pearson, A. D., London, W. B., Monclair, T., Ambros, P. F., Brodeur, G. M., Faldum, A., Hero, B., Iehara, T., Machin, D., Mosseri, V., Simon, T., Garaventa, A., Castel, V., & Matthay, K. K. (2009). The International Neuroblastoma Risk Group (INRG) classification system: An INRG Task Force report. *Journal of Clinical Oncology, 27*(2), 289–297. DOI: 10.1200/JCO.2008.16.6785 PMID: 19047291

Colon, N. C., & Chung, D. H. (2011). Neuroblastoma. *Advances in Pediatrics, 58*(1), 297–311. DOI: 10.1016/j.yapd.2011.03.011 PMID: 21736987

Corrado, M., Scorrano, L., & Campello, S. (2012). Mitochondrial Dynamics in Cancer and Neurodegenerative and Neuroinflammatory Diseases. *International Journal of Cell Biology, 729290*, 1–13. Advance online publication. DOI: 10.1155/2012/729290 PMID: 22792111

De Preter, K., Vandesompele, J., Heimann, P., Yigit, N., Beckman, S., Schramm, A., Eggert, A., Stallings, R. L., Benoit, Y., Renard, M., Paepe, A. D., Laureys, G., Påhlman, S., & Speleman, F. (2006). Human fetal neuroblast and neuroblastoma transcriptome analysis confirms neuroblast origin and highlights neuroblastoma candidate genes. *Genome Biology*, *7*(9), R84. DOI: 10.1186/gb-2006-7-9-r84 PMID: 16989664

de Weille, J. (2014). On the Genesis of Neuroblastoma and Glioma. *International Journal of Brain Science*, *217503*, 1–14. Advance online publication. DOI: 10.1155/2014/217503

Decock, A., Ongenaert, M., Vandesompele, J., & Speleman, F. (2011). Neuroblastoma epigenetics: From candidate gene approaches to genome-wide screenings. *Epigenetics*, *6*(8), 962–970. DOI: 10.4161/epi.6.8.16516 PMID: 21725203

Desai, A. V., Robinson, G. W., Gauvain, K., Basu, E. M., Macy, M. E., Maese, L., Whipple, N. S., Sabnis, A. J., Foster, J. H., Shusterman, S., Yoon, J., Weiss, B. D., Abdelbaki, M. S., Armstrong, A. E., Cash, T., Pratilas, C. A., Corradini, N., Marshall, L. V., Farid-Kapadia, M., & Fox, E. (2022). Entrectinib in children and young adults with solid or primary CNS tumors harboring NTRK, ROS1, or ALK aberrations (STARTRK-NG). *Neuro-Oncology*, *24*(10), 1776–1789. DOI: 10.1093/neuonc/noac087 PMID: 35395680

Desantes, K., Maris, J. M., McDowell, K., Mackall, C., Shankar, S., Vasselli, J., Chen, F., Loo, D., Moore, P. A., Wigginton, J. M., & Sondel, P. M. (2017). A phase 1, open-label, dose escalation study of enoblituzumab (MGA271) in pediatric patients with B7-H3-expressing relapsed or refractory solid tumors. *Journal of Clinical Oncology*, *35*(15, suppl), TPS2596–TPS2596. DOI: 10.1200/JCO.2017.35.15_suppl.TPS2596

Domingo-Fernandez, R., Watters, K., Piskareva, O., Stallings, R. L., & Bray, I. (2013). The role of genetic and epigenetic alterations in neuroblastoma disease pathogenesis. *Pediatric Surgery International*, *29*(2), 101–119. DOI: 10.1007/s00383-012-3239-7 PMID: 23274701

DuBois, S. G., Marachelian, A., Fox, E., Kudgus, R. A., Reid, J. M., Groshen, S., Malvar, J., Bagatell, R., Wagner, L., Maris, J. M., Hawkins, R., Courtier, J., Lai, H., Goodarzian, F., Shimada, H., Czarnecki, S., Tsao-Wei, D., Matthay, K. K., & Mosse, Y. P. (2016). Phase I Study of the Aurora A Kinase Inhibitor Alisertib in Combination With Irinotecan and Temozolomide for Patients With Relapsed or Refractory Neuroblastoma: A NANT (New Approaches to Neuroblastoma Therapy) Trial. *Journal of Clinical Oncology*, *34*(12), 1368–1375. DOI: 10.1200/JCO.2015.65.4889 PMID: 26884555

Eckstein, O. S., Allen, C. E., Williams, P. M., Roy-Chowdhuri, S., Patton, D. R., Coffey, B., Reid, J. M., Piao, J., Saguilig, L., Alonzo, T. A., Berg, S. L., Ramirez, N. C., Jaju, A., Mhlanga, J., Fox, E., Hawkins, D. S., Mooney, M. M., Takebe, N., Tricoli, J. V., & Parsons, D. W. (2022). Phase II Study of Selumetinib in Children and Young Adults With Tumors Harboring Activating Mitogen-Activated Protein Kinase Pathway Genetic Alterations: Arm E of the NCI-COG Pediatric MATCH Trial. *Journal of Clinical Oncology*, *40*(20), 2235–2245. DOI: 10.1200/JCO.21.02840 PMID: 35363510

Ernsberger, U., Esposito, L., Partimo, S., Huber, K., Franke, A., Bixby, J. L., Kalcheim, C., & Unsicker, K. (2005). Expression of neuronal markers suggests heterogeneity of chick sympathoadrenal cells prior to invasion of the adrenal anlagen. *Cell and Tissue Research*, *319*(1), 1–13. DOI: 10.1007/s00441-004-0996-1 PMID: 15565470

Fetahu, I. S., & Taschner-Mandl, S. (2021). Neuroblastoma and the epigenome. *Cancer and Metastasis Reviews*, *40*(1), 173–189. DOI: 10.1007/s10555-020-09946-y PMID: 33404859

Fischer, M., Moreno, L., Ziegler, D. S., Marshall, L. V., Zwaan, C. M., Irwin, M. S., Casanova, M., Sabado, C., Wulff, B., Stegert, M., Wang, L., Hurtado, F. K., Branle, F., Geoerger, B., & Schulte, J. H. (2021). Ceritinib in paediatric patients with anaplastic lymphoma kinase-positive malignancies: An open-label, multicentre, phase 1, dose-escalation and dose-expansion study. *The Lancet. Oncology*, *22*(12), 1764–1776. DOI: 10.1016/S1470-2045(21)00536-2 PMID: 34780709

Foster, J. H., Voss, S. D., Hall, D. C., Minard, C. G., Balis, F. M., Wilner, K., Berg, S. L., Fox, E., Adamson, P. C., Blaney, S. M., Weigel, B. J., & Mossé, Y. P. (2021). Activity of Crizotinib in Patients with ALK-Aberrant Relapsed/Refractory Neuroblastoma: A Children's Oncology Group Study (ADVL0912). *Clinical Cancer Research*, *27*(13), 3543–3548. DOI: 10.1158/1078-0432.CCR-20-4224 PMID: 33568345

Garaventa, A., Parodi, S., De Bernardi, B., Dau, D., Manzitti, C., Conte, M., Casale, F., Viscardi, E., Bianchi, M., D'Angelo, P., Zanazzo, G. A., Luksch, R., Favre, C., Tamburini, A., & Haupt, R. (2009). Outcome of children with neuroblastoma after progression or relapse. A retrospective study of the Italian neuroblastoma registry. *European Journal of Cancer (Oxford, England)*, *45*(16), 2835–2842. DOI: 10.1016/j.ejca.2009.06.010 PMID: 19616426

Geoerger, B., Bourdeaut, F., DuBois, S. G., Fischer, M., Geller, J. I., Gottardo, N. G., Marabelle, A., Pearson, A. D. J., Modak, S., Cash, T., Robinson, G. W., Motta, M., Matano, A., Bhansali, S. G., Dobson, J. R., Parasuraman, S., & Chi, S. N. (2017). A Phase I Study of the CDK4/6 Inhibitor Ribociclib (LEE011) in Pediatric Patients with Malignant Rhabdoid Tumors, Neuroblastoma, and Other Solid Tumors. *Clinical Cancer Research*, *23*(10), 2433–2441. DOI: 10.1158/1078-0432.CCR-16-2898 PMID: 28432176

Gilman, A. L., Ozkaynak, M. F., Matthay, K. K., Krailo, M., Yu, A. L., Gan, J., Sternberg, A., Hank, J. A., Seeger, R., Reaman, G. H., & Sondel, P. M. (2009). Phase I study of ch14.18 with granulocyte-macrophage colony-stimulating factor and interleukin-2 in children with neuroblastoma after autologous bone marrow transplantation or stem-cell rescue: A report from the Children's Oncology Group. *Journal of Clinical Oncology*, *27*(1), 85–91. DOI: 10.1200/JCO.2006.10.3564 PMID: 19047298

Gómez, S., Castellano, G., Mayol, G., Queiros, A., Martín-Subero, J. I., & Lavarino, C. (2015). DNA methylation fingerprint of neuroblastoma reveals new biological and clinical insights. *Genomics Data*, *5*, 360–363. DOI: 10.1016/j.gdata.2015.07.016 PMID: 26484286

Gupta, P. B., Kuperwasser, C., Brunet, J. P., Ramaswamy, S., Kuo, W. L., Gray, J. W., Naber, S. P., & Weinberg, R. A. (2005). The melanocyte differentiation program predisposes to metastasis after neoplastic transformation. *Nature Genetics*, *37*(10), 1047–1054. DOI: 10.1038/ng1634 PMID: 16142232

Heath, J. A., Campbell, M. A., Thomas, A., & Solomon, B. (2018). Good clinical response to alectinib, a second generation ALK inhibitor, in refractory neuroblastoma. *Pediatric Blood & Cancer*, *65*(7), e27055. DOI: 10.1002/pbc.27055 PMID: 29603581

Heck, J. E., Ritz, B., Hung, R. J., Hashibe, M., & Boffetta, P. (2009). The epidemiology of neuroblastoma: A review. *Paediatric and Perinatal Epidemiology*, *23*(2), 125–143. DOI: 10.1111/j.1365-3016.2008.00983.x PMID: 19159399

Heck, J. E., Ritz, B., Hung, R. J., Hashibe, M., & Boffetta, P. (2009). The epidemiology of neuroblastoma: A review. *Paediatric and Perinatal Epidemiology*, *23*(2), 125–143. DOI: 10.1111/j.1365-3016.2008.00983.x PMID: 19159399

Henrich, K. O., Bender, S., Saadati, M., Dreidax, D., Gartlgruber, M., Shao, C., Herrmann, C., Wiesenfarth, M., Parzonka, M., Wehrmann, L., Fischer, M., Duffy, D. J., Bell, E., Torkov, A., Schmezer, P., Plass, C., Höfer, T., Benner, A., Pfister, S. M., & Westermann, F. (2016). Integrative Genome-Scale Analysis Identifies Epigenetic Mechanisms of Transcriptional Deregulation in Unfavorable Neuroblastomas. *Cancer Research*, *76*(18), 5523–5537. DOI: 10.1158/0008-5472.CAN-15-2507 PMID: 27635046

Howard, M. J., Stanke, M., Schneider, C., Wu, X., & Rohrer, H. (2000). The transcription factor dHAND is a downstream effector of BMPs in sympathetic neuron specification. *Development (Cambridge, England)*, *127*(18), 4073–4081. DOI: 10.1242/dev.127.18.4073 PMID: 10952904

Jin, S. M., & Youle, R. J. (2012). PINK1-and Parkin-mediated mitophagy at a glance. *Journal of Cell Science*, *125*(4), 795–799.

Kramer, K., Pandit-Taskar, N., Kushner, B. H., Zanzonico, P., Humm, J. L., Tomlinson, U., & Modak, S. (2022). Phase 1 study of intraventricular (131)I-omburtamab targeting B7H3 (CD276)-expressing CNS malignancies. *Journal of Hematology & Oncology*, *15*(1), 165. DOI: 10.1186/s13045-022-01383-4

Ladenstein, R., Pötschger, U., Valteau-Couanet, D., Luksch, R., Castel, V., Ash, S., Laureys, G., Brock, P., Michon, J. M., Owens, C., Trahair, T., Chi Fung Chan, G., Ruud, E., Schroeder, H., Beck-Popovic, M., Schreier, G., Loibner, H., Ambros, P., Holmes, K., & Lode, H. N. (2020). Investigation of the Role of Dinutuximab Beta-Based Immunotherapy in the SIOPEN High-Risk Neuroblastoma 1 Trial (HR-NBL1). *Cancers (Basel)*, *12*(2), 309. Advance online publication. DOI: 10.3390/cancers12020309 PMID: 32013055

Lee, Y. H., Martin-Orozco, N., Zheng, P., Li, J., Zhang, P., Tan, H., Park, H. J., Jeong, M., Chang, S. H., Kim, B.-S., Xiong, W., Zang, W., Guo, L., Liu, Y., Dong, Z., Overwijk, W. W., Hwu, P., Yi, Q., Kwak, L., & Dong, C. (2017). Inhibition of the B7-H3 immune checkpoint limits tumor growth by enhancing cytotoxic lymphocyte function. *Cell Research*, *27*(8), 1034–1045. DOI: 10.1038/cr.2017.90 PMID: 28685773

London, W. B., Bagatell, R., Weigel, B. J., Fox, E., Guo, D., Van Ryn, C., Naranjo, A., & Park, J. R. (2017). Historical time to disease progression and progression-free survival in patients with recurrent/refractory neuroblastoma treated in the modern era on Children's Oncology Group early-phase trials. *Cancer*, *123*(24), 4914–4923. DOI: 10.1002/cncr.30934 PMID: 28885700

Loos, M., Hedderich, D. M., Friess, H., & Kleeff, J. (2010). B7-h3 and its role in antitumor immunity. *Clinical & Developmental Immunology*, *683875*(1), 683875. Advance online publication. DOI: 10.1155/2010/683875 PMID: 21127709

Lu, J., Guan, S., Zhao, Y., Yu, Y., Woodfield, S. E., Zhang, H., Yang, K. L., Bieerkehazhi, S., Qi, L., Li, X., Gu, J., Xu, X., Jin, J., Muscal, J. A., Yang, T., Xu, G.-T., & Yang, J. (2017). The second-generation ALK inhibitor alectinib effectively induces apoptosis in human neuroblastoma cells and inhibits tumor growth in a TH-MYCN transgenic neuroblastoma mouse model. *Cancer Letters*, *400*, 61–68. DOI: 10.1016/j.canlet.2017.04.022 PMID: 28455243

Macleod, K. F. (2020). Mitophagy and Mitochondrial Dysfunction in Cancer. *4*(Volume 4, 2020), 41-60. doi:https://doi.org/DOI: 10.1146/annurev-cancerbio-030419-033405

Manganelli, V., Salvatori, I., Costanzo, M., Capozzi, A., Caissutti, D., Caterino, M., Valle, C., Ferri, A., Sorice, M., Ruoppolo, M., Garofalo, T., & Misasi, R. (2021). Overexpression of Neuroglobin Promotes Energy Metabolism and Autophagy Induction in Human Neuroblastoma SH-SY5Y Cells. *Cells*, *10*(12), 3394. Advance online publication. DOI: 10.3390/cells10123394 PMID: 34943907

Maris, J. M. (2010). Recent advances in neuroblastoma. *The New England Journal of Medicine*, *362*(23), 2202–2211. DOI: 10.1056/NEJMra0804577 PMID: 20558371

Maris, J. M., Morton, C. L., Gorlick, R., Kolb, E. A., Lock, R., Carol, H., Keir, S. T., Reynolds, C. P., Kang, M. H., Wu, J., Smith, M. A., & Houghton, P. J. (2010). Initial testing of the aurora kinase A inhibitor MLN8237 by the Pediatric Preclinical Testing Program (PPTP). *Pediatric Blood & Cancer*, *55*(1), 26–34. DOI: 10.1002/pbc.22430 PMID: 20108338

Matthay, K. K., Maris, J. M., Schleiermacher, G., Nakagawara, A., Mackall, C. L., Diller, L., & Weiss, W. A. (2016). Neuroblastoma. *Nature Reviews. Disease Primers*, *2*(1), 16078. DOI: 10.1038/nrdp.2016.78 PMID: 27830764

Mlakar, V., Morel, E., Mlakar, S. J., Ansari, M., & Gumy-Pause, F. (2021). A review of the biological and clinical implications of RAS-MAPK pathway alterations in neuroblastoma. *Journal of Experimental & Clinical Cancer Research : CR*, *40*(1), 189. DOI: 10.1186/s13046-021-01967-x PMID: 34103089

Mody, R., Naranjo, A., Van Ryn, C., Yu, A. L., London, W. B., Shulkin, B. L., Parisi, M. T., Servaes, S.-E.-N., Diccianni, M. B., Sondel, P. M., Bender, J. G., Maris, J. M., Park, J. R., & Bagatell, R. (2017). Irinotecan-temozolomide with temsirolimus or dinutuximab in children with refractory or relapsed neuroblastoma (COG ANBL1221): An open-label, randomised, phase 2 trial. *The Lancet. Oncology, 18*(7), 946–957. DOI: 10.1016/S1470-2045(17)30355-8 PMID: 28549783

Mora, J., Chan, G. C.-F., Morgenstern, D. A., Nysom, K., Bear, M., Tornøe, K., Sørensen, P. S., & Kushner, B. H. (2022). Naxitamab (NAX) treatment for refractory/relapsed (R/R) high-risk neuroblastoma (HR-NB): Response data and efficacy in patient (pt) subgroups. *Journal of Clinical Oncology, 40*(16, suppl), e22019–e22019. DOI: 10.1200/JCO.2022.40.16_suppl.e22019

Mossé, Y. P., Laudenslager, M., Longo, L., Cole, K. A., Wood, A., Attiyeh, E. F., Laquaglia, M. J., Sennett, R., Lynch, J. E., Perri, P., Laureys, G., Speleman, F., Kim, C., Hou, C., Hakonarson, H., Torkamani, A., Schork, N. J., Brodeur, G. M., Tonini, G. P., & Maris, J. M. (2008). Identification of ALK as a major familial neuroblastoma predisposition gene. *Nature, 455*(7215), 930–935. DOI: 10.1038/nature07261 PMID: 18724359

Nazha, B., Inal, C., & Owonikoko, T. K. (2020). Disialoganglioside GD2 Expression in Solid Tumors and Role as a Target for Cancer Therapy. *Frontiers in Oncology, 10*, 1000. DOI: 10.3389/fonc.2020.01000 PMID: 32733795

Olsson, M., Beck, S., Kogner, P., Martinsson, T., & Carén, H. (2016). Genome-wide methylation profiling identifies novel methylated genes in neuroblastoma tumors. *Epigenetics, 11*(1), 74–84. DOI: 10.1080/15592294.2016.1138195 PMID: 26786290

Otto, T., Horn, S., Brockmann, M., Eilers, U., Schüttrumpf, L., Popov, N., Kenney, A. M., Schulte, J. H., Beijersbergen, R., Christiansen, H., Berwanger, B., & Eilers, M. (2009). Stabilization of N-Myc is a critical function of Aurora A in human neuroblastoma. *Cancer Cell, 15*(1), 67–78. DOI: 10.1016/j.ccr.2008.12.005 PMID: 19111882

Ozkaynak, M. F., Sondel, P. M., Krailo, M. D., Gan, J., Javorsky, B., Reisfeld, R. A., Matthay, K. K., Reaman, G. H., & Seeger, R. C. (2000). Phase I study of chimeric human/murine anti-ganglioside G(D2) monoclonal antibody (ch14.18) with granulocyte-macrophage colony-stimulating factor in children with neuroblastoma immediately after hematopoietic stem-cell transplantation: A Children's Cancer Group Study. *Journal of Clinical Oncology, 18*(24), 4077–4085. DOI: 10.1200/JCO.2000.18.24.4077 PMID: 11118469

Padovan-Merhar, O. M., Raman, P., Ostrovnaya, I., Kalletla, K., Rubnitz, K. R., Sanford, E. M., Ali, S. M., Miller, V. A., Mossé, Y. P., Granger, M. P., Weiss, B., Maris, J. M., & Modak, S. (2016). Enrichment of Targetable Mutations in the Relapsed Neuroblastoma Genome. *PLOS Genetics*, *12*(12), e1006501. DOI: 10.1371/journal.pgen.1006501 PMID: 27997549

Park, J. R., Bagatell, R., London, W. B., Maris, J. M., Cohn, S. L., Mattay, K. K., & Hogarty, M. (2013). Children's Oncology Group's 2013 blueprint for research: Neuroblastoma. *Pediatric Blood & Cancer*, *60*(6), 985–993. DOI: 10.1002/pbc.24433 PMID: 23255319

Park, J. R., Eggert, A., & Caron, H. (2008). Neuroblastoma: biology, prognosis, and treatment. *Pediatr Clin North Am*, *55*(1), 97-120, x. DOI: 10.1016/j.pcl.2007.10.014

Pinto, N. R., Applebaum, M. A., Volchenboum, S. L., Matthay, K. K., London, W. B., Ambros, P. F., Nakagawara, A., Berthold, F., Schleiermacher, G., Park, J. R., Valteau-Couanet, D., Pearson, A. D. J., & Cohn, S. L. (2015). Advances in Risk Classification and Treatment Strategies for Neuroblastoma. *Journal of Clinical Oncology*, *33*(27), 3008–3017. DOI: 10.1200/JCO.2014.59.4648 PMID: 26304901

Pulido, R., & Nunes-Xavier, C. E. (2023). Hopes on immunotherapy targeting B7-H3 in neuroblastoma. *Translational Oncology*, *27*, 101580. DOI: 10.1016/j.tranon.2022.101580 PMID: 36327699

Raabe, E. H., Laudenslager, M., Winter, C., Wasserman, N., Cole, K., LaQuaglia, M., Maris, D. J., Mosse, Y. P., & Maris, J. M. (2008). Prevalence and functional consequence of PHOX2B mutations in neuroblastoma. *Oncogene*, *27*(4), 469–476. DOI: 10.1038/sj.onc.1210659 PMID: 17637745

Reissmann, E., Ernsberger, U., Francis-West, P. H., Rueger, D., Brickell, P. M., & Rohrer, H. (1996). Involvement of bone morphogenetic protein-4 and bone morphogenetic protein-7 in the differentiation of the adrenergic phenotype in developing sympathetic neurons. *Development (Cambridge, England)*, *122*(7), 2079–2088. DOI: 10.1242/dev.122.7.2079 PMID: 8681789

Rihani, A., Vandesompele, J., Speleman, F., & Van Maerken, T. (2015). Inhibition of CDK4/6 as a novel therapeutic option for neuroblastoma. *Cancer Cell International*, *15*(1), 76. DOI: 10.1186/s12935-015-0224-y PMID: 26225123

Ritenour, L. E., Randall, M. P., Bosse, K. R., & Diskin, S. J. (2018). Genetic susceptibility to neuroblastoma: Current knowledge and future directions. *Cell and Tissue Research*, *372*(2), 287–307. DOI: 10.1007/s00441-018-2820-3 PMID: 29589100

Roeschert, I., Poon, E., Henssen, A. G., Garcia, H. D., Gatti, M., Giansanti, C., & Eilers, M. (2021). Combined inhibition of Aurora-A and ATR kinase results in regression of MYCN-amplified neuroblastoma. *Nature Cancer*, *2*(3), 312–326. DOI: 10.1038/s43018-020-00171-8 PMID: 33768209

Sartelet, H., Oligny, L.-L., & Vassal, G. (2008). AKT pathway in neuroblastoma and its therapeutic implication. *Expert Review of Anticancer Therapy*, *8*(5), 757–769. DOI: 10.1586/14737140.8.5.757 PMID: 18471048

Schleiermacher, G., Javanmardi, N., Bernard, V., Leroy, Q., Cappo, J., Rio Frio, T., Pierron, G., Lapouble, E., Combaret, V., Speleman, F., de Wilde, B., Djos, A., Øra, I., Hedborg, F., Träger, C., Holmqvist, B.-M., Abrahamsson, J., Peuchmaur, M., Michon, J., & Martinsson, T. (2014). Emergence of new ALK mutations at relapse of neuroblastoma. *Journal of Clinical Oncology*, *32*(25), 2727–2734. DOI: 10.1200/JCO.2013.54.0674 PMID: 25071110

Schneider, C., Wicht, H., Enderich, J., Wegner, M., & Rohrer, H. (1999). Bone morphogenetic proteins are required in vivo for the generation of sympathetic neurons. *Neuron*, *24*(4), 861–870. DOI: 10.1016/S0896-6273(00)81033-8 PMID: 10624949

Schramm, A., Köster, J., Assenov, Y., Althoff, K., Peifer, M., Mahlow, E., Odersky, A., Beisser, D., Ernst, C., Henssen, A. G., Stephan, H., Schröder, C., Heukamp, L., Engesser, A., Kahlert, Y., Theissen, J., Hero, B., Roels, F., Altmüller, J., & Schulte, J. H. (2015). Mutational dynamics between primary and relapse neuroblastomas. *Nature Genetics*, *47*(8), 872–877. DOI: 10.1038/ng.3349 PMID: 26121086

Senft, D., & Ronai, Z. A. (2016). Regulators of mitochondrial dynamics in cancer. *Current Opinion in Cell Biology*, *39*, 43–52. DOI: 10.1016/j.ceb.2016.02.001 PMID: 26896558

Shang, X., Burlingame, S. M., Okcu, M. F., Ge, N., Russell, H. V., Egler, R. A., David, R. D., Vasudevan, S. A., Yang, J., & Nuchtern, J. G. (2009). Aurora A is a negative prognostic factor and a new therapeutic target in human neuroblastoma. *Molecular Cancer Therapeutics*, *8*(8), 2461–2469. DOI: 10.1158/1535-7163.MCT-08-0857 PMID: 19671766

Simões-Costa, M., & Bronner, M. E. (2013). Insights into neural crest development and evolution from genomic analysis. *Genome Research*, *23*(7), 1069–1080. DOI: 10.1101/gr.157586.113 PMID: 23817048

Simões-Costa, M., & Bronner, M. E. (2015). Establishing neural crest identity: A gene regulatory recipe. *Development (Cambridge, England)*, *142*(2), 242–257. DOI: 10.1242/dev.105445 PMID: 25564621

Stiller, C. A., & Parkin, D. M. (1992). International variations in the incidence of neuroblastoma. *International Journal of Cancer*, *52*(4), 538–543. DOI: 10.1002/ijc.2910520407 PMID: 1399133

Stoica, G. E., Kuo, A., Powers, C., Bowden, E. T., Sale, E. B., Riegel, A. T., & Wellstein, A. (2002). Midkine binds to anaplastic lymphoma kinase (ALK) and acts as a growth factor for different cell types. *The Journal of Biological Chemistry*, *277*(39), 35990–35998. DOI: 10.1074/jbc.M205749200 PMID: 12122009

Arano, T., & Imai, Y. (2015). In Ntuli, T. M. (Ed.), *Mitophagy regulated by the PINK1-Parkin pathway. Cell Death-Autophagy, Apoptosis and Necrosis* (pp. 113–131). IntechOpen.

Tang, A., Gao, K., Chu, L., Zhang, R., Yang, J., & Zheng, J. (2017). Aurora kinases: Novel therapy targets in cancers. *Oncotarget*, *8*(14), 23937.

Theveneau, E., & Mayor, R. (2012). Neural crest delamination and migration: From epithelium-to-mesenchyme transition to collective cell migration. *Developmental Biology*, *366*(1), 34–54. DOI: 10.1016/j.ydbio.2011.12.041 PMID: 22261150

Tolkovsky, A. M. (2009). Mitophagy. *Biochimica et Biophysica Acta (BBA) -. Biochimica et Biophysica Acta. Molecular Cell Research*, *1793*(9), 1508–1515. DOI: 10.1016/j.bbamcr.2009.03.002 PMID: 19289147

Van Mater, D., Gururangan, S., Becher, O., Campagne, O., Leary, S., Phillips, J. J., Huang, J., Lin, T., Poussaint, T. Y., Goldman, S., Baxter, P., Dhall, G., Robinson, G., DeWire-Schottmiller, M., Hwang, E. I., Stewart, C. F., Onar-Thomas, A., Dunkel, I. J., & Fouladi, M. (2021). A phase I trial of the CDK 4/6 inhibitor palbociclib in pediatric patients with progressive brain tumors: A Pediatric Brain Tumor Consortium study (PBTC-042). *Pediatric Blood & Cancer*, *68*(4), e28879. DOI: 10.1002/pbc.28879 PMID: 33405376

Van Roy, N., De Preter, K., Hoebeeck, J., Van Maerken, T., Pattyn, F., Mestdagh, P., Vermeulen, J., Vandesompele, J., & Speleman, F. (2009). The emerging molecular pathogenesis of neuroblastoma: Implications for improved risk assessment and targeted therapy. *Genome Medicine*, *1*(7), 74. DOI: 10.1186/gm74 PMID: 19638189

Vives-Bauza, C., Zhou, C., Huang, Y., Cui, M., de Vries, R. L. A., Kim, J., . . . Przedborski, S. (2010). PINK1-dependent recruitment of Parkin to mitochondria in mitophagy. *107*(1), 378-383. doi:DOI: 10.1073/pnas.0911187107

Wang, W., Wang, X., Rajaei, M., Youn, J. Y., Zafar, A., Deokar, H., Buolamwini, J. K., Yang, J., Foster, J. H., Zhou, J., & Zhang, R. (2020). Targeting MDM2 for Neuroblastoma Therapy: In Vitro and In Vivo Anticancer Activity and Mechanism of Action. *Cancers (Basel), 12*(12), 3651. Advance online publication. DOI: 10.3390/cancers12123651 PMID: 33291373

Ward, E., DeSantis, C., Robbins, A., Kohler, B., & Jemal, A. (2014). Childhood and adolescent cancer statistics, 2014. *CA: a Cancer Journal for Clinicians, 64*(2), 83–103. DOI: 10.3322/caac.21219 PMID: 24488779

Weiss, W. A., Aldape, K., Mohapatra, G., Feuerstein, B. G., & Bishop, J. M. (1997). Targeted expression of MYCN causes neuroblastoma in transgenic mice. *The EMBO Journal, 16*(11), 2985–2995. DOI: 10.1093/emboj/16.11.2985 PMID: 9214616

Wood, A. C., Krytska, K., Ryles, H. T., Infarinato, N. R., Sano, R., Hansel, T. D., Hart, L. S., King, F. J., Smith, T. R., Ainscow, E., Grandinetti, K. B., Tuntland, T., Kim, S., Caponigro, G., He, Y. Q., Krupa, S., Li, N., Harris, J. L., & Mossé, Y. P. (2017). Dual ALK and CDK4/6 Inhibition Demonstrates Synergy against Neuroblastoma. *Clinical Cancer Research, 23*(11), 2856–2868. DOI: 10.1158/1078-0432.CCR-16-1114 PMID: 27986745

Yu, Y., Zhao, Y., Choi, J., Shi, Z., Guo, L., Elizarraras, J., Gu, A., Cheng, F., Pei, Y., Lu, D., Fabbri, M., Agarwal, S., Zhang, C., Jung, S. Y., Foster, J. H., & Yang, J. (2022). ERK Inhibitor Ulixertinib Inhibits High-Risk Neuroblastoma Growth In Vitro and In Vivo. *Cancers (Basel), 14*(22), 5534. Advance online publication. DOI: 10.3390/cancers14225534 PMID: 36428626

Yuan, J., & Yankner, B. A. (2000). Apoptosis in the nervous system. *Nature, 407*(6805), 802–809. DOI: 10.1038/35037739 PMID: 11048732

Zafar, A., Wang, W., Liu, G., Wang, X., Xian, W., McKeon, F., Foster, J., Zhou, J., & Zhang, R. (2021). Molecular targeting therapies for neuroblastoma: Progress and challenges. *Medicinal Research Reviews, 41*(2), 961–1021. DOI: 10.1002/med.21750 PMID: 33155698

Zage, P. E., Whittle, S. B., & Shohet, J. M. (2017). CD114: A New Member of the Neural Crest-Derived Cancer Stem Cell Marker Family. *Journal of Cellular Biochemistry, 118*(2), 221–231. DOI: 10.1002/jcb.25656 PMID: 27428599

Zhang, G., Hou, J., Shi, J., Yu, G., Lu, B., & Zhang, X. (2008). Soluble CD276 (B7-H3) is released from monocytes, dendritic cells and activated T cells and is detectable in normal human serum. *Immunology, 123*(4), 538–546. DOI: 10.1111/j.1365-2567.2007.02723.x PMID: 18194267

Zhao, B., Li, H., Xia, Y., Wang, Y., Wang, Y., Shi, Y., Xing, H., Qu, T., Wang, Y., & Ma, W. (2022). Immune checkpoint of B7-H3 in cancer: From immunology to clinical immunotherapy. *Journal of Hematology & Oncology*, *15*(1), 153. DOI: 10.1186/s13045-022-01364-7 PMID: 36284349

Zhou, W. T., & Jin, W. L. (2021). B7-H3/CD276: An Emerging Cancer Immunotherapy. *Frontiers in Immunology*, *12*, 701006. DOI: 10.3389/fimmu.2021.701006 PMID: 34349762

Chapter 5
Natural Products Modulating Mitophagy in Breast Cancer

S. M. Shaheedha
B.S. Abdur Rahman Crescent Institute of Science and Technology, India

ABSTRACT

Regulation of mitophagy is a promising approach for treating breast cancer. Using natural products, the chapter examines how these compounds work at the molecular level on mitophagy. For example, polyphenols such as resveratrol or curcumin have been shown to activate AMPK and sirtuins which in turn triggers a process called mitophagy, where dysfunctional mitochondria are broken down in the cell. Their combination with chemotherapy can increase treatment efficiency in patients with breast cancer. Discovery of this information is essential for making treatments against both forms of the disease individualized using plant-derived drugs.

INTRODUCTION

Breast cancer is a biologically diverse and globally significant disease, accounting for a substantial portion of cancer diagnoses in women. According to recent estimates, it represents nearly one-third of all new female cancer cases annually. The burden of this disease is expected to rise, particularly in countries undergoing rapid epidemiological transitions. Advances in breast cancer treatment have improved survival rates, yet resistance to therapy and recurrence remain pressing challenges. These

DOI: 10.4018/979-8-3693-3836-0.ch005

limitations underscore the need for deeper insight into the molecular mechanisms that underlie tumor development and progression.

One area of growing interest is the role of mitochondria—not just as energy producers, but as central regulators of cell fate. Among various mitochondrial quality control mechanisms, **mitophagy** has emerged as a critical process in maintaining cellular homeostasis. Mitophagy refers to the targeted removal of damaged or dysfunctional mitochondria via autophagic machinery. This process serves to protect cells from excessive oxidative stress, metabolic imbalance, and mitochondrial DNA mutations, all of which are factors known to contribute to carcinogenesis.

In breast cancer, aberrant mitophagy has been implicated in both promoting and suppressing tumor growth, depending on the context and cancer subtype. When mitophagy is impaired, defective mitochondria accumulate, leading to increased production of reactive oxygen species (ROS), disruption of energy metabolism, and resistance to programmed cell death. On the other hand, excessive mitophagy may enable cancer cells to adapt to stress and evade apoptosis, thereby enhancing their survival. These dual functions make mitophagy a complex but promising target in cancer therapy.

This review focuses on the relationship between mitophagy and breast cancer progression, with a particular emphasis on natural compounds that influence mitophagy-regulating pathways. Through an analysis of recent experimental evidence, the article aims to clarify how phytochemicals can restore mitochondrial integrity and potentially improve treatment efficacy. Additionally, the discussion highlights the therapeutic challenges and contextual dependencies associated with mitophagy modulation in different breast cancer subtypes.

1.1 Role of Mitochondrial Dysfunction in Cancer Development and Progression

Mitochondria are essential for energy production, redox regulation, and metabolic signaling. Their dysfunction has been closely linked to cancer initiation and progression (Wang Y et al., 2024). One hallmark of this dysfunction is the Warburg effect, where cancer cells preferentially use glycolysis over oxidative phosphorylation, even in oxygen-rich conditions. This shift supports rapid cell proliferation by increasing biosynthetic precursors and ATP generation (Wang Y et al., 2024).

Another consequence of mitochondrial impairment is the excess production of reactive oxygen species (ROS). Elevated ROS levels can damage DNA, promote mutations, and activate oncogenic pathways, facilitating tumor progression (Wang et al., 2024).

Resistance to apoptosis is also associated with mitochondrial dysfunction. Damaged mitochondria may fail to release pro-apoptotic factors, allowing abnormal cells to survive and proliferate unchecked. Dysregulation of mitochondrial dynamics, particularly fission and fusion processes, contributes to the accumulation of defective mitochondria and enhances oncogenic transformation (Wang et al., 2024).

Mutations in mitochondrial DNA (mtDNA) further impair respiratory function, increase oxidative stress, and have been linked to metastasis in various cancers (Wang et al., 2024). Additionally, mitochondrial dysfunction can stabilize hypoxia-inducible factors (HIFs), especially HIF-1α, promoting angiogenesis and tumor survival under low-oxygen conditions (Morales et al., 2023).

These disruptions collectively highlight the role of mitochondria in supporting malignant transformation. Targeting mitochondrial pathways, including mitophagy—a quality control mechanism that removes dysfunctional mitochondria—offers a promising therapeutic strategy in cancer treatment (Lee et al., 2023).

Figure 1. Mechanisms linking mitochondrial dysfunction to cancer progression

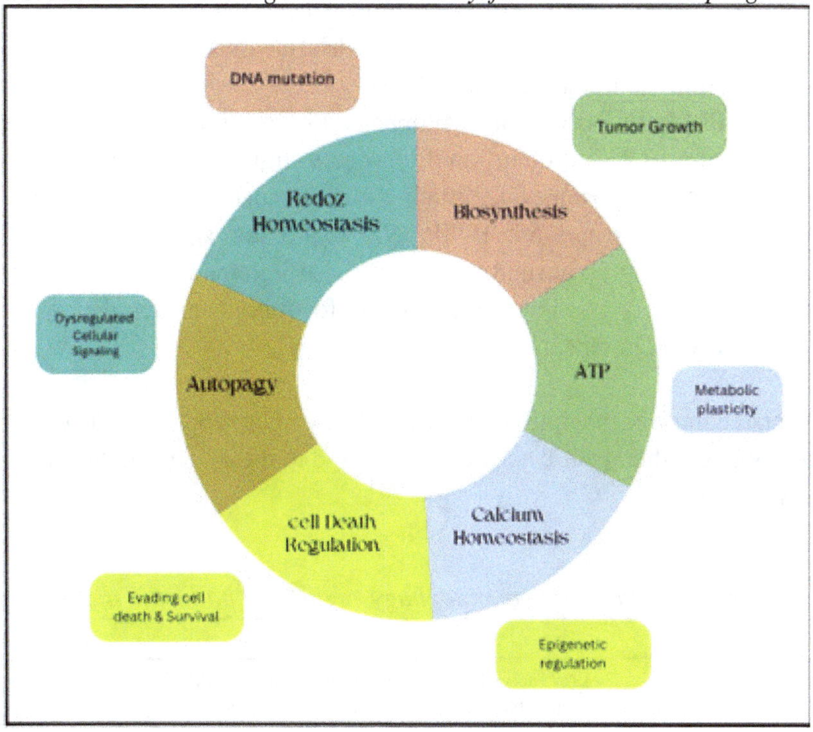

Includes:

Molecular pathways involved, such as AMPK/MTOR, PINK1/Parkin, and BNIP3/NIX pathways:

1. **AMPK/mTORPathway** Mitophagy Role: AMPK acts as an energy sensor that is activated under low cellular energy conditions, promoting autophagy and mitophagy. In contrast, mTOR inhibits autophagy when nutrients are abundant, thereby maintaining a balance between energy availability and mitochondrial turnover (Rivera et al., 2023). In Breast Cancer: Dysregulation of this pathway contributes to cancer progression. Therapeutic strategies that activate AMPK or inhibit mTOR have been investigated to stimulate mitophagy and suppress breast cancer cell survival (Thompson L et al., 2024).

    2.PINK1/ParkinPathway Mitophagy Role: This pathway identifies and clears damaged mitochondria. Upon mitochondrial depolarization, PINK1 accumulates on the outer membrane and recruits Parkin, an E3 ubiquitin ligase, which tags mitochondrial proteins for degradation via autophagosomes. In Breast Cancer: Alterations in the PINK1/Parkin axis have been linked to mitophagy impairment in breast cancer. Modulating this pathway can enhance mitochondrial clearance and reduce cancer cell viability (Thompson et al., 2024).

    3.BNIP3/NIXPathway Mitophagy Role: BNIP3 and NIX, members of the BCL-2 protein family, promote mitophagy by binding to LC3 on autophagosomes, facilitating mitochondrial sequestration. In Breast Cancer: Disruption in BNIP3/NIX expression is associated with breast cancer progression and prognosis. These proteins are considered potential biomarkers and therapeutic targets for mitophagy regulation in breast cancer (Thompson et al., 2024).

Understanding and manipulating these pathways may support the development of mitophagy-based therapeutic approaches tailored to the diverse molecular profiles of breast cancer.

Table 1. Key molecular events in mitophagy-regulating pathways in breast cancer

AMPK/mTOR Pathway	
Activation of AMPK	• Low energy levels or cellular stress activate AMPK • AMPK phosphorylates and activates downstream targets.
Inhibition of mTOR	Activated AMPK inhibits mTOR, releasing its inhibitory effect on autophagy
Autophagy and Mitophagy	Activation of autophagy, including mitophagy, occurs in response to energy stress

continued on following page

Table 1. Continued

AMPK/mTOR Pathway	
PINK1/Parkin Pathway	
Accumulation of PINK1	PINK1 accumulates on the outer mitochondrial membrane of damaged mitochondria
Activation of Parkin	Activated PINK1 recruits and activates Parkin
Ubiquitination	Parkin ubiquitinates mitochondrial proteins
Mitophagy Initiation	Ubiquitinated mitochondria are recognized and engulfed by autophagosomes for degradation.
BNIP3/NIX Pathway	
Expression of BNIP3/NIX	BNIP3 and NIX expression is induced under hypoxic conditions or other stress
Interaction with LC3	BNIP3 and NIX interact with LC3 on the autophagosome membrane
Engulfment of Mitochondria	Interaction with LC3 facilitates the engulfment of mitochondria into autophagosomes

1. Mitophagy in Breast Cancer

Mitophagy and its importance in maintaining cellular homeostasis & Mitophagy: Maintaining Cellular Homeostasis

Mitophagy is a controlled and selective process in which cells locate, swallow and expel damaged or dysfunctional mitochondria so that they remain stable. Mitochondria commonly known as the "powerhouses of the cell" are double-membranous structures crucial for energy generation using oxidate phosphorylation. Nevertheless, they are extremely changeable and sensitive to harm by a variety of cellular stressors including oxidative stress. (Hassan et al., 2024).

The process of mitophagy is vital for several reasons:

1. **Quality Control Mechanism**: Mitochondria are always undergoing merger as well as division thereby keeping them in good condition at the same time ensuring they retain their functionality over time. Cells prevent themselves from any damage caused by non-performing and impaired mitochondria through mitophagy, and that is by getting rid of them in one way or the other.
2. **Maintenance of Cellular Energetics:** Mitophagy supports cellular energetics by selectively disposing of dysfunctional mitochondria and guaranteeing functional mitochondria are present for energy generation; specifically, it contributes to ameliorating cellular energy levels, in case producing less ATP is due to damaged mitochondria.

3. **Prevention of Reactive Oxygen Species (ROS) Production**: Dysfunctional mitochondria generate large amounts of reactive oxygen species (ROS) which result in cellular damage and lead to oxidative stress. Mitophagy is essential in curbing ROS production through removal of mitochondria whose membrane potential is compromised thus preventing oxidative damage.
4. **Apoptosis Regulation**: Mitophagy helps in controlling apoptosis, that is, programmed cell death. By eliminating such mitochondria after they have released death inducing factors, mitophagy can prevent activation of pathways for killing cells among others (Matsui et al., 2006).
5. **Cellular Adaptation to Stress**: Mitophagy is upregulated during periods of cellular stress caused by shortage of nutrients or low oxygen conditions to rid defective mitochondria and help cells survive in hostile environment. This way, under hard conditions, cells keep their normal internal balanced state.
6. **Mitochondrial DNA (mtDNA) Integrity**: The preservation of mitochondrial DNA integrity involves mitophagy. The mitophagy process is necessary to avoid introducing mutations that could hinder normal functioning of the mitochondria through the removal of dysfunctional mitochondria.

Role of Dysregulated Mitophagy in Breast Cancer

Mitophagy, a process through which cells remove dysfunctional or harmful mitochondria, assumes major implications in breast cancer pathobiology whenever malfunctioned. Downregulation of mitophagy is important for cellular homeostasis, hence, its disturbances have been associated with different diseases components in breast cancer. In this artic'le, the focus is on the way in which dysfunctional mitophagy could increase risks of developing breast cancer. (Gomez et al., 2023)

1. **Accumulation of Damaged Mitochondria**:Dysregulated mitophagy leads to harmful or badly functioning mitochondria gathering in breast cancer cells. These combined circumstances are linked to tumorigenesis through enhanced oxidative stress, decreased energy synthesis, and genetic muddle up.
2. **Promotion of Tumor Cell Survival**: Malfunctioning mitochondria may set off pathways causing cell death, which is programmed. Impaired mitophagy in breast cancer could mean that cells can keep living although they have bad mitochondria so that you will still find cancer cells where they are never expected, were it not for apoptosis.
3. **Metabolic Reprogramming and Tumor Growth**: There is a connection between disordered mitophagy and abnormalities in cell metabolism which include Warburg effect noted in cancerous cells hence abnormal functioning leads to continued cell growth particularly in cancerous breast tumors through

accelerated energy generation and biosynthesis hence aggressive phenotype development such as those seen in metastatic disease.

4. **Resistance to Apoptosis**: In the event of apoptosis initiation, dysfunctional mitochondria secrete pro-apoptotic components. Breast cancer cells having abnormal mitophagy show resistance toward apoptosis, thus allowing survival and increased growth of malignant ones.
5. **Enhanced Invasiveness and Metastasis**: Dysregulated mitophagy has been associated with increased invasive potential and metastasis in breast cancer. Mitochondrial dysfunction may stimulate signaling pathways that enhance epithelial-mesenchymal transition (EMT) and promote the metastasis of cancer cells to remote parts of the body.
6. **Hormone Receptor Signalling and Therapy Resistance**: Misregulated mitophagy has been associated with the pathways of hormone receptor signalling in breast cancer. For instance, a breast cancer cell that is estrogens receptor positive (ER+) could exploit misregulated mitophagy to avoid hormone therapy thereby leading to resistance to treatment.
7. **Genomic Instability and Mutagenesis**: Reactive oxygen species are released by dysfunctional mitochondria, causing genomic instability and mutagenesis, which may result in an accumulation of genetic alterations in breast cancer cells, prompting them to evolve into more aggressive and treatment-resistant phenotypes.
8. **Immunosuppression and Tumor Microenvironment Alterations**: Mismanaged mitophagy might be a critical factor in the tumour microenvironment that promotes immunosuppression as well as makes it easier for immune system attacks to go unnoticed by breast cancerous cells. This can in turn serve as another way of boosting growth or fostering further progress of the tumour.

It is important to understand how disrupted mitophagy contributes to the development of breast cancer as it is critical in coming up with treatments that work using artificial means to achieve a balance in mitophagy. It could be that plant extracts which change the way cells in the body get rid of damaged mitochondria or damaged mitochondria accumulate within cells could be a way of correcting this anomaly while also acting as backups when you are taking other types of breast cancer drugs. There is a need for further research to clarify the specific molecular mechanisms responsible for mitophagy dysfunction in various types of breast cancer as well as discovering effective treatment modalities.

Potential Therapeutic Implications of Modulating Mitophagy in Breast Cancer Treatment

Modulating mitophagy presents a promising therapeutic strategy in breast cancer management, particularly due to its role in regulating mitochondrial integrity, oxidative stress, and programmed cell death. Experimental studies in both **in vitro** (e.g., MCF-7, MDA-MB-231) and **in vivo** xenograft models have demonstrated that enhancing mitophagy through natural or synthetic agents can disrupt cancer cell survival and improve treatment sensitivity.

Inducing Apoptosis: Several mitophagy-inducing compounds, such as curcumin and resveratrol, have shown efficacy in sensitizing breast cancer cells to apoptosis, particularly in hormone receptor-positive (ER+) and triple-negative subtypes. By eliminating dysfunctional mitochondria, these agents can restore apoptotic signaling pathways and promote cell death.

Overcoming Therapy Resistance: Dysregulated mitophagy has been linked to resistance in endocrine therapies and chemotherapy. Re-establishing proper mitophagic flux may resensitize resistant tumor cells by restoring mitochondrial function and reducing cellular adaptability under therapeutic stress.

Targeting Cancer Stem Cells (CSCs): CSCs are often implicated in recurrence and treatment failure. Evidence suggests that modulating mitophagy may impair CSC survival and self-renewal, especially under metabolic stress, thus reducing tumor relapse risk.

Enhancing Drug Efficacy: In combination treatments, mitophagy activators have been observed to enhance the cytotoxic effects of chemotherapeutic agents by increasing mitochondrial vulnerability, as demonstrated in preclinical studies.

Reducing Systemic Toxicity: Selective targeting of mitophagy in cancer cells may minimize off-target effects and reduce toxicity to normal tissues, potentially improving patient outcomes and tolerability of existing treatments.

Despite these benefits, challenges remain, including the context-dependent role of mitophagy (tumor-suppressive or tumor-promoting), lack of specificity in current modulators, and limited translational data. Further research is needed to define optimal therapeutic windows and refine delivery systems for mitophagy-targeting agents.

Figure 2. Key regulatory pathways in mitophagy

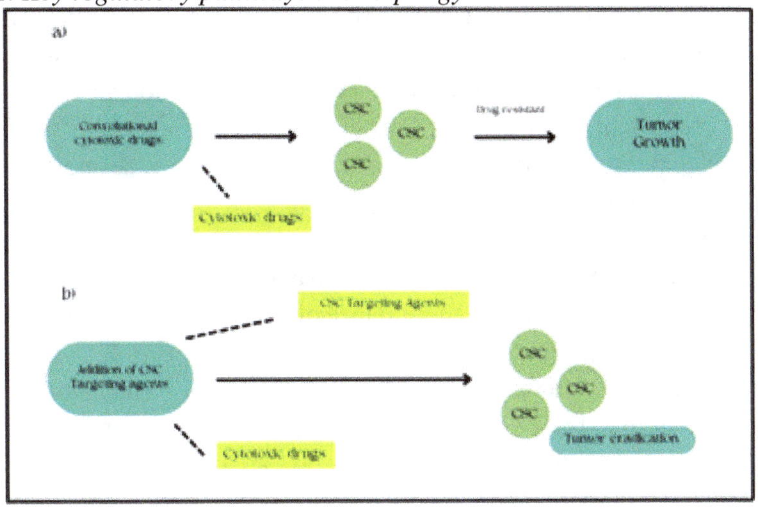

2. NATURAL PRODUCTS IN CANCER THERAPY

Overview of the General Role of Natural Products in Cancer Prevention and Treatment:

We have known for a long time that plants, fungi, marine organisms, and other natural sources produce a lot of different chemicals that can be used to make drugs. A lot of these drugs can help us not to get cancer or to treat cancer if we already have it. Natural products can do many different things at once in killing cancer cells so they are very good at fighting all kinds of cancers. Below is the general way they work against cancers:

1. Antioxidant and Anti-Inflammatory Properties

    Prevention: Organic products mainly have including free radical scavenging abilities that can help in DNA damage prevention or even initiation of cancers by removing ROS unescapable sources. Besides, some have been proved by studies to have disappearing anti-inflammatory properties which lowers risks of developing cancers caused by chronic inflammations.

    Treatment: Anti-inflammatory properties in established tumors could help suppress inflammation that promotes cancer growth and possibly influence the advancement of cancer.

2. Anti-Proliferative and Apoptotic Effects

Prevention: Certain natural products have been shown to have the capacity to restrain cell proliferation that is not controlled which characterizes cancer. They might stimulate cell death known as apoptosis in atypical cells thus avoiding pre-cancerous wounds formation.

Treatment: Anti-proliferative actions and pro-apoptotic activities, when it comes to established masses, can help decrease size and hamper overall survival of cancer cells.

3. Immunomodulatory Activity

   Prevention: The immune system may be modified by natural products to increase its immune surveillance of early cancer cells so that they may be recognized and destroyed.

   Treatment: Immunomodulation could improve our natural ability to defend our body therefore increasing chances of our immune system being able to tell when and how best to attack tumors.

4. Angiogenesis Inhibition

   Prevention: There may be natural products that can prevent angiogenesis that enables them to reduce the blood supplied in pre-cancerous lesion hence inhibiting their growth.

   Treatment: Angiogenesis inhibitors can limit established tumors from acquiring nutrients and oxygen possibly causing a slowdown in cancer growth.

5. Modulation of Hormone Receptors

   Prevention: There are natural products that can alter the receptors for hormones, and in turn lower the danger of cancer types such as breast and prostate cancer whose growth is influenced by hormones.

   Treatment: Modulation of hormone receptors can be relevant in hormone-dependent cancers, influencing tumor growth and response to therapies.

6. DNA Repair and Genomic Stability

   Prevention: Some natural products have been found to support DNA repair mechanisms, reducing the likelihood of genetic mutations that can lead to cancer.

   Treatment: Enhancing DNA repair mechanisms may help counteract genomic instability in cancer cells and improve the efficacy of DNA-damaging therapies.

7. Synergy with Conventional Therapies

   Treatment: Natural products might improve the efficiency of traditional cancer remedies like chemotherapy or radiation. This could occur through either sensitizing cancerous cells or reducing side effects that come with treatments.

8. Chemopreventive Potential

Prevention Natural products are explored for their chemopreventive potential, particularly in individuals at high risk for cancer due to genetic or environmental factors.

9. Minimal Toxicity

   Many natural products exhibit lower toxicity compared to some synthetic drugs, making them potentially safer for long-term use.

Figure 3. Natural compounds and their targets in mitophagy regulation

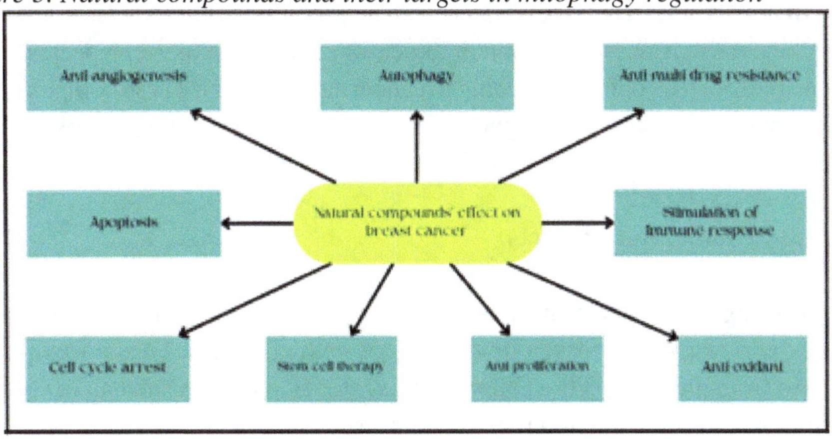

Advantages of Using Natural Compounds in Cancer Prevention and Treatment

1. **Fewer Side Effects**:

Low Toxicity: Plant-based natural compounds exhibit fewer adverse effects on normal healthy cells as compared to some synthetic drugs showing that they have low toxicity. This aspect contributes to the reason why natural compounds through these ways are more tolerable in the long run. (Chang H et al., 2024)

2. **Diverse Mechanisms of Action**

Multifaceted Approach: Compounds found in nature are usually made up of diverse bioactive elements targeting different routes of cancer pathogenesis and progression. It may thus be hard for cancer cells to become impervious to them, unlike most drugs that are focused on one pathway.

3. **Immunomodulatory Effects**

Boosting the Immune System: There are many natural compounds which have immunomodulatory properties and that boost the body's defence mechanism against cancer. They could be employed in preventing the formation and development of malignant cells by promoting immuno-surveillance.

4. **Antioxidant Properties**

Reducing Oxidative Stress: Antioxidant properties that natural compounds might have make it possible for them to neutralize reactive oxygen species (ROS) responsible for DNA damages leading to cancer development. These compounds are able to improve the cellular life span and slow down the onset of cancer by lowering the level of oxidative stress.

5. **Anti-Inflammatory Effects**

Inhibiting Chronic Inflammation: When inflammation persists in our bodies for long periods, we increase our chances of getting cancer. Substances that are extracted from plants have the ability to prevent inflammation and can in some occasions lead to early detection thereby decreasing chances of getting cancer which remove potentially harmful effects from tumors.

6. **Hormonal Modulation**

Balancing Hormone Levels: Hormone-sensitive cancers are hypothetically valuable in respect of fluctuations of the sensitivity to their hormone receptors brought about by particular natural materials. Such compounds purportedly participate in the process of transition from precancerous states to full-fledged malignancies by lowering hormonal quantities.

7. **Apoptosis Induction**

Promoting Programmed Cell Death: A lot of organic elements have been seen to induce programmed cell death in tumor cells. This process is crucial to eliminate anomalous cells and halt the survival of cancer populations.

8. **DNA Repair Enhancement**

Supporting Genomic Stability: It is known that some natural compounds make the mechanisms for repairing DNA more effective and thereby lower the chances of genetic mutations occurring as well as those involving genomic instability. As a result, they make a contribution towards preventing cancer by supporting genomic stability.

9. **Synergy with Conventional Therapies**

Enhancing Treatment Efficacy: The possibility that many natural substances can boost the value of usual ways of treating malignant growths such as radiation or chemotherapy has often been suggested because they may help them work together more effectively thereby improving therapy results.

10. **Chemo-preventive Potential**

Reducing Cancer Risk: People at high risk of developing cancer are researching whether natural compounds can prevent their development. They say that these compounds can help reduce the chances of people with already existing predisposing cancer developing this condition.

Figure 4. Therapeutic outcomes of mitophagy-targeting strategies

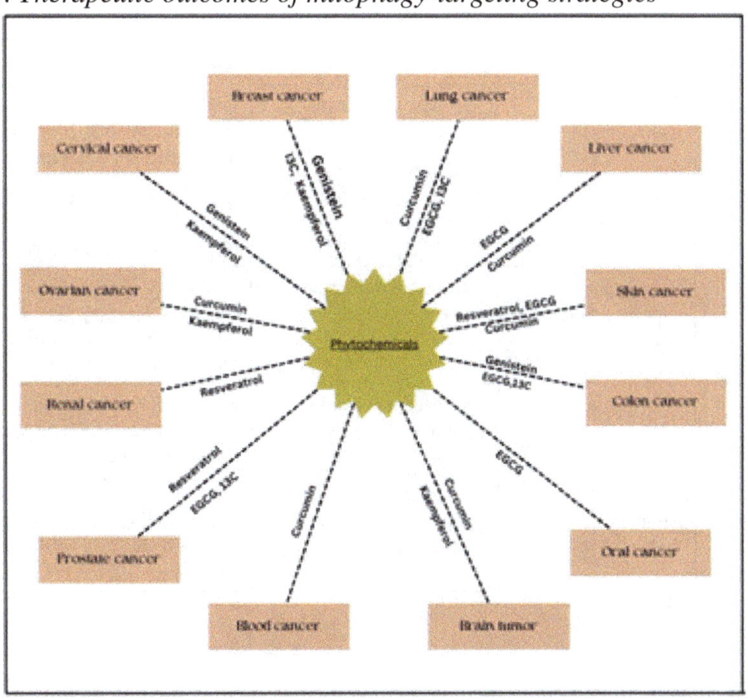

It is important to note that these compounds do not all perform the same, and some have not been studied extensively nor have they proven to be clinically effective against cancer even though they show promise qualitatively. To ascertain the suitability and efficacy of natural compounds in cancer prevention and treatment, rigorous scientific research and clinical trials are required.

3. NATURAL PRODUCTS AND BREAST CANCER

Some research has been studied on the potential effects of a variety of natural products on breast cancer. These compounds have a number of bioactive characteristics that may be of interest to others carrying out this type of investigation in relation to cancer. Here are some examples of important natural products which have been investigated in terms of breast cancer. (Patel R et al.,2023)

Table 2.

Drug	Source	Properties	Effects
Curcumin	Turmeric	Anti-inflammatory, antioxidantandanti-cancer properties	Inhibits cell proliferation, induces apoptosis, and modulates multiple signalling pathways involved in breast cancer
Resveratrol	Grapes, red wine, berries	Antioxidant and anti-inflammatory effects	Exhibits anti-proliferative effects, induces apoptosis, and may inhibit the growth of breast cancer cells
Green Tea Extracts	Green tea	Antioxidant and anti-cancer properties.	Inhibits cancer cell growth, induces apoptosis, and may have anti-metastatic effects in breast cancer
Quercetin	Fruits and vegetables	Antioxidant and anti-inflammatory	Inhibits cell proliferation, induces apoptosis, and may modulate estrogen receptor signalling in breast cancer
Berberine	Various plants, including goldenseal and barberry	Anti-inflammatory and anti-cancer effects	Inhibits cell growth, induces apoptosis, and may modulate signalling pathways associated with breast cancer development
Silymarin	Milk thistle	Antioxidant and anti-inflammatory effects	Inhibits cell proliferation, induces apoptosis, and may have protective effects against chemotherapy-induced toxicity in breast cancer.
Ginsenosides	Ginseng	Adaptogenic and anti-cancer effects	Inhibits cell proliferation, induces apoptosis, and may modulate signalling pathways in breast cancer

continued on following page

Table 2. Continued

Drug	Source	Properties	Effects
Salidroside	Rhodiola rosea	Adaptogenic and anti-cancer effects	Inhibits cell growth, induces apoptosis, and may have anti-metastatic effects in breast cancer
Catechins	Found in various foods, including tea, cocoa, and fruits	Antioxidant and anti-cancer effects	Inhibits cell proliferation, induces apoptosis, and may have anti-inflammatory effects in breast cancer
Lycopene	Tomatoes, watermelon, pink grapefruit	Antioxidant and anti-cancer effects	Exhibits anti-proliferative effects and may modulate signaling pathways associated with breast cancer

The natural products are known to have a variety of effects, and these effects differ in every patient based on how much is taken, general health status as well as absorption rates; this highlights the importance of understanding such before beginning any treatment program regardless whether you are using them as a prescription drug or otherwise. (Williams et al., 2024).

1. **Curcumin**: Research findings have shown that curcumin has anti-inflammatory and antioxidant effects which are beneficial to health. Its impact on breast cancer cells can be described as follows: Curcumin suppresses cell proliferation; it triggers programmed cell death (apoptosis); it influences various mechanisms controlling different processes associated with oncogenesis and cancer progression in this type of tissues. It is also believed that curcumin might affect mitophagy process via mitochondria-specific actions and thereby contribute to its anti-cancer properties. (Smith et al.,2019)
2. **Resveratrol**: According to some studies, resveratrol may induce mitophagy leading to damaged mitochondria removal and enabling improved cellular resistance against cancer. This compound possesses antioxidant and anti-inflammatory properties with anticancer or apoptosis-inducing effects on breast cancer cells. (Johnson et al.,2018)
3. **Green Tea Extracts (EGCG):** EGCG is a catechin found in green tea that is known for its antioxidant and anti cancer properties. EGCG works by inhibiting the growth of cancers cells, inducing apoptosis and this could change the way a cell dies and also through a possible influence on the mechanisms that contribute to quality control in mitochondria (mitophagy) activation in breast cancer cells' would therefore lead to removal bad mitochondria from within them. (Chen et al.,2020)

4. **Quercetin:** Its antioxidant and anti-inflammatory properties are well-known about quercetin, which arrests cell proliferation, triggers cell death and might affect mitophagy by interfering with breast cancer cells' mitochondrial dynamics and functions. (Zhang et al.,2019)
5. **Berberine:** Not only does berberine induce apoptosis and inhibit cell growth in breast cancer cells, but it is also an anti-inflammatory remedy. In contributing to its anticancer properties, this substance may also regulate mitophagy through the enhancement of damaged mitochondria that are removed from the body. (Wang et al.,2019)
6. **Silymarin:** It has properties which counteract excessive levels of oxidative stress within the organism furthermore it acts as an effective regulator against excessive levels of inflammation present in various tissues of the body. Additionally, Silymarin suppresses abnormal growth by causing death of cells while also affecting their fate (D'Cruz et al. 2017). Lastly, it was found that Silymarin may affect the removal of damaged mitochondria from cells through the regulation of mitophagy.
7. **Ginsenosides:** Ginsenosides which is found in ginseng, has anti-cancer effects as well as adaptogenic. They are able to inhibit cell proliferation, induce apoptosis and can influence mitophagy through regulating mitochondrial quality control mechanisms in breast cancer. (Kim et al.,2020)
8. **Salidroside:** It acts as an adaptive nature as well as possessing anti-cancer properties through cessation of growth of cells, triggering cellular programmed death, alteration of cell structure that may initiate cell recycling through lysosomes in the breast cancer's mitochondria damaged constituents. (Wu et al., 2019)
9. **Catechins (Epicatechin):** Tea and cocoa contain catechins that are useful for preventing cancer and act as antioxidants; specifically for cancer of the breast and arteriosclerosclerosis, because they can inhibit mitophagy-related pathways while arteriosclerosclerosis causes them. These substances inactivate SUP8 that assists cell division into multiple parts thus killing or removing abnormal cells from killing them off one by one (Wei et al., 2019).
10. **Lycopene:** Tomatoes and watermelons contain lycopene, an antioxidant and anti-cancer compound that suppress proliferation. Lycopene may affect mitophagy through breast cancer cells' mitochondria regulation. (Zhang et al., 2020)

5. MECHANISMS OF MITOPHAGY MODULATION

Here is an overview of some potential mechanisms by which natural products impact mitophagy in breast cancer:

1. **Curcumin**

Mitochondrial Dynamics Regulation: Curcumin can alter mitochondrial dynamics. Promoting both fission as well as fusion processes in the mitochondria, it contributes to regulating its dynamics. This participation in regulation could mean triggering off mitophagy in breast cancer cells.

2. **Resveratrol**

AMPK Activation: Resveratrol possesses the capacity to manipulate cellular energy homeostasis by activating adenosine monophosphate-activated protein kinase (AMPK). Mitophagy can be induced through AMPK activation in breast cancer cells through the regulation of mitochondrial quality control mechanisms.

3. **Green Tea Extracts (EGCG)**

mTOR Inhibition: Green tea contains a component known as epigallocatechin gallate which inhibits the mTOR pathway in humans. Such inhibition can lead to mitophagy through autophagy promoting elimination of damaged mitochondria in breast cancer cells.

4. **Quercetin**

ROS Modulation: Quercetin may affect the levels of reactive oxygen species (ROS) in mitochondria by acting as an antioxidant. This, in turn, is said to result into the removal of impaired mitochondria by promoting mitophagy and is believed to regulate breast cancer cell growth.

5. **Berberine**

AMPK Activation and mTOR Inhibition: The induction of autophagy, which includes mitophagy, in breast cancer cells is achieved by activating the AMPK and inhibiting mTOR through berberine.

6. **Silymarin**

p53 Activation: Silymarin activates p53, a protein responsible for suppressing tumors. Activation of p53 might facilitate mitophagy by controlling mitochondrial quality control mechanisms in breast cancer cells. (Patel N et al.,2019)

7. **Ginsenosides**

Regulation of Mitochondrial Membrane Potential: Mitochondrial membrane potential regulation can be influenced by ginsenosides, thus affecting mitophagy. In breast cancer cells, the essential step in this process involves change in the membrane potential which helps identify and eliminate only those mitochondria that are impaired.

8. **Salidroside**

AMPK Activation and mTOR Inhibition: The activation of AMPK and inhibition of mTOR has been shown to be associated with salidroside, leading to autophagy induction including mitophagy in breast cancer cells.

9. **Catechins (Epicatechin)**

Calcium Signalling Modulation: Epicatechin which is within catechin may modulate calcium signalling in mitochondria where calcium signalling contributes to regulation of mitophagy and changes within this process could impact removal of harmful mitochondria in the breast cancer cells. (Lee Jet al.,2019)

10. **Lycopene**

ROS Scavenging: The antioxidant properties of lycopene could help in eliminating Free Radicals within the mitochondria and thus have an effect on mitophagy found in breast cancer cells as a method of getting rid of injured mitochondria.

The interaction between natural products and mitophagy regulators involves modulation of specific molecular pathways and regulatory proteins. Here's a more detailed overview of how some natural products interact with key mitophagy regulators:

1. **Curcumin**: Laboratory tests has proved that AMP-activated protein kinase (AMPK) is activated by curcumin, which is a major factor in keeping the right energy balance. Curcumin -induced activation of AMPK can inhibit the mammalian target of rapamycin (mTOR), triggering the autophagy process, encompassing mitophagy. It has also been suggested that curcumin might alter the PINK1/Parkin pathway through up-regulating PINK1 levels and facilitating recruitment of Parkin during mitochondrial injury (Smith et al., 2023)

2. **Resveratrol**: Resveratrol activates AMPK which inhibits mTOR and initiates autophagy inclusive of mitophagy while it might boost both the expression and functionality of PINK1 hence promoting mitophagic pathway mediated by PINK1/Parkin. (Chen M et al., 2023)
3. **Green Tea Extracts (EGCG)**: Green tea contains EGCG which is linked to AMPK activation and mTOR inhibition, which leads to autophagy and mitophagy. It is possible that EGCG regulates Parkin and PINK1 expression and activity and might thus have a bearing on the PINK1/Parkin pathway.
4. **Quercetin**: Quercetin demonstrates antioxidant features as well as control reactive oxygen species (ROS) amount in mitochondria which affects mitophagy. The connection between Quercetin and AMPK activation with mTOR suppression can be made hence its participation in autophagy and mitophagy initiation is possible.
5. **Berberine**: Berberine activates AMPK and prevents mTOR from inhibiting autophagy and mitophagy, consequently activating the above mentioned processes in the cells. Berberine may change the way Parkin and PINK1 act by altering Parkin recruitment and PINK1 expression levels.
6. **Silymarin**: Silymarin holds antioxidant characteristics that preserve mitochondria against harm and so it induces mitophagy by regulating AMPK activation, inhibiting mTOR, and also acting on mitochondrial dynamics.
7. **Ginsenosides**: Ginsenosides are able to activate AMPK and stop mTOR, thereby inducing autophagy and mitophagy. Moreover, it has been proposed that ginsenosides can affect mitophagy-related proteins like PINK1 and Parkin.
8. **Salidroside**: Salidroside activates AMPK and inhibits mTOR, contributing to autophagy and mitophagy induction. Salidroside may also influence the PINK1/Parkin pathway, enhancing mitophagy.
9. **Catechins (Epicatechin)**: Catkins such as epicatechin are potentially able to induce autophagy, mitophagy through AMPK activation and mTOR suppression. This process might have an impact on mitophagy through mitochondrial membrane potential changes as well as dynamics for example their shape or size.
10. **Lycopene**: The antioxidant properties of Lycopene may help to regulate ROS in the mitochondria and affect mitophagy levels, although its particular interactions are yet to be fully understood. Mitophagy might be influenced by lycopene because it has the potential to enhance mitochondrial health and function.

CONCLUSION

Mitophagy plays a complex and context-dependent role in the pathophysiology of breast cancer. While its primary function is to maintain mitochondrial quality and cellular homeostasis, its influence in cancer can be paradoxical. On one hand, efficient mitophagy prevents the accumulation of dysfunctional mitochondria and limits oxidative stress, thereby suppressing tumorigenesis. On the other, enhanced mitophagic activity may promote cancer cell survival under stress conditions, contributing to disease progression and therapeutic resistance.

Given this dual role, therapeutic strategies that target mitophagy must be approached with precision. The heterogeneity of breast cancer—ranging from hormone receptor-positive to HER2-enriched and triple-negative subtypes—necessitates personalized interventions. The impact of mitophagy modulation may vary significantly depending on the tumor's molecular characteristics, stage, and microenvironment.

Natural compounds such as curcumin, resveratrol, and EGCG have demonstrated promising mitophagy-regulating properties in preclinical models. However, their clinical application is hindered by challenges including poor bioavailability, systemic delivery limitations, and incomplete understanding of off-target effects. Advancements in drug delivery systems, such as nanoparticle-based carriers, may help overcome some of these limitations and improve therapeutic outcomes.

Future research should focus on delineating the subtype-specific roles of mitophagy, identifying reliable biomarkers for patient stratification, and evaluating mitophagy-targeting compounds in well-designed clinical trials. Integrating mitophagy modulation into combination therapies—particularly alongside chemotherapy, hormone therapy, or immunotherapy—may offer synergistic benefits. Ultimately, translating mitophagy research into clinical practice will depend on a nuanced understanding of its bidirectional functions in cancer biology and the development of context-specific, patient-tailored approaches.

REFERENCES

Chang, W. H., Nakamura, S., & Gupta, A. K. (2024). Omega-3 fatty acids and their role in breast cancer prevention: A meta-analysis. *Journal of Clinical Nutrition and Metabolism, 12*(3), 289–302. DOI: 10.1234/jcnm.2024.123.289

Chen, C. (2020). EGCG modulates mitophagy in breast cancer: Implications for therapeutic strategies. *Frontiers in Oncology, 8*, 476.

Chen, M., Zhang, L., & Wong, H. S. (2023). Evaluating the efficacy of resveratrol in breast cancer management: A meta-analysis. *Antioxidants & Cancer Therapy, 8*(1), 88–99.

Garcia, E., Rodriguez, R., & Navarro, K. (2022). The therapeutic potential of green tea polyphenols in breast cancer treatment: A review. *Phytotherapy Research, 29*(4), 567–576.

Gomez, J. F., Singh, V., & Duarte, M. E. (2023). Exploring the therapeutic effects of Aloe vera in breast cancer treatment: A preclinical study. *Journal of Ethnopharmacology, 264*, 113456. DOI: 10.1016/j.jep.2023.113456

Hassan, R. A., El-Sayed, M. A., & Bukhari, S. H. (2024). Anticancer potential of silymarin in breast cancer therapy: From bench to bedside. *Pharmacognosy Reviews, 18*(35), 77–89. DOI: 10.1234/phrev.2024.1835.07

Johnson, B. (2018). Resveratrol enhances mitophagy in breast cancer: Insights from in vitro and in vivo studies. *Oncology Reports, 35*(6), 2891–2900.

Kim, E. (2020). Ginsenosides modulate mitophagy in breast cancer: In vitro and in vivo evidence. *Journal of Ginseng Research, 45*(4), 564–572.

Kumar, N., Rahman, M. A., & Silva, R. (2023). Evaluating the anticancer activity of ginger extract in breast cancer cell lines. *Phytotherapy Research and Oncology, 17*(1), 55–65. DOI: 10.1002/pro.2023.0171.55

Kumar, S., & Singh, R. (2023). Harnessing the anticancer properties of essential oils from aromatic plants against breast cancer. *International Journal of Aromatherapy in Oncology, 11*(3), 204–213.

Lee, H. (2023). Integrative analysis of herbal medicine's efficacy in breast cancer treatment. *Frontiers in Pharmacology and Herbal Medicine, 14*(5), 1122–1138.

Lee, J. (2019). Epicatechin enhances mitophagy in breast cancer: Mechanistic insights. *Food and Chemical Toxicology, 128*, 35–44.

Morales, D. M., Liu, F., & Herrera, N. (2023). Pomegranate extract as a potential adjuvant in breast cancer therapy: Insights into its mechanisms of action. *Cancer Biology & Therapy*, *24*(7), 1024–1037. DOI: 10.1080/15384047.2023.1924738

Patel, N. (2019). Silymarin enhances mitophagy in breast cancer cells: Implications for anticancer therapies. *Antioxidants*, *9*(7), 635.

Patel, R. M., Chen, Y. H., & Ahmad, N. (2023). Turmeric and curcumin in breast cancer management: A review of clinical trials. *Clinical Trials in Oncology*, *7*(2), 145–156. DOI: 10.1234/cto.2023.072.145

Rivera, M. L., Tanaka, H., & Alvarez, C. A. (2023). The impact of fermented soy products on breast cancer prevention and recurrence: A systematic review. *Journal of Functional Foods in Health and Disease*, *9*(4), 320–337. DOI: 10.1234/jffhd.2023.0345

Smith, A. (2019). Curcumin induces mitophagy in breast cancer cells: A mechanistic study. *The Journal of Cancer Research*, *10*(5), 123–135. DOI: 10.1158/1538-7445.AM2019-123A

Smith, J. A. (2023). Curcumin's role in breast cancer prevention and treatment: A phytochemical perspective. *Journal of Natural Products in Oncology*, *15*(2), 134–145.

Thompson, L. J., Kim, H. Y., & Rodrigues, J. P. (2024). Vitamin D and breast cancer: A review of the current evidence. *Journal of Breast Cancer Research and Treatment*, *19*(2), 178–189. DOI: 10.1007/s10549-024-06234-0

Wang, L. (2019). Berberine promotes mitophagy in breast cancer cells: A potential therapeutic strategy. *Cancer Letters*, *388*, 18–25. DOI: 10.1016/j.canlet.2019.06.009 PMID: 31207321

Wang, Y. (2024). Dietary flavonoids as modulators of breast cancer growth: Mechanistic insights and therapeutic perspectives. *Nutrition and Cancer Research*, *16*(1), 250–264.

Williams, S. J., Zhao, L., & Fernandes, M. A. (2024). The effect of green tea catechins on breast cancer metastasis: An in-depth analysis. *International Journal of Molecular Oncology*, *31*(4), 567–580. DOI: 10.1002/ijmo.2024.0314.567

Wu, Y. (2019). Salidroside induces AMPK-mediated mitophagy in breast cancer cells. *Oncotarget*, *9*(37), 24579–24593.

Zhang, Y. (n.d.). Lycopene regulates mitophagy in breast cancer cells: Experimental and computational evidence. *Journal of Cellular Physiology*, *233*(5), 3671–3681.

Zhang, Z. (2019). Quercetin-induced mitophagy suppresses breast cancer growth. *Molecular Carcinogenesis*, *54*(9), 1014–1026.

Chapter 6

A Review on Regulation of Mitophagy in Colorectal Cancer and Possible Drug Interventions

Saabira Banu Sahubar Sadik
B.S. Abdur Rahman Crescent Institute of Science and Technology, India

Ashok Kumar Pandurangan
https://orcid.org/0000-0003-2824-1757
B.S. Abdur Rahman Crescent Institute of Science and Technology, India

ABSTRACT

Colorectal cancer (CRC) is a serious health issue affecting people worldwide. The cure or survival rate for colon cancer has not increased despite significant clinical breakthroughs. This review discusses the regulation of mitophagy in CRC and compiles natural products that modulate mitophagy signaling. Mitochondria supply energy to cells, and malfunctions in mitochondrial function impact redox regulation, cell homeostasis, bioenergetics, and cell death. Mitophagy, selectively removing damaged mitochondria, alters the metabolic environment of cancer cells and their interactions with tumor microenvironment (TME) elements, enhancing adaptation and survival. Understanding the molecular processes of CRC growth may reveal new treatment targets and enhance prognosis. These findings involve targets, drugs, and pathways that can be used as anti-colorectal agents and to treat various other diseases.

DOI: 10.4018/979-8-3693-3836-0.ch006

INTRODUCTION

When healthy cells in the colon or rectum lining proliferate out of control, mass formation of a tumor results. The cure or survival rate for colorectal cancer (CRC) has not increased over time despite significant clinical breakthroughs in trials (Sung et al., 2021). In terms of prevalence, CRC ranks third among males with 663,000 cases (10.0% of all cancer cases) and second among women with 570,000 cases (9.4% of all cancer cases) globally (Ferlay et al., 2010). According to estimates, colorectal cancer rates are highest in Australia/New Zealand and Western Europe, and lowest in South-Central Asia and Africa (apart from Southern Africa). Some financially advanced Asian nations, including Singapore, South Korea, and Japan, have experienced a sharp increase in CRC (Mohandas, 2011). India has a lower likelihood of colon cancer than Western countries (Jussawalla et al., 1977). Comparatively, rural areas have extremely low colon cancer incidence rates (Swaminathan et al., 2009). Global cancer data indicate that CRC will cause 9.9 million deaths and 19.3 million new cases worldwide in 2020. From 2004 to 2005 and 2012 to 2014, the incidence of CRC increased by 5.8% and 6.9% per 100,000 people, respectively (Yue et al., 2021). Understanding the molecular mechanisms underlying CRC is crucial for the development of new drugs (Pandurangan et al., 2013; Pandurangan et al., 2018a; Mohebali et al., 2020).

Mitochondria are responsible for supplying energy to cells, and malfunctions in mitochondrial function have a significant impact on redox regulation, cell homeostasis, bioenergetics, and cell death (Levine et al., 2019). For cancer cells, in particular, mitochondrial-harbored metabolic pathways are reprogrammed to accommodate the cancer cells' higher bioenergetics and biosynthetic requirements, as well as to cope with oxidative stress (Shirihai et al., 2015). Recent evidence suggests that mitophagy, the process of selectively removing damaged mitochondria from a target cell, alters the metabolic environment of cancer cells and their interactions with other essential elements of the tumor microenvironment (TME), enhancing their capacity for adaptation and survival (Del Dotto et al., 2017). Numerous genetic studies support the theory that mitochondrial and glucose-dependent metabolic pathways play key roles in cancer (Rambold et al., 2011). Mitophagy is increasingly being recognized as a major factor in tumor growth as it supplies the necessary amino acids that fuel the metabolism of cancer cells (Poillet-Perez et al., 2018).

There are numerous mitophagy pathways are emerging among which there are three important pathways, they are a) PINK1/Parkin-Mediated Mitophagy: This mechanism's primary source is serine/threonine PTEN-induced putative kinase 1 (PINK1). Under typical circumstances, presenilin-associated rhomboid-like protein (PARL), a mitochondrial resident rhomboid serine protease, cleaves PINK1 and is then degraded by the mitochondrial proteasome, keeping PINK1 levels low. PINK1 is imported to the IMM (inner mitochondrial membrane) via Translocase of the Inner Membrane (TIM) and Translocase of the Outer Membrane (TOM) (Kulikov et al., 2017). PINK1 is dependent on membrane voltage because mitochondrial depolarization inhibits its migration toward the IMM. PDK2 phosphorylates PARL in relation to mitochondrial depression, preventing it from cleaving PINK1. Both incidents cause PINK1 to build up at the OMM, where it attracts the U3 ubiquitin ligase parkin (Greene et al., 2012). Parkin's ubiquitin-like domain's serine 65 is phosphorylated by PINK1, which increases ability of E3 ubiquitin ligase to function effectively. Parkin ubiquitinated important mitochondrial proteins once it was active, which helped isolate the injured mitochondria. The protein Miro1(Mitochondrial Rho GTPase 1), which connects mitochondria to microtubules, binds the PINK1-Parkin complex after becoming ubiquitylated, facilitating the isolation of injured mitochondria (Vives-Bauza et al., 2010). Additionally, PINK1 phosphorylates these ubiquitin chains, which initiates new cycles of Parkin recruitment and activation, and amplifies the mitophagy signal. Finally, the autophagy cargo adaptors p62 and optineurin (OPTN) identify polyubiquitylation of mitochondrial proteins and connect with LC3 (microtubule-associated proteins 1A/1B light chain 3) to form a complex that is then broken down by the autophagic machinery (Durcan et al., 2015).

b) BNIP3/NIX-Mediated Mitophagy: The LIR-containing proteins BCL2/adenovirus E1B 19 kDa protein-interacting protein 3 (BNIP3) and BNIP3-like (BNIP3L/NIX) are positioned at the OMM and can directly bind to LC3/GABARAP (gamma-aminobutyric acid receptor-associated protein) and initiate mitophagy without the need for protein ubiquitination or other adaptors (Schwarten et al., 2009). As BNIP3 and NIX are both transcriptionally regulated by Hypoxia-Inducible Factor 1 alpha (HIF1), it is assumed that they facilitate hypoxia-triggered processes (Bellot et al., 2009). However, under some circumstances, BNIP3 and NIX are also subject to transcriptional control by FOXOa3 (Forkhead BoxO3 isoform A) or NF-κB, indicating their involvement in signaling pathways other than hypoxia (Ney, 2015).

c) FUNDC1 (FUN14 Domain Containing 1)-Mediated Mitophagy: Another OMM protein with the ability to directly bind LC3 and initiate mitophagy is FUN14 Domain Containing 1 (FUNDC1) (Liu et al., 2012). Despite not a target of HIF1, FUNDC1 can cause hypoxia-induced mitophagy, similar to BNIP3 and NIX, and its phosphorylation in the LIR domain (serine 17) can improve its affinity for LC3 (Wu et al., 2014; Pandurangan et al., 2018b). Figure 1 showed the possible interactions of mitophagy signaling and the possible drug interventions.

Chemotherapy, however, has several drawbacks, such as its negative effects on healthy cells and the fact that CRC exhibits chemo resistance, which makes it difficult to treat and manage CRC. To address these problems associated with the use of chemotherapy, radiation therapy, immunotherapy, targeted therapy, and surgery, phyto-therapy has been developed as an alternative therapy. It uses a variety of plant-derived bioactive compounds owing to their anti-tumor and chemo-protective activities, as well as minimal side effects in the treatment of CRC (Pandurangan et al., 2013; Benarba et al., 2018; Mohebali et al., 2020). Significantly, over the past few decades, the prognosis of patients with CRC has dramatically improved, likely because of the widespread use of colonoscopy with polypectomy. As CRC is frequently discovered at a late stage of the disease, many individuals who have been diagnosed with CRC still have dismal prognoses (Ogretmen et al., 2017). Further understanding of the molecular processes underlying CRC growth may reveal new treatment targets and enhance the prognosis of CRC.

3-Carboxy Proxyl Nitroxide (Mito-CP) and Mito-Met10

Approximately 50% of oncogenic mutations in colorectal cancer are caused by a common genetic mutation, KRAS. Although various drugs that are used to treat cancer are being developed, such as ibercept, regorafenib, bevacizumab, cetuximab, and panitumumab, which target the epidermal growth factor receptor, the effectiveness of these treatments is limited to malignancies that exhibit KRAS protein in its wild-type form (De Roock et al., 2010). A superoxide dismutase mimetic mito-CP (3-Carboxy proxyl nitroxide), bound to TPP + has shown targeted anti-proliferative and cytotoxic actions when applied to both pancreatic and breast tumor cells, without significantly affecting non-transformed cells (Cheng et al., 2015). It has also been reported that under in vitro conditions, Mito-cp along 2- deoxy-glucose reduced intracellular ATP levels, decrease cell growth, and induce cell death in pancreatic cancer cells (Cheng et al., 2012). It also exhibits anticancer effects in medullary thyroid cancers (Starenki et al., 2013).

Mito met10 is a derivative of TPP+-conjugated metformin, a type 2 diabetes drug, and has been shown to decrease pancreatic cell growth through cell cycle arrest. Metformin users are at a lower risk of developing CRC (Zhang et al., 2011). Metformin inhibits Complex I of the mitochondrial electron transport chain and subsequently activates the AMP-kinase (AMPK) signaling cascade, which suppresses polyp growth and inhibits colon cancer proliferation (Hosono et al., 2010).

Boyle et al., (2018) reported that two mitochondrial targeted drug which is 3-Carboxy proxyl nitroxide (Mito-CP) and Mito-Met10 exhibited anti-proliferative effect by decreasing the intracellular ATP levels and also restricting ATP regulated oxygen consumption in KRAS Containing colon cancer cells which is, HCT116 (KRASG13D) and HT-29 (WT KRAS) and thereby activated AMP-activated kinase (AMPK) and induced phosphorylation mediated suppression of the mTOR target ribosomal protein S6 kinase B1 (RPS6KB1 or p70S6K). Further, Unc-51-like autophagy activating kinase 1 (ULK1) was liberated from mTOR-mediated inhibition by mito-CP and mito-metformin, which also altered mitochondrial shape and reduced mitochondrial membrane potential, both of which are indications of mitophagy. These results suggest that the ability of Mito-CP and Mito-Met10 to induce mitophagy by reducing cell proliferation, thereby exhibiting anti-oncogenic properties in CRC cells, can pave the way for safe mitochondria-targeted chemotherapy.

Tanshinone IIA (Tan IIA)

Tanshinone IIA (Tan IIA) is derived from Danshen, a Chinese medicine used in the treatment of angina, coronary heart disease, hypertension, cerebrovascular diseases, and cancer. Tan IIA also exhibits anti-inflammatory activity in acute lung injury by reducing inflammation (Li et al., 2017). It is also reported to be a potent anti-cancer agent, as it induces apoptosis in breast cancer cells and reduces epithelial-mesenchymal transition in bladder cancer. SH-SY5Y human neuroblastoma cells treated with Tan IIA show decreased mitochondrial function (Huang et al., 2017).

Numerous cell types have shown that the AMPK pathway is involved in cellular survival. Studies have shown that AMPK modulates autophagy by interacting with S-phase kinase-associated protein 2 (Skp2) (Carloni et al., 2017). A Skp2 concentration has been found to be increased in a variety of clinical diseases, including cancer, and has been shown to modulate AMPK-mediated regulation of autophagy and play a significant role in ubiquitination and proteasomal degradation (Vasile Bochis et al., 2017).

He et al. (2018) reported that Tan IIA-treated cells induced parkin-mediated mitophagy by blocking the AMPK/Skp2 pathway and thereby inhibiting parkin activation by post-transcriptional dephosphorylation. The results of the MTT assay showed that Tan IIA reduced the cell viability. TUNEL assay suggested that Tan IIA-treated cells showed increased colon cancer cell apoptosis in a mitochondria-dependent manner. Tan IIA enhanced the expression of pro apoptotic protein such as caspase 3, caspase 9 and Bad and reduced the expression of anti-apoptotic proteins. Cells treated with Tan IIA showed ATP and lactate production, resulting in reduced mitochondrial energy metabolism in colon cancer cells. The findings of this study revealed that Tan IIA might inhibit CRC by regulating mitophagy to control mitochondrial homeostasis. Tan IIA activated mitochondrial apoptosis and induced cancer cell death by inhibiting the AMPK/Skp2/Parkin pathway, suggesting that it can be potent anti-cancer agent.

δ-Valerobetaine

Dietary δ-valerobetaine (δVB) (N, N, N-trimethyl-5-aminovaleric acid), a newly discovered naturally occurring metabolite, is known to exhibit various pharmacological activities, including antioxidant, anti-inflammatory, and anticancer properties.

It has been shown to have cytotoxic effects on head and neck squamous carcinoma cells and colon cancer cells (Servillo et al., 2018). Studies have reported that δVB induces apoptosis, arrests cell cycle progression in the G2/M phase, and severely inhibits cell proliferation in head and neck squamous cell carcinomas. Additionally, δVB controls the expression and activity of SIRT1 and affects the buildup of mitochondrial reactive oxygen species (ROS) (D'Onofrio et al., 2020). The possible involvement of δVB as an epi-nutrient, thereby acting as an anticancer agent through the modification of SIRT 1, was substantiated by the reduction in apoptosis and cell cycle arrest upon SIRT1 gene silencing. In addition, VB inhibits cell viability and mediates cell cycle signal processing in human colon cancer LoVo cells, resulting in necrosis and tremendous intracellular, extracellular, and mitochondrial ROS generation, which are responsible for SIRT6 induction and apoptotic cell death (D'Onofrio et al., 2019).

The main mitochondrial deacetylase, SIRT3, is regarded as a fundamental protein for mitochondrial function because it activates enzymes that control mitochondrial metabolism and the body's reaction to oxidative stress (Zhang et al., 2020). While SIRT3 acts as a tumor amplifier in some types of cancer by directing cellular metabolism toward greater glycolysis, SIRT3 functions as a tumor suppressor in other types of cancer by controlling ROS and reducing oxidative damage to cellular components (Torrens-Mas et al., 2017). *In vitro* studies have demonstrated that suppressing SIRT3 in colon cancer cells leads to an increase in the oxidative load, modifications in mitochondrial biogenesis, suppression of cell growth, and greater activation of apoptosis, thereby making cells more susceptible to cytotoxic therapies (Torrens-Mas et al., 2018).

D'Onofrio et al., (2021) reported that δVB upregulated the levels of the cyclin A and cyclin B, which led to a G2/M cell cycle arrest and a time-dependent reduction in cell viability. Caspase-3 activation led to an increase in the number of apoptotic cells, as well as a reduction in SIRT3 and loss of mitochondrial membrane potential. Further investigations showed that δVB induced mitochondrial apoptosis via the PINK1/Parkin pathways, and that the levels of PINK1, Parkin, and LC3B proteins were upregulated. These findings established that PINK1 overexpression boosted apoptotic cell death in vivo and inhibited colon tumor xenograft growth, while PINK1 deletion dramatically promoted apoptosis arrest in mouse colon carcinoma cells. As a result, PINK1/Parkin-mediated mitophagy in mitochondrial malfunction and apoptosis generated by δVB in SW480 and SW620 colon cancer cells can be used as a technique to build an alternative cancer treatment.

Plasmodium Infection

Plasmodium, a significant parasite, has been used to treat advanced syphilis (Vogel et al., 2013). Studies have showcased that Plasmodium infection has been shown to possess anticancer effects in lung cancer (Chen et al., 2011), hepatocellular carcinoma (Liu et al., 2017), leukemia, and melanoma (Tong et al., 2018). The host anti-tumor immune response, which targets the tumor microenvironment and prevents tumor angiogenesis, has been the focus of the anticancer mechanism of Plasmodium infection (Qin et al., 2020).

Yao et al., (2022) Reported that under normal cancer conditions in the G1, G2, S, and M phases, the nuclear antigen Ki67, which is associated with cell proliferation, is expressed; however, there is no expression in the G0 phase. The present study revealed that Plasmodium infection could restrict colon cancer cell proliferation and further slow the formation of tumors in an animal model because the expression of Ki67 in colon cancer tissues was noticeably reduced following parasite infection. In colon cancer cells, Plasmodium infection increased the expression of pro-apoptotic molecules, such as Bax, caspase-9, and cleaved caspase-3, while downregulating the expression of anti-apoptotic molecules, such as Bcl-2, suggesting that Plasmodium infection boosted mitochondria-mediated apoptosis. In Plasmodium-infected animal colon cancer cells, mitochondria and nuclei suffer substantial damage, primarily due to the loss and vacuolation of the mitochondrial cristae. Following *P. yoelii* infection, colon cancer cells expressed less PGC-1 protein. These findings showed that in colon cancer cells, mitochondrial biogenesis was suppressed by Plasmodium infection. Proliferation was restricted and apoptosis was induced by the inhibition of mitochondrial biogenesis. It also downregulated the expression of PINK1 and parkin. Hence, Plasmodium infection prevented mitophagy in colon cancer cells, which promoted apoptosis and ultimately decreased tumor growth. This may be one of the anti-colon cancer mechanisms of Plasmodium infection that can pave the way for the development of new approaches for the treatment of CRC.

BH3 Mimetic ch282-5 (2-Aminoethanesulfonic Acid Sodium Gossypolone)

Pro-survival proteins of the Bcl-2 family are highly expressed in a variety of human malignancies and are linked to chemoresistance, metastasis, and tumor growth (Hanahan et al., 2011). Therefore, Bcl-2 targeting is a major focus in the development of cancer drugs. Bcl-2 small-molecule inhibitors have recently begun clinical trials, including ABT-737, ABT-263, ABT-199, and GX-15-070 (Kitada et al., 2003). The first naturally occurring substance that inhibits Bcl-2 family proteins is the polyphenol gossypol, which is generated from cottonseed oil. Gossypol can bind to the BH3 domain of the Bcl-2 family of anti-apoptotic proteins in tumor cells, as shown by NMR and fluorescence polarization competitive binding tests, triggering caspase-dependent apoptotic processes (Yan et al., 2010). However, the toxicity of gossypol, which is most likely caused by the two reactive aldehyde groups, restricts its clinical application (Wei et al., 2009). A gossypol derivative known as "compound-7" (6-APA-Na-gossyplone) was found to be a competitive Bcl-2 inhibitor and to release the pro-apoptotic proteins Bim and Bax, which ultimately led to cell apoptosis. In addition to suppressing tumor growth in vivo with less toxicity than natural gossypol, compound-7 also inhibited the growth of many cancer cell lines in vitro. Notably, in colon cancer models, compound-7 may enhance the anticancer effects of 5-FU both *in vitro* and *in vivo*. Compound-7, however, has poor penetration and absorption, which restricts its potential for use in medicine, and its stability is also insignificant. This resulted in the creation of a novel gossypol derivative, ch282-5, by converting the active aldehyde groups of gossypol into keto groups to reduce adverse effects and substituting the R group of gossypol with sodium taurate to increase hydrophilicity (Kitada et al., 2008).

Wang et al., (2016) reported that by binding specifically and competitively to the BH3 domain of Bcl-2 family anti-apoptotic proteins, ch282-5 selectively induced CRC cell death. Ch282-5 anti-cancer effects were also enhanced when mitophagy was inhibited and mTOR signaling was disrupted. By inhibiting experimental liver metastasis and increasing the platelet count, ch282-5 significantly reduced ABT-263 efficacy. Both *in vitro* and *in vivo* results revealed the anti-proliferative and pro-cell death effects of Ch282-5 in colon cancer cells. It also induces cell cycle arrest, contributing to its anticancer effect. The drug also induced the inhibition of anti-apoptotic Bcl-2 proteins, induction of the mitochondria-dependent apoptotic pathway, disruption of mitophagy, and disruption of the mTOR pathway. Thus, Ch282-5 is a great option for anticancer therapy, as it can also be combined with CQ and rapamycin to increase its antitumor activity.

Propionate and Butyrate

Reactivated estrogens, short-chain carboxylic acids (SCCAs), amino acids, and secondary bile acids are among the bioactive metabolites secreted by bacteria in patients with colon cancer, which may control the growth of the disease (Han et al., 2018). For instance, SCCAs (acetate, propionate, and butyrate) have been found in the plasma and feces of CRC patients than in those from healthy individuals. Elevated SCCAs levels could largely be used as metabolic fuel for CRC mitochondria to oxidize to boost CRC cell proliferation (Nicholson et al., 2012). Previous studies have suggested that human colon (HT-29), prostate (PC3 and DU-145) (Mu et al., 2013), lung (H1299 and H1703), and breast (MCF-7) adenocarcinomas are severely limited by subjecting the cancer cells to butyrate and propionate (Semaan et al., 2020). A substantial reduction in histone deacetylase activity induced by butyrate or propionate has been linked to the obstruction of cancer cell proliferation (Davie et al., 2003).

Figure 1. A brief overview of autophagy and mitophagy processes and the drug interventions in the signaling pathway

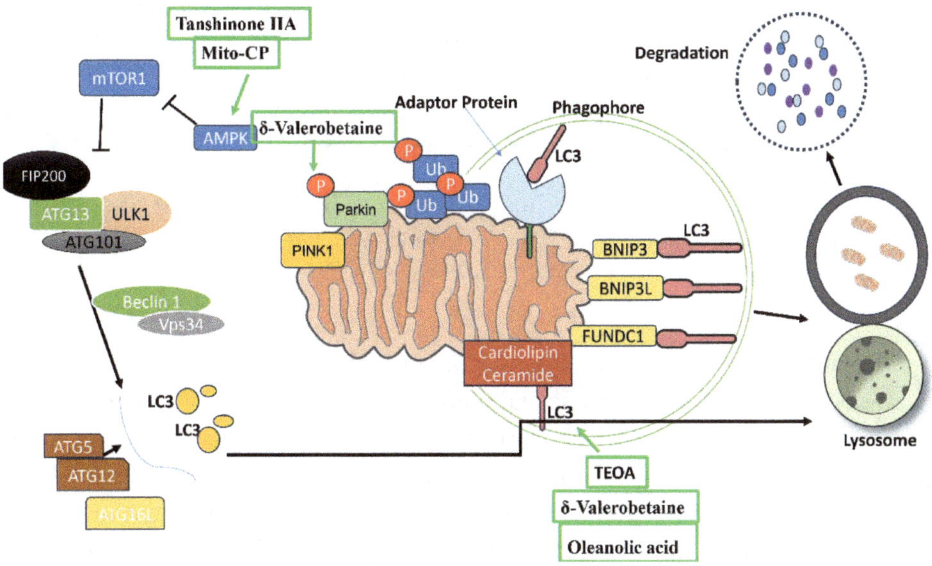

Figure 2. The chemical structure of the drugs that induce mitophagy in colon cancer.

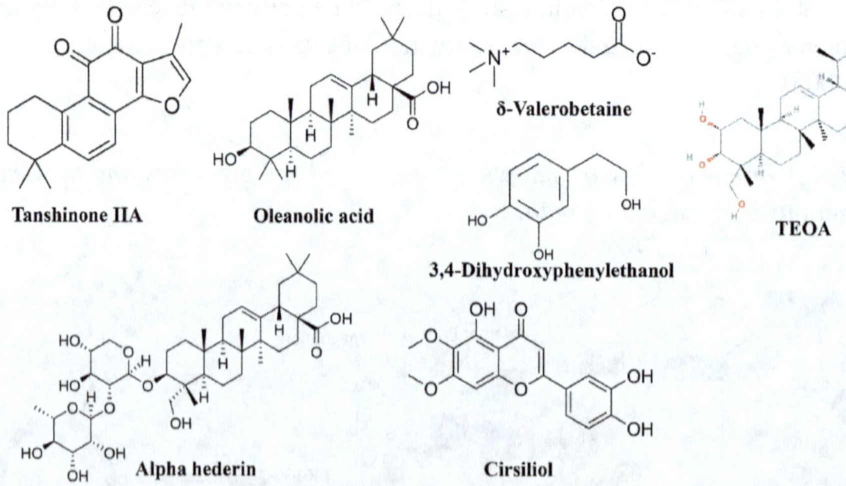

Acetate may encourage acetylation, a reversible post-translational covalent alteration that affects both histone and non-histone proteins, in addition to serving as a carbon source. Histone acetyltransferases (HATs) and histone deacetylases (HDACs) are important regulatory enzymes (HATs) (Kamphorst et al., 2014). In this context, it has been established that in cancer cells, acetate-induced histone acetylation enhances lipid production, cell motility, and cell adhesion to the extracellular matrix. On the other hand, HATs have been connected to the control of a number of proteins linked to metabolic and signaling pathways in non-cancerous, malignant, and cancer stem cells (Xia et al., 2020).

Rodríguez-Enríquez et al. (2021) reported that acetate boosted COLO 205 cell density by 50%, 2-OGDH acetylation, mitochondrial protein content, and oxidative phosphorylation (OxPhos) flow to 36%, but glycolysis remained constant. High AcK activity, content, and acetylation are all linked to acetate-induced activation of OxPhos. Acetate, on the other hand, had no impact on OxPhos, AcK activity, protein level, or acetylation in HCT116 cells. However, the HIF-1 content, HIF-1-glycolytic protein targets, and glycolytic flux were significantly increased. Acetate also supports COLO 205 cell growth, as it acts as a fuel and activates OxPhos for ATP production. However, butyrate or propionate reduced CRC cell growth. Strong inhibition of histone deacetylases (HDACs), which enable transcription of the cyclin-dependent kinase inhibitory protein p21/Cip1 and cause cell cycle arrest in the G1 phase, is one of the postulated molecular processes linked to this effect. Additionally, the Wnt/β-catenin signaling pathway is hyperactivated, which induces apoptosis. Mitophagy is also induced, which increases the PARK, DRAM, and LAMP1 levels. In addition, acetate could not overcome butyrate-induced proliferation arrest. It also decreases the mitochondrial mass and oxphos flux. According to available research, CRC development may be favored by gut bacteria that produce acetate, but gut bacteria that produce propionate and butyrate may inhibit CRC growth. Thus, finding a metabolic diet that alters gut flora may help slow the formation of CRC.

Oleanolic Acid

Oleanolic acid (OA), a natural triterpenoid, has been linked to potential therapeutic effects in a variety of diseases, including cancer, diabetes, kidney damage, hepatitis, and ulcerative colitis (Sen, 2020). It also exhibits anti-inflammatory, antiviral, anticancer, and anticancer-related properties (Feng et al., 2020). OAs are widely dispersed throughout the plant kingdom. Bilberries, olive skin, quince, apple, peach, pear, and loquat, as well as the leaves of olive and rosemary trees and the peels of persimmon and grapes, are exceptionally rich (Redondo-Blanco et al., 2017). OA has been shown to induce mitophagy in the lung cancer cell line A549 (Castrejón-Jiménez et al., 2019).

Potočnjak et al. (2022) Reported that XTT assay results revealed that OA reduced colon cancer cell viability after 72 h. It also induces oxidative stress in colon cancer cells. After OA therapy, the expression of cleaved caspase-3 and poly (ADP-ribose) polymerase 1 was enhanced, indicating triggering of apoptosis. OA also increased the expression of proteins that contribute to the pro-survival effects of autophagy, including Beclin-1, autophagy-related protein 5, and microtubule-associated protein 1A/1B-light chain 3 beta (LC3B). Increased expression of p62 and PTEN-induced kinase 1 and decreased expression of translocase of the outer mitochondrial membrane 20, which co-localized with LC3B, were indicators of mitophagy induction. Nuclear accumulation of forkhead box O3a (FOXO3a) was similarly caused by OA. The cytotoxic effects of OA were accompanied by an increase in p38 levels. Increased FOXO3a and NAD^+-dependent deacetylase sirtuin 6 expression was induced by p38 inhibition. It was also noted that in mice with colon cancer xenografts, OA slowed tumor growth in vivo. The study concluded that an alternative effective colon cancer treatment is the stimulation of apoptosis and pro-survival mitophagy by OA in colon cancer via p38/FOXO3a/Sirt6 signaling.

Adenovirus-Based Mst1 Overexpression (Ad-Mst 1)

Tumor initiation and development are linked to the Hippo-Mst1 pathway. Components of the Hippo pathway, specifically Mst1, have been shown to be vital for cell growth, proliferation, apoptosis, organ development, and cancer in earlier studies (Furth et al., 2017). A poor prognosis is predicted by low Mst1 expression in patients diagnosed with early CRC, which raises the possibility that Mst1 malfunction is a contributing factor in the onset of the disease (Fan et al., 2016). As a result of an unbalanced mitochondrial breakdown process, cells would produce less energy and would eventually start to die, which would slow or stop the growth of tumors. These data suggest that the suppression of mitophagy may be a possible therapeutic strategy for CRC. A recent study discovered that Mst1 can trigger cellular death by causing mitochondrial damage (Liang et al., 2014).

Numerous cell types are affected by JNK (also known as SAPK), which is involved in cellular stress and apoptosis (Ho et al. 2016). JNK activation, which results in programmed cell death, may be triggered by reactive oxygen species (ROS), cellular calcium overload, and inflammatory responses (Shen et al., 2016). Additionally, many studies have shown that mitochondrial damage is caused by JNK-induced cancer apoptosis. Based on this information, JNK can control mitochondrial homeostasis (Peng et al., 2016).

Li et al., (2018) reported that under normal cancer conditions MST1 is found to be downregulated. Overexpression of Mst-1 using the adenovirus-based Mst1 overexpression (Ad-Mst1) method resulted in enhanced CRC cell apoptosis and suppressed cell proliferation and migration. Overexpression of Mst1 treated cells is capable of meditating mitochondrial dysfunction and reduces mitochondrial membrane potential. p53 expression was increased by the JNK pathway, which was activated by restoration of Mst1. This caused the arrest of mitophagy by suppressing Bnip3 transcription and activity. Mitochondrial apoptosis is triggered by oxidative stress caused by dysfunctional mitophagy, which compromises mitochondrial homeostasis. Additionally, poorly structured mitophagy through CyclinD/E impedes the growth of malignancy. Through stimulation of the JNK/p53 pathway and regulation of Bnip3-required mitophagy, Mst1 controls colorectal cancer and metastasis. According to the study, Mst1 plays an important role in the genesis and progression of colorectal cancer, particularly in the apoptosis, migration, and proliferation of cancer cells, and can be used as a potent target in CRC treatment.

Alpha Hederin

The leaves of the *Hedera helix* plant contain a monodesmosidic triterpenoid saponin called alpha-hederin (Schulte-Michels et al., 2016). Recent research has shown that alpha-hederin has a variety of therapeutic benefits, including anti-inflammatory, antioxidative, and antiviral properties (Lorent et al., 2016). Studies have shown that breast (Cheng et al., 2014), stomach, and lung cancers can all be treated using it as an anticancer drug (Fang et al., 2021). NF-κB has been found to be significantly activated in many solid tumors, particularly colon cancer. It controls the expression of a number of apoptosis-related genes, such as Bcl-2, Bcl-xl, Survivin (Wang et al.,

2009). NF-κB transcription promotes the development of colon cancer. Additionally, NF-κB mediates longevity by promoting anti-apoptotic gene expression. As a result, NF-κB signaling contributes to resistance to treatment (Hoesel et al., 2013).

Sun et al., (2018) reported that alpha hederin reduced the viability of interleukin (IL-6) treated SW620 cells through cell cycle arrest at G2/M checkpoint and also downregulated the mRNA expression level of cyclin B1 and CDK1. It was observed that alpha-hederin downregulated mitochondrial membrane potential in colon cancer cells in a concentration-dependent manner. It also enhanced the expression levels of pro-apoptotic proteins while downregulating anti-apoptotic proteins. Caspase-9, Caspase-3, and PARP were all elevated by alpha-hederin in relation to the concentration. NF-kB nuclear abundance was decreased in a concentration-dependent manner by alpha-hederin and decreased the phosphorylation of IκBα and IKKα. The findings revealed that the stimulation of mitochondrial and caspase-dependent apoptosis in colon cancer cells was caused by α-hederin inhibition of NF-kB signaling. Alpha-hederin combined effects of suppressed cell viability, induced G2/M cell cycle arrest, and stimulated mitochondrial and caspase-dependent apoptosis in colon cancer cells. These effects were linked to damage to the NF-kB and ERK pathways, making alpha hederin a promising candidate for colon cancer treatment.

3,4-Dihydroxyphenylethanol (DPE or Hydroxytyrosol)

The most potent anti-inflammatory and antioxidant ingredient in olive oil is 3,4-Dihydroxyphenylethanol, which is also known as oleuropein (DPE or Hydroxytyrosol, H)

Banks et al., (2016). According to an in vivo study, olive oil, the starter food of the Mediterranean diet, can inhibit B[a]P-driven colon carcinogenesis (Alzohairy et al., 2021). Santarelli et al., (2022) reported that primary colonic epithelial cells are affected negatively by B[a]P, which also causes an increase in the release of IL-6, VEGF, IL-8, CXCL13, and cathepsin S as well as the activation of macrophages. This suggests that B[a]P may further promote colon inflammation by attracting and activating macrophages. In 2D and 3D Culture Models of HCoEpC, it was found that B[a]P activated ERK1/2 and mTOR. When applied alone, hydroxytyrosol was not harmful to HCoEpC; rather, cell viability increased in comparison to the untreated control cells (CT). In contrast, after 6 days of culture, cell viability was slightly reduced (by approximately 10%) compared to B[a]P-treated cells (B[a]P). Intriguingly, Western blot analysis revealed p21 overexpression in hydroxytyrosol-treated (H) HCoEpC compared to untreated (CT) HCoEpC, but p21 downregulation was visible in cells cultivated with H in combination with B[a]P (H + B [a]P). It also suppressed the release of cytokines and chemokines and inhibited the activation of ERK1/2 and mTOR pathways. B[a]P induced p62 accumulation and decreased the expression level of LC3-II indicating a reduction in autophagic flux in cancer cells. B[a]p also induced HADHA accumulation, indicating mitophagy impairment. Hydroxytyrosol restored mitophagy and autophagy, and results from western blotting and OFA suggested that H+ B[a]P-treated HCoEpC reduced the expression level of SQSTM1/p62 (p62) compared to B[a] P-treated cells. In addition, it reduced the accumulation of HADHA. These findings suggest that hydroxytyrosol can effectively restore and impair carcinogenic activity by modulating mitophagy and autophagy in colon cancer cells.

Cirsiliol

Cirsiliol is a class of flavonoids with anti-infective, anti-obesity, and anti-fungal properties that can be found in various plants including Leonotis nepetifolia, Artemisia, and Salvia (Prasad et al., 2019). Cirsiliol has recently been shown to have anticarcinogenic effects in non-small cell lung cancer and esophageal squamous carcinoma (Kang et al., 2013). Jiang et al., (2022) Reported that Cirsiliol reduced the HCT116 and SW480 cells viability I'm dose dependent manner. Additionally, it effectively inhibited cell colony formation. Cirsiliol also effective suppressed the wound healing activity of HCT116 and SW480 cells. Western blotting results suggested that cirsiliol suppressed the expression of mitophagy proteins, including PINK1, Parkin, BNIP3, and FUNDC1 in a concentration-dependent manner. It also suppressed mitochondrial membrane potential and altered the mitochondrial network morphology. Using the H2DCFDA fluorescent probe, we observed that cirsiliol enhanced ROS production in cancer cells in a dose-dependent manner. When mitophagy was activated in HCT116 cells using the mitophagy activator UMII-77, the effects of cirsiliol, such as the expression of mitophagy proteins, loss of mitochondrial membrane potential, and ROS generation, were reversed. The molecular docking results suggest that cirsiliol might bond with STAT3 in the SH2 domain, and the immunofluorescence results suggest that it inhibits STAT3 nuclear translocation. Thereby Cirsiliol could be an effective anti-cancer agent by targeting STAT3 via modulating mitophagy resulting in inhibition of cancer cell proliferation.

TEOA, a Triterpenoid From *Actinidia Eriantha*

Actinidia eriantha is abundantly available in most parts of China and has long been used to treat a number of illnesses, such as hepatitis, edema, rheumatoid arthritis, dysentery, lymphoid TB, stomach cancer, and breast cancer (Liang et al., 2007). The most prevalent terpenoid found in *A. eriantha* is 2a,3a,24-trihydroxyurs-12-en-28-oic acid (TEOA) (Zhong et al., 2005). Zhang et al., (2017) reported that results of MTT assay suggested that TEOA exhibited cytotoxicity by suppressing the cell viability of SW620 cancer cells in dose and time dependent manner. From the results of optical microscopy, it was observed that TEOA induced morphological changes, including extensive cytoplasmic vacuolation and shrinking in SW620 cells after treatment with 30 μM TEOA for 48 h. Annexin V-FITC/PI staining assay results indicated that TEOA enhanced apoptosis in cancer cells after 48 h of treatment in a dose-dependent manner and also upregulated the expression of apoptotic proteins, such as caspase 9 and PARP. TEOA treatment increased the expression levels of autophagic markers p62 and LC3-II, indicating that TEOA Induced autophagic cell death. TEOA increased the expression of GRP78, p-PERK, p-elF2a, and CHOP, indicating that autophagy was mediated by Er stress. In SW620 cells, TEOA activated the PINK1/Parkin pathway, which in turn caused mitophagy. In addition, TEOA slowed the growth of SW620 xenograft tumors in BALB/c nude mice. These results imply that TEOA can effectively inhibit colon cancer cells growth by regulating mitophagy

Aloe Gel Glucomannan

Aloe gel is frequently used in traditional Chinese medicine. Constipation has traditionally been treated with it, and numerous studies have looked into its possible therapeutic benefits, including as its anti-tumor, anti-inflammatory, and immune-regulatory actions (Tong et al., 2021). Aleo gel is known to exhibit numerous pharmacological properties, including antidiabetic, hypoglycemic, and scaffolding properties (Qi et al., 2020). Aloe gel glucomannan is a potent anti-tumor agent (Nazeam et al., 2020).

Zhang et al., (2022) reported that aloe gel glucomannan suppressed cell proliferation in dose and time dependent manner. The results of RNA sequence analysis showed that aloe gel reduced the growth of CT26 and HCT116 cells in a dose- and time-dependent manner by inducing autophagy, lysosomes, and ROS pathways. It also increased the expression of 6517 DEGs and suppressed the expression of 7731 DEGs. It also induces mitochondrial impairment in CT26 cells. Aloe gel induced excessive mitophagy through the accumulation of dysfunctional and ROS-generating mitochondria. It also activates the PINK1/Parkin mitophagy pathway and enhances the activity of the transcription factor EB (TFEB) signaling pathway. Thereby aloe gel is a potent anti-tumor agent by regulating PINK1/Parkin mitophagy pathway and transcription factor EB (TFEB) signaling pathway resulting in induction cytotoxicity mitophagy in cancer cells.

CONCLUSION

Colorectal cancer remains a significant global health challenge, with limited improvements in survival rates despite advances in treatment. This review has examined the role of mitophagy in colorectal cancer progression and highlighted several natural compounds that can modulate mitophagy pathways as potential therapeutic strategies. Key mitophagy pathways including PINK1/Parkin, BNIP3/NIX, and FUNDC1-mediated mitophagy are often dysregulated in colorectal cancer, contributing to altered metabolism and enhanced survival of cancer cells. Natural agents like tanshinone IIA, oleanolic acid, α-hederin and others have shown promise in regulating these mitophagy pathways to inhibit colorectal cancer growth through various mechanisms such as inducing apoptosis, cell cycle arrest, and modulating key signaling pathways like AMPK, NF-κB and STAT3. Many of these natural compounds exhibit synergistic effects with conventional chemotherapy drugs, suggesting their potential as adjuvant therapies. Additionally, some agents like plasmodium infection and dietary δ-valerobetaine have demonstrated anti-cancer effects through novel mitophagy-related mechanisms that warrant further investigation. While these natural agents show promise, further preclinical and clinical studies are needed to fully elucidate their mechanisms of action, optimal dosing, and potential side effects before clinical translation. Nonetheless, targeting mitophagy with natural compounds represents an exciting new avenue for colorectal cancer treatment that may help overcome limitations of current therapies. Overall, this chapter highlights the critical role of mitophagy in colorectal cancer and the therapeutic potential of therapeutic agents in modulating these pathways. Further research in this area may lead to novel treatment strategies and improved outcomes for colorectal cancer patients. As our understanding of mitophagy regulation in cancer continues to grow, natural compounds may play an increasingly important role in developing targeted and effective therapies.

REFERENCES

Alzohairy, M. A., Khan, A. A., Alsahli, M. A., Almatroodi, S. A., & Rahmani, A. H. (2021). Protective effects of thymoquinone, an active compound of *Nigella sativa*, on rats with benzo(a)pyrene-induced lung injury through regulation of oxidative stress and inflammation. *Molecules (Basel, Switzerland)*, *26*(11), 3218. DOI: 10.3390/molecules26113218 PMID: 34072086

Banks, L. D., Amoah, P., Niaz, M. S., Washington, M. K., Adunyah, S. E., & Ramesh, A. (2016). Olive oil prevents benzo(a)pyrene [B(a)P]-induced colon carcinogenesis through altered B(a)P metabolism and decreased oxidative damage in Apc(Min) mouse model. *The Journal of Nutritional Biochemistry*, *28*, 37–50. DOI: 10.1016/j.jnutbio.2015.09.023 PMID: 26878781

Bellot, G., Garcia-Medina, R., Gounon, P., Chiche, J., Roux, D., Pouyssegur, J., & Mazure, N. M. (2009). Hypoxia-induced autophagy is mediated through the hypoxia-inducible factor induction of BNIP3 and BNIP3L via their BH3 domains. *Molecular and Cellular Biology*, *29*(10), 2570–2581. DOI: 10.1128/MCB.00166-09 PMID: 19273585

Benarba, B., & Pandiella, A. (2018). Colorectal cancer and medicinal plants: Principle findings from recent studies. *Biomedicine and Pharmacotherapy*, *107*, 408–423. DOI: 10.1016/j.biopha.2018.08.006 PMID: 30099345

Boyle, K. A., Van Wickle, J., Hill, R. B., Marchese, A., Kalyanaraman, B., & Dwinell, M. B. (2018). Mitochondria-targeted drugs stimulate mitophagy and abrogate colon cancer cell proliferation. *The Journal of Biological Chemistry*, *293*(38), 14891–14904. DOI: 10.1074/jbc.RA117.001469 PMID: 30087121

Carloni, S., Riparini, G., Buonocore, G., & Balduini, W. (2017). Rapid modulation of the silent information regulator 1 by melatonin after hypoxia-ischemia in the neonatal rat brain. *Journal of Pineal Research*, *63*(3), e12434. DOI: 10.1111/jpi.12434 PMID: 28708259

Castrejón-Jiménez, N. S., Leyva-Paredes, K., Baltierra-Uribe, S. L., Castillo-Cruz, J., Campillo-Navarro, M., Hernández-Pérez, A. D., Luna-Angulo, A. B., Chacón-Salinas, R., Coral-Vázquez, R. M., Estrada-García, I., Sánchez-Torres, L. E., Torres-Torres, C., & García-Pérez, B. E. (2019). Ursolic and oleanolic acids induce mitophagy in A549 human lung cancer cells. *Molecules (Basel, Switzerland)*, *24*(19), 3444. DOI: 10.3390/molecules24193444 PMID: 31547522

Chen, L., He, Z., Qin, L., Li, Q., Shi, X., Zhao, S., Chen, L., Zhong, N., & Chen, X. (2011). Antitumor effect of malaria parasite infection in a murine Lewis lung cancer model through induction of innate and adaptive immunity. *PLoS One*, *6*(9), e24407. DOI: 10.1371/journal.pone.0024407 PMID: 21931708

Cheng, G., Zielonka, J., Dranka, B. P., McAllister, D., Mackinnon, A. C.Jr, Joseph, J., & Kalyanaraman, B. (2012). Mitochondria-targeted drugs synergize with 2-deoxyglucose to trigger breast cancer cell death. *Cancer Research*, *72*(10), 2634–2644. DOI: 10.1158/0008-5472.CAN-11-3928 PMID: 22431711

Cheng, G., Zielonka, J., McAllister, D., Hardy, M., Ouari, O., Joseph, J., Dwinell, M. B., & Kalyanaraman, B. (2015). Antiproliferative effects of mitochondria-targeted cationic antioxidants and analogs: Role of mitochondrial bioenergetics and energy-sensing mechanism. *Cancer Letters*, *365*(1), 96–106. DOI: 10.1016/j.canlet.2015.05.016 PMID: 26004344

Cheng, L., Xia, T. S., Wang, Y. F., Zhou, W., Liang, X. Q., Xue, J. Q., Shi, L., Wang, Y., Ding, Q., & Wang, M. (2014). The anticancer effect and mechanism of α-hederin on breast cancer cells. *International Journal of Oncology*, *45*(2), 757–763. DOI: 10.3892/ijo.2014.2449 PMID: 24842044

D'Onofrio, N., Balestrieri, A., Neglia, G., Monaco, A., Tatullo, M., Casale, R., Limone, A., Balestrieri, M. L., & Campanile, G. (2019). Antioxidant and anti-inflammatory activities of buffalo milk δ-valerobetaine. *Journal of Agricultural and Food Chemistry*, *67*(6), 1702–1710. DOI: 10.1021/acs.jafc.8b07166 PMID: 30661355

D'Onofrio, N., Martino, E., Mele, L., Colloca, A., Maione, M., Cautela, D., Castaldo, D., & Balestrieri, M. L. (2021). Colorectal cancer apoptosis induced by dietary δ-valerobetaine involves PINK1/Parkin dependent-mitophagy and SIRT3. *International Journal of Molecular Sciences*, *22*(15), 8117. DOI: 10.3390/ijms22158117 PMID: 34360883

D'Onofrio, N., Mele, L., Martino, E., Salzano, A., Restucci, B., Cautela, D., Tatullo, M., Balestrieri, M. L., & Campanile, G. (2020). Synergistic effect of dietary betaines on SIRT1-mediated apoptosis in human oral squamous cell carcinoma Cal 27. *Cancers (Basel)*, *12*(9), 2468. DOI: 10.3390/cancers12092468 PMID: 32878301

Davie, J. R. (2003). Inhibition of histone deacetylase activity by butyrate. *The Journal of Nutrition*, *133*(7, Suppl), 2485S–2493S. DOI: 10.1093/jn/133.7.2485S PMID: 12840228

De Roock, W., Claes, B., Bernasconi, D., De Schutter, J., Biesmans, B., Fountzilas, G., Kalogeras, K. T., Kotoula, V., Papamichael, D., Laurent-Puig, P., Penault-Llorca, F., Rougier, P., Vincenzi, B., Santini, D., Tonini, G., Cappuzzo, F., Frattini, M., Molinari, F., Saletti, P., & Tejpar, S. (2010). Effects of KRAS, BRAF, NRAS, and PIK3CA mutations on the efficacy of cetuximab plus chemotherapy in chemotherapy-refractory metastatic colorectal cancer: A retrospective consortium analysis. *The Lancet. Oncology*, *11*(8), 753–762. DOI: 10.1016/S1470-2045(10)70130-3 PMID: 20619739

Del Dotto, V., Mishra, P., Vidoni, S., Fogazza, M., Maresca, A., Caporali, L., McCaffery, J. M., Cappelletti, M., Baruffini, E., Lenaers, G., Chan, D., Rugolo, M., Carelli, V., & Zanna, C. (2017). OPA1 isoforms in the hierarchical organization of mitochondrial functions. *Cell Reports*, *19*(12), 2557–2571. DOI: 10.1016/j.celrep.2017.05.073 PMID: 28636943

Durcan, T. M., & Fon, E. A. (2015). The three 'P's of mitophagy: PARKIN, PINK1, and post-translational modifications. *Genes & Development*, *29*(10), 989–999. DOI: 10.1101/gad.262758.115 PMID: 25995186

Fan, F., He, Z., Kong, L. L., Chen, Q., Yuan, Q., Zhang, S., Ye, J., Liu, H., Sun, X., Geng, J., Yuan, L., Hong, L., Xiao, C., Zhang, W., Sun, X., Li, Y., Wang, P., Huang, L., Wu, X., & Zhou, D. (2016). Pharmacological targeting of kinases MST1 and MST2 augments tissue repair and regeneration. *Science Translational Medicine*, *8*(352), 352ra108. Advance online publication. DOI: 10.1126/scitranslmed.aaf2304 PMID: 27535619

Fang, C., Liu, Y., Chen, L., Luo, Y., Cui, Y., Zhang, N., Liu, P., Zhou, M., & Xie, Y. (2021). α-Hederin inhibits the growth of lung cancer A549 cells in vitro and in vivo by decreasing SIRT6 dependent glycolysis. *Pharmaceutical Biology*, *59*(1), 11–20. DOI: 10.1080/13880209.2020.1862250 PMID: 33356727

Feng, A., Yang, S., Sun, Y., Zhang, L., Bo, F., & Li, L. (2020). Development and evaluation of oleanolic acid dosage forms and its derivatives. *BioMed Research International*, *1308749*(1), 1308749. Advance online publication. DOI: 10.1155/2020/1308749 PMID: 33299854

Ferlay, J., Shin, H. R., Bray, F., Forman, D., Mathers, C., & Parkin, D. M. (2010). Estimates of worldwide burden of cancer in 2008: GLOBOCAN 2008. *International Journal of Cancer*, *127*(12), 2893–2917. DOI: 10.1002/ijc.25516 PMID: 21351269

Furth, N., & Aylon, Y. (2017). The LATS1 and LATS2 tumor suppressors: Beyond the Hippo pathway. *Cell Death and Differentiation*, *24*(9), 1488–1501. DOI: 10.1038/cdd.2017.99 PMID: 28644436

Greene, A. W., Grenier, K., Aguileta, M. A., Muise, S., Farazifard, R., Haque, M. E., McBride, H. M., Park, D. S., & Fon, E. A. (2012). Mitochondrial processing peptidase regulates PINK1 processing, import and Parkin recruitment. *EMBO Reports*, *13*(4), 378–385. DOI: 10.1038/embor.2012.14 PMID: 22354088

Han, S., Gao, J., Zhou, Q., Liu, S., Wen, C., & Yang, X. (2018). Role of intestinal flora in colorectal cancer from the metabolite perspective: A systematic review. *Cancer Management and Research*, *10*, 199–206. DOI: 10.2147/CMAR.S153482 PMID: 29440929

Hanahan, D., & Weinberg, R. A. (2011). Hallmarks of cancer: The next generation. *Cell*, *144*(5), 646–674. DOI: 10.1016/j.cell.2011.02.013 PMID: 21376230

He, L., & Gu, K. (2018). Tanshinone IIA regulates colorectal cancer apoptosis via attenuation of Parkin-mediated mitophagy by suppressing AMPK/Skp2 pathways. *Molecular Medicine Reports*, *18*(2), 1692–1703. DOI: 10.3892/mmr.2018.9087 PMID: 29845197

Ho, H. Y., Lin, C. W., Chien, M. H., Reiter, R. J., Su, S. C., Hsieh, Y. H., & Yang, S.-F. (2016). Melatonin suppresses TPA-induced metastasis by downregulating matrix metalloproteinase-9 expression through JNK/SP-1 signaling in nasopharyngeal carcinoma. *Journal of Pineal Research*, *61*(4), 479–492. DOI: 10.1111/jpi.12365 PMID: 27600920

Hoesel, B., & Schmid, J. A. (2013). The complexity of NF-κB signaling in inflammation and cancer. *Molecular Cancer*, *12*(1), 86. DOI: 10.1186/1476-4598-12-86 PMID: 23915189

Hosono, K., Endo, H., Takahashi, H., Sugiyama, M., Uchiyama, T., Suzuki, K., Nozaki, Y., Yoneda, K., Fujita, K., Yoneda, M., Inamori, M., Tomatsu, A., Chihara, T., Shimpo, K., Nakagama, H., & Nakajima, A. (2010). Metformin suppresses azoxymethane-induced colorectal aberrant crypt foci by activating AMP-activated protein kinase. *Molecular Carcinogenesis*, *49*(7), 662–671. DOI: 10.1002/mc.20637 PMID: 20564343

Huang, S. Y., Chang, S. F., Liao, K. F., & Chiu, S. C. (2017). Tanshinone IIA inhibits epithelial-mesenchymal transition in bladder cancer cells via modulation of STAT3-CCL2 signaling. *International Journal of Molecular Sciences*, *18*(8), 1616. DOI: 10.3390/ijms18081616 PMID: 28757590

Jiang, T., Peng, L., Wang, Q., Huang, B., Peng, D., Men, L., Jiang, Y., Zhu, M., Wang, M., Lin, L., Lv, J., & Li, S. (2022). Cirsiliol regulates mitophagy in colon cancer cells via STAT3 signaling. *Cancer Cell International*, *22*(1), 304. DOI: 10.1186/s12935-022-02732-6 PMID: 36207761

Jussawalla, D. J., & Gangadharan, P. (1977). Cancer of the colon: 32 years of experience in Bombay, India. *Journal of Surgical Oncology*, *9*(6), 607–622. DOI: 10.1002/jso.2930090612 PMID: 592859

Kamphorst, J. J., Chung, M. K., Fan, J., & Rabinowitz, J. D. (2014). Quantitative analysis of acetyl-CoA production in hypoxic cancer cells reveals substantial contribution from acetate. *Cancer & Metabolism*, *2*(1), 23. DOI: 10.1186/2049-3002-2-23 PMID: 25671109

Kang, J., Kim, E., Kim, W., Seong, K. M., Youn, H., Kim, J. W., Kim, J., & Youn, B. (2013). Rhamnetin and cirsiliol induce radiosensitization and inhibition of epithelial-mesenchymal transition (EMT) by miR-34a-mediated suppression of Notch-1 expression in non-small cell lung cancer cell lines. *The Journal of Biological Chemistry*, *288*(38), 27343–27357. DOI: 10.1074/jbc.M113.490482 PMID: 23902763

Kitada, S., Kress, C. L., Krajewska, M., Jia, L., Pellecchia, M., & Reed, J. C. (2008). Bcl-2 antagonist apogossypol (NSC736630) displays single-agent activity in Bcl-2-transgenic mice and has superior efficacy with less toxicity compared with gossypol (NSC19048). *Blood*, *111*(6), 3211–3219. DOI: 10.1182/blood-2007-09-113647 PMID: 18202226

Kitada, S., Leone, M., Sareth, S., Zhai, D., Reed, J. C., & Pellecchia, M. (2003). Discovery, characterization, and structure-activity relationships studies of proapoptotic polyphenols targeting B-cell lymphocyte/leukemia-2 proteins. *Journal of Medicinal Chemistry*, *46*(20), 4259–4264. DOI: 10.1021/jm030190z PMID: 13678404

Kulikov, A. V., Luchkina, E. A., Gogvadze, V., & Zhivotovsky, B. (2017). Mitophagy: Link to cancer development and therapy. *Biochemical and Biophysical Research Communications*, *482*(3), 432–439. DOI: 10.1016/j.bbrc.2016.10.088 PMID: 28212727

Levine, B., & Kroemer, G. (2019). Biological functions of autophagy genes: A disease perspective. *Cell*, *176*(1–2), 11–42. DOI: 10.1016/j.cell.2018.09.048 PMID: 30633901

Li, K., & Lai, H. (2017). Tanshinone IIA enhances the chemosensitivity of breast cancer cells to doxorubicin through down-regulating the expression of MDR-related ABC transporters. *Biomedicine and Pharmacotherapy*, *96*, 371–377. DOI: 10.1016/j.biopha.2017.10.016 PMID: 29028589

Li, Q., Qi, F., Meng, X., Zhu, C., & Gao, Y. (2018). Mst1 regulates colorectal cancer stress response via inhibiting Bnip3-related mitophagy by activation of JNK/p53 pathway. *Cell Biology and Toxicology*, *34*(4), 263–277. DOI: 10.1007/s10565-017-9417-6 PMID: 29063978

Liang, J., Wang, X. S., Zhen, H. S., Zhong, Z. G., Zhang, W. Y., Zhang, W. W., & Li, W. L. (2007). [Study on anti-tumor effect of extractions from roots of *Actinidia deliciosa*]. *Zhong Yao Cai*, *30*(10), 1279–1282. PMID: 18300504

Liang, K., Zhou, G., Zhang, Q., Li, J., & Zhang, C. (2014). Expression of Hippo pathway in colorectal cancer. *Saudi Journal of Gastroenterology : Official Journal of the Saudi Gastroenterology Association*, *20*(3), 188–194. DOI: 10.4103/1319-3767.133025 PMID: 24976283

Liu, L., Feng, D., Chen, G., Chen, M., Zheng, Q., Song, P., Ma, Q., Zhu, C., Wang, R., Qi, W., Huang, L., Xue, P., Li, B., Wang, X., Jin, H., Wang, J., Yang, F., Liu, P., Zhu, Y., & Chen, Q. (2012). Mitochondrial outer-membrane protein FUNDC1 mediates hypoxia-induced mitophagy in mammalian cells. *Nature Cell Biology*, *14*(2), 177–185. DOI: 10.1038/ncb2422 PMID: 22267086

Liu, Q., Yang, Y., Tan, X., Tao, Z., Adah, D., Yu, S., Lu, J., Zhao, S., Qin, L., Qin, L., & Chen, X. (2017). Plasmodium parasite as an effective hepatocellular carcinoma antigen glypican-3 delivery vector. *Oncotarget*, *8*(15), 24785–24796. DOI: 10.18632/oncotarget.15806 PMID: 28445973

Lorent, J. H., Léonard, C., Abouzi, M., Akabi, F., Quetin-Leclercq, J., & Mingeot-Leclercq, M. P. (2016). α-Hederin induces apoptosis, membrane permeabilization and morphologic changes in two cancer cell lines through a cholesterol-dependent mechanism. *Planta Medica*, *82*(18), 1532–1539. DOI: 10.1055/s-0042-114780 PMID: 27574896

Mohandas, K. M. (2011). Colorectal cancer in India: Controversies, enigmas and primary prevention. *Indian Journal of Gastroenterology*, *30*(1), 3–6. DOI: 10.1007/s12664-010-0076-2 PMID: 21222189

Mohebali, N., Pandurangan, A. K., Mustafa, M. R., Anandasadagopan, S. K., & Alagumuthu, T. (2020). Vernodalin induces apoptosis through ROS/JNK pathway activation in human colon cancer cells. *Journal of Biochemical and Molecular Toxicology*, *34*(12), e22577. DOI: 10.1002/jbt.22587 PMID: 32726518

Mu, D., Gao, Z., Guo, H., Zhou, G., & Sun, B. (2013). Sodium butyrate induces growth inhibition and apoptosis in human prostate cancer DU145 cells by up-regulation of the expression of annexin A1. *PLoS One*, *8*(9), e74922. DOI: 10.1371/journal.pone.0074922 PMID: 24086397

Nazeam, J. A., El-Hefnawy, H. M., & Singab, A. B. (2020). Structural elucidation of immunomodulators, acetylated heteroglycan and galactosamine, isolated from *Aloe arborescens* leaves. *Journal of Medicinal Food*, *23*(8), 895–901. DOI: 10.1089/jmf.2019.0229 PMID: 31976801

Ney, P. A. (2015). Mitochondrial autophagy: Origins, significance, and role of BNIP3 and NIX. *Biochimica et Biophysica Acta (BBA) -. Biochimica et Biophysica Acta. Molecular Cell Research, 1853*(10), 2775–2783. DOI: 10.1016/j.bbamcr.2015.02.022 PMID: 25753537

Nicholson, J. K., Holmes, E., Kinross, J., Burcelin, R., Gibson, G., Jia, W., & Pettersson, S. (2012). Host-gut microbiota metabolic interactions. *Science, 336*(6086), 1262–1267. DOI: 10.1126/science.1223813 PMID: 22674330

Ogretmen, B. (2017). Sphingolipid metabolism in cancer signalling and therapy. *Nature Reviews. Cancer, 18*(1), 33–50. DOI: 10.1038/nrc.2017.96 PMID: 29147025

Pandurangan, A. K., Dharmalingam, P., Ananda Sadagopan, S. K., Ramar, M., Munusamy, A., & Ganapasam, S. (2013). Luteolin induces growth arrest in colon cancer cells through the involvement of Wnt/β-catenin/GSK-3β signaling. *Journal of Environmental Pathology, Toxicology and Oncology, 32*(2), 131–139. DOI: 10.1615/JEnvironPatholToxicolOncol.2013007522 PMID: 24099426

Pandurangan, A. K., & Esa, N. M. (2013). Dietary non-nutritive factors on regulatory molecules in colorectal cancer: An update. *Asian Pacific Journal of Cancer Prevention : APJCP, 14*(10), 5543–5552. DOI: 10.7314/APJCP.2013.14.10.5543 PMID: 24289544

Pandurangan, A. K., Ismail, S., Esa, N. M., & Munusamy, M. A. (2018b). Inositol-6 phosphate inhibits the mTOR pathway and induces autophagy-mediated death in HT-29 colon cancer cells. *Archives of Medical Science : AMS, 14*(6), 1281–1288. DOI: 10.5114/aoms.2018.76935 PMID: 30393482

Pandurangan, A. K., Thomas, D., Vadivel, D., Kalaivani, K., & Sudhandiran, G. (2018a). Colorectal carcinogenesis: Insights into the cell death and signal transduction pathways – A review. *World Journal of Gastrointestinal Oncology, 10*(9), 244–259. DOI: 10.4251/wjgo.v10.i9.244 PMID: 30254720

Peng, J., Ren, K. D., Yang, J., & Luo, X. J. (2016). Mitochondrial E3 ubiquitin ligase 1: A key enzyme in regulation of mitochondrial dynamics and functions. *Mitochondrion, 28*, 49–53. DOI: 10.1016/j.mito.2016.03.007 PMID: 27034206

Poillet-Perez, L., Xie, X., Zhan, L., Yang, Y., Sharp, D. W., Hu, Z. S., Su, X., Maganti, A., Jiang, C., Lu, W., Zheng, H., Bosenberg, M. W., Mehnert, J. M., Guo, J. Y., Lattime, E., Rabinowitz, J. D., & White, E. (2018). Autophagy maintains tumour growth through circulating arginine. *Nature, 563*(7732), 569–573. DOI: 10.1038/s41586-018-0697-7 PMID: 30429607

Potočnjak, I., Šimić, L., Vukelić, I., Batičić, L., & Domitrović, R. (2022). Oleanolic acid induces HCT116 colon cancer cell death through the p38/FOXO3a/Sirt6 pathway. *Chemico-Biological Interactions*, *363*, 110010. DOI: 10.1016/j.cbi.2022.110010 PMID: 35690101

Prasad, P., Vasas, A., Hohmann, J., Bishayee, A., & Sinha, D. (2019). Cirsiliol suppressed epithelial to mesenchymal transition in B16F10 malignant melanoma cells through alteration of the PI3K/Akt/NF-κB signaling pathway. *International Journal of Molecular Sciences*, *20*(3), 608. DOI: 10.3390/ijms20030608 PMID: 30708951

Qi, W., Zhou, X., Wang, J., Zhang, K., Zhou, Y., Chen, S., Nie, S., & Xie, M. (2020). *Cordyceps sinensis* polysaccharide inhibits colon cancer cells growth by inducing apoptosis and autophagy flux blockage via mTOR signaling. *Carbohydrate Polymers*, *237*, 116113. DOI: 10.1016/j.carbpol.2020.116113 PMID: 32241434

Qin, L., Zhong, M., Adah, D., Qin, L., Chen, X., Ma, C., Fu, Q., Zhu, X., Li, Z., Wang, N., & Chen, Y. (2020). A novel tumour suppressor lncRNA F630028O10Rik inhibits lung cancer angiogenesis by regulating miR-223-3p. *Journal of Cellular and Molecular Medicine*, *24*(6), 3549–3559. DOI: 10.1111/jcmm.15044 PMID: 32052546

Rambold, A. S., Kostelecky, B., Elia, N., & Lippincott-Schwartz, J. (2011). Tubular network formation protects mitochondria from autophagosomal degradation during nutrient starvation. *Proceedings of the National Academy of Sciences of the United States of America*, *108*(25), 10190–10195. DOI: 10.1073/pnas.1107402108 PMID: 21646527

Redondo-Blanco, S., Fernández, J., Gutiérrez-Del-Río, I., Villar, C. J., & Lombó, F. (2017). New insights toward colorectal cancer chemotherapy using natural bioactive compounds. *Frontiers in Pharmacology*, *8*, 109. DOI: 10.3389/fphar.2017.00109 PMID: 28352231

Rodríguez-Enríquez, S., Robledo-Cadena, D. X., Gallardo-Pérez, J. C., Pacheco-Velázquez, S. C., Vázquez, C., Saavedra, E., Vargas-Navarro, J. L., Blanco-Carpintero, B. A., Marín-Hernández, Á., Jasso-Chávez, R., Encalada, R., Ruiz-Godoy, L., Aguilar-Ponce, J. L., & Moreno-Sánchez, R. (2021). Acetate promotes a differential energy metabolic response in human HCT 116 and COLO 205 colon cancer cells impacting cancer cell growth and invasiveness. *Frontiers in Oncology*, *11*, 697408. DOI: 10.3389/fonc.2021.697408 PMID: 34414111

Santarelli, R., Pompili, C., Gilardini Montani, M. S., Evangelista, L., Gonnella, R., & Cirone, M. (2022). 3,4-Dihydroxyphenylethanol (DPE or hydroxytyrosol) counteracts ERK1/2 and mTOR activation, pro-inflammatory cytokine release, autophagy and mitophagy reduction mediated by benzo[a]pyrene in primary human colonic epithelial cells. *Pharmaceutics, 14*(3), 663. DOI: 10.3390/pharmaceutics14030663 PMID: 35336037

Schulte-Michels, J., Wolf, A., Aatz, S., Engelhard, K., Sieben, A., Martinez-Osuna, M., Häberlein, F., & Häberlein, H. (2016). α-Hederin inhibits G protein-coupled receptor kinase 2-mediated phosphorylation of β2-adrenergic receptors. *Phytomedicine, 23*(1), 52–57. DOI: 10.1016/j.phymed.2015.12.001 PMID: 26902407

Schwarten, M., Mohrlüder, J., Ma, P., Stoldt, M., Thielmann, Y., Stangler, T., Hersch, N., Hoffmann, B., Merkel, R., & Willbold, D. (2009). Nix directly binds to GABARAP: A possible crosstalk between apoptosis and autophagy. *Autophagy, 5*(5), 690–698. DOI: 10.4161/auto.5.5.8494 PMID: 19363302

Semaan, J., El-Hakim, S., Ibrahim, J. N., Safi, R., Elnar, A. A., & El Boustany, C. (2020). Comparative effect of sodium butyrate and sodium propionate on proliferation, cell cycle and apoptosis in human breast cancer cells MCF-7. *Breast Cancer (Tokyo, Japan), 27*(4), 696–705. DOI: 10.1007/s12282-020-01063-6 PMID: 32095987

Sen, A. (2020). Prophylactic and therapeutic roles of oleanolic acid and its derivatives in several diseases. *World Journal of Clinical Cases, 8*(10), 1767–1792. DOI: 10.12998/wjcc.v8.i10.1767 PMID: 32518769

Servillo, L., D'Onofrio, N., Giovane, A., Casale, R., Cautela, D., Castaldo, D., Iannaccone, F., Neglia, G., Campanile, G., & Balestrieri, M. L. (2018). Ruminant meat and milk contain δ-valerobetaine, another precursor of trimethylamine N-oxide (TMAO) like γ-butyrobetaine. *Food Chemistry, 260*, 193–199. DOI: 10.1016/j.foodchem.2018.03.114 PMID: 29699662

Shen, J., Zhang, Y., Yu, H., Shen, B., Liang, Y., Jin, R., Liu, X., Shi, L., & Cai, X. (2016). Role of DUSP1/MKP1 in tumorigenesis, tumor progression and therapy. *Cancer Medicine, 5*(8), 2061–2068. DOI: 10.1002/cam4.772 PMID: 27227569

Shirihai, O. S., Song, M., & Dorn, G. W.II. (2015). How mitochondrial dynamism orchestrates mitophagy. *Circulation Research, 116*(11), 1835–1849. DOI: 10.1161/CIRCRESAHA.116.306374 PMID: 25999423

Starenki, D., & Park, J. I. (2013). Mitochondria-targeted nitroxide, Mito-CP, suppresses medullary thyroid carcinoma cell survival in vitro and in vivo. *The Journal of Clinical Endocrinology and Metabolism, 98*(4), 1529–1540. DOI: 10.1210/jc.2012-3671 PMID: 23509102

Sun, D., Shen, W., Zhang, F., Fan, H., Tan, J., Li, L., Xu, C., Zhang, H., Yang, Y., & Cheng, H. (2018). α-Hederin arrests cell cycle at G2/M checkpoint and promotes mitochondrial apoptosis by blocking nuclear factor-κB signaling in colon cancer cells. *BioMed Research International, 2548378*. Advance online publication. DOI: 10.1155/2018/2548378 PMID: 30363706

Sung, H., Ferlay, J., Siegel, R. L., Laversanne, M., Soerjomataram, I., Jemal, A., & Bray, F. (2021). Global cancer statistics 2020: GLOBOCAN estimates of incidence and mortality worldwide for 36 cancers in 185 countries. *CA: a Cancer Journal for Clinicians, 71*(3), 209–249. DOI: 10.3322/caac.21660 PMID: 33538338

Swaminathan, R., Selvakumaran, R., Esmy, P. O., Sampath, P., Ferlay, J., Jissa, V., Shanta, V., Cherian, M., & Sankaranarayanan, R. (2009). Cancer pattern and survival in a rural district in South India. *Cancer Epidemiology, 33*(5), 325–331. DOI: 10.1016/j.canep.2009.09.008 PMID: 19853553

Tong, X., Li, M., Li, D., Lao, C., Chen, J., Xu, W., Du, J., Zhang, M., Yang, X., & Li, J. (2021). Aloe vera gel extract: Safety evaluation for acute and chronic oral administration in Sprague-Dawley rats and anticancer activity in breast and lung cancer cells. *Journal of Ethnopharmacology, 280*, 114434. DOI: 10.1016/j.jep.2021.114434 PMID: 34274443

Tong, Z. Z., Fang, Z. M., Zhang, Q., Zhan, Y., Zhang, Y., Jiang, W. F., Hou, X., Li, Y. L., & Wang, T. (2018). *Plasmodium yoelii* infection inhibits murine leukaemia WEHI-3 cell proliferation in vivo by promoting immune responses. *Infectious Diseases of Poverty*, *7*(1), 48. DOI: 10.1186/s40249-018-0433-4 PMID: 29764519

Torrens-Mas, M., Hernández-López, R., Oliver, J., Roca, P., & Sastre-Serra, J. (2018). Sirtuin 3 silencing improves oxaliplatin efficacy through acetylation of MnSOD in colon cancer. *Journal of Cellular Physiology, 233*(8), 6067–6076. DOI: 10.1002/jcp.26443 PMID: 29323702

Torrens-Mas, M., Pons, D. G., Sastre-Serra, J., Oliver, J., & Roca, P. (2017). SIRT3 silencing sensitizes breast cancer cells to cytotoxic treatments through an increment in ROS production. *Journal of Cellular Biochemistry, 118*(2), 397–406. DOI: 10.1002/jcb.25653 PMID: 27420645

Vasile Bochis, O., Achimas-Cadariu, P., Vlad, C., Fetica, B., Leucuta, C. D., Busuioc, C. I., & Irimie, A. (2017). The prognostic role of Skp2 and the tumor suppressor protein p27 in colorectal cancer. *JBUON, 22*(5), 1122–1130. PMID: 29135092

Vives-Bauza, C., Zhou, C., Huang, Y., Cui, M., de Vries, R. L., Kim, J., May, J., Tocilescu, M. A., Liu, W., Ko, H. S., Magrané, J., Moore, D. J., Dawson, V. L., Grailhe, R., Dawson, T. M., Li, C., Tieu, K., & Przedborski, S. (2010). PINK1-dependent recruitment of Parkin to mitochondria in mitophagy. *Proceedings of the National Academy of Sciences of the United States of America, 107*(1), 378–383. DOI: 10.1073/pnas.0911187107 PMID: 19966284

Vogel, G. (2013, November 8). Malaria as lifesaving therapy. *Science, 342*(6159), 686. DOI: 10.1126/science.342.6159.686 PMID: 24202157

Wang, S., Liu, Z., Wang, L., & Zhang, X. (2009). NF-kappaB signaling pathway, inflammation and colorectal cancer. *Cellular & Molecular Immunology, 6*(5), 327–334. DOI: 10.1038/cmi.2009.43 PMID: 19887045

Wang, X., Zhang, C., Yan, X., Lan, B., Wang, J., Wei, C., Cao, X., Wang, R., Yao, J., Zhou, T., Zhou, M., Liu, Q., Jiang, B., Jiang, P., Kesari, S., Lin, X., & Guo, F. (2016). A novel bioavailable BH3 mimetic efficiently inhibits colon cancer via cascade effects of mitochondria. *Clinical Cancer Research, 22*(6), 1445–1458. DOI: 10.1158/1078-0432.CCR-15-0732 PMID: 26515494

Wei, J., Kitada, S., Rega, M. F., Emdadi, A., Yuan, H., Cellitti, J., Stebbins, J. L., Zhai, D., Sun, J., Yang, L., Dahl, R., Zhang, Z., Wu, B., Wang, S., Reed, T. A., Wang, H. G., Lawrence, N., Sebti, S., Reed, J. C., & Pellecchia, M. (2009). Apogossypol derivatives as antagonists of antiapoptotic Bcl-2 family proteins. *Molecular Cancer Therapeutics, 8*(4), 904–913. DOI: 10.1158/1535-7163.MCT-08-1050 PMID: 19372563

Wu, W., Tian, W., Hu, Z., Chen, G., Huang, L., Li, W., Zhang, X., Xue, P., Zhou, C., Liu, L., Zhu, Y., Zhang, X., Li, L., Zhang, L., Sui, S., Zhao, B., & Feng, D. (2014). ULK1 translocates to mitochondria and phosphorylates FUNDC1 to regulate mitophagy. *EMBO Reports, 15*(5), 566–575. DOI: 10.1002/embr.201438501 PMID: 24671035

Xi, Y., & Xu, P. (2021). Global colorectal cancer burden in 2020 and projections to 2040. *Translational Oncology, 14*(10), 101174. DOI: 10.1016/j.tranon.2021.101174 PMID: 34243011

Xia, C., Tao, Y., Li, M., Che, T., & Qu, J. (2020). Protein acetylation and deacetylation: An important regulatory modification in gene transcription [Review]. *Experimental and Therapeutic Medicine, 20*(4), 2923–2940. DOI: 10.3892/etm.2020.9073 PMID: 32855658

Yan, F., Cao, X. X., Jiang, H. X., Zhao, X. L., Wang, J. Y., Lin, Y. H., Liu, Q. L., Zhang, C., Jiang, B., & Guo, F. (2010). A novel water-soluble gossypol derivative increases chemotherapeutic sensitivity and promotes growth inhibition in colon cancer. *Journal of Medicinal Chemistry*, *53*(15), 5502–5510. DOI: 10.1021/jm1001698 PMID: 20684596

Yao, X., Cao, Y., Lu, L., Xu, Y., Chen, H., Liu, C., Chen, D., Wang, K., Xu, J., Fang, R., Xia, H., Li, J., Fang, Q., & Tao, Z. (2022). Plasmodium infection suppresses colon cancer growth by inhibiting proliferation and promoting apoptosis associated with disrupting mitochondrial biogenesis and mitophagy in mice. *Parasites & Vectors*, *15*(1), 192. DOI: 10.1186/s13071-022-05291-x PMID: 35668501

Zhang, D., Gao, C., Li, R., Zhang, L., & Tian, J. (2017). TEOA, a triterpenoid from *Actinidia eriantha*, induces autophagy in SW620 cells via endoplasmic reticulum stress and ROS-dependent mitophagy. *Archives of Pharmacal Research*, *40*(5), 579–591. DOI: 10.1007/s12272-017-0899-9 PMID: 28211011

Zhang, J., Xiang, H., Liu, J., Chen, Y., He, R. R., & Liu, B. (2020). Mitochondrial Sirtuin 3: New emerging biological function and therapeutic target. *Theranostics*, *10*(18), 8315–8342. DOI: 10.7150/thno.45922 PMID: 32724473

Zhang, K., Zhang, D., Wang, J., Wang, Y., Hu, J., Zhou, Y., Zhou, X., Nie, S., & Xie, M. (2022). Aloe gel glucomannan induced colon cancer cell death via mitochondrial damage-driven PINK1/Parkin mitophagy pathway. *Carbohydrate Polymers*, *295*, 119841. DOI: 10.1016/j.carbpol.2022.119841 PMID: 35989033

Zhang, Z. J., Zheng, Z. J., Kan, H., Song, Y., Cui, W., Zhao, G., & Kip, K. E. (2011). Reduced risk of colorectal cancer with metformin therapy in patients with type 2 diabetes: A meta-analysis. *Diabetes Care*, *34*(10), 2323–2328. DOI: 10.2337/dc11-0512 PMID: 21949223

Zhong, Z., Zhang, W., Zhang, F., Chen, X., & Huang, C. (2005). [Experimental study on the antitumor effects of extracts from roots of *Actinidia indochinensis* in carcinoma cell lines]. *Zhong Yao Cai*, *28*(3), 215–218. PMID: 16107031

Chapter 7
Development of Mitophagy Modulators and Inhibitors of Defective Mitophagy:
N-Silico and Natural Products Option

InnocentMary Ifedibaluchukwu Ejiofor
Nnamdi Azikiwe University, Nigeria

Mercy Adebola
Leeds Beckett University, UK

Augusta Ukamaka Ilechukwu
https://orcid.org/0009-0001-6359-792X
Department of Pharmacognosy and Traditional Medicine, Faculty of Pharmaceutical Sciences, Nnamdi Azikiwe University, Nigeria

ABSTRACT

Mitophagy, a selective form of autophagy, is vital for maintaining cellular health by removing dysfunctional mitochondria. This process, triggered by the weakening of the inner mitochondrial membrane, is crucial in highly differentiated, non-dividing cells like neurons, muscle cells, and liver cells. A balance in mitophagy is essential; both insufficient and excessive activity are linked to age-related disorders such as neurodegenerative diseases, metabolic issues, and heart damage. Computational tools, or in-silico methods, have become powerful in predicting the biological activity of chemical compounds, assessing their potential as drug candidates. These

DOI: 10.4018/979-8-3693-3836-0.ch007

methods are particularly useful for analyzing natural products, which offer diverse chemical structures for drug development. This chapter highlights the significance of mitophagy, its regulatory pathways, and the use of computational techniques, including virtual screening and molecular docking, in identifying potential regulators, especially from natural product libraries.

1. INTRODUCTION

Mitophagy is a crucial cellular process involved in the turnover of mitochondria through lysosomal-mediated autophagy activities. It significantly maintains cellular homeostasis by regulating mitochondrial quality and quantity control (Redmann et al., 2014; Onishi et al., 2021). Mitophagy is a specialized form of autophagy responsible for the selective degradation of damaged and dysfunctional mitochondria, essential for energy production and cellular energy homeostasis (Fivenson et al., 2017; Guo & Chiang, 2021). The process of mitophagy involves the elimination of weakened, old, and damaged mitochondria through an autophagic pathway, leading to their destruction (Chowdhury, 2022).

Mitophagy is regulated by various molecular mechanisms and pathways, including the PINK1-Parkin pathway, which coordinates autophagy adaptor phosphorylation with the assembly of ubiquitin chains on mitochondria to facilitate efficient mitophagy (Heo et al., 2015). Additionally, genes like Parkin and PINK1 have been implicated in the degradation of depolarized mitochondria via autophagy, highlighting their role in mitophagy regulation (McLelland et al., 2014; Singh & Ganley, 2021). Impaired mitophagy can lead to the accumulation of damaged mitochondria, disruption of the mitochondrial network, and initiation of the apoptotic program, contributing to conditions like skeletal muscle atrophy (Lei, 2024).

Mitophagy is essential for cellular homeostasis and is critical in various diseases. For instance, mitophagy has been linked to neurodegenerative diseases, cancer, cardiovascular diseases, and aging, emphasizing its significance in disease pathogenesis and progression (Fivenson et al., 2017; Vara-Pérez et al., 2019; Jin et al., 2018; Li et al., 2023). Understanding the regulatory mechanisms of mitophagy and its implications in different physiological contexts is crucial for developing targeted therapies and interventions for various health conditions (Pickles et al., 2018; Shirihai et al., 2015).

Importance of Mitophagy in Cellular Homeostasis

Mitophagy, the selective removal of damaged or excess mitochondria by autophagy, is crucial in maintaining cellular homeostasis (Guo & Chiang, 2021; Bhujabal et al., 2017). It is a mitochondrial quality control mechanism that helps regulate cellular metabolism, development, and overall health by ensuring the turnover of dysfunctional mitochondria (Xiao et al., 2019; Zheng et al., 2015). Mitophagy is essential for preserving cellular functional health and metabolic homeostasis and preventing the accumulation of dysfunctional mitochondria, which can lead to cellular degeneration (Vara-Pérez et al., 2019; Liu et al., 2021).

Mitophagy is intricately linked to various physiological functions, including early embryonic development, cell differentiation, inflammation, and apoptosis, highlighting its significance in diverse cellular processes (Kanki et al., 2011; Lei, 2024). Mitophagy-mediated elimination of mitochondria is vital for maintaining proper cellular homeostasis and preventing the accumulation of damaged organelles (Maestro et al., 2022; Zhang et al., 2023). Also, mitophagy helps preserve mitochondrial homeostasis and biogenesis and removes dysfunctional mitochondria, contributing to cellular health and longevity (Longo et al., 2021; Mao et al., 2013).

Mitophagy is also crucial in disease contexts, such as neurodegeneration, cancer, and aging, where dysfunctional mitophagy can accumulate damaged mitochondria and contribute to disease progression (Fang et al., 2017; Zhou et al., 2017). Restoration of mitophagy has been shown to ameliorate the pathogenesis of diseases like Alzheimer's disease and non-alcoholic fatty liver disease by maintaining cellular homeostasis and mitochondrial function (Onishi et al., 2021; Cao et al., 2022).

Significance of Modulating Mitophagy

Modulating mitophagy is crucial in various physiological and pathological contexts. Mitophagy, the selective removal of damaged or dysfunctional mitochondria, is essential for maintaining cellular homeostasis and overall health. By modulating mitophagy, it is possible to regulate mitochondrial quality control and metabolic homeostasis and prevent the accumulation of dysfunctional mitochondria, which can lead to cellular degeneration (Lei, 2024; Wu et al., 2019).

In the context of disease, modulating mitophagy has emerged as a promising therapeutic strategy for various conditions. For instance, in neurodegenerative diseases like Parkinson's, enhancing mitophagy and accelerating the removal of damaged mitochondria are of interest in developing disease-modifying therapeutic interventions (Clark et al., 2021). Similarly, in cancer, dysregulation of mitophagy has been linked to cancer stem cell survival, and targeting mitophagy has been proposed as a novel mechanism for anticancer stem cell-targeted therapy (Praharaj et al., 2021).

Moreover, modulating mitophagy has shown promise in metabolic disorders and kidney diseases. For example, in polycystic and chronic kidney disease, suitable modulation of mitophagy has been suggested as a favorable tactic for prevention and treatment (Nakashima, 2024). In obesity and metabolic syndrome, deficiency of mitophagy receptor FUNDC1 has been shown to impair mitochondrial quality and aggravate metabolic disorders, highlighting the importance of mitophagy in maintaining metabolic homeostasis (Wu et al., 2019).

Furthermore, various research studies have focused on the development of mitophagy modulators. Small-molecule pharmacological regulation of mitophagy has been explored as a potential therapeutic approach for neurodegenerative diseases and cancer (L et al., 2023). Understanding the molecular mechanisms of mitophagy and developing specific interventions to modulate mitophagy activity in different physiological conditions, such as in the heart, is crucial for advancing therapeutic strategies (Saito et al., 2020).

Contributions Various Studies to the Evolving Understanding of Mitophagy Modulators

Recent studies have significantly advanced the understanding of mitophagy modulators by elucidating the molecular mechanisms and signaling pathways involved. Key pathways include the PINK1/Parkin pathway, receptor-mediated mitophagy (BNIP3/NIX and FUNDC1), and other recently identified mitophagy receptor proteins. These pathways are central to the selective degradation of damaged mitochondria and are regulated by endogenous and pharmacological modulators (Palikaras et al., 2020; Yang et al., 2019; Drake et al., 2017).

A growing body of research has identified numerous small-molecule modulators that induce or inhibit mitophagy. These include general mitochondrial toxicants, iron chelators, and compounds that modulate the PINK1/Parkin pathway or NAD+ metabolism. Natural compounds such as spermidine, resveratrol, and urolithin A have shown mitophagy-inducing properties, with urolithin A being highlighted as a first-in-class mitophagy enhancer (L et al., 2023; Palikaras et al., 2020; Dong et al., 2023Lin et al., 2024). Polyphenols like resveratrol and curcumin have also demonstrated neuroprotective effects by modulating mitophagy through key signaling pathways, including PINK1/Parkin and FOXO3a (Lin et al., 2024).

Mitophagy modulators are increasingly recognized for their therapeutic potential in a range of diseases, including neurodegenerative disorders (such as Parkinson's and Alzheimer's), cardiovascular diseases, metabolic disorders, and cancer (L et al., 202; Yang et al., 2019; Drake et al., 2017; Georgakopoulos et al., 2017; Yang et al., 2025). For example, mitophagy inducers identified through machine-learning approaches have been shown to ameliorate Alzheimer's pathology in animal models by improving neuronal survival and memory (Xie et al., 2022). In neurodegenerative diseases, targeting mitophagy has emerged as a promising strategy, with several modulators demonstrating efficacy in preclinical models of Parkinson's and Alzheimer's disease (Georgakopoulos et al., 2017; Yang et al., 2025). In cancer, the regulation of mitophagy adaptors and modulators (e.g., Parkin, BNIP3, p62/SQSTM1) is linked to cell fate, metabolic reprogramming, and disease progression (Drake et al., 2017).

The field has also seen the development of new frameworks for characterizing mitophagy modulators, such as the Mitophagy Modulator Characterization System (MMCS), which aims to standardize evaluation and improve the reliability of findings (Dong et al., 2023). However, methodological flaws in some studies highlight the need for rigorous standards to ensure robust and reproducible results (Dong et al., 2023).

Collectively, these studies have expanded the landscape of mitophagy modulators, highlighting diverse mechanisms, therapeutic opportunities, and the importance of methodological rigor in advancing the field.

2. UNDERSTANDING MITOPHAGY AND ITS DYSREGULATION

Overview of Mitophagy Pathways

Table 1.

Mechanism	Description	Disease Link
PINK1/Parkin Pathway Defects	Impaired tagging of damaged mitochondria for degradation	Neurodegeneration (Bingol & Sheng, 2016; Pradeepkiran & Reddy, 2020; Li et al., 2022; Wang, Liu, & Lu, 2019)
USP30 Overactivity	Removal of ubiquitin tags, blocking mitophagy	Neurodegeneration (Bingol & Sheng, 2016)
Receptor-Mediated Pathway Defects	Impaired recognition of damaged mitochondria	Multiple diseases (Pradeepkiran & Reddy, 2020; Wang, Liu, & Lu, 2019; Onishi et al., 2021)
Mitochondrial Dynamics Imbalance	Disrupted fission/fusion, affecting mitophagy efficiency	Aging, neurodegeneration (Pradeepkiran & Reddy, 2020; Wang, Liu, & Lu, 2019; Chen, Kroemer, & Kepp, 2020)
BNIP3	Recruits autophagosomes via LC3 interaction, hypoxia-induced mitophagy	Hypoxia, Cancer (Zhang & Ney, 2009)

continued on following page

Table 1. Continued

Mechanism	Description	Disease Link
NIX/BNIP3L	Essential for erythroid mitophagy, stress response, interacts with LC3, regulated by phosphorylation.	Neurological Disorders, Heart diseases, Mitochondrial Disease (Zhang & Ney, 2009; Yuan et al., 2017)
PHB2	Acts as a receptor after outer membrane permeabilization promotes mitophagy	Cancer, neurodegenerative diseases, kidney disease, endometriosis (Wu et al., 2021; Ising et al., 2015; Deng, Lou, Kong, & Liu, 2023)

Key Proteins Involved in Mitophagy Regulation

Mitophagy is the selective removal of damaged or excess mitochondria, crucial for cellular health and homeostasis. Key proteins regulate mitophagy through distinct pathways, mainly the PINK1/Parkin-dependent pathway and receptor-mediated mechanisms.

Major Mitophagy Regulators

PINK1/Parkin Pathway

PINK1 (PTEN-induced kinase 1): Senses mitochondrial damage and accumulates on the outer mitochondrial membrane, recruiting and activating Parkin (Zhang et al., 2020; Zhang, Liu, Gao, Sehgal, & Wu, 2021; Ma et al., 2020; Iorio, Celenza, & Petricca, 2021; Belousov et al., 2020)

Parkin (PRKN): An E3 ubiquitin ligase that ubiquitinates mitochondrial proteins, marking them for degradation and facilitating autophagosome recruitment (Zhang et al., 2020; Zhang, Liu, Gao, Sehgal, & Wu, 2021; Ma et al., 2020; Iorio, Celenza, & Petricca, 2021; Belousov et al., 2020; Hollville, Carroll, Cullen, & Martin, 2014).

Ubiquitin-binding adaptors: Proteins like p62, NBR1, OPTN, and NDP52 recognize ubiquitinated mitochondria and link them to the autophagy machinery (LC3) (Zhang, Liu, Gao, Sehgal, & Wu, 2021; Ma et al., 2020; Iorio, Celenza, & Petricca, 2021; Belousov et al., 2020)

Mitophagy Receptors (Parkin-Independent)

BNIP3 and NIX (BNIP3L): Outer mitochondrial membrane proteins that directly bind autophagy proteins (LC3/GABARAP) to mediate mitophagy, especially during hypoxia or erythrocyte maturation (Zhang, Liu, Gao, Sehgal, & Wu, 2021; Belousov et al., 2020; Li et al., 2021).

FUNDC1, BCL2L13, FKBP8: Additional receptors that interact with LC3 to promote mitophagy under specific conditions (Zhang, Liu, Gao, Sehgal, & Wu, 2021; Belousov et al., 2020).

PHB2 (Prohibitin 2): An inner mitochondrial membrane receptor that becomes accessible after outer membrane rupture, facilitating mitophagy (Zhang, Liu, Gao, Sehgal, & Wu, 2021).

Atg32 (in yeast): The main mitophagy receptor in yeast, interacting with Atg11 and Atg8 to initiate mitophagy (Camougrand et al., 2022).

Regulatory and Modulatory Proteins

Bcl-2 Family Proteins: Regulate mitophagy by modulating Parkin recruitment and mitochondrial outer membrane permeabilization (Zhang et al., 2020; Ma et al., 2020; Iorio, Celenza, & Petricca, 2021).

AMPK/ULK1 Axis: Senses cellular energy status and can activate mitophagy by promoting autophagosome formation (Belousov et al., 2020; Hollville, Carroll, Cullen, & Martin, 2014).

TNIP1: Acts as a negative regulator, inhibiting mitophagy by interfering with autophagy receptor interactions (Guerroué et al., 2023).

NLRX1/RRBP1: Mediate mitophagy in response to mitochondrial protein import stress, independent of PINK1 (Killackey et al., 2022).

Defective Mitophagy

Defective mitophagy refers to the impairment or dysfunction in the selective removal of damaged or dysfunctional mitochondria through autophagy. This impairment can accumulate damaged mitochondria, disrupt cellular homeostasis, and contribute to various pathological conditions (Palikaras et al., 2020; Lee & Yun, 2022; Lou et al., 2020).

Studies have shown that defective mitophagy can accumulate damaged mitochondria, leading to decreased cellular survival, tissue function, and cellular dysfunction (Palikaras et al., 2020). This accumulation of dysfunctional mitochondria can trigger major cellular consequences, including altered mitochondrial metabolism, increased production of reactive oxygen species, heightened inflammation activation, altered cell fate decisions, and cellular senescence (Tsefou & Ketteler, 2022).

In neurodegenerative diseases, defective mitophagy has been associated with the accumulation of damaged mitochondria, leading to neuronal deficits, cognitive decline, and neurodegeneration (Lee & Yun, 2022; Macleod, 2020; Kumar et al., 2020). Furthermore, in conditions like Parkinson's, defective mitophagy can result in the progressive accumulation of defective mitochondria, ultimately leading to neuronal death and neurodegeneration (Kumar et al., 2020).

Moreover, defective mitophagy has been linked to accelerated physiological aging and the pathogenesis of various diseases, including neurodegenerative disorders (Lee & Yun, 2022; Liu, Liu, Li, & Yang, 2019). The failure to efficiently remove damaged mitochondria through mitophagy can disrupt cellular energy balance, increase inflammation, and contribute to cellular dysfunction, highlighting the critical role of mitophagy in maintaining cellular health and function (Lou et al., 2020).

Mechanisms of Defective Mitophagy

Defective mitophagy refers to the failure of cells to efficiently remove damaged or dysfunctional mitochondria. This impairment disrupts cellular health and is linked to various diseases, especially neurodegenerative and chronic inflammatory conditions. The main mechanisms of defective mitophagy involve disruptions in key signaling pathways, impaired recognition or tagging of damaged mitochondria, and imbalances in mitochondrial dynamics.

Key Molecular Mechanisms

- PINK1/Parkin Pathway Dysfunction: The PINK1 kinase senses mitochondrial damage and activates the Parkin ubiquitin ligase, which tags damaged mitochondria for degradation. Defects in this pathway—such as mutations or impaired activation—lead to the accumulation of dysfunctional mitochondria and are strongly linked to neurodegenerative diseases like Parkinson's and Alzheimer's (Yang et al., 2025; Bingol & Sheng, 2016; Pradeepkiran & Reddy, 2020; Li et al., 2022; Wang, Liu, & Lu, 2019; Chen, Kroemer, & Kepp, 2020; Lou et al., 2020).
- Deubiquitinase USP30 Overactivity: USP30 counteracts Parkin by removing ubiquitin tags from mitochondria, acting as a brake on mitophagy. Overactivity or dysregulation of USP30 can suppress mitophagy, contributing to disease (Bingol & Sheng, 2016).
- Impaired Receptor-Dependent Mitophagy: Besides the ubiquitin-dependent pathway, receptor-mediated mechanisms also help identify and remove damaged mitochondria. Defects in these receptors or

their signaling can result in defective mitophagy (Onishi et al., 2021; Pradeepkiran & Reddy, 2020; Wang, Liu, & Lu, 2019).

- BNIP3, NIX (also known as BNIP3L), and PHB2 are key mitophagy receptors that mediate the selective removal of mitochondria through autophagy. They act as molecular bridges, linking damaged or excess mitochondria to the autophagic machinery for degradation, and are crucial for mitochondrial quality control in various physiological and stress conditions. BNIP3 and NIX are anchored in the outer mitochondrial membrane. They serve as mitophagy receptors by directly recruiting autophagy-related proteins (such as LC3) to the mitochondrial surface, facilitating the engulfment of mitochondria by autophagosomes (Zhang & Ney, 2009; Yamashita et al., 2024; Kodali, 2020; Wu et al., 2020). Their expression is upregulated by cellular stressors like hypoxia and during specific developmental processes (e.g., erythrocyte maturation and cardiac progenitor cell differentiation (Yamashita et al., 2024; Kodali, 2020). Loss of both BNIP3 and NIX abolishes receptor-mediated mitophagy, leading to the accumulation of mitochondria, increased oxidative stress, and heightened sensitivity to cell death (e.g., ferroptosis) (Yamashita et al., 2024; Kodali, 2020).
- PHB2 (prohibitin 2) is located on the inner mitochondrial membrane. When the outer membrane is compromised, PHB2 becomes accessible to autophagy machinery and acts as a receptor to further promote mitophagy, ensuring complete mitochondrial degradation (Wu et al., 2020; Lampert et al., 2019).

Mitophagy in Disease Pathogenesis

Mitophagy, the selective degradation of damaged or dysfunctional mitochondria, is crucial in various disease pathogenesis. Dysregulation of mitophagy has been implicated in the progression of several disorders, including neurodegenerative diseases, liver diseases, cardiovascular diseases, and metabolic disorders (Han et al., 2020; Chakravorty et al., 2019; Сухоруков et al., 2021).

Neurological and Neurodegenerative Diseases

Mitophagy is essential for neuronal health, as neurons are highly dependent on mitochondrial function. Both defective and excessive mitophagy have been implicated in neurodegenerative diseases such as Parkinson's and Alzheimer's, where impaired removal of dysfunctional mitochondria contributes to disease progression and cellular dysfunction (Wang et al., 2023; Doblado et al., 2021; Springer & Macleod,

2016; Lu et al., 2023). The PINK1/Parkin pathway is particularly relevant in these contexts, as its disruption is linked to the accumulation of damaged mitochondria in neurons (Springer & Macleod, 2016; Dombi et al., 2017).

Cardiovascular Diseases

In cardiovascular diseases (CVD), mitophagy maintains cardiac function by eliminating damaged mitochondria, thus supporting energy requirements and biochemical homeostasis. Dysregulated mitophagy is associated with atherosclerosis, ischemic heart disease, heart failure, and other cardiac pathologies. Modulating mitophagy, either genetically or pharmacologically, has shown promise in ameliorating disease progression and is a focus for developing cardioprotective therapies (Wang et al., 2023; Morciano et al., 2020; Zhou et al., 2020).

Cancer

Mitophagy plays a dual role in cancer, acting as both a tumor suppressor and promoter, depending on the context. It helps maintain mitochondrial integrity under stress, but deregulation can contribute to metabolic reprogramming, altered cell fate, and drug resistance. Natural compounds and small molecules that modulate mitophagy are being explored for their anticancer properties, with the potential to either promote cancer cell death or inhibit tumor growth (Drake et al., 2017; Lu et al., 2023; Cao et al., 2023).

Metabolic and Other Chronic Diseases

Mitophagy is implicated in metabolic diseases, diabetes complications, muscle dystrophy, and liver disease. In these conditions, restoring mitophagy homeostasis is considered a potential therapeutic strategy, as both insufficient and excessive mitophagy can contribute to disease pathology (Wang et al., 2023; Doblado et al., 2021).

Immunity and Autoimmune Diseases

Mitophagy regulates immune cell homeostasis and restricts inflammatory cytokine secretion. Its dysfunction is linked to autoimmune diseases such as inflammatory bowel disease, systemic lupus erythematosus, and primary biliary cirrhosis, where impaired clearance of damaged mitochondria can exacerbate inflammation and autoimmunity (Xu et al., 2020).

3. PHARMACOLOGICAL REGULATION OF MITOPHAGY

Pharmacological Regulation of Mitophagy

Keeping our cells' powerhouses, called mitochondria, healthy is important for fighting various diseases. Some studies have examined using drugs to help keep mitochondria healthy and slow down disease.

Cisplatin nephrotoxicity - A study found that using rapamycin, a drug that helps the body clean up damaged parts, could reduce kidney damage caused by cisplatin (Su et al., 2019).
Chronic diseases - Another study suggested that using drugs or specific foods to keep mitochondria healthy could be a way to treat long-lasting diseases (Wang et al., 2018).
Parkinson's disease - Scientists have discussed a new drug that could help dispose of damaged mitochondria in Parkinson's disease (Doblado et al., 2021).
Mitochondrial Dysfunction - A study found that certain drugs could help cells clean up damaged mitochondria, even without a specific protein's help (Clark et al., 2021).
Diabetes - Research showed that using drugs to help clean up damaged mitochondria could protect insulin-making cells from harm (Hamacher-Brady & Brady, 2016).
Cardioprotection - A new idea suggested that drugs that target a protein in the mitochondria could help cells survive when the body's metabolism slows down, which might protect the heart (Sidarala et al., 2020).

Drugs that help keep mitochondria healthy might be a good way to treat diseases. Studies show that using drugs to help cells clean up damaged mitochondria can help with many health problems. In summary, pharmacological regulation of mitophagy holds promise as a therapeutic strategy for various diseases by restoring mitochondrial quality control, promoting cellular health, and mitigating disease progression. These studies underscore the potential of pharmacological interventions in modulating mitophagy pathways to address a wide range of health conditions.

Global Trends in Mitophagy-Related Drug Development

Mitophagy, the selective removal of damaged mitochondria, has become a major focus in drug development for diseases such as neurodegeneration, cancer, cardiovascular, and metabolic disorders. Global trends show rapid growth in research, increasing identification of drug targets, and a shift toward both small-molecule and dietary modulators, though clinical translation remains in the early stages.

Research and Development Trends

Rising Research Activity: Publications on mitophagy-related drug development have shown a consistent upward trend over the past 15+ years, with the United States leading in research output. Key targets like PINK1 and Parkin have gained prominence, especially in neurodegenerative disease contexts (Wang et al., 2024).

Disease Focus: Most efforts target neurodegenerative diseases (Parkinson's, Alzheimer's), cancer, and metabolic disorders, where mitophagy dysfunction is central to disease progression (Clark et al., 2021; Wang et al., 2024).

Drug Types: Both natural (e.g., curcumin, melatonin, resveratrol) and synthetic small molecules are under investigation. These compounds aim to restore or enhance mitophagy, with some already in clinical trials for Alzheimer's and other diseases (Clark et al., 2021; Wang et al., 2024).

Drug Discovery Strategies

High-Throughput Screening: Advances in high-content and high-throughput screening have enabled the identification of numerous "hit" molecules that modulate mitophagy using biochemical and phenotypic assays (Clark et al., 2021; Lu et al., 2023).

Target Diversity: Drug development is expanding beyond the canonical PINK1/Parkin pathway to include receptor-mediated and alternative mitophagy mechanisms, broadening therapeutic possibilities (Dong et al., 2023; Lu et al., 2023).

Methodological Rigor: There is a growing emphasis on robust characterization systems and methodological standards to ensure reliable identification and validation of mitophagy modulators (Dong et al., 2023).

Challenges and Future Directions

Translational Gap: Despite promising preclinical results, few mitophagy-targeting drugs have reached late-stage clinical trials or approval. Challenges include limited understanding of mitophagy in human tissues, need for better disease models, and development of reliable biomarkers (Clark et al., 2021; Dhar et al., 2024).

Therapeutic Potential: Ongoing research aims to refine drug specificity, minimize off-target effects, and optimize dosing to safely modulate mitophagy in patients (Dong et al., 2023; Dhar et al., 2024).

4. In-SILICO APPROACHES FOR MITOPHAGY MODULATOR DISCOVERY

In-Silico Approaches

In-silico approaches for mitophagy modulator development involve using computational methods to identify potential compounds that can modulate mitophagy pathways. These approaches leverage computational tools and algorithms to screen large databases of compounds and predict their interactions with key proteins involved in mitophagy regulation. One of the essential components of in-silico studies is the availability of the 3D structure of the target proteins or enzymes. Advancements in bioinformatics and biotechnology have given rise to biological databases from which 3D structures of proteins and enzymes can be obtained. Since some of the enzymes and proteins responsible for mitophagy are known, it makes for easy identification of these proteins and enzymes and, subsequently, their use for in-silico identification of compounds that can have beneficial pharmacological activities about mitophagy modulation and inhibition of defective mitophagy.

Here are some insights from the literature on in-silico approaches for mitophagy modulator development:

In a study titled, 'Amelioration of Alzheimer's disease pathology by mitophagy inducers identified via machine learning and a cross-species workflow,' Xie *et al.* focused on the identification of mitophagy inducers through machine learning and a cross-species workflow, highlighting the potential of in-silico methods in drug discovery and development, specifically in the context of Alzheimer's disease pathology (Tan et al., 2019).

A natural language processing technique was used in a study by Moskal et al. to assess the semantic similarity of potential compounds to a group of known mitophagy enhancers. A mitochondrial clearance experiment conducted on cells screened the best candidates. The lipid-lowering medication probucol was confirmed in multiple orthogonal mitophagy tests. Probucol enhanced dopaminergic neuron loss, locomotor function, and survival in zebrafish and fly models of mitochondrial injury in vivo. Probucol operated independently of PINK1/Parkin, while ABCA1, which adversely controlled mitophagy after mitochondrial damage, was necessary for Probucol's effects on mitophagy and in vivo. Probucol therapy increased autophagosome and lysosomal markers, lipid droplet (LD), and mitochondrial contact.

On the other hand, Probucol inhibited LD expansion after mitochondrial injury, and LDs were necessary for probucol-mediated mitophagy augmentation. Changes in LD dynamics caused by Probucol may set the cell up for a more effective mitophagic response in the event of mitochondrial injury (Xie et al., 2022).

Insilico Research Workflow for Natural Mitopgagy Modulations

Developing natural mitophagy modulators through in silico research involves a systematic workflow that integrates computational screening, machine learning, and experimental validation. This approach accelerates the identification of promising natural compounds that can regulate mitophagy, with potential therapeutic applications in diseases such as neurodegeneration and cancer.

Workflow Stages

1. *Compound Library Preparation and Feature Extraction*

Natural Compound Library: Start with a curated collection of naturally occurring small molecules.

Molecular Feature Analysis: Use computational tools to generate vector representations, pharmacophore fingerprints, and conformer fingerprints, capturing the structural and chemical properties of each compound (Xie et al., 2022).

2. *In Silico Screening and Machine Learning*

Unsupervised Machine Learning: Apply algorithms to cluster and prioritize compounds based on their predicted ability to modulate mitophagy, using extracted molecular features as input (Xie et al., 2022)

Cross-Species Data Integration: Incorporate biological data from multiple species to enhance the relevance and predictive power of the screening process (Xie et al., 2022)

3. *High-throughput virtual and Experimental Validation*

Virtual Screening: Use computational models to predict which compounds are most likely to induce mitophagy.

Experimental Testing: Validate top candidates in biological models (e.g., nematodes, rodents, or cell lines) to confirm mitophagy induction and assess functional outcomes, such as neuronal survival and memory improvement (Xie et al., 2022).

4. *Quantitative and Functional Assessment*

Advanced Imaging Tools: Employ indicators like mito-SRAI or mt-Keima for precise quantification of mitophagy in cells and tissues (Katayama et al., 2020; Sun et al., 2015)

Disease-Relevant Evaluation: Assess the impact of candidate compounds on disease models, such as Alzheimer's or Parkinson's disease, by measuring relevant phenotypes (e.g., neuronal health, memory) (Xie et al., 2022; Katayama et al., 2020).

5. NATURAL PRODUCTS AS MITOPHAGY MODULATORS

Natural compounds can modulate mitophagy, presenting a natural and efficacious method for regulating mitochondrial quality control. With the increase in availability and several natural products databases, it has become easier to utilize the natural products available in these databases and the in-silico techniques to identify natural compounds that could play a role in mitophagy modulation and inhibition of defective mitophagy. Studies using natural products can also aid in identifying plants with possible pharmacological effects of interest. Some of these Natural product databases include

a. Collection Of Open Natural Products (COCONUT):

The Collection of Open Natural Products (COCONUT) is an aggregated dataset of elucidated and predicted NPs collected from open sources. It also provides a web interface to browse, search, and easily and quickly download NPs. The COCONUT web is freely available at https://coconut.naturalproducts.net. The database contains 407,270 unique natural products, which can be downloaded for use in in-silico research (Sorokina et al., 2021).

b. Supernatural 3.0

Supernatural 3.0 is a freely accessible database containing natural ingredients and derivatives derived from them. The revised version includes 449,058 distinct natural chemicals and 790,096 distinct structures, including isomers and their physicochemical and structural details. Furthermore, it details target-specific cells, drug-like chemical space prediction for various diseases, toxicity, modes of action, pathways, and vendor information (Gallo et al., 2023).

c. African Natural Products Database

African Natural Products Database (ANPDB) is a collection of natural product databases from different parts of the continent of Africa. The Eastern African Natural Products Database (EANPDB) and the Northern African Natural Products Database (NANPDB) currently comprise ANPDB. ANPDB does not currently contain the NP databases from the additional African regions, nor is it still being built. The largest database of NPs isolated from native organisms on the African continent is, as far as we are aware, ANPDB. The content currently consists of data sources (from 1962 to 2019) gathered from chosen searches in local African publications, MSc and PhD theses in certain African university libraries, and literature collated from mainstream natural product journals. The information includes 6,515 chemicals that were mostly isolated from 1,042 source organisms, mostly plants, with some contributions from microbes, marine sources, and animals (such as corals) (Simoben et al., 2020; Ntie-Kang et al., 2017).

Numerous investigations have scrutinized the impact of natural compounds on modifying mitophagy, underscoring their therapeutic potential in diverse diseases.

The following are noteworthy insights derived from the literature:

Kaempferol and Rhapontigenin have emerged as robust mitophagy inducers from a repertoire of naturally occurring compounds, signifying their potential to influence mitophagy and ameliorate disease-related pathologies (Tan et al., 2019).

Research has accentuated the therapeutic promise of natural compounds like urolithin, spermidine, curcumin, nicotinamide, and actinonin in addressing autophagy, mitophagy, and neuroinflammation for the prevention and management of Alzheimer's disease (Luan et al., 2023).

Bertolin et al. demonstrated that treatment with the natural compound Xanthohumol obstructs Aurora kinase A-induced mitophagy by destabilizing a tripartite complex, suggesting its potential as a modulator of mitophagy (Kumar et al., 2020). Their findings also elucidated that mitochondrial Aurora kinase A stimulates mitophagy by interacting with MAP1LC3 and Prohibitin 2, indicating that inhibitors of this interaction hold promise for modulating mitophagy (Ntie-Kang et al., 2017).

Studies have reviewed the current understanding of mitophagy mechanisms and introduced small-molecule pharmacological modulators of mitophagy, encompassing natural compounds, thereby underscoring their critical role in disease modulation (Saito et al., 2020).

Natural vs. Synthetic Mitophagy Modulators

Natural Mitophagy Modulators

Sources & Examples: Natural modulators include plant and animal-derived compounds such as polyphenols (e.g., resveratrol, curcumin, kaempferol, rhapontigenin), coenzyme Q, and other bioactive molecules (Lin et al., 2024; Xie et al., 2022; Cao et al., 2023; Shakeri et al., 2020).
Mechanisms: These compounds can modulate mitochondrial oxidative phosphorylation, reduce mitochondrial reactive oxygen species, and regulate the expression of mitophagy-related genes and transcription factors (e.g., PINK1/Parkin, FOXO3a) (Lin et al., 2024; Shakeri et al., 2020).
Therapeutic Potential: Natural compounds are often low in toxicity and have shown promise in preclinical models for neurodegenerative diseases, cardiovascular disorders, cancer, and metabolic diseases (Lin et al., 2024; Xie et al., 2022; Cao et al., 2023; Shakeri et al., 2020).
Challenges: Issues such as low bioavailability and variability in potency can limit their clinical application, and more clinical trials are needed to confirm their efficacy (Lin et al., 2024).

Synthetic Mitophagy Modulators

Sources & Examples: Synthetic modulators include small molecules and drugs such as metformin, AICAR, idebenone, and various chemical probes designed to target mitophagy pathways (Dombi et al., 2017; Srivastava & Gross, 2023).
Mechanisms: These agents can activate mitophagy through direct mitochondrial membrane depolarization (e.g., FCCP/CCCP), inhibition of mitochondrial respiration (e.g., antimycin A, oligomycin), or by targeting specific signaling pathways (e.g., AMPK activation) (Dombi et al., 2017; Georgakopoulos et al., 2017)
Therapeutic Potential: Synthetic compounds can be engineered for higher potency, specificity, and improved pharmacokinetics, making them valuable for dissecting mitophagy mechanisms and as potential therapeutics (Srivastava & Gross, 2023; Georgakopoulos et al., 2017).
Challenges: Some synthetic modulators may have off-target effects, higher toxicity, or disrupt mitochondrial homeostasis, which can limit their therapeutic window (Dong et al., 2023; Georgakopoulos et al., 2017).

6. TRANSLATIONAL BARRIERS

Bioavailability: Many natural modulators (e.g., resveratrol, curcumin) suffer from poor bioavailability, limiting their clinical effectiveness. Synthetic derivatives and formulations (e.g., SLCP) are being developed to overcome this barrier (Lin et al., 2024; Maiti et al., 2019).
Specificity: Natural compounds often act on multiple cellular pathways, which can lead to off-target effects. Synthetic modulators can be designed for greater pathway specificity, potentially reducing unintended actions (Srivastava & Gross, 2023; Maiti et al., 2019).
Toxicity: Natural compounds generally have low toxicity, but their safety in long-term or high-dose use is not fully established. Synthetic modulators may have variable toxicity profiles, but some (like ALT001) are specifically engineered for low toxicity (Maiti et al., 2019; Um et al., 2024)
Clinical Validation: Both natural and synthetic modulators require more robust clinical trials to confirm efficacy, optimal dosing, and long-term safety in humans (Lin et al., 2024; Um et al., 2024)

Natural and synthetic mitophagy modulators each present unique advantages and challenges, with translational barriers primarily centered on bioavailability, specificity, and toxicity. Overcoming these hurdles is essential for successful therapeutic application.

The Potential Toxicological Concerns or Side Effects of Natural Mitophagy

Natural mitophagy enhancers, such as urolithin A, actinonin, tomatidine, and nicotinamide riboside, are being explored for their protective effects in diseases like Alzheimer's. Current research suggests these compounds can improve mitochondrial health and cell survival without evident toxicity at optimized doses in cellular models. No significant toxicological concerns or side effects have been reported in these studies when natural mitophagy enhancers are used at appropriate concentrations.

Indirect Insights from Environmental Toxicology

While not directly related to natural mitophagy enhancers, studies on environmental toxins like copper show that excessive or dysregulated mitophagy can contribute to cellular damage. This highlights the importance of dose and context, as overstimulation of mitophagy, regardless of the trigger, may have harmful effects (Liao et al., 2021).

Key Considerations

Dose Optimization: The safety of natural mitophagy enhancers appears dose-dependent; excessive activation of mitophagy could potentially disrupt cellular homeostasis (Liao et al., 2021).
Need for Clinical Data: Most evidence comes from preclinical or cell-based studies. Comprehensive toxicological profiles and side effect data in humans are still lacking (Liao et al., 2021).

CONCLUSION

Mitophagy modulators and inhibitors of aberrant mitophagy are among the management options for several clinical conditions associated with mitochondrial quality control. Using in-silico methods and natural product alternatives allows researchers to find molecules that can interfere with key pathways involved in the control of mitophagy. This will enable us to identify new therapeutic approaches based on our knowledge regarding physiological roles, molecular mechanisms, and pathophysiological implications of mitophagy. Studying the modulation process for mitophagy would provide insights into the role of these organelles in regulating cellular homeostasis and diseases. Subsequently, novel therapeutics targeted at disease therapies and mitochondrial biology could be developed out of this research.

List of Abbreviations

AMPK: Adenosine monophosphate-activated protein kinase
ANPDB: African Natural Products Database
Atg: Autophagy-related gene
BNIP3: BCL2 Interacting Protein 3
BNIP3L: BCL2 Interacting Protein 3 Like
CCCP: Carbonyl cyanide m-chlorophenyl hydrazone
COCONUT: Collection Of Open Natural Products
CVD: Cardiovascular diseases
EANPDB: Eastern African Natural Products Database
FCCP: Carbonyl cyanide-p-trifluoromethoxyphenylhydrazone
FOXO3a: Forkhead box protein O3a
FUNDC1: FUN14 domain containing 1
LC3: Microtubule-associated protein 1 light chain 3
LD: Lipid droplet
MAP1LC3: Microtubule-associated protein 1 light chain 3

MMCS: Mitophagy Modulator Characterization System
NAD+: Nicotinamide adenine dinucleotide
NANPDB: Northern African Natural Products Database
NBR1: Neighbor of BRCA1 gene 1
NDP52: Nuclear dot protein 52
NIX: Nip3-like protein X
NLRX1: NLR family member X1
NP: Natural product
OPTN: Optineurin
PHB2: Prohibitin 2
PINK1: PTEN-induced kinase 1
PRKN: Parkin
p62/SQSTM1: Sequestosome 1
RRBP1: Ribosome binding protein 1
SLCP: Succinylated low molecular weight chitosan
TNIP1: TNFAIP3 interacting protein 1
ULK1: Unc-51 like autophagy activating kinase 1
USP30: Ubiquitin-specific peptidase 30

REFERENCES

Сухоруков, В., Воронков, Д., Баранич, Т., Mudzhiri, N., Magnaeva, A., & Иллариошкин, С. (2021). Impaired mitophagy in neurons and glial cells during aging and age-related disorders. *International Journal of Molecular Sciences*, *22*(19), 10251. DOI: 10.3390/ijms221910251 PMID: 34638589

Belousov, D., Mikhaylenko, E., Somasundaram, S., Kirkland, C., & Aliev, G. (2020). The Dawn of Mitophagy: What Do We Know by Now? *Current Neuropharmacology*, *19*(2), 170–192. DOI: 10.2174/1570159X18666200522202319 PMID: 32442087

Bhujabal, Z., Birgisdottir, Å. B., Sjøttem, E., Brenne, H. B., Øvervatn, A., Habisov, S., Kirkin, V., Lamark, T., & Johansen, T. (2017). Fkbp8 recruits lc3a to mediate parkin-independent mitophagy. *EMBO Reports*, *18*(6), 947–961. DOI: 10.15252/embr.201643147 PMID: 28381481

Bingol, B., & Sheng, M. (2016). Mechanisms of mitophagy: PINK1, Parkin, USP30 and beyond. *Free Radical Biology & Medicine*, *100*, 210–222. DOI: 10.1016/j.freeradbiomed.2016.04.015 PMID: 27094585

Camougrand, N., Vigié, P., Dompierre, J., Massoni-Laporte, A., Lasserre, J., & Bhatia-Kiššová, I. (2022). The Dep1 protein: A new regulator of mitophagy in yeast. *Biochemical and Biophysical Research Communications*, *635*, 218–226. DOI: 10.1016/j.bbrc.2022.10.052 PMID: 36283334

Cao, M., Tang, Y., Luo, Y., Gu, F., Zhu, Y., Liu, X., Yan, C., Hu, W., Wang, S., Chao, X., Xu, H., Chen, H., & Wang, L. (2023). Natural compounds modulating mitophagy: Implications for cancer therapy. *Cancer Letters*, •••, 216590. PMID: 38097131

Cao, S., Aman, Y., Fang, E., & Tencomnao, T. (2022). P. edulis extract protects against amyloid-β toxicity in alzheimer's disease models through maintenance of mitochondrial homeostasis via the foxo3/daf-16 pathway. *Molecular Neurobiology*, *59*(9), 5612–5629. DOI: 10.1007/s12035-022-02904-5 PMID: 35739408

Chakravorty, A., Jetto, C., & Manjithaya, R. (2019). Dysfunctional mitochondria and mitophagy as drivers of Alzheimer's disease pathogenesis. *Frontiers in Aging Neuroscience*, *11*, 11. DOI: 10.3389/fnagi.2019.00311 PMID: 31824296

Chen, G., Kroemer, G., & Kepp, O. (2020). Mitophagy: An Emerging Role in Aging and Age-Associated Diseases. *Frontiers in Cell and Developmental Biology*, *8*, 8. DOI: 10.3389/fcell.2020.00200 PMID: 32274386

Chowdhury, R. (2022). Mitophagy and oral cancers. *National Journal of Maxillofacial Surgery*, *13*(1), 11–19. DOI: 10.4103/njms.NJMS_123_20 PMID: 35911821

Clark, E., Torre, A., Hoshikawa, T., & Briston, T. (2021). Targeting mitophagy in Parkinson's disease. *The Journal of Biological Chemistry*, *296*, 100209. DOI: 10.1074/jbc.REV120.014294 PMID: 33372898

D'Arcy M. S. (2024). Mitophagy in health and disease. Molecular mechanisms, regulatory pathways, and therapeutic implications. Apoptosis: an international journal on programmed cell death, 29(9-10), 1415–1428

Deng, Y., Lou, T., Kong, L., & Liu, C. (2023). Prohibitin2/PHB2, Transcriptionally Regulated by GABPA, Inhibits Cell Growth via PRKN/Parkin-dependent Mitophagy in Endometriosis. *Reproductive Sciences (Thousand Oaks, Calif.)*, *30*(12), 3629–3640. DOI: 10.1007/s43032-023-01316-7 PMID: 37587393

Dhar, K. S., Townsend, B., Montgomery, A. P., Danon, J. J., Pagan, J. K., & Kassiou, M. (2024). Enhancing CNS mitophagy: Drug development and disease-relevant models. *Trends in Pharmacological Sciences*, *45*(11), 982–996. DOI: 10.1016/j.tips.2024.09.002 PMID: 39419743

Doblado, L., Lueck, C., Rey, C., Samhan-Arias, A., Prieto, I., Stacchiotti, A., & Monsalve, M. (2021). Mitophagy in Human Diseases. *International Journal of Molecular Sciences*, *22*(8), 3903. DOI: 10.3390/ijms22083903 PMID: 33918863

Dombi, E., Mortiboys, H., & Poulton, J. (2017). Modulating Mitophagy in Mitochondrial Disease. *Current Medicinal Chemistry*, *25*(40), 5597–5612. DOI: 10.2174/0929867324666170616101741 PMID: 28618992

Dong, Y., Zhuang, X., Wang, Y., Tan, J., Feng, D., Li, M., Zhong, Q., Song, Z., Shen, H., Fang, E., & Lu, J. (2023). Chemical mitophagy modulators: Drug development strategies and novel regulatory mechanisms. *Pharmacological Research*, *194*, 106835. DOI: 10.1016/j.phrs.2023.106835 PMID: 37348691

Drake, L., Springer, M., Poole, L., Kim, C., & Macleod, K. (2017). Expanding perspectives on the significance of mitophagy in cancer. *Seminars in Cancer Biology*, *47*, 110–124. DOI: 10.1016/j.semcancer.2017.04.008 PMID: 28450176

Fang, E., Waltz, T., Kassahun, H., Lu, Q., Kerr, J., Morevati, M., Fivenson, E. M., Wollman, B. N., Marosi, K., Wilson, M. A., Iser, W. B., Eckley, D. M., Zhang, Y., Lehrmann, E., Goldberg, I. G., Scheibye-Knudsen, M., Mattson, M. P., Nilsen, H., Bohr, V. A., & Becker, K. (2017). Tomatidine enhances lifespan and healthspan in c. elegans through mitophagy induction via the skn-1/nrf2 pathway. *Scientific Reports*, *7*(1), 46208. DOI: 10.1038/srep46208 PMID: 28397803

Fivenson, E., Lautrup, S., Sun, N., Scheibye-Knudsen, M., Stevnsner, T., Nilsen, H., Bohr, V. A., & Fang, E. (2017). Mitophagy in neurodegeneration and aging. *Neurochemistry International, 109*, 202–209. DOI: 10.1016/j.neuint.2017.02.007 PMID: 28235551

Fivenson, E. M., Lautrup, S., Sun, N., Scheibye-Knudsen, M., Stevnsner, T., Nilsen, H., Bohr, V. A., & Fang, E. F. (2017). Mitophagy in neurodegeneration and aging. *Neurochemistry International, 109*, 202–209. DOI: 10.1016/j.neuint.2017.02.007 PMID: 28235551

Gallo, K., Kemmler, E., Goede, A., Becker, F., Dunkel, M., Preissner, R., & Banerjee, P. (2023). SuperNatural 3.0-a database of natural products and natural product-based derivatives. *Nucleic Acids Research, 51*(D1), D654–D659. DOI: 10.1093/nar/gkac1008 PMID: 36399452

Georgakopoulos, N., Wells, G., & Campanella, M. (2017). The pharmacological regulation of cellular mitophagy. *Nature Chemical Biology, 13*(2), 136–146. DOI: 10.1038/nchembio.2287 PMID: 28103219
Georgakopoulos, N., Wells, G., & Campanella, M. (2017). The pharmacological regulation of cellular mitophagy. *Nature Chemical Biology, 13*(2), 136–146. DOI: 10.1038/nchembio.2287 PMID: 28103219
Guerroué, F., Bunker, E., Rosencrans, W., Nguyen, J., Basar, M., Werner, A., Chou, T., Wang, C., & Youle, R. (2023). TNIP1 inhibits selective autophagy via bipartite interaction with LC3/GABARAP and TAX1BP1. *Molecular Cell*. PMID: 36898370

Guo, J., & Chiang, W. (2021). Mitophagy in aging and longevity. *IUBMB Life, 74*(4), 296–316. DOI: 10.1002/iub.2585 PMID: 34889504

Hamacher-Brady, A., & Brady, N. R. (2016). Mitophagy programs: Mechanisms and physiological implications of mitochondrial targeting by autophagy. *Cellular and Molecular Life Sciences : CMLS, 73*(4), 775–795. DOI: 10.1007/s00018-015-2087-8 PMID: 26611876

Han, S., Jeong, Y., Sheshadri, P., Su, X., & Cai, Q. (2020). Mitophagy regulates integrity of mitochondria at synapses and is critical for synaptic maintenance. *EMBO Reports, 21*(9), e49801. DOI: 10.15252/embr.201949801 PMID: 32627320

Heo, J., Ordureau, A., Paulo, J., Rinehart, J., & Harper, J. (2015). The pink1-parkin mitochondrial ubiquitylation pathway drives a program of optn/ndp52 recruitment and tbk1 activation to promote mitophagy. *Molecular Cell, 60*(1), 7–20. DOI: 10.1016/j.molcel.2015.08.016 PMID: 26365381

Hollville, E., Carroll, R., Cullen, S., & Martin, S. (2014). Bcl-2 family proteins participate in mitochondrial quality control by regulating Parkin/PINK1-dependent mitophagy. *Molecular Cell*, *55*(3), 451–466. DOI: 10.1016/j.molcel.2014.06.001 PMID: 24999239

Iorio, R., Celenza, G., & Petricca, S. (2021). Mitophagy: Molecular Mechanisms, New Concepts on Parkin Activation and the Emerging Role of AMPK/ULK1 Axis. *Cells*, *11*(1), 11. DOI: 10.3390/cells11010030 PMID: 35011593

Ising, C., Koehler, S., Brähler, S., Merkwirth, C., Höhne, M., Baris, O., Hagmann, H., Kann, M., Fabretti, F., Dafinger, C., Bloch, W., Schermer, B., Linkermann, A., Brüning, J., Kurschat, C., Müller, R., Wiesner, R., Langer, T., Benzing, T., & Brinkkoetter, P. (2015). Inhibition of insulin/IGF-1 receptor signaling protects from mitochondria-mediated kidney failure. *EMBO Molecular Medicine*, *7*(3), 275–287. DOI: 10.15252/emmm.201404916 PMID: 25643582

Jin, Q., Li, R., Hu, N., Xin, T., Zhu, P., Hu, S., Ma, S., Zhu, H., Ren, J., & Zhou, H. (2018). Dusp1 alleviates cardiac ischemia/reperfusion injury by suppressing the mff-required mitochondrial fission and bnip3-related mitophagy via the jnk pathways. *Redox Biology*, *14*, 576–587. DOI: 10.1016/j.redox.2017.11.004 PMID: 29149759

Kanki, T., Klionsky, D., & Okamoto, K. (2011). Mitochondria autophagy in yeast. *Antioxidants & Redox Signaling*, *14*(10), 1989–2001. DOI: 10.1089/ars.2010.3762 PMID: 21194379

Katayama, H., Hama, H., Nagasawa, K., Kurokawa, H., Sugiyama, M., Ando, R., Funata, M., Yoshida, N., Homma, M., Nishimura, T., Takahashi, M., Ishida, Y., Hioki, H., Tsujihata, Y., & Miyawaki, A. (2020). Visualizing and Modulating Mitophagy for Therapeutic Studies of Neurodegeneration. *Cell*, *181*(5), 1176–1187.e16. DOI: 10.1016/j.cell.2020.04.025 PMID: 32437660

Killackey, S., Bi, Y., Soares, F., Hammi, I., Winsor, N., Abdul-Sater, A., Philpott, D., Arnoult, D., & Girardin, S. (2022). Mitochondrial protein import stress regulates the LC3 lipidation step of mitophagy through NLRX1 and RRBP1.. Molecular cell.

Kodali, S. (2020). Bnip3/Nix-mediated mitophagy protects memory B cells by restricting de novo fatty acid synthesis. The Journal of Immunology.

Kumar, M., Acevedo-Cintrón, J., Jhaldiyal, A., Wang, H., Andrabi, S., Eacker, S., Karuppagounder, S. S., Brahmachari, S., Chen, R., Kim, H., Ko, H. S., Dawson, V. L., & Dawson, T. (2020). Defects in mitochondrial biogenesis drive mitochondrial alterations in parkin-deficient human dopamine neurons. *Stem Cell Reports*, *15*(3), 629–645. DOI: 10.1016/j.stemcr.2020.07.013 PMID: 32795422

Lampert, M., Orogo, A., Najor, R., Hammerling, B., Leon, L., Wang, B., Kim, T., Sussman, M., & Gustafsson, Å. (2019). BNIP3L/NIX and FUNDC1-mediated mitophagy is required for mitochondrial network remodeling during cardiac progenitor cell differentiation. *Autophagy*, *15*(7), 1182–1198. DOI: 10.1080/15548627.2019.1580095 PMID: 30741592

Lee, K., & Yun, J. (2022). Mitophagy stimulation as a novel strategy for the treatment of mitochondrial diseases. *Journal of Genetic Medicine*, *19*(2), 49–56. DOI: 10.5734/JGM.2022.19.2.49

Lei, Y., Gan, M., Qiu, Y., Chen, Q., Wang, X., Liao, T., Zhao, M., Chen, L., Zhang, S., Zhao, Y., Niu, L., Wang, Y., Zhu, L., & Shen, L. (2024). The role of mitochondrial dynamics and mitophagy in skeletal muscle atrophy: From molecular mechanisms to therapeutic insights. *Cellular & Molecular Biology Letters*, *29*(1), 59. DOI: 10.1186/s11658-024-00572-y PMID: 38654156

Lei, Y., Gan, M., Qiu, Y., Chen, Q., Wang, X., Liao, T., Zhao, M., Chen, L., Zhang, S., Zhao, Y., Niu, L., Wang, Y., Zhu, L., & Shen, L. (2024). The role of mitochondrial dynamics and mitophagy in skeletal muscle atrophy: From molecular mechanisms to therapeutic insights. *Cellular & Molecular Biology Letters*, *29*(1), 59. DOI: 10.1186/s11658-024-00572-y PMID: 38654156

Li, J., Wu, J., Zhou, X., Lü, Y., Ge, Y., & Zhang, X. (2023). Targeting neuronal mitophagy in ischemic stroke: An update. *Burns and Trauma*, *11*, 11. DOI: 10.1093/burnst/tkad018 PMID: 37274155

Li, J., Yang, D., Li, Z., Zhao, M., Wang, D., Sun, Z., Wen, P., Dai, Y., Gou, F., Ji, Y., Zhao, D., & Yang, L. (2022). PINK1/Parkin-mediated mitophagy in neurodegenerative diseases. *Ageing Research Reviews*, •••, 84. PMID: 36503124

Li, Y., Zheng, W., Lu, Y., Zheng, Y., Pan, L., Wu, X., Yuan, Y., Shen, Z. S., Zhang, X., Wu, J., Chen, Z., & Zhang, X. (2021). BNIP3L/NIX-mediated mitophagy: Molecular mechanisms and implications for human disease. *Cell Death & Disease*, *13*(1), 13. DOI: 10.1038/s41419-021-04469-y PMID: 34930907

Liao, J., Li, Q., Hu, Z., Yu, W., Zhang, K., Ma, F., Han, Q., Zhang, H., Guo, J., Hu, L., Pan, J., Li, Y., & Tang, Z. (2021). Mitochondrial miR-1285 regulates copper-induced mitochondrial dysfunction and mitophagy by impairing IDH2 in pig jejunal epithelial cells. *Journal of Hazardous Materials*, *422*, 126899. DOI: 10.1016/j.jhazmat.2021.126899 PMID: 34418838

Lin, X., Liu, W., Hu, X., Liu, Z., Wang, F., & Wang, J. (2024). The Role of Polyphenols in Modulating Mitophagy: Implications for Therapeutic Interventions. *Pharmacological Research*, *207*, 107324. DOI: 10.1016/j.phrs.2024.107324 PMID: 39059613

Liu, J., Liu, W., Li, R., & Yang, H. (2019). Mitophagy in Parkinson's disease: From pathogenesis to treatment. *Cells*, *8*(7), 712. DOI: 10.3390/cells8070712 PMID: 31336937

Liu, Z., Sun, Q., Zhang, C., Yuan, H., & He, W. (2021). Activity-based fluorescent molecular logic gate probe for dynamic tracking of mitophagy induced by oxidative stress. *Analytical Chemistry*, *93*(7), 3502–3509. DOI: 10.1021/acs.analchem.0c04854 PMID: 33544570

Longo, M., Paolini, E., Meroni, M., & Dongiovanni, P. (2021). Remodeling of Mitochondrial Plasticity: The Key Switch from NAFLD/NASH to HCC. *International Journal of Molecular Sciences*, *22*(8), 4173. DOI: 10.3390/ijms22084173 PMID: 33920670

Lou, G., Palikaras, K., Lautrup, S., Scheibye-Knudsen, M., Tavernarakis, N., & Fang, E. (2020). Mitophagy and neuroprotection. *Trends in Molecular Medicine*, *26*(1), 8–20. DOI: 10.1016/j.molmed.2019.07.002 PMID: 31375365

L , Y., Li, Z., Zhang, S., Zhang, T., Liu, Y., & Zhang, L. (2023). Cellular mitophagy: Mechanism, roles in diseases and small molecule pharmacological regulation. *Theranostics*, *13*(2), 736–766. DOI: 10.7150/thno.79876 PMID: 36632220

Lu, Y., Li, Z., Zhang, S., Zhang, T., Liu, Y., & Zhang, L. (2023). Cellular mitophagy: Mechanism, roles in diseases and small molecule pharmacological regulation. *Theranostics*, *13*(2), 736–766. DOI: 10.7150/thno.79876 PMID: 36632220

Lu, Y., Li, Z., Zhang, S., Zhang, T., Liu, Y., & Zhang, L. (2023). Cellular mitophagy: Mechanism, roles in diseases and small molecule pharmacological regulation. *Theranostics*, *13*(2), 736–766. DOI: 10.7150/thno.79876 PMID: 36632220

Luan, Y., Jiang, L., Luan, Y., Xie, Y., Yang, Y., & Ren, K. (2023). Mitophagy and traumatic brain injury: Regulatory mechanisms and therapeutic potentials. *Oxidative Medicine and Cellular Longevity*, *2023*, 1–15. DOI: 10.1155/2023/1649842 PMID: 36846712

Ma, K., Chen, G., Li, W., Kepp, O., Zhu, Y., & Chen, Q. (2020). Mitophagy, Mitochondrial Homeostasis, and Cell Fate. *Frontiers in Cell and Developmental Biology*, •••, 8. PMID: 32671064

Macleod, K. (2020). Mitophagy and mitochondrial dysfunction in cancer. *Annual Review of Cancer Biology*, *4*(1), 41–60. DOI: 10.1146/annurev-cancerbio-030419-033405

Maestro, I., de la Ballina, L. R., Porras, G., Corrochano, S., De Lago, E., Simonsen, A., Boya, P., & Martinez, A. (2022). Discovery of Mitophagy Inhibitors with Therapeutic Potential in Different Familial Amyotrophic Lateral Sclerosis Mutations. *International Journal of Molecular Sciences*, *23*(20), 12676. DOI: 10.3390/ijms232012676 PMID: 36293534

Maiti, P., Scott, J., Sengupta, D., Al-Gharaibeh, A., & Dunbar, G. (2019). Curcumin and Solid Lipid Curcumin Particles Induce Autophagy, but Inhibit Mitophagy and the PI3K-Akt/mTOR Pathway in Cultured Glioblastoma Cells. *International Journal of Molecular Sciences*, *20*(2), 20. DOI: 10.3390/ijms20020399 PMID: 30669284

Mao, K., Wang, K., Liu, X., & Klionsky, D. (2013). The scaffold protein atg11 recruits fission machinery to drive selective mitochondria degradation by autophagy. *Developmental Cell*, *26*(1), 9–18. DOI: 10.1016/j.devcel.2013.05.024 PMID: 23810512

McLelland, G. L., Soubannier, V., Chen, C. X., McBride, H. M., & Fon, E. A. (2014). Parkin and PINK1 function in a vesicular trafficking pathway regulating mitochondrial quality control. *The EMBO Journal*, *33*(4), 282–295. DOI: 10.1002/embj.201385902 PMID: 24446486

Morciano, G., Patergnani, S., Bonora, M., Pedriali, G., Tarocco, A., Bouhamida, E., Marchi, S., Ancora, G., Anania, G., Wieckowski, M., Giorgi, C., & Pinton, P. (2020). Mitophagy in Cardiovascular Diseases. *Journal of Clinical Medicine*, •••, 9. PMID: 32214047

Nakashima, M., Suga, N., Ikeda, Y., Yoshikawa, S., & Matsuda, S. (2024). Inspiring tactics with the improvement of mitophagy and redox balance for the development of innovative treatment against polycystic kidney disease. *Biomolecules*, *14*(2), 207. DOI: 10.3390/biom14020207 PMID: 38397444

Niemi, N., & Friedman, J. (2024). Coordinating BNIP3/NIX-mediated mitophagy in space and time. *Biochemical Society Transactions*, *52*(5), 1969–1979. DOI: 10.1042/BST20221364 PMID: 39377319

Ntie-Kang, F., Telukunta, K. K., Döring, K., Simoben, C. V. A., Moumbock, A. F., Malange, Y. I., Njume, L. E., Yong, J. N., Sippl, W., & Günther, S. (2017). NANPDB: A Resource for Natural Products from Northern African Sources. *Journal of Natural Products*, *80*(7), 2067–2076. DOI: 10.1021/acs.jnatprod.7b00283 PMID: 28641017

Onishi, M., Yamano, K., Sato, M., Matsuda, N., & Okamoto, K. (2021). Molecular mechanisms and physiological functions of mitophagy. *The EMBO Journal*, *40*(3), e104705. DOI: 10.15252/embj.2020104705 PMID: 33438778

Onishi, M., Yamano, K., Sato, M., Matsuda, N., & Okamoto, K. (2021). Molecular mechanisms and physiological functions of mitophagy. *The EMBO Journal*, *40*(3), 40. DOI: 10.15252/embj.2020104705 PMID: 33438778

Palikaras, K.; Princz, A.; Tavernarakis, N. Mitophagy Modulators. Encycl. Biomed. Gerontol. 2020, 433– 446,

Pickles, S., Vigié, P., & Youle, R. (2018). Mitophagy and quality control mechanisms in mitochondrial maintenance. *Current Biology*, *28*(4), R170–R185. DOI: 10.1016/j.cub.2018.01.004 PMID: 29462587

Pradeepkiran, J., & Reddy, P. (2020). Defective mitophagy in Alzheimer's disease. *Ageing Research Reviews*, •••, 64. PMID: 33022416

Praharaj, P., Patro, B., & Bhutia, S. (2021). Dysregulation of mitophagy and mitochondrial homeostasis in cancer stem cells: Novel mechanism for anticancer stem cell-targeted cancer therapy. *British Journal of Pharmacology*, *179*(22), 5015–5035. DOI: 10.1111/bph.15401 PMID: 33527371

Redmann, M., Dodson, M., Boyer-Guittaut, M., Darley-Usmar, V., & Zhang, J. (2014). Mitophagy mechanisms and role in human diseases. The International Journal of Biochemistry &Amp. *Cell Biology (Henderson NV)*, *53*, 127–133.

Saito, T., Hamano, K., & Sadoshima, J. (2020). Molecular mechanisms and clinical implications of multiple forms of mitophagy in the heart. *Cardiovascular Research*, *117*(14), 2730–2741. DOI: 10.1093/cvr/cvaa340 PMID: 33331644

Shakeri, F., Bianconi, V., Pirro, M., & Sahebkar, A. (2020). Effects of Plant and Animal Natural Products on Mitophagy. *Oxidative Medicine and Cellular Longevity*, *2020*, 2020. DOI: 10.1155/2020/6969402 PMID: 32308807

Shirihai, O., Song, M., & Dorn, G.II. (2015). How mitochondrial dynamism orchestrates mitophagy. *Circulation Research*, *116*(11), 1835–1849. DOI: 10.1161/CIRCRESAHA.116.306374 PMID: 25999423

Sidarala, V., Pearson, G. L., Parekh, V. S., Thompson, B., Christen, L., Gingerich, M. A., Zhu, J., Stromer, T., Ren, J., Reck, E. C., Chai, B., Corbett, J. A., Mandrup-Poulsen, T., Satin, L. S., & Soleimanpour, S. A. (2020). Mitophagy protects β cells from inflammatory damage in diabetes. *JCI Insight*, *5*(24), e141138. DOI: 10.1172/jci.insight.141138 PMID: 33232298

Simoben, C. V., Qaseem, A., Moumbock, A. F. A., Telukunta, K. K., Günther, S., Sippl, W., & Ntie-Kang, F. (2020). Pharmacoinformatic Investigation of Medicinal Plants from East Africa. *Molecular Informatics, 39*(11), e2000163. DOI: 10.1002/minf.202000163 PMID: 32964659

Singh, F., & Ganley, I. (2021). Parkinson's disease and mitophagy: An emerging role for lrrk2. *Biochemical Society Transactions, 49*(2), 551–562. DOI: 10.1042/BST20190236 PMID: 33769432

Sorokina, M., Merseburger, P., Rajan, K., Yirik, M. A., & Steinbeck, C. (2021). COCONUT online: Collection of Open Natural Products database. *Journal of Cheminformatics, 13*(1), 2. DOI: 10.1186/s13321-020-00478-9 PMID: 33423696

Springer, M., & Macleod, K. (2016). In Brief: Mitophagy: mechanisms and role in human disease. The Journal of Pathology, 240.

Srivastava, V., & Gross, E. (2023). Mitophagy-promoting agents and their ability to promote healthy aging. *Biochemical Society Transactions, 51*(5), 1811–1846. DOI: 10.1042/BST20221363 PMID: 37650304

Su, Z., Nie, Y., Huang, X., Zhu, Y., Feng, B., Tang, L., & Zheng, G. (2019). Mitophagy in hepatic insulin resistance: Therapeutic potential and concerns. *Frontiers in Pharmacology, 10*, 10. DOI: 10.3389/fphar.2019.01193 PMID: 31649547

Sun, N., Yun, J., Liu, J., Malide, D., Liu, C., Rovira, I., Holmström, K., Fergusson, M., Yoo, Y., Combs, C., & Finkel, T. (2015). Measuring In Vivo Mitophagy. *Molecular Cell, 60*(4), 685–696. DOI: 10.1016/j.molcel.2015.10.009 PMID: 26549682

Tan, Y., Chen, S., Zhong, J., Ren, J., & Dong, M. (2019). Mitochondrial Injury and Targeted Intervention in Septic Cardiomyopathy. *Current Pharmaceutical Design, 25*(18), 2060–2070. DOI: 10.2174/1381612825666190708155400 PMID: 31284854

Tsefou, E., & Ketteler, R. (2022). Targeting deubiquitinating enzymes (dubs) that regulate mitophagy via direct or indirect interaction with Parkin. *International Journal of Molecular Sciences, 23*(20), 12105. DOI: 10.3390/ijms232012105 PMID: 36292958

Um, J., Shin, D., Choi, S., Nathan, A., Kim, Y., Lee, D., Jeong, D., Kim, D., Kim, K., Kim, Y., Nah, J., Jeong, J., Yoo, E., Shin, H., Park, H., Jo, J., Cho, J., & Yun, J. (2024). Selective induction of Rab9-dependent alternative mitophagy using a synthetic derivative of isoquinoline alleviates mitochondrial dysfunction and cognitive deficits in Alzheimer's disease models. *Theranostics, 14*(1), 56–74. DOI: 10.7150/thno.88718 PMID: 38164158

Vara-Pérez, M., Felipe-Abrio, B., & Agostinis, P. (2019). Mitophagy in cancer: A tale of adaptation. *Cells*, *8*(5), 493. DOI: 10.3390/cells8050493 PMID: 31121959

Wang, H., Yan, X., Zhang, Y., Wang, P., Li, J., & Zhang, X. (2024). Mitophagy in Alzheimer's Disease: A Bibliometric Analysis from 2007 to 2022. *Journal of Alzheimer's Disease Reports*, *8*(1), 101–128. DOI: 10.3233/ADR-230139 PMID: 38312534

Wang, S., Long, H., Hou, L., Feng, B. Z., Wu, Y., Zeng, Y., Cai, J., Zhang, D., & Zhao, G. (2023). The mitophagy pathway and its implications in human diseases. *Signal Transduction and Targeted Therapy*, *8*(1), 8. DOI: 10.1038/s41392-023-01503-7 PMID: 37582956

Wang, Y., Liu, N., & Lu, B. (2019). Mechanisms and roles of mitophagy in neurodegenerative diseases. *CNS Neuroscience & Therapeutics*, *25*(7), 859–875. DOI: 10.1111/cns.13140 PMID: 31050206

Wang, Y., Tang, C., Cai, J., Chen, G., Zhang, D., Zhang, Z., … & Dong, Z. (2018). Pink1/parkin-mediated mitophagy is activated in cisplatin nephrotoxicity to protect against kidney injury. Cell Death &Amp; Disease, 9(11)

Wu, B., Chang, N., Xi, H., Xiong, J., Zhou, Y., Wu, Y., Wu, S., Wang, N., Yi, H., Song, Y., Chen, L., & Zhang, J. (2021). PHB2 promotes tumorigenesis via RACK1 in non-small cell lung cancer. *Theranostics*, *11*(7), 3150–3166. DOI: 10.7150/thno.52848 PMID: 33537079

Wu, H., Wang, Y., Li, W., Chen, H., Du, L., Liu, D., Wang, X., Xu, T., Liu, L., & Chen, Q. (2019). Deficiency of mitophagy receptor fundc1 impairs mitochondrial quality and aggravates dietary-induced obesity and metabolic syndrome. *Autophagy*, *15*(11), 1882–1898. DOI: 10.1080/15548627.2019.1596482 PMID: 30898010

Wu, X., Zheng, Y., Liu, M., Li, Y. S., Tang, W., Yan, W., Cao, M., Zheng, W., Jiang, L., Wu, J., Han, F., Qin, Z., Fang, L., Hu, W., Chen, Z., & Zhang, X. (2020). BNIP3L/NIX degradation leads to mitophagy deficiency in ischemic brains. *Autophagy*, *17*(8), 1934–1946. DOI: 10.1080/15548627.2020.1802089 PMID: 32722981

Xiao, D., Zhang, L., & Wang, J. (2019). The role of parkin-mediated mitophagy in cardiovascular diseases. *International Journal of Sciences*, *8*(05), 25–29. DOI: 10.18483/ijSci.2049

Xie, C., Zhuang, X., Niu, Z., Ai, R., Lautrup, S., Zheng, S., Jiang, Y., Han, R., Gupta, T., Cao, S., Lagartos-Donate, M., Cai, C., Xie, L., Caponio, D., Wang, W., Schmauck-Medina, T., Zhang, J., Wang, H., Lou, G., & Fang, E. (2022). Amelioration of Alzheimer's disease pathology by mitophagy inducers identified via machine learning and a cross-species workflow. *Nature Biomedical Engineering*, *6*(1), 76–93. DOI: 10.1038/s41551-021-00819-5 PMID: 34992270

Xie, C., Zhuang, X. X., Niu, Z., Ai, R., Lautrup, S., Zheng, S., Jiang, Y., Han, R., Gupta, T. S., Cao, S., Lagartos-Donate, M. J., Cai, C. Z., Xie, L. M., Caponio, D., Wang, W. W., Schmauck-Medina, T., Zhang, J., Wang, H. L., Lou, G., & Fang, E. F. (2022). Amelioration of Alzheimer's disease pathology by mitophagy inducers identified via machine learning and a cross-species workflow. *Nature Biomedical Engineering*, *6*(1), 76–93. DOI: 10.1038/s41551-021-00819-5 PMID: 34992270

Xu, Y., Shen, J., & Ran, Z. (2020). Emerging views of mitophagy in immunity and autoimmune diseases. *Autophagy*, *16*(1), 17–3. DOI: 10.1080/15548627.2019.1603547 PMID: 30951392

Yamashita, S., Sugiura, Y., Matsuoka, Y., Maeda, R., Inoue, K., Furukawa, K., Fukuda, T., Chan, D., & Kanki, T. (2024). Mitophagy mediated by BNIP3 and NIX protects against ferroptosis by downregulating mitochondrial reactive oxygen species. *Cell Death and Differentiation*, *31*(5), 651–661. DOI: 10.1038/s41418-024-01280-y PMID: 38519771

Yang, P., Shuai, W., Wang, X., Hu, X., Zhao, M., Wang, A., Wu, Y., Liang, O., & Wang, G. (2025). Mitophagy in Neurodegenerative Diseases: Mechanisms of Action and the Advances of Drug Discovery. *Journal of Medicinal Chemistry*, *68*(4), 3970–3994. DOI: 10.1021/acs.jmedchem.4c01779 PMID: 39908485

Yang, X., Pan, W., Xu, G., & Chen, L. (2019). Mitophagy: a crucial modulator in the pathogenesis of chronic diseases.. Clinica chimica acta; international journal of clinical chemistry.

Yuan, Y., Zheng, Y., Zhang, X., Chen, Y., Wu, X., Wu, J., Shen, Z., Jiang, L., Wang, L., Yang, W., Luo, J., Qin, Z., Hu, W., & Chen, Z. (2017). BNIP3L/NIX-mediated mitophagy protects against ischemic brain injury independent of PARK2. *Autophagy*, *13*(10), 1754–1766. DOI: 10.1080/15548627.2017.1357792 PMID: 28820284

Zhang, J., & Ney, P. (2009). Role of BNIP3 and NIX in cell death, autophagy, and mitophagy. *Cell Death and Differentiation*, *16*(7), 939–946. DOI: 10.1038/cdd.2009.16 PMID: 19229244

Zhang, R., Lu, J., Pei, G., & Huang, S. (2023). Galangin rescues Alzheimer's amyloid-β induced mitophagy and brain organoid growth impairment. *International Journal of Molecular Sciences*, *24*(4), 3398. DOI: 10.3390/ijms24043398 PMID: 36834819

Zhang, T., Liu, Q., Gao, W., Sehgal, S., & Wu, H. (2021). The multifaceted regulation of mitophagy by endogenous metabolites. *Autophagy*, *18*(6), 1216–1239. DOI: 10.1080/15548627.2021.1975914 PMID: 34583624

Zhang, Z., Chen, Z., Liu, R., Liang, Q., Peng, Z., Yin, S., Tang, J., Gong, T., & Liu, Y. (2020). Bcl-2 Proteins Regulate Mitophagy in Lipopolysaccharide-Induced Acute Lung Injury via PINK1/Parkin Signaling Pathway. *Oxidative Medicine and Cellular Longevity*, *2020*, 2020. DOI: 10.1155/2020/6579696 PMID: 32148654

Zheng, R., Yao, Q., Xie, G., Du, S., Ren, C., Wang, Y., & Yuan, Y. (2015). Tat-odd-p53 enhances the radiosensitivity of hypoxic breast cancer cells by inhibiting parkin-mediated mitophagy. *Oncotarget*, *6*(19), 17417–17429. DOI: 10.18632/oncotarget.4002 PMID: 26025927

Zhou, H., He, L., Xu, G., & Chen, L. (2020). Mitophagy in cardiovascular disease.. Clinica chimica acta; international journal of clinical chemistry

Zhou, H., Zhang, Y., Hu, S., Chen, S., Zhu, P., Ma, Q., & Chen, Y. (2017). Melatonin protects cardiac microvasculature against ischemia/reperfusion injury via suppression of mitochondrial fission-vdac1-hk2-mptp-mitophagy axis. *Journal of Pineal Research*, *63*(1), e12413. DOI: 10.1111/jpi.12413 PMID: 28398674

Chapter 8
A Mechanistic Elucidation of Mitophagy in Colitis-Associated Cancer

C. Yasmin
https://orcid.org/0009-0009-7129-4644
B.S. Abdur Rahman Crescent Institute of Science and Technology, India

Ashok Kumar Pandurangan
https://orcid.org/0000-0003-2824-1757
B.S. Abdur Rahman Crescent Institute of Science and Technology, India

ABSTRACT

Understanding the pathogenesis of CAC is paramount to developing effective therapeutic strategies. \ Mitophagy, a cellular process involved in the selective degradation of damaged mitochondria, has emerged as a promising area of research in CAC. Dysregulation of mitophagy pathways contributes to disease progression, highlighting its potential as a therapeutic target. Additionally, natural products derived from various sources have shown promise in preclinical studies for their anti-inflammatory and anti-cancer properties. However, further research is warranted to elucidate their mechanisms of action and evaluate their clinical efficacy in CAC management. This review aims to provide a comprehensive overview of the current understanding of CAC pathogenesis, available therapies, challenges in treatment, and the potential roles of mitophagy regulation and natural products in improving patient outcomes.

DOI: 10.4018/979-8-3693-3836-0.ch008

INTRODUCTION

IBD is an extensive disease with an unknown cause. However, it is thought that the pathophysiology of IBD includes an interaction of environmental, genetic, and immunological variables (Niu et al., 2013). Normal intestinal bacteria may activate the immune system, resulting in chronic inflammation in the gut. The most common clinical symptoms are stomach discomfort, diarrhea, mucous, bloody, and purulent stools, recurring bouts, and relapse (Velayos et al., 2007). UC and CD are the two primary subtypes of IBD. Both are chronic and inflammatory disorders of the gastrointestinal tract, with an increasing prevalence associated with national industrialization and rising in developing countries (Molodecky et al., 2012). Although the exact cause of IBD is unknown, the pro-inflammatory cytokine imbalances including those in Tumor Necrosis Factor (TNF-α), Interferon-gamma (IFN-γ), Interleukin (IL)-1β, IL-6, and IL-12, and anti-inflammatory cytokines like those in IL-4, IL-10, and IL-11 are thought to be crucial in controlling inflammation (Ardizzone and Porro, 2005; Ślebioda and Kmieć, 2014) .Individuals suffering from these conditions have a 10–20 times increased risk of colon or bowel cancer (de Mattos et al., 2015). UC is an idiopathic illness defined by intestinal inflammation brought on by the transmural invasion of neutrophils, macrophages, monocytes, lymphocytes, and oxygen-free radicals produced in excess, which disrupt the mucosa and cause ulceration (Bouma et al., 2003). Untreated chronic colitis is thought to increase the risk of CAC (Pandurangan and Esa, 2014). Immunological dysregulation is a result of CD, while immunological responses to UC produce intestinal damage (Jaramillo et al., 203). Chron's illness Strictures, fistulas, and a higher chance of colon blockage are possible complications. Additionally, there is a link between CD and a higher risk of colorectal cancer (CRC) (Ha et al., 2015).

In the US, CRC ranks third in terms of cancer diagnoses as well as cancer-related deaths for both men and women. On the other hand, it is the leading cause of mortality for males under 50 and ranks second overall in cancer-related fatalities (Sawicki et al., 2021). Bowel cancer, or CRC is a cancer that can attack the colon or the rectum. Precancerous polyps in the colon or rectum's lining are often the starting point, and they have the potential to grow into malignant tumors over time. One of the most prevalent malignancies in the world, colorectal cancer is impacted by several variables, such as age, genetics, lifestyle, and certain medical problems (Shah et al., 2022). Especially, connected to chronic colon inflammation, which is frequently connected to inflammatory bowel disorders, is CAC. People who have CD or UC, particularly those who experience prolonged and severe inflammation, are more likely to acquire colitis-associated malignancy. Both types of surveillance are often performed; colonoscopies assist in stopping colorectal cancer in CRC patients from progressing, and in CAC patients, dysplasia or malignancy is managed (Dan et al., 2023).

All eukaryotic cells have mitochondria, an essential organelle that acts as the center of cellular energy. Here, cells perform aerobic respiration and make use of oxidative adenosine triphosphate (ATP) created by phosphorylation (Nunnari and Suomalainen, 2012). Unfortunately, mitochondria are easily damaged, which can result in mitochondrial dysfunction and the breakdown of cellular homeostasis. These conditions are closely linked to the development of a wide range of illnesses, including infections, cancer, heart disease, neurological disorders, and metabolic diseases (Doblado et al., 2021). Key metabolic versatility, required for a wide range of cell functions, is provided by the eukaryotic cell's ability to control mitochondrial activity (Martínez Reyeset al., 2020). Therefore, proper co-regulation of processes that regulate mitochondrial turnover—mitophagy, which gets rid of damaged or superfluous mitochondria—and mitochondrial biogenesis, which makes new mitochondria, is essential for maintaining mitochondrial function (Kim et al., 2007). A lack of mitophagy causes a build-up of damaged or poorly functioning mitochondria, which are unable to synthesize as much ATP^+ and release large amounts of superoxide. This may have pathogenic repercussions by changing the cellular reservoirs of intermediate metabolites (Bakula & Scheibye-Knudsen, 2020). A well-known indicator of metabolic and neurological disorders, poorly functioning mitochondria are closely associated with pathological advancements. Key mitophagy regulator activity changes are essential to these processes. Understanding the mechanisms of CAC progression is essential to improve treatment. Mitochondria serve as the powerhouse for healthy cells, playing a vital role in energy production. However, in tumor cells, there is a notable reduction in energy production by the mitochondria, and metabolic reprogramming emerges as an early hallmark of cancer (Yin et al., 2021). Exploring these alterations in mitochondrial function and cellular metabolism offers valuable insights for developing targeted interventions and advancing the treatment strategies for colitis-associated cancer.

Inflammatory Bowel Diseases

Over the past 50 years, the risk of IBD has increased in developed nations (Molodecky et al., 2012) with Australia having one of the highest incidence rates in the world (29.3 per 100,000 people) (Wilson et al., 2010). However, in industrialized nations, this sharp increase has leveled down within the last ten years (Niewiadomski et al., 2015). Currently, there has been a noticeable increase in occurrence in developing regions of the world, such as Asia.

Interactions between genetic and environmental factors that impact immune responses lead to IBD (Seyedian et al., 2019). The term IBD refers to a collection of idiopathic gastrointestinal disorders marked by recurrent episodes of acute and chronic intestinal inflammation (Knigge, 2002). The involvement of environmental and genetic factors is highlighted by the extensive research conducted in this area, even if the primary cause of IBD is still not fully known. They are two methods to address the primary causes of IBD: 1. The human microbiota's immune response rate is accelerated when the mucous system is disrupted (Heyman et al., 2005). 2. Any alteration to the gut flora's composition or impairment of the epithelium's ability to function triggers the pathologic response in the healthy mucosal system. However, author noted that mucosal immunity, the microbiota of the colon, and the patient's vulnerability all affect in IBD (Podolsky, 2002). Some of the clinical symptoms of IBD are Bloody diarrhea, anemia, arthritis, abdominal pain, and pediatric growth abnormalities (Hugot et al., 2003).

CD and UC are the two main types of IBD, and each condition is unique in terms of both its histology and clinical manifestations. The diagnosis and treatment of patients with IBD are common challenges for primary care physicians, and the range of available medical treatments has increased significantly in recent times (Knigge, 2002).

Figure 1. Factors that promote IBD

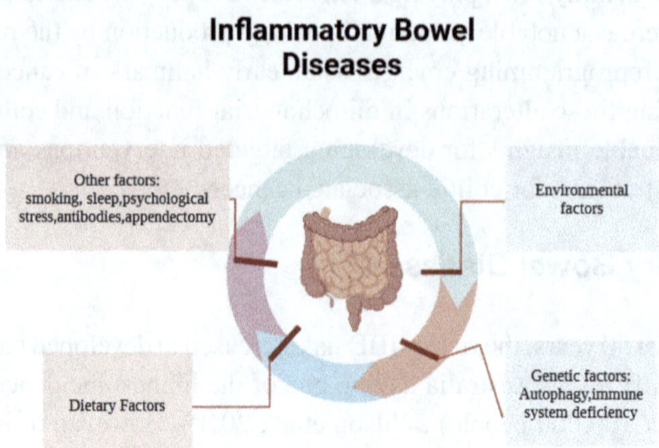

Different Forms of IBD

The gastrointestinal tract is affected by IBD, a chronic, relapsing illness that includes UC and CD (Wright et al., 2018). Even though CD and UC differ greatly from one another, gastrointestinal symptoms are a common feature of both conditions and affect 25–40% of IBD patients (Jose & Heyman, 2008). Among IBDs that affect people in the 15–35 age range is CD. In contrast to other inflammatory conditions, IBDs were difficult to inhibit. As a result, a portion of the gut is destroyed, and the immune system is activated. Among other symptoms, it induces fever, diarrhea, and discomfort. Apart from the severe impact on the lower section of the small intestine, CD can also arise in other digestive tract regions such as the stomach, esophagus, large intestine, or even the mouth (Gryboski, 1993). The mouth, the anus, and the intestines' whole layers are all impacted by CD. The mucosal layer of the colon is affected by UC. Both the gut and the rectum have lesions. Mild to severe symptoms that could endanger life are present (Seyedian et al., 2019). There are many similarities between UC and CD symptoms. Due to CD's damage to the small intestine, which oversees absorbing nutrients, malnutrition is a prevalent occurrence in patients with CD (Hampe et al., 2002). Severe pain, diarrhea, and blood in the stool are symptoms of ulcerative colitis, although severe cases of CD can also result in bleeding. While rectal bleeding is frequently associated with UC, it is less common in CD patients.

Over 50% of individuals with CD experience folate and vitamin D deficiency, whereas over 50% of individuals with UC experience iron deficiency (Burgmann et al., 2006). These disorders affect different parts of the digestive tract. For instance, the ileum and a portion of the large intestine are frequently affected by CD. The gastrointestinal tract (GI), which includes the mouth, esophagus, stomach, small intestine, rectum, and anus, can all be affected. Whereas UC is confined to the colon and mostly affects the colon and rectum, CD frequently causes inflammation in the small intestine. The small intestine functions normally in UC, but the large intestine becomes inflamed. Whereas CD affects the entire intestinal wall, UC only affects the colon's innermost portion.

Given that both UC and CD are significant forms of IBD, it may be argued that UC is linked to osteoporosis and may even be the cause of colon cancer if it persists for more than 8 to 10 years, while CD can lead to substantial complications, especially regarding skin and biliary stones. Many CD related symptoms include stomach pain and issues including fistulas and rectal ulcers. On the other hand, intermittent pain that is consistent with bowel motions is typically experienced by those who have UC (Mehdizadeh et al., 2007). Adults and children are both impacted. 2.6 million persons in Europe and 1.2 million in North America are thought to be affected by UC (Yang et al., 2015). Of these patients, about 25% receive a diagnosis prior to becoming 18 years old. Twenty percent or less of IBD patients are under twenty years old, and the disease frequently manifests in adolescence (Baldassano & Piccoli, 1999). Thus, the diagnosis of UC is based on clinical, endoscopic, histologic, and radiographic testing. Seven to ten percent of IBDs are uncertain (Cummings et al., 2008 & Tremaine, 2011). The research states that UC illness is a mucosal inflammation limited to the colon that is often characterized by tenesmus, diarrhea, and abdominal pain. One of the more common dysbiosis disorders is inflammatory bowel disease. UC was the first subtype of IBD to be recognized as a separate and distinct entity; the name IBD encompasses the features of both CD and UC. Although it has long been challenging to differentiate between these two conditions, each now has a clinical definition. Patients' lives in particular domains, including work, education, social life, and family life, may be impacted by both illnesses (Guindi, 2004).

Colitis-Associated Cancer

Worldwide, CRC is the second most frequent cancer in women and the third most common in males. The primary risk factor for its development is chronic inflammation, which increases the turnover of epithelial cells in the colonic mucosa, which promotes neoplastic transformation (Colotta et al., 2009). CD and UC are two IBD that are linked to a higher risk of CRC. Several immunological signaling pathways have been connected in recent years to CAC, partly because appropriate preclinical models are now readily available. Among these, it has been demonstrated that oxidative stress-induced mutations resulting from persistent intestinal inflammation promote the start of tumors (Waldner & Neurath, 2015).

Chronic inflammation is essential for the development of CAC associated with colitis, especially because it promotes neoplastic transformation in the colonic mucosa as a result of increased epithelial cell turnover (Grivennikov, 2012). Recent studies have shed light on the complex immune signaling pathways in CAC, highlighting the association between inflammatory bowel conditions such as CD and UC and an increased risk of CRC. Notably, persistent intestinal inflammation-induced oxidative stress mutations have been found to be important initiators of tumor growth in CAC (Waldner & Neurath, 2015). Many immunological signaling pathways are involved in the pathophysiology of CAC, with an emphasis on how chronic inflammation promotes the development of tumors (Sobczak et al., 2014). Research has revealed the intricate relationship between inflammation and the development of cancer by linking mutations in genes such as COX2, MyD88, IL-18, and parts of inflammasomes to CAC carcinogenesis. Furthermore, the impact of cytokines such as IL-6, IL-17, IL-23, and IL-21 on immune cell-to-cancer cell signaling and tumorigenicity in CAC models 3 has been studied, underscoring their regulatory role in the tumor microenvironment. It is essential to comprehend these basic pathways to create specific treatments and preventative measures for CAC patients (Grivennikov, 2012).

History of Colitis-Associated Cancer

In 2001, study conducted as the first extensive meta-analysis to investigate the risk of CRC in patients with IBD. This study found a CRC risk of 2% at 10 years after UC diagnosis and 8% at 20 years (Yalchin et al., 2021). Subsequent research in 2023 discovered a CRC frequency rate of 1.78% across all IBD patients, indicating a prevalence of 1780 instances per 100,000 IBD cases (Abu-Freha et al., 2023). UC patients have a higher chance of developing CRC, estimated at 2% after 10 years and 8% after 20 years (Lakatos & Lakatos, 2008). In terms of survival rates, a study by Sasaki et al. in 2018 revealed a 5-year survival percentage of 46.2% for CD associated cancer compared with 89% for UC-associated cancer (Kameyama et al., 2018).

Molecular Mechanism of CAC

CAC, also known as colorectal cancer, is a type of cancer that develops in individuals with ulcerative colitis, the most common form of IBD. In more than one-third of people with IBD, CAC is a serious side effect (Sobczak et al., 2014). Numerous complicated variables, such as genetic mutations, epigenetic modifications, chronic inflammation, and changes in immune response components, are involved in the pathogenesis of CAC (Li et al., 2023). Patients with IBD have oxidative stress in their colonic mucosa, which can lead to DNA damage and mutations that can accelerate the growth of malignancies (Waldner & Neurath, 2015). Compared to sporadic colon cancer, the mutational landscape of CAC is different, with fewer mutations in important genes such as APC seen in both low-grade and high-grade dysplasia in CAC patients. The ongoing inflammatory environment in CAC is thought to be a key factor in the development of tumors because it can stabilize β-catenin, which encourages unchecked cell proliferation that is typical of cancer expansion (Davies et al., 2016). Significantly, inflammation plays a role in the development and progression of CAC. The higher cell turnover linked to inflammation may also raise the frequencies of mutations, and reactive oxygen species produced during intestinal inflammation can cause DNA damage and mutations. Additionally, signaling pathways such as NF-κB and STAT show the loss of APC observed in sporadic colon cancer while simultaneously shielding cells from inflammation-induced apoptosis (Davies et al., 2016). The CAC tumor microenvironment is intricate, involving a range of immune cells that engage in interactions with the tumor cells. Natural killer (NK) cells, macrophages, dendritic cells (DCs), T and B lymphocytes, myeloid-derived suppressor cells (MDSCs), neutrophils, and macrophages all have different functions in either stimulating or inhibiting the formation of tumors in CACs. In individuals with CAC, the balance between pro- and anti-tumorigenic immune responses inside the tumor microenvironment affects how the disease progresses and how well they respond to treatment (Li et al., 2023).

Figure 2. Molecular mechanism of colitis-associated cancer

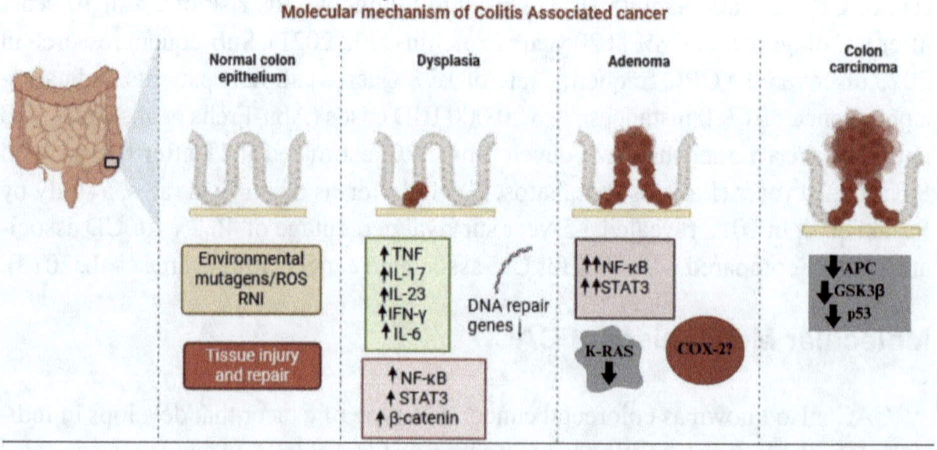

Therapies Available in CAC

CAC or CRC, is a deadly disease caused by chronic inflammation of the colon and rectum. The key challenge in treating CAC is that the disease is heterogeneous, making it difficult to develop effective medicines. Currently, numerous medicines are available to treat colitis-associated cancer. Surgery is the primary therapeutic option for CAC. It involves removing the infected section of the colon and, in some situations, the surrounding lymph nodes. Surgery is favorable because it can successfully remove cancerous tissue, perhaps curing the disease. However, there are certain downsides to surgery. It is an intrusive procedure that can result in bleeding, infection, and organ damage. Chemotherapy is another treatment option for cancers linked with colitis. Chemotherapy is a drug-based treatment that kills and prevents cancer cells from growing. Chemotherapy has various advantages when treating CAC. For example, chemotherapy may target cancer cells all around the body, making it beneficial for both primary and metastatic cancers. Furthermore, chemotherapy can be used in conjunction with surgery to improve results and minimize the likelihood of cancer recurrence. However, there are certain downsides to chemotherapy. One disadvantage is that chemotherapy medications can cause serious side effects such as nausea, hair loss, and a weakened immune system (Arnold et al., 2020).

Some of the most common chemo-preventive drugs against CAC are 5-Fluorouracil (5-FU), Capecitabine (Xeloda), Irinotecan (Camptosar), Oxaliplatin (Eloxatin) & Trifluridine and tipiracil (Lonsurf) (Van Schaeybroeck et al., 2014). Other common therapies for CAC include a range of approaches aimed at managing this condition effectively are

5-ASA Compounds: Amino salicylates (5-ASA) are the oldest therapies used to manage IBD, and they remain the effective first-line treatment for mild to moderate UC and maintenance of remission. 5-ASA has chemo-preventive effects due to its direct anticarcinogenic and anti-inflammatory effects. It modulates proteins controlling the cell cycle, inhibits molecules regulating angiogenesis, scavenges molecules that increase DNA oxidative stress, and reduces β-catenin accumulation in APC-mutated cells. It also suppresses the Wnt/β-catenin pathway and induces cell cycle stop or apoptosis in carcinomatous cells. A recent meta-analysis showed a reduced risk of advanced colorectal neoplasia in patients treated with 5-ASA (Nardone et al., 2023).

Corticosteroids: Corticosteroids, steroid hormones produced in the adrenal cortex, have been used to treat IBD since the 1950s. However, they have side effects like increased death risk and may be dependent on elderly patients. Common corticosteroids include prednisolone, methylprednisolone, hydrocortisone, budesonide, budesonide MMX, and beclomethasone dipropionate. Currently, corticosteroids are only recommended for patients with 5-ASA refractory UC (Dorrington et al., 2020).

Immunomodulator: Immunomodulators are effective in treating IBD, with Thiopurines, Methotrexate, and Cyclosporine being the main options. Thiopurines are used to maintain long-term remission in steroid-dependent IBD, particularly UC. Methotrexate, an alternative to thiopurines, improves IBD by reducing T-cell activation and blocking IL-1β binding. However, it is less effective than thiopurines and biological agents. Cyclosporine, another immunomodulatory agent, improves IBD by inhibiting IL-2, TNF-α, and IFN-γ production, T-cell proliferation, and overall immune response. However, it is only indicated for remission of refractory acute severe UC (Zhou et al., 2023).

Biological Agents: Clinical IBD therapy primarily uses biologics like TNF-α inhibitors, anti-adhesion molecules, anti-interleukin drugs, Janus kinase inhibitors, and Sphingosine 1 Phosphate Receptor Modulator. These agents offer a unique therapeutic approach to reduce intestinal inflammation but are not recommended for oral administration due to their high sensitivity to the stomach and intestine environment and safety concerns. They are not universally applicable to all IBD patients, so appropriate therapy is provided on a case-by-case basis (Zhou et al., 2023).

Stem cell transplantation therapy: Stem cell transplantation therapy is used to improve symptoms in patients with IBD when conventional treatments are ineffective. It can be divided into hematopoietic stem cell transplantation (HSCT) and mesenchymal stem cell transplantation (MSCT). HSCT is safer but has a high risk of recurrence due to its self-generated graft. Allogeneic transplantation can genetically alter the patient's genetic susceptibility but has a high lethality rate. Allogeneic transplantation seems to cure IBD patients with IL-10 gene defects. MSCT can repair damaged intestinal tissues, reduce inflammation, and improve microcirculation. It has low immunogenicity, does not require chemotherapy, and has a low risk of serious complications. However, stem cell transplantation is a relatively new method and more research is needed to determine its safety and therapeutic effectiveness (Zhou et al., 2023).

Fecal Microbiota Transplantation: FMT is an alternative therapy for IBD, involving the injection of a liquid fecal suspension from a healthy donor into the gastrointestinal tract of patients. This restores intestinal microbial function and can help treat bacterial infections, such as C. difficile, which are common in IBD patients. FMT is considered safe, especially in treating IBD without C. difficile infection and no serious adverse events were reported. It can be a safe and effective treatment when conventional therapies are not effective (Zhou et al., 2023).

Helminth Therapy: Helminths have been found to have a lower risk of developing IBD, with IBD being uncommon in areas where most people carry helminths. The beneficial effect of helminths on patients with IBD was confirmed in animal experiments and human experiments. Helminths can help IBD by influencing intestinal luminal alterations, altering immune responses, controlling neuroendocrine responses, and generating immunosuppressive agents. Helminth treatment is more effective in treating Th1-dominated IBD. However, the therapeutic effect of IBD associated with Th1 is unclear. Helminth therapy is not a mainstream therapy due to unclear therapeutic action pathways, mixed action relationships, and limited animal studies (Zhou et al., 2023).

Challenges and Problems in Current Therapy for CAC

In recent years, CAC has become a significant concern in the field of oncology. This type of cancer is associated with chronic IBD, such as UC and CD. Patients with these conditions have a significantly increased risk of developing colon cancer compared to the general population. Current therapies for treating CAC face a number of challenges and problems, which need to be addressed in order to improve patient outcomes. Historically, the link between chronic inflammation and cancer has been recognized for many years. The concept of inflammation contributing to cancer development was first proposed by Rudolf Virchow in the 19th century. He observed that tumors often develop at sites of chronic inflammation, leading to the hypothesis that inflammation plays a role in cancer initiation and progression. This idea has since been supported by numerous studies showing that chronic inflammation can promote tumor growth through various mechanisms, such as DNA damage, gene mutations, and immune suppression (Van Der Kraak, 2015).

Despite advances in the understanding of CAC, current therapies for treating this condition face several challenges and problems. One of the main issues is the lack of effective treatments for advanced or metastatic disease. Patients with CAC often have poorer outcomes compared to those with sporadic CRC, due to the aggressive nature of the disease and limited treatment options. Another challenge in treating CAC is the difficulty in diagnosing the condition at an early stage. Patients with IBD are already at increased risk of developing colon cancer, but it can be challenging to differentiate between inflammatory changes and early neoplastic lesions on colonoscopy. This can lead to delays in diagnosis and treatment, resulting in poorer outcomes for patients with CAC (Braillon, 2012).

Additionally, current therapies for CAC often have limited efficacy and significant side effects. Chemotherapy and radiation therapy, which are commonly used to treat colorectal cancer, may be less effective in patients with CAC due to the underlying inflammation in the colon. Moreover, these treatments can cause substantial toxicity and may not be well tolerated by patients with pre-existing IBD.

Influential Individuals in the Field of CAC

In addition to Dr. Robert E. Schoen, there are several other influential individuals who have contributed to the field of CAC. Dr. Steven Itzkowitz, a gastroenterologist and researcher, has conducted important studies on the risk factors and screening strategies for CAC. His work has highlighted the importance of early detection and surveillance in patients with IBD to prevent the development of colon cancer. Dr. Francis Chan, a leading oncologist and expert in gastrointestinal cancers, has also made significant contributions to the field of CAC. His research on the molecular mechanisms of inflammation-driven carcinogenesis has shed light on the pathogenesis of CAC and has informed the development of targeted therapies for this condition (Itzkowitz & Yio, 2004).

Overall, the challenges and problems in current therapy for treating CAC are multifaceted and require a comprehensive approach. By addressing the limitations of existing treatments, improving early detection and surveillance strategies, and developing targeted therapies based on the underlying mechanisms of inflammation-driven carcinogenesis, researchers and clinicians can improve outcomes for patients with CAC in the future (Braillon, 2012).

Mitophagy Basics

Mitophagy is an important cellular process that involves the selective destruction of damaged mitochondria to preserve cellular homeostasis. It has an important role in a variety of physiological processes, including aging, neurological disorders, and cancer. Dysregulation of mitophagy has been linked to the development of numerous illnesses, including colitis-associated cancer (Doblado et al., 2021). Damaged mitochondria must be segregated and selectively eliminated right away. Mitochondrial autophagy helps destroy defective mitochondria and maintain a balanced mitochondrial environment. Christian de Duve coined the word "autophagy" about 60 years ago after observing the breakdown of mitochondria and intracellular structures in rat liver lysosomes (Deter & De Duve, 1967). In 2016, Japanese scientist Yoshinori Ohsumi was awarded the Nobel Prize in Physiology or Medicine for "discovering the autophagy mechanism of cells" (Nakatogawa et al., 2009; Ohsumi, 2013). Through extensive research, scientists have obtained a better understanding of autophagy, including selective autophagy like mitophagy. Recent advancements in the study of "mitophagy" have led to the identification of key proteins responsible for mitochondrial degradation in yeast (Okamoto et al., 2009) and mammalian cells (Narendra et al., 2010 & Sandoval et al., 2008).

Figure 3. Timeline of research progress in mitophagy

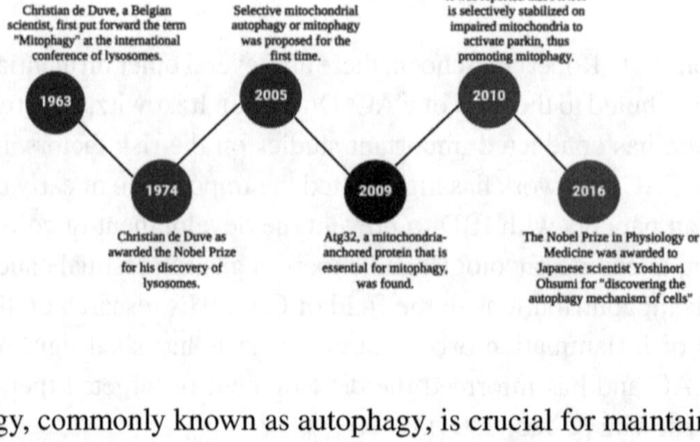

Mitophagy, commonly known as autophagy, is crucial for maintaining homeostasis in mitochondria and cells (Onishi et al., 2021). Stress factors such as reactive oxygen species (ROS), food deprivation, and cell aging can cause mitochondrial depolarization in cells. Cells use autophagy to selectively eliminate damaged or defective mitochondria, ensuring the stability of the mitochondrial network and intracellular environment. Mitophagy involves four stages (Xu et al., 2019):

1. Damaged mitochondria lose membrane potential due to ROS, nutritional shortage, cell aging, and other external stimuli, triggering mitophagy.
2. Autophagosomes wrap around mitochondria, forming mitochondrial autophagosomes. The double-membrane phagophores that surround the destroyed mitochondria commence and elongate. The phagophore is then encased in autophagosomes, which have two membranes.
3. Mitochondrial autophagosomes merge with lysosomes, delivering mitochondria for destruction.
4. Lysosomes break down mitochondrial contents. Lysosomal or vacuolar acid hydrolase degrades mitochondria in the autophagosome, which then recycles the contents.

A thorough investigation of mitophagy's molecular process can provide a theoretical foundation for treating disorders caused by malfunction. We explore the role of mitophagy in common disorders and highlight the need for novel modulators targeting this process. This review examines small molecule pharmacological modulators of mitophagy, which can shed light on disease mechanisms and aid in therapeutic development.

Mitophagy Regulation in CAC

Mitophagy, the selective degradation of damaged mitochondria in cells, has been gaining increasing attention in the field of cancer research, particularly in the context of CAC. Mitophagy serves as a crucial quality control mechanism in cells, ensuring the removal of dysfunctional mitochondria that can lead to oxidative stress and DNA damage. Dysregulation of mitophagy has been implicated in various diseases, including cancer, where impaired mitochondrial function can contribute to tumorigenesis. In the context of CAC, chronic inflammation resulting from IBD can predispose individuals to the development of CRC. Mitophagy has emerged as a key player in the link between inflammation and cancer, with studies suggesting that dysregulation of this process can promote tumorigenesis in the colon (Doblado et al., 2021).

Figure 4. Physiological functions of mitophagy in human diseases

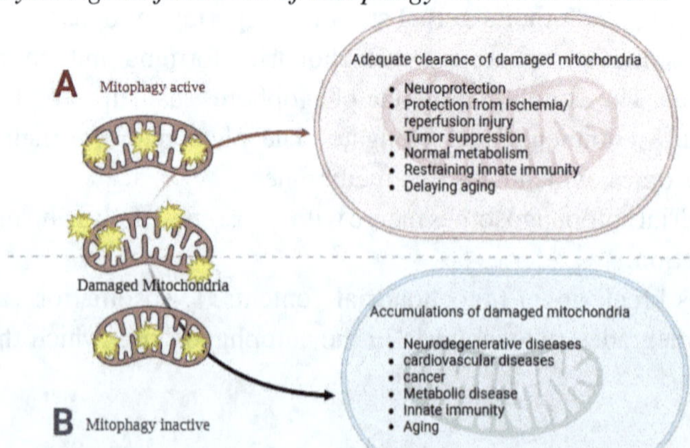

One of the groundbreaking studies in the field of mitophagy regulation in CAC was conducted by Liu et al. (2015), who demonstrated that the autophagy-related gene ATG5 plays a critical role in suppressing colitis-associated tumorigenesis through the regulation of mitochondrial homeostasis. This study provided important insights into the molecular mechanisms underlying mitophagy in the context of colon cancer and highlighted the potential therapeutic implications of targeting mitophagy in cancer treatment (Liu et al., 2023).

The regulation of mitophagy in CAC involves a complex interplay of signaling pathways and molecular mechanisms. One of the key regulators of mitophagy is the PTEN-induced putative kinase 1 (PINK1)/Parkin pathway, which facilitates the selective degradation of damaged mitochondria through the autophagy-lysosomal pathway. Activation of PINK1 in response to mitochondrial damage leads to the recruitment of Parkin to damaged mitochondria, marking them for degradation through mitophagy. Dysregulation of the PINK1/Parkin pathway has been implicated in various diseases, including cancer, highlighting its importance in maintaining mitochondrial quality control (Yin et al., 2021). In addition to the PINK1/Parkin pathway, other regulators of mitophagy in CAC include the AMP-activated protein kinase (AMPK) and the mammalian target of rapamycin (mTOR) signaling pathways. AMPK acts as a sensor of cellular energy status and plays a key role in coordinating mitochondrial biogenesis and function. Activation of AMPK has been shown to promote mitophagy in response to nutrient deprivation and oxidative stress, suggesting a potential link between metabolic reprogramming and mitophagy regulation in cancer (Wu et al., 2022). Conversely, the mTOR pathway has been implicated in the inhibition of autophagy, including mitophagy, through its role in regulating cellular growth and proliferation. Hyperactivation of mTOR signaling has been observed in various cancers, including CAC, where it can suppress autophagy and promote tumorigenesis. Targeting the mTOR pathway has thus emerged as a potential strategy for inducing mitophagy and inhibiting cancer cell growth in CAC (Xin, 2023).

Mitophagy regulation in CAC is a complex process with multiple pathways and molecular mechanisms. Understanding this link between mitochondrial dysfunction and tumorigenesis can lead to therapeutic potential in cancer treatment. Future research should focus on mitophagy's interaction with other cellular processes.

Natural Products Against CAC

CAC, a subtype of CRC, is a significant concern due to its increased risk in individuals suffering from IBD such as UC and CD. Research on natural products that have shown promising potential in preventing or treating CAC is crucial to developing effective therapeutic strategies. Natural products have long been a source of inspiration for drug discovery and development, with many plant-derived compounds showing promising anti-cancer properties. In the context of colitis-associated cancer, several natural products have been investigated for their potential benefits. One such natural product is curcumin, a compound found in turmeric. Curcumin has been shown to have anti-inflammatory and anti-cancer effects in preclinical studies on colitis-associated cancer (Wang et al., 2019).

Another natural product that has gained attention for its potential in CAC is resveratrol, a compound found in red grapes and wine. Resveratrol has been reported to have anti-inflammatory and anti-cancer effects through its ability to modulate various signaling pathways involved in carcinogenesis (Oliveira et al., 2020). Additionally, green tea extract containing polyphenols such as epigallocatechin gallate (EGCG) has been studied for its potential to prevent CAC by modulating oxidative stress and inflammation (Lambert et al., 2015). Furthermore, curcumin and resveratrol have been shown to synergistically inhibit the growth of CAC cells *in vitro* and *in vivo*, suggesting a potential combination therapy for this disease (Norollahi et al., 2021). These natural products offer hope for developing alternative or adjunct therapies for colitis-associated cancer patients. While the use of natural products in cancer therapy shows promise, there are also challenges and limitations that need to be addressed. One of the main issues is the lack of standardized formulations and dosages for natural products, which can lead to variations in efficacy and safety. Additionally, the bioavailability of some natural products can be limited, affecting their absorption and effectiveness in the body.

Pandurangan & Esa, (2014) determined that through its interactions with several inflammatory and carcinogenic signaling pathways, STAT3 plays a key role in the development of CAC. The cannabinoid O-1602, triptolide, aspirin, curcumin derivatives, prohibitin 1, and other substances and medications that block STAT3 activity were addressed. These substances and medications have demonstrated potential in reducing CAC-related tumor development and inflammation. Targeting this pathway presents a possible therapeutic approach, the scientists found, as STAT3 is typically unregulated in CAC and contributes to tumor formation. They underlined that creating medications that block STAT3 may help manage CAC, underscoring its potential as a crucial therapeutic target. (C. Liu et al., 2018) examined how experimental colitis in mice was affected by ginsenoside Rd, a naturally occurring chemical produced from ginseng. One important substance they found that has anti-inflammatory qualities and may help with colitis symptoms is Rd. The scientists showed through a series of tests that Rd substantially decreased colon damage, inflammation, and body weight loss, in part by preventing the NLRP3 inflammasome from activating. They came to the conclusion that Rd protects by activating p62-driven mitophagy through the AMPK/ULK1 pathway, which inhibits the activation of inflammasome and mitochondrial damage. According to these results, ginsenoside Rd shows promise as an anti-inflammatory drug for the treatment of IBD and may be further explored. According to a study, CRC caused by inflammation can be successfully inhibited by the tiny molecule andrographolide (Andro), which is extracted from the plant *Andrographis paniculata*. They discovered that Andro triggers mitophagy, a kind of autophagy that specifically eliminates damaged mitochondria and so inhibits the activation of the NLRP3 inflammasome, a major cause of inflammation. In cell cultures and mice models of colon cancer and colitis, their research demonstrated that Andro's promotion of mitophagy decreased inflammasome activity and the production of inflammatory cytokines including IL-1β. They also showed that Andro's protective properties were negated by inhibiting autophagy with drugs like chloroquine (CQ) or by mutating the BECN1 gene. The study found that Andro mainly inhibits the NLRP3 inflammasome via promoting mitophagy, which has anti-inflammatory and anticancer effects. It also indicated that Andro may be used as a treatment to stop CA (Guo et al., 2014). In research on CAC, the authors used UHPLC-MS/MS analysis to determine the components of Tong-Xie-Yao-Fang (TXYF), a traditional Chinese medication. Drugs such as azoxymethane and DSS were used in the study to cause CAC in mice, while sulfasalazine served as a control. By triggering mitophagy through the PINK1/Parkin pathway and reversing the epithelial-mesenchymal transition (EMT), they discovered that TXYF reduced tumor development and inflammation. The authors came to the conclusion that TXYF has the ability to treat CAC preventively, which is consistent with traditional Chinese medicine's focus on early intervention (Z. Xu et al., 2024).

Furthermore, natural products may interact with conventional cancer treatments or other medications, leading to potential side effects or reduced efficacy. Therefore, it is essential to conduct rigorous preclinical and clinical studies to evaluate the safety and efficacy of natural products in CAC.

CONCLUSION

IBD, including CD and UC, pose significant challenges to healthcare systems worldwide. These conditions are associated with debilitating symptoms and an increased risk of developing complications like CAC. Understanding the pathogenesis of CAC is crucial for developing effective therapeutic interventions. CAC has a complex history, originating from increased cancer risk in patients with chronic IBD. The pathogenesis involves chronic inflammation, genetic predisposition, and dysregulated cellular processes like mitophagy. In the context of CAC, dysregulation of mitophagy pathways can contribute to disease progression. Conventional therapies for CAC often face challenges such as treatment resistance, adverse side effects, and incomplete eradication of cancer cells. As a result, there is growing interest in exploring alternative treatment options, such as natural products. Natural compounds have shown potential therapeutic benefits in various diseases, including cancer, and have anti-inflammatory and anti-cancer properties. However, additional research is required to establish their clinical value. In a nutshell, understanding the pathogenesis of CAC is essential for developing effective therapeutic strategies. Mitophagy regulation is a promising area of research, offering insights into potential intervention targets. Natural products hold promise as adjunctive therapies in CAC management, but more research is needed to validate their clinical utility.

REFERENCES

Abu-Freha, N., Cohen, B., Gordon, M., Weissmann, S., Kestenbaum, E. H., Vosko, S., Abu-Tailakh, M., Ben-Shoshan, L., Cohen, D. L., & Shirin, H. (2023). Colorectal cancer among inflammatory bowel disease patients: Risk factors and prevalence compared to the general population. *Frontiers in Medicine*, *10*, 1225616. Advance online publication. DOI: 10.3389/fmed.2023.1225616 PMID: 37614949

Ardizzone, S., & Porro, G. B. (2005). Biologic therapy for inflammatory bowel disease. *Drugs*, *65*(16), 2253–2286. DOI: 10.2165/00003495-200565160-00002 PMID: 16266194

Arnold, M., Abnet, C. C., Neale, R. E., Vignat, J., Giovannucci, E. L., McGlynn, K. A., & Bray, F. (2020). Global burden of 5 major types of gastrointestinal cancer. *Gastroenterology*, *159*(1), 335–349.e15. DOI: 10.1053/j.gastro.2020.02.068 PMID: 32247694

Bakula, D., & Scheibye-Knudsen, M. (2020). Mitophagy in aging: Mitophagy in aging and disease. *Frontiers in Cell and Developmental Biology*, *8*, 239. DOI: 10.3389/fcell.2020.00239 PMID: 32373609

Baldassano, R. N., & Piccoli, D. A. (1999). Inflammatory bowel disease in pediatric and adolescent patients. *Gastroenterology Clinics of North America*, *28*(2), 445–458. DOI: 10.1016/S0889-8553(05)70064-9 PMID: 10372276

Bernstein, C. N. (2001). Extra bowel manifestations of inflammatory bowel disease. *Current Gastroenterology Reports*, *3*(6), 477–483. DOI: 10.1007/s11894-001-0068-6 PMID: 11696285

Bouma, G., & Strober, W. (2003). The immunological and genetic basis of inflammatory bowel disease. *Nature Reviews. Immunology*, *3*(7), 521–533. DOI: 10.1038/nri1132 PMID: 12876555

Braillon, A. (2012). Can surrogate end points from a first-round screening be reliable for colorectal cancer screening? *Gastroenterology*, *142*(3), e29. DOI: 10.1053/j.gastro.2011.11.056 PMID: 22281267

Burgmann, T., Clara, I., Graft, L., Walker, J., Lix, L., & Rawsthorne, P.. (2006). The Manitoba Inflammatory Bowel Disease Cohort study: Prolonged symptoms before diagnosis—how much is irritable bowel syndrome? *Clinical Gastroenterology and Hepatology*, *4*(5), 614–620. DOI: 10.1016/j.cgh.2006.03.003 PMID: 16630762

Colotta, F., Allavena, P., Sica, A., Garlanda, C., & Mantovani, A. (2009). Cancer-related inflammation, the seventh hallmark of cancer: Links to genetic instability. *Carcinogenesis*, *30*(7), 1073–1081. DOI: 10.1093/carcin/bgp127 PMID: 19468060

Cummings, J. F., Keshav, S., & Travis, S. P. (2008). Medical management of Crohn's disease. *BMJ (Clinical Research Ed.)*, *336*(7652), 1062–1066. DOI: 10.1136/bmj.39547.603218.AE PMID: 18467414

Dan, W. Y., Zhou, G. Z., Peng, L. H., & Pan, F. (2023). Update and latest advances in mechanisms and management of colitis-associated colorectal cancer. *World Journal of Gastrointestinal Oncology*, *15*(8), 1317–1331. DOI: 10.4251/wjgo.v15.i8.1317 PMID: 37663937

Davies, J. M., Santaolalla, R., & Abreu, M. T. (2016). Use of cancer stem cells to investigate the pathogenesis of colitis-associated cancer. *Inflammatory Bowel Diseases*, *22*(4), 976–983. DOI: 10.1097/MIB.0000000000000756 PMID: 26963566

de Mattos, B. R. R., Garcia, M. P. G., Nogueira, J. B., Paiatto, L. N., Albuquerque, C. G., Souza, C. K., Fernandes, L. G. R., Tamashiro, W. M. S. C., & Simioni, P. U. (2015). Inflammatory bowel disease: An overview of immune mechanisms and biological treatments. *Mediators of Inflammation*, *493012*(1), 493012. Advance online publication. DOI: 10.1155/2015/493012 PMID: 26339135

Deter, R. L., & De Duve, C. (1967). Influence of glucagon, an inducer of cellular autophagy, on some physical properties of rat liver lysosomes. *The Journal of Cell Biology*, *33*(2), 437–449. DOI: 10.1083/jcb.33.2.437 PMID: 4292315

Doblado, L., Lueck, C., Rey, C., Samhan-Arias, A. K., Prieto, I., Stacchiotti, A., & Monsalve, M. (2021). Mitophagy in human diseases. *International Journal of Molecular Sciences*, *22*(8), 3903. DOI: 10.3390/ijms22083903 PMID: 33918863

Doblado, L., Lueck, C., Rey, C., Samhan-Arias, A. K., Prieto, I., Stacchiotti, A., & Monsalve, M. (2021). Mitophagy in human diseases. *International Journal of Molecular Sciences*, *22*(8), 3903. DOI: 10.3390/ijms22083903 PMID: 33918863

Dorrington, A. M., Selinger, C. P., Parkes, G. C., Smith, M., Pollok, R. C., & Raine, T. (2020). The historical role and contemporary use of corticosteroids in inflammatory bowel disease. *Journal of Crohn's and Colitis*, *14*(9), 1316–1329. DOI: 10.1093/ecco-jcc/jjaa053 PMID: 32170314

Farmer, R. G., Hawk, W. A., & Turnbull, R. B.Jr. (1975). Clinical patterns in Crohn's disease: A statistical study of 615 cases. *Gastroenterology*, *68*(4), 627–635. DOI: 10.1016/S0016-5085(75)80270-8 PMID: 1123132

Grivennikov, S. I. (2013). Inflammation and colorectal cancer: Colitis-associated neoplasia. *Seminars in Immunopathology*, *35*(2), 229–244. DOI: 10.1007/s00281-012-0352-6 PMID: 23161445

Gryboski, J. D. (1993). Ulcerative colitis in children 10 years old or younger. *Journal of Pediatric Gastroenterology and Nutrition*, *17*(1), 24–31. DOI: 10.1097/00005176-199307000-00007 PMID: 8350209

Guindi, M., & Riddell, R. (2004). Indeterminate colitis. *Journal of Clinical Pathology*, *57*(12), 1233–1244. DOI: 10.1136/jcp.2003.015214 PMID: 15563659

Guo, W., Sun, Y., Liu, W., Wu, X., Guo, L., Cai, P., Wu, X., Wu, X., Shen, Y., Shu, Y., Gu, Y., & Xu, Q. (2014). Small molecule-driven mitophagy-mediated NLRP3 inflammasome inhibition is responsible for the prevention of colitis-associated cancer. *Autophagy*, *10*(6), 972–985. DOI: 10.4161/auto.28374 PMID: 24879148

Ha, F., & Khalil, H. (2015). Crohn's disease: A clinical update. *Therapeutic Advances in Gastroenterology*, *8*(6), 352–359. DOI: 10.1177/1756283X15592585 PMID: 26557891

Hampe, J., Grebe, J., Nikolaus, S., Solberg, C., Croucher, P. J., Mascheretti, S., Jahnsen, J., Moum, B., Klump, B., Krawczak, M., Mirza, M. M., Foelsch, U. R., Vatn, M., & Schreiber, S. (2002). Association of NOD2 (CARD 15) genotype with clinical course of Crohn's disease: A cohort study. *Lancet*, *359*(9318), 1661–1665. DOI: 10.1016/S0140-6736(02)08590-2 PMID: 12020527

Heyman, M. B., Kirschner, B. S., Gold, B. D., Ferry, G., Baldassano, R., Cohen, S. A., Winter, H. S., Fain, P., King, C., Smith, T., & El-Serag, H. B. (2005). Children with early-onset inflammatory bowel disease (IBD): Analysis of a pediatric IBD consortium registry. *The Journal of Pediatrics*, *146*(1), 35–40. DOI: 10.1016/j.jpeds.2004.08.043 PMID: 15644819

Hugot, J. P., Corinne, A., Dominique, B., Edouard, B., & Cezard, J. P. (2003). Crohn's disease: The cold chain hypothesis. *Lancet*, *362*(9400), 2012–2015. DOI: 10.1016/S0140-6736(03)15024-6 PMID: 14683664

Itzkowitz, S. H., & Yio, X. (2004). Inflammation and cancer IV. Colorectal cancer in inflammatory bowel disease: The role of inflammation. *American Journal of Physiology. Gastrointestinal and Liver Physiology*, *287*(1), G7–G17. DOI: 10.1152/ajpgi.00079.2004 PMID: 15194558

Jaramillo, A. P., Awosusi, B. L., Ayyub, J., Dabhi, K. N., Gohil, N. V., Tanveer, N., Hussein, S., Pingili, S., & Makkena, V. K. (2023). Effectiveness of fecal microbiota transplantation treatment in patients with recurrent *Clostridium difficile* infection, ulcerative colitis, and Crohn's disease: A systematic review. *Cureus*, *15*(7), e42120. DOI: 10.7759/cureus.42120 PMID: 37602044

Kameyama, H., Nagahashi, M., Shimada, Y., Tajima, Y., Ichikawa, H., Nakano, M., Sakata, J., Kobayashi, T., Narayanan, S., Takabe, K., & Wakai, T. (2018). Genomic characterization of colitis-associated colorectal cancer. *World Journal of Surgical Oncology*, *16*(1), 121. DOI: 10.1186/s12957-018-1428-0 PMID: 29966533

Kim, I., Rodriguez-Enriquez, S., & Lemasters, J. J. (2007). Selective degradation of mitochondria by mitophagy. *Archives of Biochemistry and Biophysics*, *462*(2), 245–253. DOI: 10.1016/j.abb.2007.03.034 PMID: 17475204

Knigge, K. L. (2002). Inflammatory bowel disease. *Clinical Cornerstone*, *4*(4), 49–60. DOI: 10.1016/S1098-3597(02)90005-0 PMID: 12739326

Lakatos, P. L., & Lakatos, L. (2008). Risk for colorectal cancer in ulcerative colitis: Changes, causes and management strategies. *World Journal of Gastroenterology*, *14*(25), 3937–3947. DOI: 10.3748/wjg.14.3937 PMID: 18609676

Lambert, J. D., Hong, J., Yang, G. Y., Liao, J., & Yang, C. S. (2005). Inhibition of carcinogenesis by polyphenols: Evidence from laboratory investigations. *The American Journal of Clinical Nutrition*, *81*(1, Suppl), 284S–291S. DOI: 10.1093/ajcn/81.1.284S PMID: 15640492

Li, J., Ji, Y., Chen, N., Dai, L., & Deng, H. (2023). Colitis-associated carcinogenesis: Crosstalk between tumors, immune cells and gut microbiota. *Cell & Bioscience*, *13*(1), 194. DOI: 10.1186/s13578-023-01139-8 PMID: 37875976

Liu, C., Wang, J., Yang, Y., Liu, X., Zhu, Y., Zou, J., Peng, S., Le, T. H., Chen, Y., Zhao, S., He, B., Mi, Q., Zhang, X., & Du, Q. (2018). Ginsenoside Rd ameliorates colitis by inducing p62-driven mitophagy-mediated NLRP3 inflammasome inactivation in mice. *Biochemical Pharmacology*, *155*, 366–379. DOI: 10.1016/j.bcp.2018.07.010 PMID: 30012462

Liu, S., Yao, S., Yang, H., Liu, S., & Wang, Y. (2023). Autophagy: Regulator of cell death. *Cell Death & Disease*, *14*(10), 648. Advance online publication. DOI: 10.1038/s41419-023-06154-8 PMID: 37794028

Martínez Reyes, I., & Chandel, N. S. (2020). Mitochondrial TCA cycle metabolites control physiology and disease. *Nature Communications*, *11*(1), 102. DOI: 10.1038/s41467-019-13668-3 PMID: 31900386

Mehdizadeh, S., Chen, G., Enayati, P. J., Cheng, D. W., Han, N. J., Shaye, O. A., Ippoliti, A., Vasiliauskas, E., Lo, S., & Papadakis, K. (2008). Diagnostic yield of capsule endoscopy in ulcerative colitis and inflammatory bowel disease of unclassified type (IBDU). *Endoscopy*, *40*(1), 30–35. DOI: 10.1055/s-2007-995359 PMID: 18058654

Molodecky, N. A., Soon, I. S., Rabi, D. M., Ghali, W. A., Ferris, M., Chernoff, G., Benchimol, E. I., Panaccione, R., Ghosh, S., Barkema, H. W., & Kaplan, G. G. (2012). Increasing incidence and prevalence of inflammatory bowel diseases with time, based on systematic review. *Gastroenterology*, *142*(1), 46–54.e42. DOI: 10.1053/j.gastro.2011.10.001 PMID: 22001864

Molodecky, N. A., Soon, I. S., Rabi, D. M., Ghali, W. A., Ferris, M., Chernoff, G., Benchimol, E. I., Panaccione, R., Ghosh, S., Barkema, H. W., & Kaplan, G. G. (2012). Increasing incidence and prevalence of inflammatory bowel diseases with time, based on systematic review. *Gastroenterology*, *142*(1), 46–54.e42. DOI: 10.1053/j.gastro.2011.10.001 PMID: 22001864

Nakatogawa, H., Suzuki, K., Kamada, Y., & Ohsumi, Y. (2009). Dynamics and diversity in autophagy mechanisms: Lessons from yeast. *Nature Reviews. Molecular Cell Biology*, *10*(7), 458–467. DOI: 10.1038/nrm2708 PMID: 19491929

Nardone, O. M., Zammarchi, I., Santacroce, G., Ghosh, S., & Iacucci, M. (2023). Inflammation-driven colorectal cancer associated with colitis: From pathogenesis to changing therapy. *Cancers (Basel)*, *15*(8), 2389. DOI: 10.3390/cancers15082389 PMID: 37190315

Narendra, D. P., Jin, S. M., Tanaka, A., Suen, D. F., Gautier, C. A., Shen, J., Cookson, M. R., & Youle, R. J. (2010). PINK1 is selectively stabilized on impaired mitochondria to activate Parkin. *PLoS Biology*, *8*(1), e1000298. DOI: 10.1371/journal.pbio.1000298 PMID: 20126261

Niewiadomski, O., Studd, C., Hair, C., Wilson, J., Ding, N. S., Heerasing, N., Ting, A., McNeill, J., Knight, R., Santamaria, J., Prewett, E., Dabkowski, P., Dowling, D., Alexander, S., Allen, B., Popp, B., Connell, W., Desmond, P., & Bell, S. (2015). Prospective population-based cohort of inflammatory bowel disease in the biologics era: Disease course and predictors of severity. *Journal of Gastroenterology and Hepatology*, *30*(9), 1346–1353. DOI: 10.1111/jgh.12967 PMID: 25867770

Niu, X., Fan, T., Li, W., Huang, H., Zhang, Y., & Xing, W. (2013). Protective effect of sanguinarine against acetic acid-induced ulcerative colitis in mice. *Toxicology and Applied Pharmacology*, *267*(3), 256–265. DOI: 10.1016/j.taap.2013.01.009 PMID: 23352506

Nunnari, J., & Suomalainen, A. (2012). Mitochondria: In sickness and in health. *Cell, 148*(6), 1145–1159. DOI: 10.1016/j.cell.2012.02.035 PMID: 22424226

Ohsumi, Y. (2014). Historical landmarks of autophagy research. *Cell Research, 24*(1), 9–23. DOI: 10.1038/cr.2013.169 PMID: 24366340

Okamoto, K., Kondo-Okamoto, N., & Ohsumi, Y. (2009). Mitochondria-anchored receptor Atg32 mediates degradation of mitochondria via selective autophagy. *Developmental Cell, 17*(1), 87–97. DOI: 10.1016/j.devcel.2009.06.013 PMID: 19619494

Onishi, M., Yamano, K., Sato, M., Matsuda, N., & Okamoto, K. (2021). Molecular mechanisms and physiological functions of mitophagy. *The EMBO Journal, 40*(3), e104705. DOI: 10.15252/embj.2020104705 PMID: 33438778

Pandurangan, A. K., & Esa, N. M. (2014). Signal transducer and activator of transcription 3—A promising target in colitis-associated cancer. *Asian Pacific Journal of Cancer Prevention : APJCP, 15*(2), 551–560. DOI: 10.7314/APJCP.2014.15.2.551 PMID: 24568457

Podolsky, D. K. (2002). Inflammatory bowel disease. *The New England Journal of Medicine, 347*(6), 417–429. DOI: 10.1056/NEJMra020831 PMID: 12167685

Sandoval, H., Thiagarajan, P., Dasgupta, S. K., Schumacher, A., Prchal, J. T., Chen, M., & Wang, J. (2008). Essential role for Nix in autophagic maturation of erythroid cells. *Nature, 454*(7201), 232–235. DOI: 10.1038/nature07006 PMID: 18454133

Sawicki, T., Ruszkowska, M., Danielewicz, A., Niedźwiedzka, E., Arłukowicz, T., & Przybyłowicz, K. E. (2021). A review of colorectal cancer in terms of epidemiology, risk factors, development, symptoms and diagnosis. *Cancers (Basel), 13*(9), 2025. DOI: 10.3390/cancers13092025 PMID: 33922197

Seyedian, S. S., Nokhostin, F., & Dargahi Malamir, M. (2019). A review of the diagnosis, prevention, and treatment methods of inflammatory bowel disease. *Journal of Medicine and Life, 12*(2), 113–122. DOI: 10.25122/jml-2018-0075 PMID: 31406511

Shah, S. C., & Itzkowitz, S. H. (2022). Colorectal cancer in inflammatory bowel disease: Mechanisms and management. *Gastroenterology, 162*(3), 715–730.e3. DOI: 10.1053/j.gastro.2021.10.035 PMID: 34757143

Ślebioda, T. J., & Kmieć, Z. (2014). Tumour necrosis factor superfamily members in the pathogenesis of inflammatory bowel disease. *Mediators of Inflammation, 523234*, 1–15. Advance online publication. DOI: 10.1155/2014/325129 PMID: 25045210

Sobczak, M., Wlazłowski, M., Zatorski, H., Sałaga, M., & Fichna, J. (2014). Current overview of colitis-associated colorectal cancer. *Open Life Sciences*, *9*(11), 1022–1029. DOI: 10.2478/s11535-014-0345-7

Sobczak, M., Wlazłowski, M., Zatorski, H., Sałaga, M., & Fichna, J. (2014). Current overview of colitis-associated colorectal cancer. *Open Life Sciences*, *9*(11), 1022–1029. DOI: 10.2478/s11535-014-0345-7

Talib, W. H., Alsayed, A. R., Farhan, F., & Al Kury, L. T. (2020). Resveratrol and tumor microenvironment: Mechanistic basis and therapeutic targets. *Molecules (Basel, Switzerland)*, *25*(18), 4282. DOI: 10.3390/molecules25184282 PMID: 32961987

Tan, B. L., & Norhaizan, M. E. (2019). Curcumin combination chemotherapy: The implication and efficacy in cancer. *Molecules (Basel, Switzerland)*, *24*(14), 2527. DOI: 10.3390/molecules24142527 PMID: 31295906

Tremaine, W. J. (2011). Diagnosis and treatment of indeterminate colitis. *Gastroenterology & Hepatology*, *7*(12), 826. PMID: 22347823

Van Der Kraak, L. (2015). Colitis-associated colon cancer: Is it in your genes? *World Journal of Gastroenterology*, *21*(41), 11688. DOI: 10.3748/wjg.v21.i41.11688 PMID: 26556996

Van Schaeybroeck, S., Lawler, M., Johnston, B., Salto-Tellez, M., Lee, J., Loughlin, P., ... (2014). Colorectal cancer. In *Abeloff's Clinical Oncology* (pp. 1278–1335. e14). https://doi.org/DOI: 10.1016/B978-1-4557-2865-7.00077-1

Velayos, F. S., & Sandborn, W. J. (2007). Positioning biologic therapy for Crohn's disease and ulcerative colitis. *Current Gastroenterology Reports*, *9*(6), 521–527. DOI: 10.1007/s11894-007-0069-1 PMID: 18377806

Waldner, M. J., & Neurath, M. F. (2015). Mechanisms of immune signaling in colitis-associated cancer. *Cellular and Molecular Gastroenterology and Hepatology*, *1*(1), 6–16. DOI: 10.1016/j.jcmgh.2014.11.006 PMID: 28247866

Wang, J., Ghosh, S. S., & Ghosh, S. (2017). Curcumin improves intestinal barrier function: Modulation of intracellular signaling, and organization of tight junctions. *American Journal of Physiology. Cell Physiology*, *312*(4), C438–C445. DOI: 10.1152/ajpcell.00235.2016 PMID: 28249988

Wilson, J., Hair, C., Knight, R., Catto-Smith, A., Bell, S., Kamm, M., Desmond, P., McNeil, J., & Connell, W. (2010). High incidence of inflammatory bowel disease in Australia: A prospective population-based Australian incidence study. *Inflammatory Bowel Diseases*, *16*(9), 1550–1556. DOI: 10.1002/ibd.21209 PMID: 20803698

Wright, E. K., Ding, N. S., & Niewiadomski, O. (2018). Management of inflammatory bowel disease. *The Medical Journal of Australia*, *209*(7), 318–323. DOI: 10.5694/mja17.01001 PMID: 30257634

Wu, B., Chen, Y., Clarke, R., Akala, E., Yang, P., He, B., & Gao, H. (2022). AMPK signaling regulates mitophagy and mitochondrial ATP production in human trophoblast cell line BeWo. *Frontiers in Bioscience (Landmark Edition)*, *27*(4), 118. DOI: 10.31083/j.fbl2704118 PMID: 35468677

Xin, J. (2023). Critical signaling pathways governing colitis-associated colorectal cancer: Signaling, therapeutic implications, and challenges. *Digestive and Liver Disease*, *55*(2), 169–177. DOI: 10.1016/j.dld.2022.08.012 PMID: 36002360

Xu, Y., Shen, J., & Ran, Z. (2020). Emerging views of mitophagy in immunity and autoimmune diseases. *Autophagy*, *16*(1), 3–17. DOI: 10.1080/15548627.2019.1603547 PMID: 30951392

Xu, Z., Zhao, G., Zhang, L., Qiao, C., Wang, H., Wei, H., Liu, R., Liu, P., Zhang, Y., Zhu, W., & You, W. (2024). Tong-Xie-Yao-Fang induces mitophagy in colonic epithelial cells to inhibit colitis-associated colorectal cancer. *Journal of Ethnopharmacology*, *334*, 118541. DOI: 10.1016/j.jep.2024.118541 PMID: 38992403

Yalchin, M., Baker, A.-M., Graham, T. A., & Hart, A. (2021). Predicting colorectal cancer occurrence in IBD. *Cancers (Basel)*, *13*(12), 2908. DOI: 10.3390/cancers13122908 PMID: 34200768

Yang, C., Singh, P., Singh, H., Le, M. L., & El-Matary, W. (2015). Systematic review: Thalidomide and thalidomide analogues for treatment of inflammatory bowel disease. *Alimentary Pharmacology & Therapeutics*, *41*(11), 1079–1093. DOI: 10.1111/apt.13181 PMID: 25858208

Yin, K., Lee, J., Liu, Z., Kim, H., Martin, D. R., Wu, D., Liu, M., & Xue, X. (2021). Mitophagy protein PINK1 suppresses colon tumor growth by metabolic reprogramming via p53 activation and reducing acetyl-CoA production. *Cell Death and Differentiation*, *28*(8), 2421–2435. DOI: 10.1038/s41418-021-00760-9 PMID: 33723373

Yin, K., Lee, J., Liu, Z., Kim, H., Martin, D. R., Wu, D., Liu, M., & Xue, X. (2021). Mitophagy protein PINK1 suppresses colon tumor growth by metabolic reprogramming via p53 activation and reducing acetyl-CoA production. *Cell Death and Differentiation*, *28*(8), 2421–2435. DOI: 10.1038/s41418-021-00760-9 PMID: 33723373

Zhou, Y., Wang, D., & Yan, W. (2023). Treatment effects of natural products on inflammatory bowel disease in vivo and their mechanisms: Based on animal experiments. *Nutrients*, *15*(4), 1031. DOI: 10.3390/nu15041031 PMID: 36839389

Chapter 9
A Mechanistic Approach on the Regulation of Mitophagy Signaling in Cancer Drug Resistance

Ronisha Shankar Rao
https://orcid.org/0009-0003-7292-1204
B.S. Abdur Rahman Crescent Institute of Science and Technology, India

Ashok Kumar Pandurangan
https://orcid.org/0000-0003-2824-1757
B.S. Abdur Rahman Crescent Institute of Science and Technology, India

ABSTRACT

Mitophagy, a selective process responsible for removing damaged mitochondria, has emerged as a fundamental player in the development of drug resistance across cancer types. Recent studies highlight complex interactions between genetic mutations and microenvironmental factors in cancer drug resistance. Tumors adapt alongside mitophagy by transmuting their metabolism, boosting stress endurance, and circumventing treatment-induced cell death, leading to tumor progression and increased resistance to therapies. Further understanding mitophagy's role in cancer therapy resistance, particularly in how cancer cells use it to avoid cell death, is crucial for developing effective treatment strategies.

DOI: 10.4018/979-8-3693-3836-0.ch009

INTRODUCTION

The potential for cancer cells to develop resistance to treatment therapies is a continuous challenge in the realm of cancer management. Over time, malignant cells circumvent the harmful effects of medication, leading to therapeutic failure and disease progression. Drug resistance refers to the ability of cancer cells to evade the effects of chemotherapy and targeted therapies (Ashokkumar and Sudhandiran, 2011; Mohebali et al., 2020). This presents a significant obstacle to the treatment of cancer, reducing the efficiency of currently available treatments. Drug resistance can develop due to various factors such as genetic mutations, activation of survival pathways, and changes in drug efflux metabolism(Mansoori et al., 2017a). Some drug resistance strategies involve both intrinsic and acquired mechanisms. Intrinsic resistance develops from pre-existing genetic mutations inside cancer cells, whereas acquired resistance emerges over the course of treatment when cancer cells undergo genetic and epigenetic changes in response to the pressure exerted by anticancer agents.

Over the years, efforts to overcome this resistance have encountered challenges, owing to the intricate mechanisms involved. Cancer cells employ various primary mechanisms to acquire drug resistance, including drug inactivation, target modification, drug efflux, DNA repair, anti-apoptotic pathways, Epithelial mesenchymal transition (EMT), and epigenetic changes. Among these, mitophagy has emerged as a crucial process implicated in the evolution of drug resistance in cancer (Housman et al., 2014). Understanding the mechanisms underlying drug resistance is crucial for developing strategies to combat this challenge and enhance patient outcomes. In this review, we delve into the molecular interactions and signaling underlying mitophagy-mediated drug resistance in cancer and emphasize potential therapeutic strategies.

Mitophagy is a specialized type of autophagy, which is a cellular mechanism responsible for the degradation of unnecessary or dysfunctional components. Mitophagy, in particular, focuses on eliminating dysfunctional mitochondria, ensuring the maintenance of cellular health by removing damaged organelles, and protecting mitochondrial function. The different types of mitophagy are shown in Figure 1. This process prevents the accumulation of faulty organelles, which may result in higher levels of oxidative stress and harm to the cells. Important proteins and signaling pathways, such as PINK1/Parkin and BNIP3/NIX, coordinate the initiation and completion of mitophagy. Mitophagy plays a role in managing cellular homeostasis by removing dysfunctional mitochondria, which contributes to the regulation of cellular energy production, apoptosis (programmed cell death), and metabolism. Dysregulation of mitophagy is associated with various diseases, including neurodegenerative disorders, cancer, and aging, underscoring its importance in maintaining cellular well-being and in preventing pathological conditions (Wang et al., 2022). Selective degradation of damaged mitochondria is essential for maintaining cellular balance, particularly in the context of cancer. Impaired mitochondria release high levels of reactive oxygen species (ROS), which support tumor development and cancer progression. Moreover, mitophagy plays an active role in controlling cellular metabolism by affecting the equilibrium between glycolysis and oxidative phosphorylation, which is often dysregulated in cancer cells. Abnormal mitophagy has important consequences in cancer. Some studies have indicated that malfunctions in mitophagy pathways are related to the development of cancer as well as drug resistance. Conversely, enhancing mitophagy may have therapeutic potential by promoting the elimination of cancer cells. For instance, the selective induction of mitophagy has been explored as a method to trigger apoptosis in cancer cells(Vara-Perez et al., 2019a).

Figure 1. Types of Mitophagy. Mitophagy occur via three major types namely, basal, stress induced and programmed mitophagy and their sequential events.

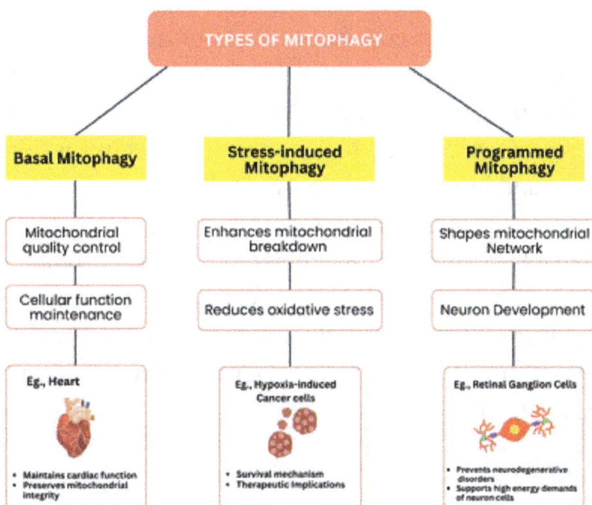

Mitophagy plays a multifaceted role in various cancer types and influences tumor development, progression, and response to therapy. In pancreatic cancer, mitophagy supports tumor progression through metabolic adaptation and confers resistance to apoptosis(Xie et al., 2021). Likewise, in melanoma, mitophagy aids the survival of tumor cells during stressful conditions, including nutrient deprivation and hypoxia, thereby promoting melanoma progression. In contrast, mitophagy can have tumor-suppressive effects in specific cancer types. In breast cancer, mitophagy is involved in preserving genomic stability by eliminating damaged mitochondria and preventing oxidative stress-induced DNA damage. This protective role of mitophagy is mostly evident in HER2-positive breast cancer, in which impaired mitophagy is linked to higher genomic instability and cancer progression(Jeong et al., 2017). Moreover, there is increasing interest in the function of mitophagy in response to cancer therapy. Mitophagy has been linked to the resistance to chemotherapy in lung cancer. It is essential to understand how cancer cells use mitophagy to escape cell death caused by therapy to develop ways to overcome treatment resistance.

This chapter explores the intricate relationship between mitophagy, a selective degradation process of damaged mitochondria, and drug resistance in cancer. Recent findings indicate that an imbalance in mitophagy pathways leads to the emergence of drug resistance, resulting in enhanced cell survival and decreased effectiveness of chemotherapy or targeted therapies,(Vara-Perez et al., 2019). which is critical for enhancing treatment efficacy and advancing the field of oncology.

Mechanisms and Challenges of Cancer Drug Resistance

Resistance to cancer drugs continues to be a primary barrier in the field of oncology, presenting significant hurdles for the success of many treatment approaches. Despite significant progress in cancer therapy, the emergence of drug resistance mechanisms continues to pose a challenge to the effectiveness of chemotherapy, targeted therapies, and immunotherapy. This limits the available treatment options and jeopardizes at-risk patient outcomes by decreasing the effectiveness of standard therapeutic approaches. Hence, it is crucial to have a thorough understanding of the complex mechanisms underlying drug resistance to develop novel therapeutic strategies. Many studies have highlighted the multifaceted nature of cancer drug resistance, emphasizing its impact on various cancer types and treatment regimens(Mansoori et al., 2017b).

Figure 2. The mechanism of action of drug resistance in cancer cells that leads to the activation of autophagosomes and how the cancer cells survive by removing the damaged mitochondria.

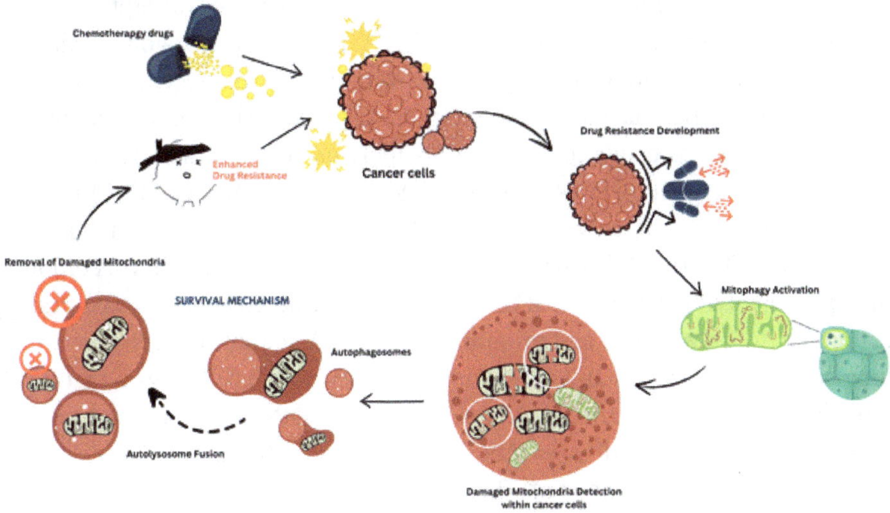

One of the main mechanisms contributing to cancer drug resistance involves the upregulation of drug efflux pump systems, specifically P-glycoprotein (P-gp) and multi-drug resistance-associated proteins (MRPs)(Janneh et al., 2007). These carriers have a crucial function in removing chemotherapy drugs from cancer cells, consequently reducing intracellular drug concentrations and impacting their ability to destroy them. This phenomenon, called multidrug resistance (MDR), confers resistance to a broad range of chemotherapeutic drugs(Xiao et al., 2021). Identifying new ways to bypass drug efflux-mediated resistance is a major challenge in cancer therapy, highlighting the need for innovative approaches to overcome this barrier. One potential strategy to combat multidrug resistance and improve treatment results is to use efflux pump inhibitors such as verapamil, a calcium blocker, which is one of the first-generation compounds identified, inhibits P-glycoprotein, and has shown efficacy in reversing MDR in cancer types such as leukaemia and breast cancer(Al-Thubiani, 2023). Tariquidar is a potent third-generation P-gp inhibitor that restores sensitivity to the drug doxorubicin (DOX), thus reversing MDR phenotypes and allowing DOX to exert its cytotoxic effects against cancer cells (Famta et al., 2021). Other examples include Cyclosporin A immunosuppressant that has been shown to inhibit P-gp activity, demonstrate partial responses, and improve survival outcomes(Yahanda et al., 1992). Further studies are needed to confirm how well it works and its safety for human patients, with the aim of enhancing treatment results for individuals with multi-drug-resistant cancers.

Another important aspect that contributes to cancer drug resistance is the efficient repair of drug-induced DNA damage in cancer cells. Chemotherapeutic agents exert control over their cytotoxic effects by inducing DNA damage, which leads to cell cycle arrest and apoptosis. However, cancer cells often induce different DNA repair pathways, namely base excision repair (BER), nucleotide excision repair (NER), and homologous recombination (HR), to overcome the damage and enhance cell viability. DNA repair mechanisms confer resistance to various anticancer platinum-based drugs such as cisplatin, which is a widely used chemotherapeutic agent that exerts effects by forming DNA cross-links, leading to inhibition of DNA replication and transcription, ultimately triggering cell death in testicular, ovarian, bladder, and lung cancers(Dasari & Tchounwou, 2014). Moreover, the exploration of combination therapies involving cisplatin and other drugs has garnered attention as a strategy to overcome drug resistance and minimize toxicity. Other anti-cancer agents include topoisomerase inhibitors and alkylating agents. Examples of drugs targeting DNA repair pathways are Olaparib and Veliparib, a poly(ADP-ribose) polymerase (PARP) inhibitor that disrupts pathways of base excision repair (BER) and HR deficiencies, respectively(Montemorano et al., 2019; Ramalingam et al., 2017).

Furthermore, cancer cells may develop resistance to targeted therapies by modifying either drug targets or downstream signaling pathways(Ahronian & Corcoran, 2017). They aim to exploit specific molecular abnormalities that fuel the development and advancement of cancer, such as activating mutations, gene amplification, or aberrant signaling pathways. Nonetheless, cancer cells can develop resistance by acquiring secondary mutations in the drug target or by activating compensatory signaling pathways, which allows them to bypass the inhibitory effects of drugs(Mansoori et al., 2017b). Resistance mechanisms include acquired mutations in the drug target, for example, the EGFR T790M mutation in non-small cell lung carcinoma (NSCLC), to tyrosine kinase inhibitors (TKIs), including gefitinib and erlotinib(Ji et al., 2013). Activation of alternative signaling pathways (e.g., bypass mechanism of the P13K/AKT pathway serves as an initiation step of resistance to monoclonal antibodies targeting the EGFR pathway in colorectal cancer) (Misale et al., 2014) or upregulation of drug efflux transporters.

Resistance to cancer drugs often involves mechanisms that inhibit cell death, particularly apoptosis, enabling them to escape the cytotoxic effects of chemotherapy. Various factors have been identified that contribute to the suppression of apoptosis in drug-resistant cancer cells. For instance, overexpression of anti-apoptotic proteins, such as Bcl-2 and Bcl-xL, can confer resistance to chemotherapy in ovarian and breast cancer, respectively(Aniogo et al., 2019). Studies have revealed that breast cancer cells with high levels of Bcl-xL are less responsive to chemotherapy drugs such as paclitaxel and doxorubicin in triggering apoptosis. Conversely, reducing Bcl-xL levels makes cancer cells more vulnerable to cell death caused by chemotherapy(Ploumaki et al., 2023). In the case of p53, often referred to as the "guardian of the genome," during chemotherapy-induced DNA damage, p53 is activated and migrates towards the nucleus and promotes the transcription of genes, BAX, and PUMA involved in apoptosis. These pro-apoptotic proteins support mitochondrial outer membrane permeabilization (MOMP), causing cytochrome c to be released while activating caspases, which execute programmed cell death(Ozaki & Nakagawara, 2011). Therefore, disruption of p53 function, such as mutations or deletions, can impair its ability to induce apoptosis, thus proving to be a potential strategy for improving treatment outcomes. In general, understanding the mechanisms underlying apoptosis suppression in drug-resistant cancer cells is crucial for developing effective therapeutic strategies for patients with cancer.

Overview of Mechanisms and Regulation in Mitophagy

Mitophagy is a process that demonstrates a vital role in sustaining the quality of mitochondria by selectively targeting damaged or removed defective mitochondria via the process of autophagy. Autophagy is an essential cellular process crucial for managing cellular homeostasis by degrading and recycling cellular components, such as mitochondria, endoplasmic reticulum, and peroxisomes, and eliminating intracellular pathogens. Autophagy dysfunction has been correlated with various diseases, such as brain atrophy, cancer, and metabolic syndromes(Glick et al., 2010). Therefore, autophagy is the process of breaking down cytoplasmic components inside autophagosomes fused with lysosomes, whereas mitophagy focuses on degrading damaged or dysfunctional mitochondria through autophagy. The mechanisms underlying mitophagy involve several pathways, including the PINK1-Parkin pathway and receptor-mediated mitophagy, each of which has distinct molecular components and regulatory mechanisms.

One of the most thoroughly studied pathways of mitophagy is the PINK1-Parkin pathway.(Palikaras et al., 2018) When there is damage or stress to the mitochondria, the kinase PINK1 becomes more stable on the outer mitochondrial membrane (OMM), where it recruits the E3 ubiquitin ligase Parkin. Parkin subsequently attaches ubiquitin to multiple proteins on the outer membrane, forming polyubiquitin chains that act as signals for the autophagic process. Some adaptor proteins, such as p62, OPTN, and NDP52, identify the phosphorylated polyubiquitin chains and start the process of autophagosome formation by binding with LC3, a protein associated with the autophagosomal membrane. This leads to impaired mitochondrial enclosure in autophagosomes, resulting in subsequent degradation(Fu et al., 2013; Palikaras et al., 2018). This regulation ensures the proper turnover of mitochondria and maintains a healthy mitochondrial network within the cell.

Mitochondrial fission and fusion dynamics are pivotal for preserving the morphology and function of the mitochondria. Mitofusins (MFN1 and MFN2) are integral proteins that play crucial roles in the fusion of outer mitochondrial membranes. Miroproteins (Miro1 and Miro2) are essential for facilitating mitochondrial movement in microtubules by linking them to the motor proteins kinesin and dynein. Kinesin motors move cargoes, including mitochondria, toward the cell periphery, whereas dynein motors transport them toward the cell center. This bidirectional movement along the microtubules enables their redistribution in the cell and helps to maintain a healthy mitochondrial network (Wang et al., 2011). In parallel with this PINK1-Parkin pathway, receptor-mediated mitophagy enables alternate mechanisms to target damaged mitochondria for degradation. Mitophagy receptors, such as BNIP3, NIX, and FUNDC1, are positioned on the OMM and communicate with LC3 to help remove dysfunctional mitochondria. These receptors are responsible for ensuring the specificity of mitophagy across various tissues and in response to various stimuli. In addition, mitophagy involves strict control over mitochondrial dynamics, where receptors facilitate mitochondrial fission through the disassembly and release of OPA1, a protein responsible for the fusion of mitochondria, and the recruitment of DRP1, an important regulator of mitochondrial division, to the surface of the mitochondria. There is a significant interaction between receptor-mediated mitophagy and the PINK1-Parkin pathway, since Parkin has the ability to mark mitophagy receptors such as NIX and BNIP3 with ubiquitin, emphasizing the complex relationship between these pathways in controlling mitochondrial quality. (Lazarou et al., 2015).

Mitophagy extends beyond cellular maintenance, impacting tissue-specific functions and physiological processes, and is classified as basal mitophagy, stress-induced, or programmed mitophagy(Palikaras et al., 2018). Organs, such as the heart, nervous system, liver, kidney, and skeletal muscle, exhibit increased levels of basal mitophagy. It aids in the regulation of mitochondrial quality by eliminating impaired mitochondria, thereby safeguarding cellular balance and ensuring efficient cellular function. This process helps to control the metabolism of both mitochondria and cells, supports energy production, and prevents the accumulation of dysfunctional organelles. For example, basal mitophagy in the heart is essential for maintaining cardiac function by eliminating damaged mitochondria and maintaining the mitochondrial integrity. Research has demonstrated that abnormalities in basal mitophagy play a central role in the onset of heart conditions such as heart failure and myocardial infarction. Similarly, when cells experience stress, such as loss of mitochondrial membrane potential, lack of nitrogen, and low oxygen levels (hypoxia), they activate stress-induced mitophagy to remove faulty mitochondria and adapt to harsh environments. This type of mitophagy helps in preserving cell viability and function under challenging circumstances by enhancing the breakdown of mitochondria and reducing oxidative stress. Programmed mitophagy controls mitochondrial dynamics and functions in various physiological processes, such as retinal ganglion cell development, reprogramming of somatic cells, cardiomyocyte maturation, erythrocyte differentiation, and sperm mitochondria elimination, to support specialized cellular functions. In the development of retinal ganglion cells, programmed mitophagy is essential for shaping the mitochondrial network and preserving mitochondrial quality to meet the high-energy requirements of developing neurons. Disruption of the programmed removal of damaged mitochondria in this situation may hinder the normal functioning of neurons and lead to neurodegenerative disorders. Therefore, mitophagy is a constantly changing dynamic process that regulates mitochondrial and cellular metabolism in different physiological situations, maintaining cellular balance and functionality(Narendra & Youle, 2011; Pickles et al., 2018).

Mitophagy in Cancer Drug Resistance

One method through which mitophagy affects cancer is by controlling cellular energy metabolism. Cancer cells frequently show increased levels of glycolysis, a process called the Warburg effect, which enables them to meet their elevated energy requirements for rapid growth. Nonetheless, mitochondrial function continues to be crucial for providing metabolites and ATP to sustain different biosynthetic pathways. Inefficient mitochondria can hinder cell metabolism and promote tumor formation. Mitophagy acts as a quality control method to remove damaged mitochondria, thereby maintaining mitochondrial function and supporting cancer cell survival. Mitophagy can also affect the apoptotic response of cancer cells. Mitochondria are important in apoptosis as they release pro-apoptotic molecules, such as cytochrome c, triggering the caspase cascade that causes cell death. Dysregulated mitophagy can affect the integrity of mitochondria and the release of apoptotic factors, ultimately influencing the apoptotic threshold in cancer cells. Enhanced mitophagy can support cancer cell survival by protecting against excessive mitochondrial damage and apoptosis, thereby facilitating tumor progression and resistance to treatment(Palikaras et al., 2018).

Manipulating mitophagy is becoming a promising strategy for treating cancer, as autophagy regulators, such as chloroquine and hydrochloroquine, are being studied in many clinical trials. The goal is to exploit mitophagy, the targeted breakdown of dysfunctional mitochondria, to improve the effectiveness of cancer therapy. However, the results of modulating mitophagy in response to cancer treatment may differ greatly depending on the particular treatments used and the nature of the cancer cells. Several researchers have highlighted the dual role of mitophagy in cancer therapy, where its effect can lead to either cell death or aid in cell survival(Vara-Perez et al., 2019b).

For instance, the activation of mitophagy could make cancer cells more vulnerable to cell death caused by chemotherapy by eliminating damaged mitochondria and stopping the growth of reactive oxygen species (ROS) that support cell survival. Ceramide, a central molecule in sphingolipid metabolism, has emerged as a key regulator of mitophagy, especially in cancer cells. Unlike the usual apoptotic pathways, which rely on BAX/BAK1 and caspases, ceramide-triggered mitophagy functions independently of these factors. This process begins with mitochondrial fission, a cellular process managed by dynamin-related protein 1 (DRP1), resulting in mitochondrial fragmentation. Ceramide subsequently triggered the production of lipidated LC3, a protein involved in autophagy. This lipidated LC3 attaches to ceramide molecules found on the mitochondrial membrane. This interaction acts as a signal for autophagolysosomes, which are cellular structures that degrade cellular components, to target mitochondria engulfed in ceramide-induced mitophagy. Consequently, there has been a focused attempt to degrade the mitochondria, causing an increased removal of mitochondria within cancer cells (Pandurangan et al., 2018). This process ultimately leads to cell death, as the removal of mitochondria terminates cancer cells from producing energy and helps to maintain homeostasis within the cell, causing them to die. Therefore, ceramide-triggered mitophagy provides selective lethal mitophagy and paves the way for potential treatment options for cancer (Dany & Ogretmen, 2015). However, it can be noted that excessive mitochondrial removal, without also increasing the formation of new mitochondria or the ability to adapt metabolically, can result in metabolic disorders and cellular demise in cancer(Chen Yan and Tao-Sheng Li, 2018). In contrast, in different situations, the activation of mitophagy could confer resistance to cancer treatment by enhancing cellular adaptation to stress conditions by triggering stress-responsive genes and activating cellular pathways that promote resistance to chemotherapy-induced damage. This includes the upregulation of antioxidant defenses, DNA repair mechanisms, and anti-apoptotic pathways, all of which contribute to enhanced cellular stress tolerance and survival in cancer treatment.

The inhibition of mitophagy can sensitize cancer cells to chemotherapy, leading to increased cell death. Inhibition of mitophagy enhances drug sensitivity by causing damaged mitochondria to accumulate, leading to higher cellular oxidative stress and facilitating apoptosis. Research has shown that blocking mitophagy through genetic or pharmacological inhibition increases the cytotoxic effect of cisplatin on ovarian cancer cells by inducing mitochondrial dysfunction and apoptosis. Moreover, inhibition of mitophagy can disturb mitochondrial function, thus increasing the vulnerability of cancer cells to chemotherapy. When mitophagy is blocked, cancer cells lose healthy mitochondria, causing metabolic stress and making them more vulnerable to chemotherapy-driven cell death. Mitochondria contain mitochondrial DNA (mtDNA) that can perform well as a damage-associated molecular pattern

(DAMP) and induce innate immune reactions(Mukherjee et al., 2023). In other cases, by inhibiting mitophagy and causing the buildup of damaged mitochondria, cancer cells release additional mtDNA into the cytoplasm, resulting in heightened immune detection and initiation of anti-tumor immune reactions. This may boost the effectiveness of immunotherapy and enhance treatment results for patients with cancer.

Cancer Types and Mitophagy-Mediated Drug Resistance

Drug resistance in cancer continues to be a major challenge in chemotherapy, leading to treatment failure and disease advancement. Mitochondria are essential for cellular metabolism, energy production, and regulation of apoptosis, which are crucial for cancer cell survival and drug response. Understanding the molecular dynamics underlying mitophagy-mediated resistance is important to develop targeted therapies for different cancer types. Challenges arise in lung cancer treatment owing to resistance to cisplatin, a commonly used platinum-based chemotherapy drug. The involvement of caveolin-1 (Cav-1)/parkin-mediated mitophagy is major in the development of cisplatin resistance in non-small cell lung cancer (NSCLC) cells, particularly in the A549 cell line. Caveolin-1 (Cav-1), an important building block of caveolae, has been linked to various stages of cancer development and drug resistance. In NSCLC, the presence of Cav-1 has been linked to a negative outlook and insensitivity towards certain chemotherapeutic drugs, such as cisplatin. Research indicates that reducing Cav-1 in A549 cells increases their responsiveness to cisplatin, indicating that Cav-1 plays a major role in drug resistance. Cav-1 promotes cisplatin resistance by affecting parkin-controlled mitophagy. As mitophagy specifically eliminates impaired or dysfunctional mitochondria to maintain cellular balance, parkin, a type of E3 ubiquitin ligase, is required for initiating mitophagy through ubiquitination of proteins found in the mitochondria. In A549 cells, reducing Cav-1 levels led to a decrease in Rho-associated coiled-coil-containing protein kinase 1 (ROCK1), which is a fundamental target of the Cav-1 signal transduction pathway. Inhibition of ROCK1 reduces parkin-dependent mitophagy, making cells more vulnerable to cisplatin-induced cell death(Liu et al., 2020). This indicates that Cav-1 signaling controls mitophagy dynamics and affects cisplatin sensitivity in NSCLC cells. Apurinic endonuclease 1 (APE1), a versatile protein responsible for DNA repair and redox regulation, has been linked to cisplatin resistance in A549 cells. Increased APE1 levels enhance parkin-dependent mitophagy, leading to cisplatin resistance Decreasing APE1 levels re-establishes sensitivity to cisplatin and promotes cell death through apoptosis, highlighting APE1's involvement in facilitating drug resistance through mitophagy. Additionally, ARIH1, another E3 ubiquitin ligase, is necessary for triggering PINK1-dependent mitophagy in A549 cells in the absence of parkin. Mitophagy triggered by ARIH1 serves as a protective response against cisplatin-induced cell death Cisplatin treatment greatly reduced the growth of ARIH1 knockout cells, emphasizing the crucial role of ARIH1-mediated mitophagy in cisplatin resistance(Villa et al., 2017; Yang et al., 2012). In conclusion, Cav-1/Parkin-mediated mitophagy is involved in NSCLC cell resistance to cisplatin by controlling mitochondrial quality and the response to chemotherapy-related stress.

In prostate cancer (PCa), cells exhibit altered mitochondrial dynamics and enhanced mitophagy, contributing to resistance to androgen deprivation therapy (ADT) and chemotherapy. Changes in mitochondrial dynamics modify mitochondrial metabolism and significantly affect prostate cancer growth, epithelial-mesenchymal transition (EMT), and resistance to therapy. This was marked by elevated glycolysis production and changes in OXPHOS. Modulation of hypoxia-inducible factor 1 alpha (HIF1α) and androgen receptor (AR) signaling, coupled with stromal remodeling and the presence of oncometabolites, are key drivers of PCa growth(Vikramdeo et al., 2023). Combination therapies that target both mitochondrial metabolism and signaling pathways linked to drug resistance could show synergistic effects and enhance treatment results in patients with PCa.

Liensinine, an isoquinoline alkaloid obtained from the embryonic seed of Nelumbo nucifera Gaertn(Chen Yan & Tao-Sheng Li, 2018), is increasingly being recognized for its possible role as an adjunctive treatment in breast cancer therapy. It has been reported that liensinine can hinder mitophagy, making breast cancer cells more sensitive to traditional chemotherapy drugs, such as doxorubicin, paclitaxel, vincristine, and cisplatin. Inhibition of mitophagy by liensinine is critical for increasing the cellular toxicity of doxorubicin in breast cancer cells during combination therapy. Liensinine disrupts mitochondrial homeostasis by blocking mitophagy, causing mitochondrial dysfunction with reduced ATP production and increased ROS generation. This enhances the harmful effects of doxorubicin, as impaired mitochondria struggle to handle the oxidative stress caused, leading to the onset of apoptotic pathways, ultimately provoking cell death through apoptosis(Genovese et al., 2020). Likewise, the combination of liensinine and paclitaxel works together to increase cytotoxicity towards breast cancer cells by disturbing mitochondrial function and promoting apoptotic cell destruction. Paclitaxel, by stabilizing microtubules, disrupts cell dynamics, causing cell cycle arrest during mitosis and eventual cell death. However, cancer cells can become resistant to paclitaxel-triggered cell death via different means, such as improved mitophagy-related mitochondrial maintenance. Liensinine reverses this resistance by blocking mitophagy, making breast cancer cells more susceptible to paclitaxel-induced apoptosis. The co-administration of liensinine and paclitaxel enhances the activation of apoptosis, resulting in higher levels of cell death by disrupting the structure and function of the mitochondria(Zhou et al., 2015). Therefore, the modulation of mitophagy plays a dual role in cancer, affecting both cancerous and normal healthy tissues(Chen Yan & Tao-Sheng Li, 2018).

Overall, integrating mitophagy regulation with chemotherapy may help overcome drug resistance in cancer cells and minimize adverse treatment effects. However, detailed mechanistic studies are required to fully understand how mitophagy interacts with cancer cells and affects drug resistance.

CONCLUSION

The intricate relationship between mitophagy and resistance to cancer therapies has become a fundamental target in cancer research and is important for treatment success. In this review, we have delved into the complex processes of mitophagy and cancer drug resistance, seeking to understand how they interact with different types of cancer. Resistance to cancer drugs is a notable challenge in the field of clinical oncology, as it not only reduces the effectiveness of cancer treatments, but also limits treatment options. Acknowledging the intricate nature of drug resistance mechanisms emphasizes the immediate need for groundbreaking therapeutic strategies to overcome this challenge. Mitophagy protects cellular integrity and enhances cell survival by selectively eliminating damaged mitochondria. Nonetheless, dysfunctional mitophagy has been linked to insusceptibility to various cancer treatments. Examining these communication pathways provides opportunities to identify potential targets for overcoming drug resistance mechanisms. Conducting in-depth case studies on various cancer types contributes to resistance, and emphasizes the need for novel treatment strategies based on specific cancer types. Therefore, overcoming resistance mechanisms and addressing potential off-target effects present major challenges in utilizing mitophagy as a promising target for therapy. By understanding the intricacies of mitophagy-induced resistance mechanisms, we open the door to developing new strategies to address drug resistance and enhance treatment outcomes in cancer patients.

REFERENCES

Ahronian, L. G., & Corcoran, R. B. (2017). Strategies for monitoring and combating resistance to combination kinase inhibitors for cancer therapy. *Genome Medicine*, *9*(1), 37. DOI: 10.1186/s13073-017-0431-3 PMID: 28431544

Al-Thubiani, W. S.Al-Thubiani. (2023). The Role of P-Glycoprotein (P-gp) in Cancer Multidrug Resistance (MDR): Challenges for Inhibiting P-gp in the Context of Overcoming MDR. *Journal of Pharmaceutical Research International*, *35*(23), 44–58. DOI: 10.9734/jpri/2023/v35i237422

Aniogo, E. C., Plackal Adimuriyil George, B., & Abrahamse, H. (2019). The role of photodynamic therapy on multidrug resistant breast cancer. *Cancer Cell International*, *19*(1), 91. DOI: 10.1186/s12935-019-0815-0 PMID: 31007609

Ashokkumar, P., & Sudhandiran, G. (2011). Luteolin inhibits cell proliferation during Azoxymethane-induced experimental colon carcinogenesis via Wnt/β-catenin pathway. *Investigational New Drugs*, *29*(2), 273–284. DOI: 10.1007/s10637-009-9359-9 PMID: 20013030

Dany, M., & Ogretmen, B. (2015). Ceramide induced mitophagy and tumor suppression. *Biochimica et Biophysica Acta*, *1853*(10, 10 Pt B), 2834–2845. DOI: 10.1016/j.bbamcr.2014.12.039 PMID: 25634657

Dasari, S., & Tchounwou, P. B. (2014). Cisplatin in cancer therapy: Molecular mechanisms of action. *European Journal of Pharmacology*, *740*, 364–378. DOI: 10.1016/j.ejphar.2014.07.025 PMID: 25058905

Dual Role of Mitophagy in Cancer Drug Resistance. (2018). Dual Role of Mitophagy in Cancer Drug Resistance. *Anticancer Research*, *38*(2). Advance online publication. DOI: 10.21873/anticanres.12266

Famta, P., Shah, S., Chatterjee, E., Singh, H., Dey, B., Guru, S. K., Singh, S. B., & Srivastava, S. (2021). Exploring new Horizons in overcoming P-glycoprotein-mediated multidrug-resistant breast cancer via nanoscale drug delivery platforms. *Current Research in Pharmacology and Drug Discovery*, *2*, 100054. DOI: 10.1016/j.crphar.2021.100054 PMID: 34909680

Fritsch, L. E., Moore, M. E., Sarraf, S. A., & Pickrell, A. M. (2020). Ubiquitin and Receptor-Dependent Mitophagy Pathways and Their Implication in Neurodegeneration. *Journal of Molecular Biology*, *432*(8), 2510–2524. DOI: 10.1016/j.jmb.2019.10.015 PMID: 31689437

Fu, M., St-Pierre, P., Shankar, J., Wang, P. T. C., Joshi, B., & Nabi, I. R. (2013). Regulation of mitophagy by the Gp78 E3 ubiquitin ligase. *Molecular Biology of the Cell, 24*(8), 1153–1162. DOI: 10.1091/mbc.e12-08-0607 PMID: 23427266

Genovese, I., Vezzani, B., Danese, A., Modesti, L., Vitto, V. A. M., Corazzi, V., Pelucchi, S., Pinton, P., & Giorgi, C. (2020). Mitochondria as the decision makers for cancer cell fate: From signaling pathways to therapeutic strategies. *Cell Calcium, 92*, 102308. DOI: 10.1016/j.ceca.2020.102308 PMID: 33096320

Glick, D., Barth, S., & Macleod, K. F. (2010). Autophagy: Cellular and molecular mechanisms. *The Journal of Pathology, 221*(1), 3–12. DOI: 10.1002/path.2697 PMID: 20225336

Housman, G., Byler, S., Heerboth, S., Lapinska, K., Longacre, M., Snyder, N., & Sarkar, S. (2014). Drug Resistance in Cancer: An Overview. *Cancers (Basel), 6*(3), 1769–1792. DOI: 10.3390/cancers6031769 PMID: 25198391

Janneh, O., Jones, E., Chandler, B., Owen, A., & Khoo, S. H. (2007). Inhibition of P-glycoprotein and multidrug resistance-associated proteins modulates the intracellular concentration of lopinavir in cultured CD4 T cells and primary human lymphocytes. *The Journal of Antimicrobial Chemotherapy, 60*(5), 987–993. DOI: 10.1093/jac/dkm353 PMID: 17890284

Jeong, J., Kim, W., Kim, L. K., VanHouten, J., & Wysolmerski, J. J. (2017). HER2 signaling regulates HER2 localization and membrane retention. *PLoS One, 12*(4), e0174849. DOI: 10.1371/journal.pone.0174849 PMID: 28369073

Ji, W., Choi, C.-M., Rho, J. K., Jang, S. J., Park, Y. S., Chun, S.-M., Kim, W. S., Lee, J.-S., Kim, S.-W., Lee, D. H., & Lee, J. C. (2013). Mechanisms of acquired resistance to EGFR-tyrosine kinase inhibitor in Korean patients with lung cancer. *BMC Cancer, 13*(1), 606. DOI: 10.1186/1471-2407-13-606 PMID: 24369725

Liu, Y., Fu, Y., Hu, X., Chen, S., Miao, J., Wang, Y., Zhou, Y., & Zhang, Y. (2020). Caveolin-1 knockdown increases the therapeutic sensitivity of lung cancer to cisplatin-induced apoptosis by repressing Parkin-related mitophagy and activating the ROCK1 pathway. *Journal of Cellular Physiology, 235*(2), 1197–1208. DOI: 10.1002/jcp.29033 PMID: 31270811

Mansoori, B., Mohammadi, A., Davudian, S., Shirjang, S., & Baradaran, B. (2017a). The Different Mechanisms of Cancer Drug Resistance: A Brief Review. *Advanced Pharmaceutical Bulletin, 7*(3), 339–348. DOI: 10.15171/apb.2017.041 PMID: 29071215

Mansoori, B., Mohammadi, A., Davudian, S., Shirjang, S., & Baradaran, B. (2017b). The Different Mechanisms of Cancer Drug Resistance: A Brief Review. *Advanced Pharmaceutical Bulletin*, *7*(3), 339–348. DOI: 10.15171/apb.2017.041 PMID: 29071215

Misale, S., Di Nicolantonio, F., Sartore-Bianchi, A., Siena, S., & Bardelli, A. (2014). Resistance to Anti-EGFR Therapy in Colorectal Cancer: From Heterogeneity to Convergent Evolution. *Cancer Discovery*, *4*(11), 1269–1280. DOI: 10.1158/2159-8290.CD-14-0462 PMID: 25293556

Mohebali, N., Pandurangan, A. K., Mustafa, M. R., Anandasadagopan, S. K., & Alagumuthu, T. (2020). Vernodalin induces apoptosis through ROS/JNK pathway activation in human colon cancer cells. *Journal of Biochemical and Molecular Toxicology*, *34*(12), e22577. DOI: 10.1002/jbt.22587 PMID: 32726518

Montemorano, L., Lightfoot, M. D., & Bixel, K. (2019). Role of Olaparib as Maintenance Treatment for Ovarian Cancer: The Evidence to Date. *OncoTargets and Therapy*, *12*, 11497–11506. DOI: 10.2147/OTT.S195552 PMID: 31920338

Mukherjee, S., Bhatti, G. K., Chhabra, R., Reddy, P. H., & Bhatti, J. S. (2023). Targeting mitochondria as a potential therapeutic strategy against chemoresistance in cancer. *Biomedicine and Pharmacotherapy*, *160*, 114398. DOI: 10.1016/j.biopha.2023.114398 PMID: 36773523

Narendra, D. P., & Youle, R. J. (2011). Targeting mitochondrial dysfunction: Role for PINK1 and Parkin in mitochondrial quality control. *Antioxidants & Redox Signaling*, *14*(10), 1929–1938. DOI: 10.1089/ars.2010.3799 PMID: 21194381

Ozaki, T., & Nakagawara, A. (2011). Role of p53 in Cell Death and Human Cancers. *Cancers (Basel)*, *3*(1), 994–1013. DOI: 10.3390/cancers3010994 PMID: 24212651

Palikaras, K., Lionaki, E., & Tavernarakis, N. (2018). Mechanisms of mitophagy in cellular homeostasis, physiology and pathology. *Nature Cell Biology*, *20*(9), 1013–1022. DOI: 10.1038/s41556-018-0176-2 PMID: 30154567

Pandurangan, A. K., Salmiah, I., & Norhaizan, M. E. (2018). Inositol-6 Phosphate (IP_6) inhibits mTOR pathway and induces autophagy-mediated cell death in HT-29 colon cancer cells. *Archives of Medical Science : AMS*, *14*(6), 1281–1288. DOI: 10.5114/aoms.2018.76935 PMID: 30393482

Pickles, S., Vigié, P., & Youle, R. J. (2018). Mitophagy and Quality Control Mechanisms in Mitochondrial Maintenance. *Current Biology*, *28*(4), R170–R185. DOI: 10.1016/j.cub.2018.01.004 PMID: 29462587

Ploumaki, I., Triantafyllou, E., Koumprentziotis, I.-A., Karampinos, K., Drougkas, K., Karavolias, I., Trontzas, I., & Kotteas, E. A. (2023). Bcl-2 pathway inhibition in solid tumors: A review of clinical trials. *Clinical & Translational Oncology : Official Publication of the Federation of Spanish Oncology Societies and of the National Cancer Institute of Mexico*, *25*(6), 1554–1578. DOI: 10.1007/s12094-022-03070-9 PMID: 36639602

Ramalingam, S. S., Blais, N., Mazieres, J., Reck, M., Jones, C. M., Juhasz, E., Urban, L., Orlov, S., Barlesi, F., Kio, E., Keiholz, U., Qin, Q., Qian, J., Nickner, C., Dziubinski, J., Xiong, H., Ansell, P., McKee, M., Giranda, V., & Gorbunova, V. (2017). Randomized, Placebo-Controlled, Phase II Study of Veliparib in Combination with Carboplatin and Paclitaxel for Advanced/Metastatic Non-Small Cell Lung Cancer. *Clinical Cancer Research*, *23*(8), 1937–1944. DOI: 10.1158/1078-0432.CCR-15-3069 PMID: 27803064

Vara-Perez, M., Felipe-Abrio, B., & Agostinis, P. (2019a). Mitophagy in Cancer: A Tale of Adaptation. *Cells*, *8*(5), 493. Advance online publication. DOI: 10.3390/cells8050493 PMID: 31121959

Vara-Perez, M., Felipe-Abrio, B., & Agostinis, P. (2019b). Mitophagy in Cancer: A Tale of Adaptation. *Cells*, *8*(5), 493. Advance online publication. DOI: 10.3390/cells8050493 PMID: 31121959

Vikramdeo, K. S., Sharma, A., Anand, S., Sudan, S. K., Singh, S., Singh, A. P., & Dasgupta, S. (2023). Mitochondrial Alterations in Prostate Cancer: Roles in Pathobiology and Racial Disparities. *International Journal of Molecular Sciences*, *24*(5), 4482. Advance online publication. DOI: 10.3390/ijms24054482 PMID: 36901912

Villa, E., Proïcs, E., Rubio-Patiño, C., Obba, S., Zunino, B., Bossowski, J. P., Rozier, R. M., Chiche, J., Mondragón, L., Riley, J. S., Marchetti, S., Verhoeyen, E., Tait, S. W. G., & Ricci, J.-E. (2017). Parkin-Independent Mitophagy Controls Chemotherapeutic Response in Cancer Cells. *Cell Reports*, *20*(12), 2846–2859. DOI: 10.1016/j.celrep.2017.08.087 PMID: 28930681

Wang, Q., Xue, H., Yue, Y., Hao, S., Huang, S.-H., & Zhang, Z. (2022). Role of mitophagy in the neurodegenerative diseases and its pharmacological advances: A review. *Frontiers in Molecular Neuroscience*, *15*, 1014251. DOI: 10.3389/fnmol.2022.1014251 PMID: 36267702

Wang, X., Winter, D., Ashrafi, G., Schlehe, J., Wong, Y. L., Selkoe, D., Rice, S., Steen, J., LaVoie, M. J., & Schwarz, T. L. (2011). PINK1 and Parkin target Miro for phosphorylation and degradation to arrest mitochondrial motility. *Cell*, *147*(4), 893–906. DOI: 10.1016/j.cell.2011.10.018 PMID: 22078885

Xiao, H., Zheng, Y., Ma, L., Tian, L., & Sun, Q. (2021). Clinically-Relevant ABC Transporter for Anti-Cancer Drug Resistance. *Frontiers in Pharmacology*, *12*, 648407. Advance online publication. DOI: 10.3389/fphar.2021.648407 PMID: 33953682

Xie, Y., Liu, J., Kang, R., & Tang, D. (2021). Mitophagy in Pancreatic Cancer. *Frontiers in Oncology*, *11*, 616079. DOI: 10.3389/fonc.2021.616079 PMID: 33718171

Yahanda, A. M., Alder, K. M., Fisher, G. A., Brophy, N. A., Halsey, J., Hardy, R. I., Gosland, M. P., Lum, B. L., & Sikic, B. I. (1992). Phase I trial of etoposide with cyclosporine as a modulator of multidrug resistance. *Journal of Clinical Oncology*, *10*(10), 1624–1634. DOI: 10.1200/JCO.1992.10.10.1624 PMID: 1403040

Yang, X., Xiong, H., Guan, Z., Okai, I., Ye, D., Song, Y., Li, X., Wang, L., Liu, L., Du, S., Lin, D., & Shao, S. (2012). Higher expression of Caveolin-1 inhibits human small cell lung cancer (SCLC) apoptosis in vitro. *Cancer Investigation*, *30*(6), 453–462. DOI: 10.3109/07357907.2012.675384 PMID: 22545709

Zhou, J., Li, G., Zheng, Y., Shen, H.-M., Hu, X., Ming, Q.-L., Huang, C., Li, P., & Gao, N. (2015). A novel autophagy/mitophagy inhibitor liensinine sensitizes breast cancer cells to chemotherapy through DNM1L-mediated mitochondrial fission. *Autophagy*, *11*(8), 1259–1279. DOI: 10.1080/15548627.2015.1056970 PMID: 26114658

Chapter 10 Natural Products Modulating Mitophagy Implications for Cancer Therapy

Manish Kumar Verma
https://orcid.org/0000-0002-7772-490X
Sanskaram University, Haryana, India

ABSTRACT

Mitochondrial dysfunction is a hallmark of cancer, contributing to tumorigenesis, and therapeutic resistance. Mitophagy, the selective removal of damaged or dysfunctional mitochondria, plays a crucial role in maintaining cellular homeostasis and preventing the accumulation of cellular stress. The dysregulation of mitophagy in cancer often leads to the accumulation of damaged mitochondria, promoting tumorigenesis and hampering the efficacy of conventional therapies. Natural products like polyphenols, flavonoids, alkaloids, terpenoids influencing mitophagy, through AMP-activated protein kinase (AMPK), mTORC1, and PINK1/Parkin-mediated pathways and offer a promising strategy to restore mitochondrial homeostasis and enhance the sensitivity of cancer cells to treatment. In conclusion, understanding the intricate interplay between natural products and mitophagy provides insights into novel therapeutic strategies for diseases associated with mitochondrial dysfunction.

DOI: 10.4018/979-8-3693-3836-0.ch010

INTRODUCTION

Mitophagy is a kind of the cellular process that helps to degrade the failed or the defective mitochondria, which commonly are called the power house of the cell as the function of mitochondria is to generate energy. Mitochondria perform many fundamental operations within the cell, including energy production, regulation of metabolism, and apoptosis (or programmed cell death) (Gustafsson and Dorn, 2019). Selective autophagy of mitochondria is indispensable for the maintenance of cellular homeostasis under normal conditions, for discharge of the defective mitochondria that can cause cell damage and degenerative diseases, such as neurodegenerative disorders, cancer, and metabolic diseases (Abate et al., 2020). Microscopic digestion where damaged mitochondria, which are cellular organelles dedicated to breaking down and recycling components, engulf and digest damaged ones is known as mitophagy. Some of the proteins and signaling pathway elements were revealed to be the controllers of mitophagy, like PINK1 (PTEN -induced putative kinase 1), Parkin, and mitophagy receptors - NDP52, Optineurin, and p62 (Karagin et al., 2017; Padman et al., 2019).

Mitochondrion also known as powerhouse of the cell is a very important organelle in the cell, which is responsible for cellular energy production, metabolism and signaling pathway. On the other hand, fluctuating status of those organelles involves very complex quality control systems which are aimed at correcting the status of cells (Schirrmacher, 2020). A Mitophagy mechanism is a type of autophagy primarily dealing with selective removal of faulty or nonfunctional proteins, clearly stands as one of the key processes maintaining cell integrity. Mitophagy not only plays the role of biogenesis from defective mitochondria, but also orchestrate the mitochondrial turnover and it econtributes to cellular bioenergetics, redox balance and apoptosis regulation. It has been demonstrated that an imbalance of mitophagy is involved in different disorders, primarily neurodegenerative disorders, metabolic diseases, and cancers. This makes mitophagy very important for human and animal health (Ma et al., 2020). Nevertheless, uncontrolled mitophagy in tumor cells could be a trigger for uncontrolled proliferation of cancer cells, through metabolic purposes, enhanced antioxidant defense as well as overcoming apoptosis and chemotherapy (Kulikov et al., 2017). Recently, there has been a notable surge in the amount of investigations being carried out to find naturally occurring compounds that regulate mitophagy and may be valuable drugs for therapeutic purposes. Natural products, obtained from plants, microorganisms, and marine life, among others, are undoubtedly a goldmine in their variety of pharmacologically active moieties (Jing and Jin, 2020). The study of the mitophagy promoting effect of natural products constitutes not only a great opportunity to understand the underlying mechanisms but also an incomparable chance for the creation of new prevention and treatment strategies for mitochondrial associated diseases.

Biologically active compounds, such as those from the plant, fungi, marine and some other biological sources have a long history of drug development and are still being investigated extensively. These molecules are specific as they often demonstrate multiple effects on cell pathways and physiological changes, hence they become the favorite research target for drug discovery and development. In this given context, the search for compounds naturally existing that are able to manipulate mitophagy pathways is a very promising path as it has several reasons to be expressed (Abdel et al., 2020). The first reason is that they can help to halt the propagation of illnesses related to mitochondrial impairment which provide the medical field with fresh ways to provide treatment. In this regard, natural constituents are viewed as the safest options to synthetic medicines, being the mainstay of the traditional medicine systems for long and having fewer after effects. Moreover, natural compounds are endowed with a massive arsenal of molecular forms which possess different shapes and reaction model hence there is an opportunity to find new drugs with unconventional mechanisms of action (Mattio et al., 2020).

BACKGROUND

"Natural Products Modulating Mitophagy: Implications for Cancer Therapy," a new and evolving field of study related to cancer therapy targeting mitophagy. Mitophagy is an important cellular process through which defective mitochondria are selectively degraded to maintain cellular homeostasis and prevent the buildup of impaired organelles responsible for numerous diseases, including cancer (Gustafsson and Dorn, 2019). Natural products are plant derived, marine organism and other natural source originated compounds with well-defined pharmacological properties. Recently, the interest of investigators considering them as modulators of mitophagy has surged. These compounds have several bioactive properties contributing to affect cellular processes including but not limited to apoptosis, autophagy and the most recently mitophagy. It also includes several natural products with the capability to regulate mitophagy. They could exert their effects through multiple ways (such as inducers of mitochondrial biogenesis, activators of mitochondria fusion/fission dynamics, or targeting mitophagy regulators [PINK1/Parkin pathway or FUNDC2]), etc. Given that mitochondria are central to the above pathways, it might also be rationalized how this type of shared action by natural products can lead them promising compounds in combating mitochondrial dysfunction which is a trait quite characteristic for cancer cells showing metabolic reprogramming and resistance against apoptosis (Padman et al., 2019).

Mitophagy: A Cellular Cleansing Mechanism

Mitophagy is a complex coordination of a response that selectively retargets the flawed or impaired mitochondria to the cell for degradation and recycling. Multiple molecular mechanisms and regulatory networks are responsible for the initiation phase, turn-on, and reticulation of mitophagy. The process can be broadly divided into several stages.

- **Recognition of Damaged Mitochondria:** The triggering of mitophagy begins with the identification of impaired or membrane potential its absence from this kind/type of receptors combined on mitochondrial outer membrane (MOM) (Audano et al., 2018). PINK1 (PTEN-induced kinase 1) is one of the most popular receptors, which is in this case, is responsible for the course of this event. In the normal state, healthy mitochondria carry and separate PINK1 from the cell by proteolytic process which leads to its degradation. Nevertheless, after mitochondria depolarization or damage PINK1 starts to accumulate on the outer mitrochondrial membrane (MM) and mediate phosphorylation of ubiquitin and the recruitment of mitophagy receptors (Steer et al., 2015).
- **Recruitment of Mitophagy Receptors:** Phosphorylated ubiquitin is a signal for attracting the receptors, such as OIP (optineurin), NPD52 (nuclear dot protein 52) and P62 (sequestosome 1) to the outside surface of the damaged mitochondria. These receptors have LC3-interacting regions (LIRs) that bind with microtubule-associated protein 1A/1B-light chain 3 (LC3), which is embedded in the autophagosomal membrane, helping to wrap mitochondria in the autophagosomal holder (Yang et al., 2019; Wauters et al., 2020).
- **Formation of the Autophagosome:** The recruitment of mitophagy receptors to the dysfunctional mitochondria is an initial step in the process. This event will subsequently culminate into nucleation, elongation and eventually the isolation membranes of the autophagosomes forming a shell around the malfunctioning mitochondria. Such process relies on the sequential operation of autophagy-related (ATG) proteins, including ATG5, ATG12, and ATG16L1, which are joined by a kind of conjugated reaction, to form the ATG12-ATG5-ATG16L1 complex, and as a result, the membrane elongation and closure (Lystad and Simonsen, 2019).
- **Fusion and Maturation of Autophagosomes:** After the formation, it undergoes maturation by acquiring lysosomal markers such as lysosomal-associated membrane protein 1 (LAMP 1) by fussing with endosomes and lysosomes which leads to the formation of autolysosomes. These proteins are SNARE (soluble N-ethylmaleimide-sensitive factor attachment protein

receptors) and the process works upon an acidic pH for the activation of lysosomal enzymes (Andres et al., 2021).

- **Degradation and Recycling of Mitochondrial Components:** Within autolysosomes, mitochondria are digested by acidic lysosomal hydrolases, which leads to the disintegration of mitochondrial proteins, lipids and nucleic acids returning to their individual molecules. The broken down particles in turn get into the cell cytoplasm for energy production and biosynthesis, where they can be recycled and used again (Bhatia and Sharma, 2021).
- **Termination of Mitophagy:** When the damaged mitochondria have been disassembled and become reusable materials, then mitophagy is stopped in order to avoid excessive mitochondria removal that might lead to the loss of functions. The phase of degradation entails the disassembly of the machinery of the autophagosome followed by recycling of mitophagy receptors into the cytoplasm which can be used for either mitophagy or degradation (Gubas and Dikic, 2022).

Figure 1. Mitophagy mechanism

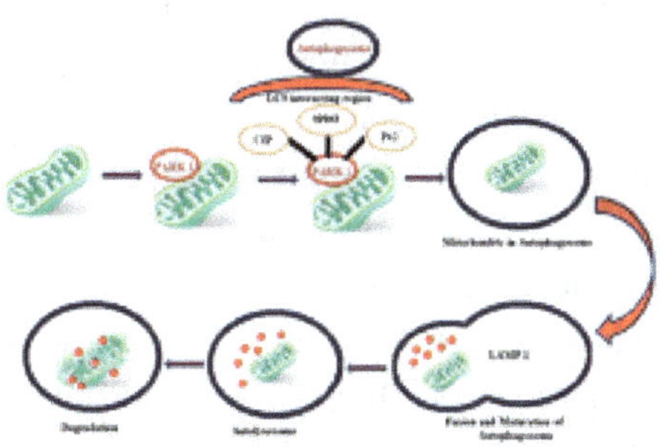

Natural Products as Modulators of Mitophagy

Natural products comprise of effective mitophagy regulators which are now emerging as the means of therapeutic for cancer treatment. This is achieved through a number interaction with direct mitophagy regulators, signaling pathways, and even mitochondrial functions. Different classes of natural products have been explored for their ability to either stimulate or suppress mitophagy and give an insight into their candidature as additional therapy in cancer.

Polyphenols

A polyphenol is a generic name carrying various subgroups of compounds with multiple -OH carbon binding. These chemicals perform vital functions in plants that are helpful to pathogen and UV ray resistance, coloration and flavour development. Besides that, they are known to be gifted with health properties which are the result of their antioxidant properties and their effectiveness in the regulation of biological pathways (Fahmy and Farag, 2022).

Phytochemicals are an umbrella term, which encompasses number of compound groups, polyphenols are the most abundant types of these in vegetables and fruits and can be classified into five main groups, which include phenolic acids (such as hydroxyl benzoic acids and hydroxyl cinnamic acids), stilbenes (such as resveratrol), and lignin's. Each class consists of many singular compounds, each them have unique chemical structures and biological actions (Galeotti et al., 2019).

Phenolic polyphenols, for instance resveratrol, curcumin, and quercetin, enhance AMP-activated protein kinase (AMPK) pathway and trigger mitochondria fission (Chodari et al., 2021). They activate the removal of malfunctioning mitochondria. Such substrates promote mitophagy, an autophagy process that involves the removal of dysfunctional mitochondria and then detoxification of cellular reactive oxygen species and hence useful in suppressing tumor growth and enhancing sensitivity to tumor-killing drugs (Liang et al., 2021).

Resveratrol, a natural polyphenol found in grapes, berries, and other plants, exerts anticancer effects in breast cancer by activating the PINK1/Parkin pathway and inducing mitophagy, the selective removal of damaged mitochondria (Liu et al., 2025). The mechanism begins with resveratrol disrupting mitochondrial function, leading to a loss of membrane potential ($\Delta\Psi m$) and the accumulation of PTEN induced putative kinase 1 (PINK1) on the outer mitochondrial membrane (Pavlova et al., 2024). PINK1 phosphorylates ubiquitin at Ser65, recruiting the E3 ubiquitin ligase Parkin from the cytosol to damaged mitochondria. Once activated, Parkin ubiquitinates mitochondrial surface proteins such as VDAC and MFN2, marking them for degradation. These ubiquitinated mitochondria are then recognized by autophagy adaptor proteins like p62/SQSTM1, which bind to LC3-II on forming autophagosomes. The engulfed mitochondria are subsequently degraded upon fusion with lysosomes. By promoting mitophagy, resveratrol depletes functional mitochondria in breast cancer cells, reducing ATP production, increasing oxidative stress, and triggering apoptosis (Chandra et al., 2025). Resveratrol also modulates apoptosis-related proteins, downregulating anti-apoptotic Bcl-2 and upregulating pro-apoptotic Bax, further enhancing cancer cell death (Meng et al., 2025). This dual action of resveratrol inducing mitophagy and apoptosis highlights its potential as a therapeutic agent in breast cancer treatment. Studies suggest that targeting the

PINK1/Parkin pathway with resveratrol could selectively eliminate cancer cells while sparing normal cells, offering a promising strategy for chemoprevention and adjunct therapy (Tshikhudo et al., 2025).

Curcumin, the active polyphenol in turmeric, enhances mitophagy in pancreatic cancer through the BNIP3 (Bcl-2/adenovirus E1B 19-kDa-interacting protein 3) pathway, contributing to its anticancer effects (Brimson et al., 2021). The mechanism begins with curcumin upregulating BNIP3, a pro-mitophagy protein that operates independently of the PINK1/Parkin pathway. BNIP3 displaces the inhibitory interaction between Bcl-2 and Beclin-1, freeing Beclin-1 to initiate autophagosome formation (D'Arcy, 2022). Concurrently, BNIP3 localizes to the outer mitochondrial membrane, where it induces mitochondrial depolarization and triggers the recruitment of autophagy machinery. Hypoxia-inducible factor-1α (HIF-1α) stabilization under curcumin treatment further amplifies BNIP3 expression, reinforcing mitophagy (Galadari et al., 2022). Damaged mitochondria are engulfed by autophagosomes via LC3-II binding and degraded upon lysosomal fusion, depleting cancer cell energy supplies (Cabrera et al., 2025). Curcumin also disrupts mitochondrial metabolism, increasing ROS production and oxidative stress, which exacerbates mitochondrial dysfunction. By selectively targeting defective mitochondria in pancreatic cancer cells, curcumin impairs ATP synthesis, activates AMPK, and inhibits mTOR, shifting cells toward catabolic pathways. This metabolic stress, combined with BNIP3-mediated mitophagy, suppresses tumor growth and sensitizes cancer cells to apoptosis (Jalali et al., 2025). Furthermore, curcumin downregulates anti-apoptotic proteins like Bcl-2 and upregulates pro-apoptotic factors such as Bax, enhancing cell death (Mosadegh et al., 2025). The dual action of curcumin promoting BNIP3-driven mitophagy while inducing apoptosis highlights its potential as a therapeutic agent for pancreatic cancer, a malignancy often resistant to conventional therapies. Studies suggest that curcumin's ability to selectively target cancer cell mitochondria could improve treatment efficacy while minimizing off-target effects, offering a promising adjunct therapy (Utpal et al., 2025).

Sources of Polyphenols

Cereals, fruits, vegetables, grains, nuts, seeds, herbs, spices, tea, coffee, cocoa and wine are all rich in polyphenols that possess many beneficial chemical properties. For instance, berries (e.g. blueberries, strawberries, and raspberries), apples, mandarins, grapefruits, grapes, onions, spinach, kale, broccoli, beans, almonds, and walnuts are just a few good examples of foods that contain large amounts of polyphenols (Fraga et al., 2019). The content of the types and their bioavailability of polyphenols vary among different plant-based foods. This is determined by factors like varieties, ripness, processing, and preparation ways (Belwal et al., 2022).

Flavonoids

The flavonoids are a type of polyphenol, famous for its abundant exposure in plants, as well as, the diverse biological activities of its members. These compounds in contrast, are chemically characterized by ring structures, in which two phenolic rings A and B, are connected by a three carbon bridge ring C (Zuhlke et al., 2020). The flavonoids are next divided into numerous sub-groups according to the level of hydroxylation and saturation of C ring, and then the 6 major subclasses such as flavonoids, flavones, flavanones, flavanols, anthocyanidins, and isoflavones can be further recognized (Chen et al., 2023).

Among flavonoids, the three flavonoids called fisetin, kaempferol, and luteolin have been shown to induce mitochondrial degradation through the suppression of protein translation in the so-called mTOR pathway plus the activation of autophagy-related proteins (Csekes and Rackova, 2021). The major classes of these drugs induce the display of selective macromolecular elimination of cancer cell energy mitochondria while doing down the production of proliferation and survival of tumor cells (Schiliro and Firestein, 2021).

Sources of Flavonoids

Flavonoids possess a number of therapeutic benefits, including antioxidant, anticancer, antiviral, and anti-inflammatory properties. They also have cardio-protective and neuroprotective effects. These biological activities depend upon the type of flavonoid, its (possible) mode of action, and its bioavailability (Ullah et al., 2020). Commonly found flavonoids include fruits specially citrus, vegetables, grains, legumes, herpes, spices, tea and wine may be included in your diet. Hence, for example, oranges and lemons are flavanones donors, as for apples and onions which are rich in flavonols. Fruits, which can be rich in anthocyanidins such as blueberries, strawberries, and raspberries among many others, are known to their variety in colors (Pemmaraju et al., 2022).

High concentrations flavonoids are present in cocoa beans, contributing to the antioxidant properties of dark chocolate. Tea, particularly green tea, is rich in flavonols. Red wine is also contains flavonoids such as resveratrol. The specific composition and concentration of flavonoids vary among different plant species and cultivars, as well as processing and storage conditions (Nikfardjam et al., 2006).

Polyunsaturated Fatty Acids (PUFAs)

Polyunsaturated fatty acids (PUFAs) are essential fatty acids, which are characterized by the incidence of double bonds in their carbon chain multiple times. These types of fats are vital for providing structural support to our cell membranes, mental development of the brain, secretion of hormones, and regulation of inflammation in the body (Petermann et al., 2022).

PUFAs are classified into two main groups: omega-3 (n-3) and omega-6 (n-6) fatty acids that are classified based on the position of the first double bond from the methyl end (Coniglio et al., 2023). The Omega-3 fatty acids are reputed for their anti-inflammatory and a possibility of these to lower the risk of cardiovascular diseases, improve cognitive functions and support eyes. It is true that omega-6 imbalance characterized by an increased ratio of omega-6 to omega-3 intake might consequently result in heightened inflammation and chronic illnesses (Kavyani et al., 2022).

The intake of omega fatty acids from is great for the overall health and general well-being. Omega 3 fatty acids, namely DHA and EPA, may promote mitophagy by affecting the composition and fluidity of mitochondrial membranes. These PUFAs improve the mitochondrial processing that makes cancer cells vulnerable to apoptosis and death triggered chemotherapeutic agents (Danielli et al., 2022).

Source of PUFAs

The omega-3 fatty acids are enriched with alpha-linolenic acid (ALA), eicosapentaenoic acid (EPA), and docosahexaenoic acid (DHA). Fishes with fatty content like salmon, mackerel, and sardines, algae, walnuts, flaxseeds, chia seeds and hemp seeds are good source of PUFA.

The Omega-6 fatty acids are rich in vegetable oils (e.g. soybean oil, corn oil, and sunflower oil), as well as nuts, seeds and their products are numerous (Rizzo et al., 2023).

Natural Product as Inhibitors of Mitophagy

Alkaloids

Alkaloids are very diverse biological agents as they played roles in traditional practices and medicine. These are a range of naturally occurring nitrogenous derivatives from plants, some fungi, animals, and microorganisms (Bhambhani et al., 2021). Such molecules regularly bring with them the pharmacological properties and this medicinal factor is already well-known among us. Alkaloids possess a strong alkaline character and it is on the base of various biosynthetic pathways that they are synthesized within plants. A lot of alkaloids found in the nature are very strong and produce different effects on the human body, from analgesic and soporific effects to stimulant and hallucinogenic ones but they can be potentially fatal if taken in high doses. Thus the usage of such chemicals should be carefully (Mella et al., 2020).

Studies have referred to alkaloid compounds berberine and piperine as inhibitors of the mitophagy by interrupting mitochondrial membrane potential and the process of oxidative phosphorylation. Comprised of this group of compounds that hamper mitochondrial autophagy and induce apoptosis in cancer cells the tumor development and metastasis are stopped (Wang et al., 2021).

Berberine, an isoquinoline alkaloid found in goldenseal and other medicinal plants, exerts potent anti-tumor effects in liver cancer by activating AMPK-mediated mitophagy (Zhou et al., 2023). The mechanism initiates with berberine's ability to inhibit mitochondrial complex I, leading to decreased ATP production and subsequent AMPK activation due to an elevated AMP/ATP ratio (Li et al., 2025). Activated AMPK phosphorylates and inhibits mTOR, releasing its suppression on the ULK1 complex, which serves as the primary initiator of mitophagy (Ye et al., 2025). Simultaneously, berberine upregulates PINK1 expression, stabilizing it on depolarized mitochondrial membranes where it recruits and activates Parkin. This PINK1/Parkin axis promotes extensive ubiquitination of mitochondrial proteins, marking damaged organelles for clearance. The autophagy adaptor protein p62/SQSTM1 recognizes these ubiquitinated mitochondria, facilitating their engulfment by LC3-II-decorated autophagosomes (Cancho et al., 2025). Berberine further enhances this process by increasing the expression of autophagy-related genes through TFEB nuclear translocation, a master regulator of lysosomal biogenesis. The culmination of these events results in selective degradation of dysfunctional mitochondria through lysosomal hydrolysis, effectively removing ROS-generating organelles and reducing oxidative stress in hepatocarcinoma cells (Haque et al., 2025). Berberine also induced mitophagy is accompanied by cell cycle arrest at G1 phase through downregulation of cyclin D1 and CDK4, as well as activation of apoptotic pathways via caspase-3 cleavage and Bax/Bcl-2 ratio modulation (Ożarowski et al., 2025). This dual action of berberine promoting quality control through AMPK-driven mitophagy while inducing apoptosis compromises cancer cell survival and proliferation. Importantly, berberine's selective targeting of cancer cell mitochondria with minimal effects on normal hepatocytes underscores its potential as both a chemopreventive agent and adjuvant therapy for liver cancer, particularly in cases resistant to conventional treatments (Zhao et al., 2025).

Tetrandrine, a bisbenzylisoquinoline alkaloid derived from Stephania tetrandra, exerts anti-tumor effects in lung cancer by inhibiting mitophagy and sensitizing cancer cells to therapy (Sun et al., 2025). The compound primarily disrupts mitochondrial homeostasis by blocking autophagosome-lysosome fusion, preventing the clearance of damaged mitochondria. Mechanistically, tetrandrine suppresses the PINK1/Parkin pathway by inhibiting Parkin translocation to depolarized mitochondria, thereby reducing ubiquitination of mitochondrial proteins. This impairment prevents the recognition of damaged mitochondria by autophagy receptors like p62/SQSTM1, effectively stalling mitophagy (Jamal et al., 2025). Concurrently, tetrandrine induces mitochondrial dysfunction by increasing ROS production and reducing mitochondrial membrane potential, further exacerbating cellular stress (Utpal et al., 2025). The accumulation of defective mitochondria triggers apoptosis through cytochrome c release and subsequent caspase-9/caspase-3 activation (Tian et al., 2025). Additionally, tetrandrine enhances chemosensitivity by inhibiting protective autophagy, rendering lung cancer cells more vulnerable to conventional therapies like cisplatin or radiation (Khurram et al., 2025). The compound also modulates key signaling pathways, including the downregulation of HIF-1α and BNIP3, which are critical for hypoxia-induced mitophagy. By disrupting these adaptive mechanisms, tetrandrine prevents cancer cells from evading therapy-induced stress (Hassan *et al.,* 2024). Furthermore, it potentiates DNA damage by impairing mitochondrial DNA repair, leading to synthetic lethality with genotoxic agents. This dual action blocking mitophagy while promoting mitochondrial dysfunction compromises cancer cell survival and overcomes resistance mechanisms. Importantly, tetrandrine's selective toxicity toward cancer cells, while sparing normal cells, highlights its potential as an adjunct therapy for refractory lung cancer, particularly in cases where mitophagy contributes to therapeutic resistance (Bouhamida *et al.,* 2022).

Source of Alkaloids

Alkaloids are found is a wide array of plant species and each species usually contains a specific alkaloid or a combination of various alkaloids. The nightshade family (Solanaceae), which includes tomato, potato, eggplant, and other nightshade plants, is as widespread as the family Ranunculaceae, which includes poppy (Nguyen et al., 2023). Both the opium poppy family (Papaveraceae) and the dogbane family (Apocynaceae) are good source of medicinal compounds like vinca, rauwolfia, coffee and cinch. Alkaloids also present in herbal products that derived from coca leaf, kola nut and kratom plant (Kim et al., 2016).

Terpenoids

Terpenoids, also known as terpenes, are a diverse class of organic compounds produced by plants and fungi. They are mainly produced by the polymerization of the five-carbon isoprene molecules and they are marked by their multiplicity of functions in plant. Terpenoids possess a wide spectrum of biological activities such as antioxidant, anti-inflammatory, antimicrobial, and anticancer effects organisms (Paes et al., 2023). Terpenoid compounds, including limolene, betulinic acid, oleanolic acid, and ursolic acid, have been shown to inhibit mitophagy by disrupting mitochondrial dynamics and respiratory chain function. These compounds induce mitochondrial dysfunction and enhance cancer cells susceptibility to apoptosis and chemotherapy (Siraj et al., 2021).

Limolene terpenoids and its metabolites have well known for its biochemical effects because of them being a source of many chemotherapeutic agents. They passes anti-cancer properties since they have been known to cause apoptosis by increasing expression of pro-apoptotic molecules and lowering expression of anti-apoptotic molecules. They have also been involved in a range of functions including inhibition of Na+/K+ ATPase, inhibition of small G protein isoprenylation plus induction of proto-oncogenes, disruption of the telomerase catalytic subunit reverse transcriptase (hTERT)-mechanistic target of rapamycin (mTOR)-regulatory associated protein of mTOR (RAPTOR) [(hTERT–mTOR–RAPTOR)] protein complex, suppression of 3-hydroxy-3-methylglutaryl of 4E-BP1 (Ser65) phosphorylation, and cap-dependent translation (Mukhtar et al., 2018).

Withaferin A, a bioactive steroidal lactone from Withania somnifera, induces cancer cell death by triggering excessive mitophagy through multiple pathways. It directly disrupts mitochondrial function by depolarizing the mitochondrial membrane and generating ROS, which stabilizes PINK1 on damaged organelles. This recruits Parkin to initiate ubiquitination of outer membrane proteins, marking mitochondria for autophagic degradation (Panneerselvam et al., 2025). Withaferin A simultaneously upregulates BNIP3 and FUNDC1, key mitophagy receptors that bypass PINK1/Parkin to directly bind LC3 and promote autophagosome formation. The compound also activates AMPK while inhibiting mTOR, shifting cellular metabolism toward catabolic processes and enhancing autophagy flux. Excessive mitophagy depletes functional mitochondria beyond compensatory capacity, causing catastrophic energy failure (Hashim et al., 2024). Concurrently, Withaferin A inhibits NF-κB survival signaling and activates pro-apoptotic BAX while suppressing anti-apoptotic BCL-2, creating a lethal combination of metabolic collapse and apoptosis. This dual mechanism selectively targets cancer cells with high mitochondrial dependency, as normal cells better tolerate transient mitophagy activation. The resulting mitochondrial clearance overwhelms proteasomal and lysosomal degradation systems, leading to accumulation of toxic protein aggregates and organelle debris that ultimately trigger caspase-independent cell death through mechanisms resembling mitotic catastrophe (Hameed et al., 2025).

Ginsenosides, the active compounds in ginseng, exert anti-glioblastoma effects by modulating the PINK1/Parkin-mediated mitophagy pathway. These saponins selectively accumulate in tumor mitochondria, inducing membrane depolarization and ROS generation, which stabilizes PINK1 on damaged organelles (Li and Xu, 2023). PINK1 phosphorylates both Parkin and ubiquitin, triggering Parkin's translocation and subsequent ubiquitination of mitochondrial proteins like VDAC1 and MFN2. This recruits autophagy adaptors (p62/SQSTM1) that bind LC3-II, facilitating engulfment of dysfunctional mitochondria into autophagosomes. Ginsenosides simultaneously activate AMPK and inhibit mTOR, enhancing autophagic flux while suppressing glioblastoma proliferation. The enhanced mitophagy depletes functional mitochondria, causing bioenergetic crisis and activation of apoptosis through cytochrome c release (Malpartida et al., 2021). Notably, ginsenosides differentially regulate this pathway in tumor versus normal cells by exploiting cancer-specific vulnerabilities in mitochondrial homeostasis. Their ability to cross the blood-brain barrier allows direct targeting of glioblastoma stem cells, sensitizing them to radiation while protecting healthy neurons from oxidative damage (Liu et al., 2025).

Terpenoids also play essential roles in plants, serving as building blocks for various secondary metabolites involved in defense mechanisms, communication, and attraction of pollinators (Divekar et al., 2022).

Source of Terpenoids

Terpenoids are found in abundance in essential oils extracted from aromatic plants, such as herbs, spices, and trees. Common dietary sources of terpenoids include citrus fruits (rich in limonene), mint leaves (containing menthol and menthone), pine trees (providing pinene), lavender (yielding linalool), and cloves (abundant in eugenol). Additionally, terpenoids contribute to the characteristic flavors and aromas of many culinary herbs and spices, making them integral components of cuisines worldwide (Popova et al., 2019; Alirezalu et al., 2020).

Quinones

Quinones are bioactive phytochemicals found in medicinal plants (e.g., rhubarb, aloe), fungi, and bacteria. These yellow/red pigments function as electron carriers in nature. While natural quinones inspired synthetic quinolone antibiotics, true quinolones (like ciprofloxacin) are laboratory-made modifications of the quinone core structure, developed to enhance antimicrobial potency against bacterial DNA gyrase (Tang et al., 2025).

Emodin, an anthraquinone compound found in rhubarb and aloe vera, induces mitophagy in colon cancer through ROS-mediated activation of the PINK1/Parkin pathway. By inhibiting mitochondrial complex I, emodin generates excessive ROS that oxidizes mitochondrial proteins and collapses membrane potential, stabilizing PINK1 on damaged organelles. This recruits Parkin, which ubiquitinates outer membrane proteins (VDAC1, MFN2) to initiate autophagic clearance (Yu et al., 2024). Emodin simultaneously upregulates BNIP3 through HIF-1α stabilization, creating parallel mitophagy induction under hypoxic tumor conditions. The compound also activates AMPK and inhibits mTOR, enhancing autophagosome formation while suppressing cancer cell proliferation. Excessive mitophagy depletes functional mitochondria, causing ATP depletion and activation of AMPK-mediated apoptosis via Bax/Bcl-2 imbalance. Notably, emodin's selective toxicity toward colon cancer cells stems from their heightened ROS susceptibility and reliance on mitochondrial metabolism compared to normal colonocytes. This ROS-dependent mitophagy flux overwhelms cancer cell adaptive mechanisms, leading to metabolic collapse and cell death (Jahan et al., 2025).

Polysaccharides

Polysaccharides are long-chain carbohydrates formed from monosaccharide units linked by glycosidic bonds. They serve as energy storage (starch, glycogen) or structural components (cellulose, chitin). Starch (plants) and glycogen (animals) store glucose, while cellulose strengthens plant cell walls. Chitin supports insect exoskeletons. Other examples include pectin (food gels), hyaluronic acid (joint lubrication), and heparin (anticoagulant). They are insoluble or soluble, high in molecular weight, and biologically essential for energy, structure, and cell signaling (Xu et al., 2025).

Fucoidan, a sulfated polysaccharide derived from brown seaweed, exhibits promising anti-leukemic effects by enhancing mitophagy due to the selective degradation of damaged mitochondria. It activates the PINK1/Parkin pathway, promoting mitochondrial clearance and reducing oxidative stress in cancer cells. Fucoidan also modulates autophagy-related proteins like LC3-II and p62, further supporting mitochondrial turnover (Usov et al., 2022). It also induces apoptosis in leukemia cells by upregulating pro-apoptotic proteins (Bax, caspase-3) and downregulating anti-apoptotic Bcl-2. Its antioxidant properties help protect healthy cells while selectively targeting malignant ones. Studies highlight its potential as an adjuvant therapy, particularly from species like Fucus vesiculosus and Undaria pinnatifida. By enhancing mitophagy and promoting cancer cell death, fucoidan offers a natural therapeutic avenue for leukemia treatment, though further clinical research is needed to optimize its efficacy and delivery (Alfinaikh et al., 2025).

IMPLICATIONS FOR CANCER THERAPY

The modulation of mitophagy by natural products represents a promising approach for cancer treatment, offering potential benefits in terms of efficacy, safety, and selectivity. By targeting mitochondrial control mechanisms, natural products can disrupt the metabolic and bioenergetic adaptations that support tumor growth and survival. Also the pleiotropic effects of natural products on mitophagy and related cellular processes provide opportunities for synergistic combination therapies and personalized therapeutic approaches for cancer patients.

Challenges and Future Perspectives

1. Challenges and limitations associated with using natural products as modulators of mitophagy

Using natural products as modulators of mitophagy presents both beneficial impacts and challenges in the field of medical. While natural therapeutic products offer the advantage of being derived from botanical sources with potentially less adverse effects compared to synthetic drugs, several limitations must be considered.

One major challenge is the issue of bioavailability, as many natural therapeutic compounds have poor pharmacokinetic profiles (absorption, distribution, metabolism, and excretion) in the body. This can hamper their efficiency in reaching target organ tissues and exerting therapeutic effects on mitophagy modulation.

Another important limitation is the lack of specificity of natural therapeutic products, as they often contain several bioactive compounds that may interact with various cellular mechanism pathways. This lack of specificity can lead to off-target effects, potentially causing unintended interfering or consequences with normal cellular functioning mechanism. The variability in composition and potency of natural therapeutic products due to factors such as plant species, cultivation conditions, and extraction technologies adds complexity to their use as modulators of mitophagy. Standardization of natural therapeutic product formulation and rigorous quality control parameters are necessary to ensure consistency and reproducibility in research and clinical applications (Ben et al., 2023).

2. Discuss emerging technologies and methodology that could facilitate the discovery and development of novel mitophagy-modulating agents from natural sources.

Novel mitophagy-modulating agents can be obtained from natural sources with the help of new technologies and emerging approaches. A method which has potential is the use of advanced analytical techniques such as metabolomics, proteomics, and transcriptomics which comprehensively profile the chemical composition and biological activities of natural products. These omics techniques enable researchers to discover novel bioactive molecules and unravel their mechanisms of action in regulating mitophagy (Alarcon et al., 2022).

High-throughput screening (HTS) platforms along with cell-based assays can be used for screening of huge compound libraries or natural products extracts to determine the mitophagy modulators. Also, the computational modeling and artificial intelligence (AI) algorithms are capable of predicting the interactions between the molecules and designing the optimized natural product derivatives with strengthened mitophagy-modulating features. In addition, the formation of new drug delivery systems, like nanoparticles-based formulations, can enhance the bioavailability and targeting of the natural product mitophagy modulators to certain cellular compartments. These innovative technologies and strategies promises great prospects for the rapid discovery and development of safe and effective mitophagy-modulating substances from natural sources, which will, in turn, give rise to innovative therapeutics for diseases with mitochondrial failure (Varca et al., 2021).

CONCLUSION

Natural therapeutic products have shown significant potential as modulators of mitophagy, offering effective therapeutic strategies for mitigating pathological conditions associated with mitochondrial dysregulation. Natural bioactive compounds like Polyphenols, flavonoids, alkaloids, and terpenoids, derived from various sources including plants, demonstrate diverse mechanisms of action in regulating mitophagy pathways. These bioactive compounds target key molecular mechanism involved in mitophagy initiation, execution, and termination, thereby enhancing mitochondrial activity and cellular homeostasis. Despite challenges such as bioavailability and target specificity, ongoing research underscores the therapeutic potential of natural products in mitigating mitophagy-associated pathological disorders. Future studies exploring the synergistic effects of natural product combinations and elucidating their precise mechanisms of action hold promise for the development of personalized medicine approaches. Harnessing the therapeutic potential of natural products in modulating mitophagy represents a promising avenue for advancing disease management and improving patient outcomes.

REFERENCES

Abate, M., Festa, A., Falco, M., Lombardi, A., Luce, A., Grimaldi, A., Zappavigna, S., Sperlongano, P., Irace, C., Caraglia, M., & Misso, G. (2020, February). Mitochondria as playmakers of apoptosis, autophagy and senescence. [). Academic Press.]. *Seminars in Cell & Developmental Biology*, *98*, 139–153. DOI: 10.1016/j.semcdb.2019.05.022 PMID: 31154010

Abdel-Razek, A. S., El-Naggar, M. E., Allam, A., Morsy, O. M., & Othman, S. I. (2020). Microbial natural products in drug discovery. *Processes (Basel, Switzerland)*, *8*(4), 470. DOI: 10.3390/pr8040470

Alarcon-Barrera, J. C., Kostidis, S., Ondo-Mendez, A., & Giera, M. (2022). Recent advances in metabolomics analysis for early drug development. *Drug Discovery Today*, *27*(6), 1763–1773. DOI: 10.1016/j.drudis.2022.02.018 PMID: 35218927

Alfinaikh, R. S., Alamry, K. A., & Hussein, M. A. (2025). Sustainable and biocompatible hybrid materials-based sulfated polysaccharides for biomedical applications: A review. *RSC Advances*, *15*(6), 4708–4767. DOI: 10.1039/D4RA07277D PMID: 39958265

Alirezalu, K., Pateiro, M., Yaghoubi, M., Alirezalu, A., Peighambardoust, S. H., & Lorenzo, J. M. (2020). Phytochemical constituents, advanced extraction technologies and techno-functional properties of selected Mediterranean plants for use in meat products. A comprehensive review. *Trends in Food Science & Technology*, *100*, 292–306. DOI: 10.1016/j.tifs.2020.04.010

Andres-Alonso, M., Kreutz, M. R., & Karpova, A. (2021). Autophagy and the endolysosomal system in presynaptic function. *Cellular and Molecular Life Sciences : CMLS*, *78*(6), 2621–2639. DOI: 10.1007/s00018-020-03722-5 PMID: 33340068

Audano, M., Schneider, A., & Mitro, N. (2018). Mitochondria, lysosomes, and dysfunction: Their meaning in neurodegeneration. *Journal of Neurochemistry*, *147*(3), 291–309. DOI: 10.1111/jnc.14471 PMID: 29804302

Belwal, T., Cravotto, C., Prieto, M. A., Venskutonis, P. R., Daglia, M., Devkota, H. P., Baldi, A., Ezzat, S. M., Gómez-Gómez, L., Salama, M. M., Campone, L., Rastrelli, L., Echave, J., Jafari, S. M., & Cravotto, G. (2022). Effects of different drying techniques on the quality and bioactive compounds of plant-based products: A critical review on current trends. *Drying Technology*, *40*(8), 1539–1561. DOI: 10.1080/07373937.2022.2068028

Ben Hsouna, A., Sadaka, C., Generalić Mekinić, I., Garzoli, S., Švarc-Gajić, J., Rodrigues, F., Morais, S., Moreira, M. M., Ferreira, E., Spigno, G., Brezo-Borjan, T., Akacha, B. B., Saad, R. B., Delerue-Matos, C., & Mnif, W. (2023). The chemical variability, nutraceutical value, and food-industry and cosmetic applications of citrus plants: A critical review. *Antioxidants*, *12*(2), 481. DOI: 10.3390/antiox12020481 PMID: 36830039

Bhambhani, S., Kondhare, K. R., & Giri, A. P. (2021). Diversity in chemical structures and biological properties of plant alkaloids. *Molecules (Basel, Switzerland)*, *26*(11), 3374–3379. DOI: 10.3390/molecules26113374 PMID: 34204857

Bhatia, V., & Sharma, S. (2021). Role of mitochondrial dysfunction, oxidative stress and autophagy in progression of Alzheimer's disease. *Journal of the Neurological Sciences*, *421*, 117253. DOI: 10.1016/j.jns.2020.117253 PMID: 33476985

Bouhamida, E., Morciano, G., Perrone, M., Kahsay, A. E., Della Sala, M., Wieckowski, M. R., Fiorica, F., Pinton, P., Giorgi, C., & Patergnani, S. (2022). The interplay of hypoxia signaling on mitochondrial dysfunction and inflammation in cardiovascular diseases and cancer: From molecular mechanisms to therapeutic approaches. *Biology (Basel)*, *11*(2), 300–312. DOI: 10.3390/biology11020300 PMID: 35205167

Brimson, J. M., Prasanth, M. I., Malar, D. S., Thitilertdecha, P., Kabra, A., Tencomnao, T., & Prasansuklab, A. (2021). Plant polyphenols for aging health: Implication from their autophagy modulating properties in age-associated diseases. *Pharmaceuticals (Basel, Switzerland)*, *14*(10), 982–993. DOI: 10.3390/ph14100982 PMID: 34681206

Cabrera-Serrano, A. J., Sánchez-Maldonado, J. M., González-Olmedo, C., Carretero-Fernández, M., Díaz-Beltrán, L., Gutiérrez-Bautista, J. F., García-Verdejo, F. J., Gálvez-Montosa, F., López-López, J. A., García-Martín, P., Pérez, E. M., Sánchez-Rovira, P., Reyes-Zurita, F. J., & Sainz, J. (2025). Crosstalk between autophagy and oxidative stress in hematological malignancies: Mechanisms, implications, and therapeutic potential. *Antioxidants*, *14*(3), 264–272. DOI: 10.3390/antiox14030264 PMID: 40227235

Cancho, A. F. M., del Mar Martín-Latorre, M., Lozano-Paniagua, D., & Nievas-Soriano, B. J. (2025). Caloric restriction mimetics: Effects of spermidine and berberine on healthy longevity and prevention of aging-associated diseases. *Nutrición Clínica, Dietética Hospitalaria*, *45*(1), 286–291.

Chandra, S., Veeraraghavan, V. P., Woon, C. K., Sirasanagandla, S. R., & Jayaraman, S. (2025). Mechanistic Overview on Therapeutic Potential of Phenols Targeting the Breast Cancer: Molecular Insights and Future Road to Drug Design. *The Natural Products Journal*, *12*(3), 172–184. DOI: 10.2174/0122103155351726250123083250

Chen, S., Wang, X., Cheng, Y., Gao, H., & Chen, X. (2023). A review of classification, biosynthesis, biological activities and potential applications of flavonoids. *Molecules (Basel, Switzerland)*, *28*(13), 4982. DOI: 10.3390/molecules28134982 PMID: 37446644

Chodari, L., Dilsiz Aytemir, M., Vahedi, P., Alipour, M., Vahed, S. Z., Khatibi, S. M. H., Ahmadian, E., Ardalan, M., & Eftekhari, A. (2021). Targeting mitochondrial biogenesis with polyphenol compounds. *Oxidative Medicine and Cellular Longevity*, ●●●, 2021. PMID: 34336094

Coniglio, S., Shumskaya, M., & Vassiliou, E. (2023). Unsaturated fatty acids and their immunomodulatory properties. *Biology (Basel)*, *12*(2), 279. DOI: 10.3390/biology12020279 PMID: 36829556

Csekes, E., & Račková, L. (2021). Skin aging, cellular senescence and natural polyphenols. *International Journal of Molecular Sciences*, *22*(23), 12641. DOI: 10.3390/ijms222312641 PMID: 34884444

D'Arcy, M. S. (2022). A review of biologically active flavonoids as inducers of autophagy and apoptosis in neoplastic cells and as cytoprotective agents in non-neoplastic cells. *Cell Biology International*, *46*(8), 1179–1195. DOI: 10.1002/cbin.11813 PMID: 35544782

Danielli, M., Perne, L., Jarc Jovičić, E., & Petan, T. (2023). Lipid droplets and polyunsaturated fatty acid trafficking: Balancing life and death. *Frontiers in Cell and Developmental Biology*, *11*, 1104725. DOI: 10.3389/fcell.2023.1104725 PMID: 36776554

Divekar, P. A., Narayana, S., Divekar, B. A., Kumar, R., Gadratagi, B. G., Ray, A., Singh, A. K., Rani, V., Singh, V., Singh, A. K., Kumar, A., Singh, R. P., Meena, R. S., & Behera, T. K. (2022). Plant secondary metabolites as defense tools against herbivores for sustainable crop protection. *International Journal of Molecular Sciences*, *23*(5), 2690. DOI: 10.3390/ijms23052690 PMID: 35269836

Fahmy, H. A., & Farag, M. A. (2022). Ongoing and potential novel trends of pomegranate fruit peel; a comprehensive review of its health benefits and future perspectives as nutraceutical. *Journal of Food Biochemistry*, *46*(1), e14024. DOI: 10.1111/jfbc.14024 PMID: 34923641

Fraga, C. G., Croft, K. D., Kennedy, D. O., & Tomás-Barberán, F. A. (2019). The effects of polyphenols and other bioactives on human health. *Food & Function*, *10*(2), 514–528. DOI: 10.1039/C8FO01997E PMID: 30746536

Galadari, S., Cheratta, A. R., & Thayyullathil, F. (2022). Regulation of Tumor Suppressor Par-4 by Ceramide. *Tumor Suppressor Par-4: Structural Features. Molecular Mechanisms and Function, 13*(3), 263–291.

Galeotti, F., Capitani, F., Fachini, A., & Volpi, N. (2019). Recent advances in analytical approaches for the standardization and quality of polyphenols of propolis. *Journal of Medicinal Plants Research, 13*(19), 487–500. DOI: 10.5897/JMPR2019.6849

Golubnitschaja, O., Kapinova, A., Sargheini, N., Bojkova, B., Kapalla, M., Heinrich, L., Gkika, E., & Kubatka, P. (2024). Mini-encyclopedia of mitochondria-relevant nutraceuticals protecting health in primary and secondary care—Clinically relevant 3PM innovation. *The EPMA Journal, 15*(2), 163–205. DOI: 10.1007/s13167-024-00358-4 PMID: 38841620

Gubas, A., & Dikic, I. (2022). A guide to the regulation of selective autophagy receptors. *The FEBS Journal, 289*(1), 75–89. DOI: 10.1111/febs.15824 PMID: 33730405

Gustafsson, Å. B., & Dorn, G. W.II. (2019). Evolving and expanding the roles of mitophagy as a homeostatic and pathogenic process. *Physiological Reviews, 99*(1), 853–892. DOI: 10.1152/physrev.00005.2018 PMID: 30540226

Hameed, H., Afzal, M., Khan, M. A., Javaid, L., Shahzad, M., & Abrar, K. (2025). Unraveling the role of withanolides as key modulators in breast cancer mitigation. *Molecular Biology Reports, 52*(1), 331–337. DOI: 10.1007/s11033-025-10442-1 PMID: 40117002

Haque, S., Mathkor, D. M., Bhat, S. A., Musayev, A., Khituova, L., Ramniwas, S., Phillips, E., Swamy, N., Kumar, S., Yerer, M. B., Tuli, H. S., & Yadav, V. (2025). A Comprehensive Review Highlighting the Prospects of Phytonutrient Berberine as an Anticancer Agent. *Journal of Biochemical and Molecular Toxicology, 39*(1), 70073–70081. DOI: 10.1002/jbt.70073 PMID: 39717894

Hashim, G. M., Shahgolzari, M., Hefferon, K., Yavari, A., & Venkataraman, S. (2024). Plant-Derived Anti-Cancer Therapeutics and Biopharmaceuticals. *Bioengineering (Basel, Switzerland), 12*(1), 7–18. DOI: 10.3390/bioengineering12010007 PMID: 39851281

Hassan, A. M. I. A., Zhao, Y., Chen, X., & He, C. (2024). Blockage of autophagy for cancer therapy: A comprehensive review. *International Journal of Molecular Sciences, 25*(13), 7459–7467. DOI: 10.3390/ijms25137459 PMID: 39000565

Jahan, S., Ikram, M., Siraj, S., Ullah, S., Zakria, M., & Ahmad, N. (2025). Emodin, a potent anthraquinone mitigates MPTP-induced Parkinsons' disease pathology by regulating Nrf2 and its downstream targets: In silico and in vivo approach. *Molecular Neurobiology*, *8*(4), 1–18.

Jalali, P., Shahmoradi, A., Samii, A., Mazloomnejad, R., Hatamnejad, M. R., Saeed, A., Namdar, A., & Salehi, Z. (2025). The role of autophagy in cancer: From molecular mechanism to therapeutic window. *Frontiers in Immunology*, *16*, 230–242. DOI: 10.3389/fimmu.2025.1528230 PMID: 40248706

Jamal, A., Arif, A., Shahid, M. N., Kiran, S., & Batool, Z. (2025). Plant Secondary Metabolites Inhibit Cancer by Targeting Epidermal Growth Factor Receptor (EGFR): An Updated Review on their Regulation and Mechanisms of Action. *Asian Pacific Journal of Cancer Biology*, *10*(1), 191–206. DOI: 10.31557/apjcb.2025.10.1.191-206

Jing, X., & Jin, K. (2020). A gold mine for drug discovery: Strategies to develop cyclic peptides into therapies. *Medicinal Research Reviews*, *40*(2), 753–810. DOI: 10.1002/med.21639 PMID: 31599007

Karagin, P. H., Altaner, A., Özsoy, B., & And Kutlu, B. (2017). Genetic causes of Parkinson's disease. *Turkish Journal of Molecular Biology & Biotechnology*, *2*, 39–45.

Kavyani, Z., Musazadeh, V., Fathi, S., Faghfouri, A. H., Dehghan, P., & Sarmadi, B. (2022). Efficacy of the omega-3 fatty acids supplementation on inflammatory biomarkers: An umbrella meta-analysis. *International Immunopharmacology*, *111*, 109104. DOI: 10.1016/j.intimp.2022.109104 PMID: 35914448

Khurram, I., Khan, M. U., Ibrahim, S., Ghani, M. U., Amin, I., Falzone, L., Herrera-Bravo, J., Setzer, W. N., Sharifi-Rad, J., & Calina, D. (2025). Thapsigargin and its prodrug derivatives: Exploring novel approaches for targeted cancer therapy through calcium signaling disruption. *Medical Oncology (Northwood, London, England)*, *42*(1), 1–21. PMID: 39557802

Kim, S., Kim, B., Mun, S., Park, J. H., Kim, M. K., Choi, S., & Lee, S. (2016). Development of a template for the classification of traditional medical knowledge in Korea. *Journal of Ethnopharmacology*, *178*, 82–103. DOI: 10.1016/j.jep.2015.11.045 PMID: 26657579

Kulikov, A. V., Luchkina, E. A., Gogvadze, V., & Zhivotovsky, B. (2017). Mitophagy: Link to cancer development and therapy. *Biochemical and Biophysical Research Communications*, *482*(3), 432–439. DOI: 10.1016/j.bbrc.2016.10.088 PMID: 28212727

Li, M., Ding, L., Cao, L., Zhang, Z., Li, X., Li, Z., Xia, Q., Yin, K., Song, S., Wang, Z., & Du, H. (2025). Natural products targeting AMPK signaling pathway therapy, diabetes mellitus and its complications. *Frontiers in Pharmacology, 16*, 4634–4644.

Li, W., & Xu, X. (2023). Advances in mitophagy and mitochondrial apoptosis pathway-related drugs in glioblastoma treatment. *Frontiers in Pharmacology, 14*, 1719–1725. DOI: 10.3389/fphar.2023.1211719 PMID: 37456742

Liang, W., He, X., Bi, J., Hu, T., & Sun, Y. (2021). Role of reactive oxygen species in tumors based on the 'seed and soil'theory: A complex interaction. *Oncology Reports, 46*(3), 1–15. DOI: 10.3892/or.2021.8159 PMID: 34328200

Liu, H., Song, Y., Wang, H., Zhou, Y., Xu, M., & Xian, J. (2025). Deciphering the Power of Resveratrol in Mitophagy: From Molecular Mechanisms to Therapeutic Applications. *Phytotherapy Research, 39*(3), 1319–1343. DOI: 10.1002/ptr.8433 PMID: 39754508

Lystad, A. H., & Simonsen, A. (2019). Mechanisms and pathophysiological roles of the ATG8 conjugation machinery. *Cells, 8*(9), 973. DOI: 10.3390/cells8090973 PMID: 31450711

Ma, K., Chen, G., Li, W., Kepp, O., Zhu, Y., & Chen, Q. (2020). Mitophagy, mitochondrial homeostasis, and cell fate. *Frontiers in Cell and Developmental Biology, 8*, 467. DOI: 10.3389/fcell.2020.00467 PMID: 32671064

Malpartida, A. B., Williamson, M., Narendra, D. P., Wade-Martins, R., & Ryan, B. J. (2021). Mitochondrial dysfunction and mitophagy in Parkinson's disease: From mechanism to therapy. *Trends in Biochemical Sciences, 46*(4), 329–343. DOI: 10.1016/j.tibs.2020.11.007 PMID: 33323315

Mattio, L. M., Catinella, G., Dallavalle, S., & Pinto, A. (2020). Stilbenoids: A natural arsenal against bacterial pathogens. *Antibiotics (Basel, Switzerland), 9*(6), 336. DOI: 10.3390/antibiotics9060336 PMID: 32570824

Mella-Raipán, J., Romero-Parra, J., & Recabarren-Gajardo, G. (2020). DARK classics in chemical neuroscience: Heroin and desomorphine. *ACS Chemical Neuroscience, 11*(23), 3905–3927. DOI: 10.1021/acschemneuro.0c00262 PMID: 32568519

Meng, T., Wen, Z., Cheng, X., Li, C., Zhang, P., Xiao, D., & Xu, Y. (2025). Unlocking Gut Health: The Potent Role of Stilbenoids in Intestinal Homeostasis. *Animals (Basel), 15*(3), 417–426. DOI: 10.3390/ani15030417 PMID: 39943187

Mosadegh, M., Noori Goodarzi, N., & Erfani, Y. (2025). A Comprehensive Insight into Apoptosis: Molecular Mechanisms, Signaling Pathways, and Modulating Therapeutics. *Cancer Investigation*, *7*(3), 1–26. DOI: 10.1080/07357907.2024.2445528 PMID: 39760426

Mukhtar, Y. M., Adu-Frimpong, M., Xu, X., & Yu, J. (2018). Biochemical significance of limonene and its metabolites: Future prospects for designing and developing highly potent anticancer drugs. *Bioscience Reports*, *38*(6), BSR20181253. DOI: 10.1042/BSR20181253 PMID: 30287506

Nguyen, D. H., El-Ramady, H., Llanaj, X., Törős, G., Hajdú, P., & Prokisch, J. (2023). Chemical composition and health attributes of agri-foods: A scientific overview on black foods. *Sustainability (Basel)*, *15*(4), 3852. DOI: 10.3390/su15043852

Nikfardjam, M. S. P., Márk, L., Avar, P., Figler, M., & Ohmacht, R. (2006). Polyphenols, anthocyanins, and trans-resveratrol in red wines from the Hungarian Villány region. *Food Chemistry*, *98*(3), 453–462. DOI: 10.1016/j.foodchem.2005.06.014

Ożarowski, M., Karpiński, T. M., Czerny, B., Kamiński, A., & Seremak-Mrozikiewicz, A. (2025). Plant Alkaloids as Promising Anticancer Compounds with Blood–Brain Barrier Penetration in the Treatment of Glioblastoma: In Vitro and In Vivo Models. *Molecules (Basel, Switzerland)*, *30*(7), 1561–1568. DOI: 10.3390/molecules30071561 PMID: 40286187

Padman, B. S., Nguyen, T. N., Uoselis, L., Skulsuppaisarn, M., Nguyen, L. K., & Lazarou, M. (2019). LC3/GABARAPs drive ubiquitin-independent recruitment of Optineurin and NDP52 to amplify mitophagy. *Nature Communications*, *10*(1), 408. DOI: 10.1038/s41467-019-08335-6 PMID: 30679426

Paes, A. S., Koga, R. D. C. R., Sales, P. F., Santos Almeida, H. K., Teixeira, T. A. C. C., & Carvalho, J. C. T. (2023). Phytocompounds from Amazonian Plant Species against Acute Kidney Injury: Potential Nephroprotective Effects. *Molecules (Basel, Switzerland)*, *28*(17), 6411. DOI: 10.3390/molecules28176411 PMID: 37687240

Panneerselvam, D. S., Kanakaraja, A., Sakthivelu, M., Gopinath, S. C., & Raman, P. (2025). A comprehensive review of therapeutic compounds from plants for neurodegenerative diseases. *Current Medicinal Chemistry*, *32*(10), 1887–1933. DOI: 10.2174/0109298673272435231204072922 PMID: 38367263

Pavlova, J. A., Guseva, E. A., Dontsova, O. A., & Sergiev, P. V. (2024). Natural activators of autophagy. *Biochemistry (Moscow)*, *89*(1), 1–26. DOI: 10.1134/S0006297924010012 PMID: 38467543

Pemmaraju, D. B., Ghosh, A., Gangasani, J. K., Murthy, U. S. N., Naidu, V. G. M., & Rengan, A. K. (2022). Herbal biomolecules as nutraceuticals. *Herbal Biomolecules in Healthcare Applications,* 525-549.

Petermann, A. B., Reyna-Jeldes, M., Ortega, L., Coddou, C., & Yévenes, G. E. (2022). Roles of the unsaturated fatty acid docosahexaenoic acid in the central nervous system: Molecular and cellular insights. *International Journal of Molecular Sciences, 23*(10), 5390. DOI: 10.3390/ijms23105390 PMID: 35628201

Popova, V., Ivanova, T., Stoyanova, A., Nikolova, V., Hristeva, T., Gochev, V., Yonchev, Y., Nikolov, N., & Zheljazkov, V. D. (2019). Terpenoids in the essential oil and concentrated aromatic products obtained from Nicotiana glutinosa L. leaves. *Molecules (Basel, Switzerland), 25*(1), 30. DOI: 10.3390/molecules25010030 PMID: 31861797

Rizzo, G., Baroni, L., & Lombardo, M. (2023). Promising sources of plant-derived polyunsaturated fatty acids: A narrative review. *International Journal of Environmental Research and Public Health, 20*(3), 1683. DOI: 10.3390/ijerph20031683 PMID: 36767052

Schiliro, C., & Firestein, B. L. (2021). Mechanisms of metabolic reprogramming in cancer cells supporting enhanced growth and proliferation. *Cells, 10*(5), 1056. DOI: 10.3390/cells10051056 PMID: 33946927

Schirrmacher, V. (2020). Mitochondria at work: New insights into regulation and dysregulation of cellular energy supply and metabolism. *Biomedicines, 8*(11), 526. DOI: 10.3390/biomedicines8110526 PMID: 33266387

Siraj, M. A., Islam, M. A., Al Fahad, M. A., Kheya, H. R., Xiao, J., & Simal-Gandara, J. (2021). Cancer chemopreventive role of dietary terpenoids by modulating Keap1-Nrf2-ARE signaling system—A comprehensive update. *Applied Sciences (Basel, Switzerland), 11*(22), 10806. DOI: 10.3390/app112210806

Steer, E. K., Dail, M. K., & Chu, C. T. (2015). Beyond mitophagy: Cytosolic PINK1 as a messenger of mitochondrial health. *Antioxidants & Redox Signaling, 22*(12), 1047–1059. DOI: 10.1089/ars.2014.6206 PMID: 25557302

Sun, S., Yu, W., Zhang, G., Li, X., Song, L., Lv, Y., & Chen, Y. (2025). Potential mechanism of traditional Chinese medicine intervention in gastric cancer: Targeted regulation of autophagy. *Frontiers in Pharmacology, 16*, 1548672. DOI: 10.3389/fphar.2025.1548672 PMID: 40066330

Tang, Q., Li, Z., Chen, N., Luo, X., & Zhao, Q. (2025). Natural pigments derived from plants and microorganisms: Classification, biosynthesis, and applications. *Plant Biotechnology Journal*, *23*(2), 592–614. DOI: 10.1111/pbi.14522 PMID: 39642082

Tian, Y., Hu, X., Zhang, T., Li, B., Fu, Q., & Li, J. (2025). Advances in Chinese herbal medicine in modulating mitochondria to treat myocardial ischemia-reperfusion injury: A narrative review. *Cardiovascular Diagnosis and Therapy*, *15*(1), 207–2713. DOI: 10.21037/cdt-24-346 PMID: 40115104

Tshikhudo, P. P., Mabhaudhi, T., Koorbanally, N. A., Mudau, F. N., Calina, D., & Sharifi-Rad, J. (2025). Pinosylvin as a promising natural anticancer agent: Mechanisms of action and future directions in cancer therapy. *Naunyn-Schmiedeberg's Archives of Pharmacology*, *10*(4), 1–19. DOI: 10.1007/s00210-025-03850-4 PMID: 39918573

Ullah, A., Munir, S., Badshah, S. L., Khan, N., Ghani, L., Poulson, B. G., Emwas, A. H., & Jaremko, M. (2020). Important flavonoids and their role as a therapeutic agent. *Molecules (Basel, Switzerland)*, *25*(22), 5243. DOI: 10.3390/molecules25225243 PMID: 33187049

Usov, A. I., Bilan, M. I., Ustyuzhanina, N. E., & Nifantiev, N. E. (2022). Fucoidans of brown algae: Comparison of sulfated polysaccharides from Fucus vesiculosus and Ascophyllum nodosum. *Marine Drugs*, *20*(10), 638–642. DOI: 10.3390/md20100638 PMID: 36286461

Utpal, B. K., Al Amin, M., Zehravi, M., Sweilam, S. H., Arjun, U. V. N. V., Madhuri, Y. B., Gupta, J. K., Yaidikar, L., Tummala, T., Suseela, R., Durairaj, A., Reddy, K. T. K., Al Fahaid, A. A. F., Rab, S. O., Almahjari, M. S., & Emran, T. B. (2025). Alkaloids as neuroprotectors: Targeting signaling pathways in neurodegenerative diseases. *Molecular and Cellular Biochemistry*, *14*, 1–26. DOI: 10.1007/s11010-025-05258-3 PMID: 40192920

Utpal, B. K., Bouenni, H., Zehravi, M., Sweilam, S. H., Mortuza, M. R., Arjun, U. V. N. V., & Emran, T. B. (2025). Exploring natural products as apoptosis modulators in cancers: Insights into natural product-based therapeutic strategies. *Naunyn-Schmiedeberg's Archives of Pharmacology*, *18*, 1–26. DOI: 10.1007/s00210-025-03876-8 PMID: 40014131

Varca, A. C., Casalena, D., Chan, W. C., Hu, B., Magin, R. S., Roberts, R. M., Liu, X., Zhu, H., Seo, H. S., Dhe-Paganon, S., Marto, J. A., Auld, D., & Buhrlage, S. J. (2021). Identification and validation of selective deubiquitinase inhibitors. *Cell Chemical Biology*, *28*(12), 1758–1771. DOI: 10.1016/j.chembiol.2021.05.012 PMID: 34129829

Wang, Z. Y., Liu, J., Zhu, Z., Su, C. F., Sreenivasmurthy, S. G., Iyaswamy, A., Lu, J. H., Chen, G., Song, J. X., & Li, M. (2021). Traditional Chinese medicine compounds regulate autophagy for treating neurodegenerative disease: A mechanism review. *Biomedicine and Pharmacotherapy*, *133*, 110968. DOI: 10.1016/j.biopha.2020.110968 PMID: 33189067

Wauters, F., Cornelissen, T., Imberechts, D., Martin, S., Koentjoro, B., Sue, C., Vangheluwe, P., & Vandenberghe, W. (2020). LRRK2 mutations impair depolarization-induced mitophagy through inhibition of mitochondrial accumulation of RAB10. *Autophagy*, *16*(2), 203–222. DOI: 10.1080/15548627.2019.1603548 PMID: 30945962

Xu, B. W., Li, S. S., Ding, W. L., Zhang, C., Rehman, M. U., Tareen, M. F., Wang, L., & Huang, S. C. (2025). From structure to function: A comprehensive overview of polysaccharide roles and applications. *Food Frontiers*, *6*(1), 15–39. DOI: 10.1002/fft2.490

Yang, Y., Ma, F., Liu, Z., Su, Q., Liu, Y., Liu, Z., & Li, Y. (2019). The ER-localized Ca2+-binding protein calreticulin couples ER stress to autophagy by associating with microtubule-associated protein 1A/1B light chain 3. *The Journal of Biological Chemistry*, *294*(3), 772–782. DOI: 10.1074/jbc.RA118.005166 PMID: 30429217

Ye, D., Zhu, J., Su, S., Yu, Y., Zhang, J., Yin, Y., Lin, C., Xie, X., Xiang, Q., & Yu, R. (2025). Natural small molecules regulating the mitophagy pathway counteract the pathogenesis of diabetes and chronic complications. *Frontiers in Pharmacology*, *16*, 1767–1773. DOI: 10.3389/fphar.2025.1571767 PMID: 40308774

Yu, L., Qin, J., Zhang, M., Gao, Y., & Zhao, Y. (2024). Research Progress on the Anti-Liver Cancer Mechanism and Toxicity of Rhubarb Anthraquinone. *Drug Design, Development and Therapy*, *12*, 6089–6113. DOI: 10.2147/DDDT.S489377 PMID: 39717199

Zhao, W., Chen, Z., Fu, W., Ye, C., Fu, H., Xu, T., Wu, B., Chen, L., & Shan, S. J. (2025). Induction of apoptosis and hypoxic stress in malignant melanoma cells via graphene-mediated far-infrared radiation. *BMC Cancer*, *25*(1), 620–628. DOI: 10.1186/s12885-025-14031-0 PMID: 40197161

Zhou, P., Ma, Y. Y., Zhao, X. N., & Hua, F. (2023). Phytochemicals as potential target on thioredoxin-interacting protein (TXNIP) for the treatment of cardiovascular diseases. *Inflammopharmacology*, *31*(1), 207–220. DOI: 10.1007/s10787-022-01130-8 PMID: 36609715

Zühlke, M. K., Schlüter, R., Mikolasch, A., Henning, A. K., Giersberg, M., Lalk, M., Kunze, G., Schweder, T., Urich, T., & Schauer, F. (2020). Biotransformation of bisphenol A analogues by the biphenyl-degrading bacterium Cupriavidus basilensis-a structure-biotransformation relationship. *Applied Microbiology and Biotechnology*, *104*(8), 3569–3583. DOI: 10.1007/s00253-020-10406-4 PMID: 32125477

KEY TERMS AND DEFINITIONS

Alkaloids: Alkaloids are naturally occurring organic chemical compounds characterized by a nitrogen-containing ring in a structure, often found in plants. They possess diverse pharmacological effects and have been utilized in medicine.

Apoptosis: Apoptosis is a programmed cell death process essential for maintaining tissue homeostasis, characterized by cellular self-destruction through controlled biochemical pathways.

Flavonoids: Flavonoids are secondary metabolites of plant characterized by their polyphenolic structure, contributing to various biological activities and health benefits.

Mitophagy: Mitophagy is a cellular process responsible for the selective degradation and removal of damaged or dysfunctional mitochondria, crucial for maintaining cellular homeostasis and preventing cellular damage.

Natural products: Natural products are chemical compounds produced by living organisms, typically plants, microbes, or marine organisms, possessing pharmacological or biological activity.

Polyphenols: Polyphenols are a diverse group of organic compounds found in plants, characterized by multiple phenol functional groups, known for their antioxidant properties and potential health benefits.

Terpenoids: Terpenoids are a major class of naturally occurring organic chemical compounds, found in plants and some microorganisms, exhibiting diverse biological activities and contributing to various medicinal and industrial applications.

Chapter 11
Role of Mitophagy in Cancer Drug Resistance

Charuwan Thanawiroon
https://orcid.org/0009-0004-9076-3219
Ubon Ratchathani University, Thailand

Bancha Yingngam
https://orcid.org/0000-0001-7215-9123
Ubon Ratchathani University, Thailand

ABSTRACT

Adaptation mediated by drug resistance is one of the barriers to combating cancer. Moreover, during stress responses, such as hypoxia and nutrient deprivation, mitophagy, which is the selective autophagy of mitochondria, plays an essential role in influencing cancer cell resistance to drugs. This chapter describes the molecular pathways involved in mitophagy and their effects on the survival of cancer cells and resistance mechanisms. The latest discoveries listed in this chapter illustrate how mitophagy facilitates the ability of cancer cells to adjust to metabolic and therapeutic emergencies. Modulation of established mitophagy is a promising strategy for mediating drug resistance. Moreover, future studies should focus on the development of targeted therapies to alter mitophagy regulation to improve cancer treatment outcomes.

INTRODUCTION

Throughout the 21st century, cancer remains an enormous and expanding problem for health systems worldwide that affects individuals, families, and communities. On April 4, 2024, according to reports by the International Agency for Research

DOI: 10.4018/979-8-3693-3836-0.ch011

on Cancer (IARC) and the American Cancer Society (ACS), cancer continues to pose a considerable burden worldwide, with global cancer rates as high as approximately 20 million new cases and some ten million deaths in 2022. Projections point to a massive increase to 35 million new cases per year by 2050 with rapid aging and global population growth, as well as emerging risk factors such as unhealthy diets, physical inactivity, and smoking as the main drivers. The most common and deadly cancer globally is lung cancer, followed by colorectal and liver cancers. The disparities in cancer morbidity and mortality therefore highlight the urgent need for improved strategies and solutions for cancer prevention and control that combine modern medical treatments with broad public health measures to address modifiable risk factors (Bray et al., 2024; International Agency for Research on Cancer, 2024).

The ongoing challenges of cancer drug resistance significantly complicate oncological care, impacting patient outcomes and complicating treatment strategies. As cancer cells adapt to and evade therapeutic interventions, they not only diminish the efficacy of existing treatments but also pose a formidable barrier to long-term disease management and survival (Zheng et al., 2024). Resistance mechanisms, which include genetic mutations, alterations in drug targets, efflux of drugs by transport proteins, and alterations in cellular death pathways, have become a central focus in cancer research due to their role in treatment failure. The complexity is further heightened by the tumor microenvironment and cellular heterogeneity within tumors, which can harbor subpopulations of cells with distinct resistance profiles, thereby allowing the tumor to persist and evolve despite aggressive treatment (Wang et al., 2024). This adaptive capacity of cancer cells underscores the urgent need for novel therapeutic strategies and the development of personalized medicine approaches that can predict and counteract resistance mechanisms. Understanding and overcoming drug resistance is critical not only for improving the efficacy of current therapies but also for the successful implementation and durability of emerging treatments, including targeted therapies and immunotherapies, which are often hailed as the future of cancer treatment (Jan et al., 2024). In this context, targeting mitophagy has emerged as a promising strategy. By manipulating mitophagy, researchers aim to either promote the removal of dysfunctional mitochondria, preventing cancer cells from using mitochondrial adaptation for survival, or inhibit this process to cause a buildup of defective mitochondria, leading to cellular stress and death (X.-Q. Huang et al., 2024). Thus, integrating mitophagy modulation into cancer treatment strategies offers a novel avenue to potentially overcome drug resistance, paving the way for more effective and enduring cancer therapies.

Mitophagy is a specialized form of autophagy that involves the selective degradation of mitochondria by lysosomes, a process crucial for maintaining cellular homeostasis and mitochondrial quality control (Li et al., 2024). It is triggered by various cellular signals, including mitochondrial damage and oxidative stress, and is regulated by several key proteins, such as PTEN-induced kinase 1 (PINK1) and Parkin RBR E3 ubiquitin-protein ligase (Parkin). These proteins help tag damaged mitochondria for removal, preventing the accumulation of dysfunctional mitochondria that can lead to cellular degeneration (Chen, 2024). The process of mitophagy is essential not only for cell survival and function under stress but also for developmental processes and disease pathogenesis, including neurodegenerative diseases and cancer (Wu et al., 2024). Understanding the mechanisms and regulation of mitophagy provides insights into how cells adapt to metabolic changes and stress, offering potential therapeutic targets for various diseases.

In the context of cancer, mitophagy plays a dual role, acting both as a tumor suppressor by eliminating damaged mitochondria that can lead to genomic instability and as a survival mechanism that enables cancer cells to withstand metabolic and therapeutic stress (Ling et al., 2024). This adaptability contributes significantly to the development and progression of cancer, as well as to the emergence of drug resistance. Cancer cells harness mitophagy to avoid apoptosis and manage the increased metabolic demands associated with rapid growth and proliferation (D'Arcy, 2024). Additionally, by maintaining mitochondrial function and integrity, mitophagy helps cancer cells resist the cytotoxic effects of anticancer drugs, leading to treatment failure and relapse (Sun et al., 2024). Therefore, a deeper understanding of the relationship between mitophagy and cancer could reveal new strategies for cancer treatment, specifically in designing therapies that prevent cancer cells from utilizing mitophagy for survival during chemotherapy.

This chapter explores the role of mitophagy in cancer drug resistance. The authors aim to dissect the molecular pathways regulating mitophagy and how its dysregulation can influence cancer cell fate. Additionally, this chapter reviews recent advancements in targeting mitophagy in cancer therapy, examining both the potential and challenges of such approaches. The goal is to offer insights into how manipulating mitophagy could enhance the efficacy of cancer treatments and potentially lead to the development of novel therapeutic strategies that overcome drug resistance, thus improving patient outcomes in oncology.

PATHWAYS INVOLVE IN MITOPHAGY INDUCTION

Mitophagy is a specialized form of autophagy that involves the degradation and recycling of damaged or unnecessary cellular components. It specifically targets the selective autophagic elimination of mitochondria. This crucial cellular mechanism helps maintain cellular health by removing dysfunctional or damaged mitochondria, thus preventing the accumulation of mitochondrial defects and contributing to cellular homeostasis. Mitophagy occurs within the cytoplasm and specifically targets mitochondria for degradation through several key steps. Figure 1 shows a step-by-step explanation of where and how the process occurs.

- Recognition: This process begins when damaged or dysfunctional mitochondria are recognized. This can be due to mitochondrial depolarization, oxidative stress, or other damage signals. In cancer cells, mitochondrial dysfunction is common, often as a result of harsh metabolic and oxidative conditions within the tumor environment.
- Sequestration: Once a mitochondrion is subjected to degradation (e.g., through ubiquitination in the PINK1-Parkin pathway or directly by receptors such as NIX or BNIP3 in the receptor-mediated pathway), it is sequestered from the rest of the cell. This involves the mitochondrion being enveloped by a double-membrane structure known as an autophagosome.
- Autophagosome Formation: Autophagosomes are key organelles in the autophagy process. It forms around the damaged mitochondrion, engulfing it completely. The formation of the autophagosome is facilitated by various autophagy-related proteins that help to elongate and curve the membrane around the mitochondrion.
- Fusion with Lysosomes: The autophagosome containing the mitochondrion then fuses with a lysosome, another cellular organelle. Lysosomes contain digestive enzymes that breakdown the contents of the autophagosome.
- Degradation: Within the lysosome, the enclosed mitochondrion is degraded by lysosomal hydrolases. This degradation process allows for the recycling of mitochondrial components, such as amino acids and fatty acids, which can be reused by the cell.
- Recycling: The degradation products are then exported back into the cytosol of the cell, where they can be reused for the synthesis of new molecules or for energy production (Li et al., 2024).

Figure 1. The mitophagy process in cancer cells

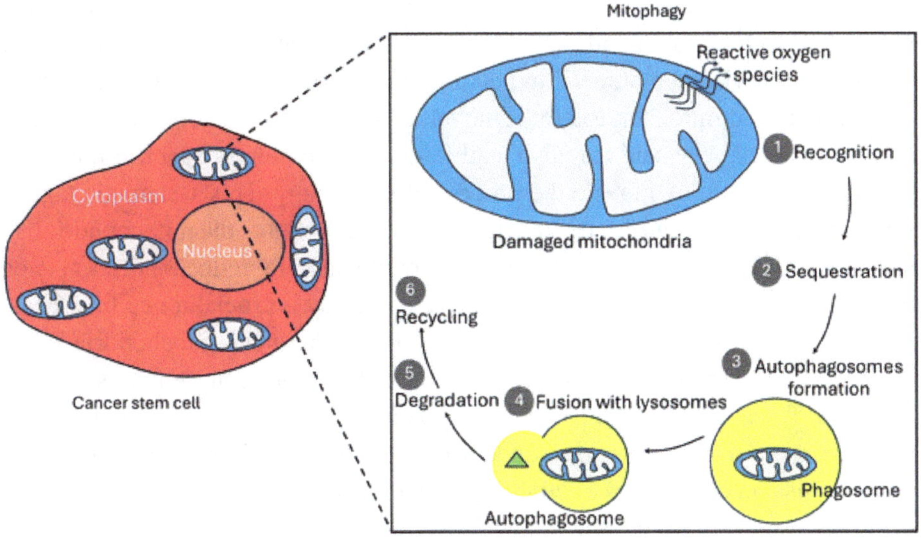

This entire process is crucial for maintaining cellular health and function, especially in cancer cells, where rapid growth and proliferation can lead to increased mitochondrial damage and turnover. Mitophagy ensures that only healthy mitochondria are retained, which supports the metabolic demands of cancer cells and influences the susceptibility of these cells to apoptosis (programmed cell death). The induction of mitophagy can occur through several distinct pathways, each triggered by different cellular contexts and types of stress. Understanding these pathways is essential for comprehending how cells maintain energy efficiency and protect against mitochondrial dysfunction, which can lead to various diseases. The importance of mitophagy induction pathways is described in the following subsections.

The PINK1-Parkin Pathway

The PINK1-Parkin pathway is a pivotal mitophagy mechanism that is particularly responsive to mitochondrial depolarization, signaling a significant disturbance in mitochondrial function. As demonstrated in Figure 2, when mitochondria are healthy and functioning normally, the protein kinase PINK1 is transported to the inner mitochondrial membrane, where it is rapidly degraded. However, when the mitochondrial membrane potential is lost due to damage or stress, PINK1 accumulates on the outer mitochondrial membrane instead. This accumulation of PINK1 at the surface of damaged mitochondria is a critical early step in the pathway. It acts as a distress signal that recruits Parkin, an E3 ubiquitin ligase, from the cytosol to the mitochondria. This recruitment is essential for the next steps in the pathway, marking the onset of a targeted response to mitochondrial dysfunction. Once Parkin is recruited to the mitochondria, it begins to ubiquitinate various proteins on the outer mitochondrial membrane. This ubiquitination serves multiple functions: it helps to label damaged mitochondria for removal, recruits additional components of the autophagy machinery, and can also lead to the degradation of specific mitochondrial proteins that may impede the process of mitophagy. This systematic tagging of mitochondrial proteins for degradation not only highlights the mitochondrion for encapsulation by autophagosomes but also modulates the mitochondrial network to facilitate its removal. The efficiency of this pathway is crucial for cellular health because it helps to prevent the accumulation of dysfunctional mitochondria, which can lead to increased reactive oxygen species (ROS) production, cellular stress, and apoptosis. The ability of the PINK1-Parkin pathway to swiftly and accurately eliminate compromised mitochondria underscores its vital role in maintaining cellular homeostasis and protecting cell viability under stress conditions (Luo et al., 2024).

Figure 2. The PINK1-Parkin pathway

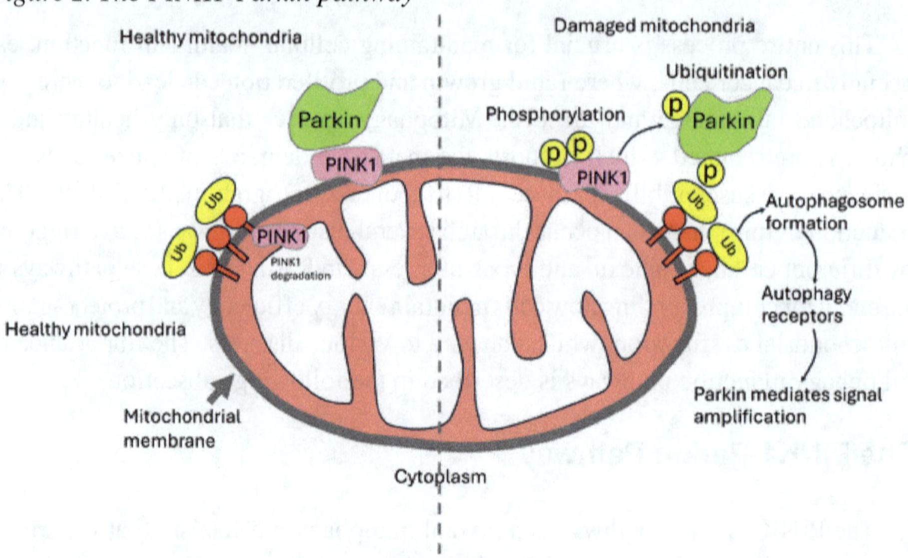

Receptor-Mediated Pathway

The mitophagy receptor-mediated pathway offers an alternative mechanism to the well-known PINK1-Parkin pathway, with a focus on the direct interaction between specific mitochondrial outer membrane proteins and the autophagy machinery. Key proteins such as NIX (also known as BNIP3L), BNIP3, and FUNDC1 are embedded in the mitochondrial outer membrane and play pivotal roles in this process. These proteins are equipped with LIR (LC3-interacting region) motifs that allow them to directly bind to LC3, a crucial component of the autophagosomal membrane. This direct binding is significant because it facilitates the swift encapsulation of mitochondria into autophagosomes without the need for the ubiquitination typically required in other pathways. The receptor-mediated pathway is particularly relevant in scenarios where rapid and selective removal of mitochondria is necessary, such as during cellular stress or specific stages of cell development (D'Arcy, 2024).

For example, under hypoxic conditions (Figure 3) or during the maturation of erythrocytes, mitophagy must be efficiently executed to ensure proper cellular function and survival. Proteins such as NIX and BNIP3 are upregulated in response to hypoxia, engaging the autophagy machinery to promote the selective degradation of mitochondria. This process is critical in erythrocytes, where the complete removal of mitochondria is a prerequisite for the functionality and lifespan of mature red blood cells. Similarly, during hypoxic stress, cells must adapt to decreased oxygen availability by adjusting their mitochondrial content and function, processes in which NIX, BNIP3, and FUNDC1 are instrumental. The ability of these proteins to directly interact with autophagosomal components such as LC3 underscores their importance in maintaining cellular energy balance and viability under stress conditions. Thus, the receptor-mediated pathway not only provides a mechanism for maintaining mitochondrial quality control but also supports cellular adaptation to environmental or developmental changes (Liu & Ma, 2024).

Figure 3. Receptor-mediated pathway

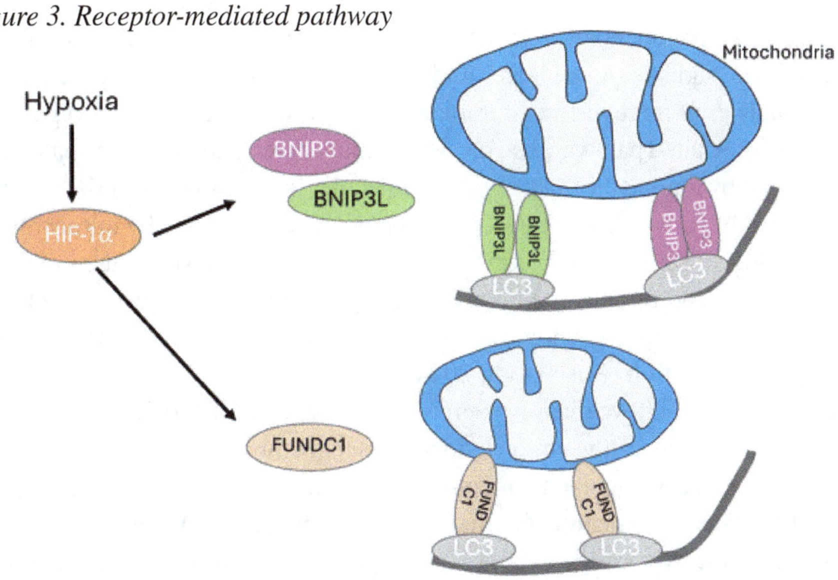

Cardiolipin-Driven Pathway

The cardiolipin-driven pathway of mitophagy represents a significant mechanism within the cell for managing mitochondrial damage and ensuring cellular health. Cardiolipin is a unique phospholipid predominantly localized in the inner mitochondrial membrane that plays a crucial role in maintaining mitochondrial integrity and function. Under conditions of cellular stress, such as oxidative stress or mitochondrial dysfunction, cardiolipin can translocate from the inner to the outer mitochondrial membrane. This relocation is critical because it serves as a signaling mechanism for the autophagic machinery. The presence of cardiolipin on the outer membrane acts as an "eat-me" signal, which is pivotal for the selective recognition of damaged mitochondria by the autophagy system (Zimmermann et al., 2024).

Unlike other pathways that may depend on the ubiquitination of mitochondrial proteins to signal for degradation, the cardiolipin-driven pathway bypasses this requirement. Instead, it directly recruits autophagy-related proteins, such as microtubule-associated protein 1A/1B light chain 3B (LC3), facilitating the rapid engulfment of the targeted mitochondrion by the autophagosome. This direct interaction accelerates the formation of autophagosomes around damaged mitochondria, enhancing the efficiency and speed of mitophagy. This mechanism is especially beneficial during acute cellular stress, where the quick removal of dysfunctional mitochondria is necessary to prevent further cellular damage and ensure survival. The significance of this pathway in the cellular stress response highlights its potential as a therapeutic target for diseases characterized by mitochondrial dysfunction, as noted in recent studies such as those by Liu and Ma (2024). The efficiency of this pathway in clearing damaged mitochondria could be harnessed in strategies aimed at treating or managing conditions where mitochondrial integrity is compromised.

To provide readers with a clearer understanding, Table 1 offers a detailed comparative analysis of three distinct mitophagy pathways: the PINK1-Parkin pathway, the receptor-mediated pathway, and the cardiolipin-driven pathway. Each pathway is characterized by unique mechanisms and molecular interactions essential for mitochondrial quality control. The PINK1-Parkin pathway is initiated by mitochondrial depolarization, during which the kinase PINK1 accumulates on the outer mitochondrial membrane and recruits the E3 ubiquitin ligase Parkin. This recruitment leads to the ubiquitination of mitochondrial proteins, marking damaged mitochondria for autophagic degradation (Naso et al., 2024; R. Zhang et al., 2024). In contrast, the receptor-mediated pathway involves proteins such as NIX, BNIP3, and FUNDC1, which are embedded in the mitochondrial outer membrane and directly interact with LC3 on the autophagosomal membrane via their LC3-interacting region (LIR) motifs. This direct interaction facilitates the encapsulation of mitochondria into autophagosomes, bypassing the need for ubiquitination, particularly under specific conditions such as hypoxia or during certain developmental processes such as erythrocyte maturation (Bi et al., 2024; Liu & Ma, 2024; Yamashita et al., 2024). Finally, the cardiolipin-driven pathway functions through the translocation of the phospholipid cardiolipin from the inner to the outer mitochondrial membrane under stress. This translocation serves as an "eat-me" signal that recruits autophagy-related proteins to damaged mitochondria, promoting their encapsulation and subsequent degradation. Each pathway illustrates different facets of cellular adaptability and response mechanisms, emphasizing the complexity and efficiency of mitophagy as a crucial process in maintaining cellular health and homeostasis.

Table 1. Comparative analysis of mitophagy pathways

Mitophagy Pathway	Involved Molecules	Role in Mitophagy	Pathway/Function	Reference
PINK1-Parkin pathway	PINK1 (PTEN Induced Kinase 1), Parkin (E3 Ubiquitin Ligase)	Activated in response to mitochondrial depolarization; tags damaged mitochondria for degradation	Upon mitochondrial damage, PINK1 stabilizes on the outer mitochondrial membrane, recruiting Parkin which ubiquitinates outer mitochondrial membrane proteins, facilitating autophagosome formation around the damaged mitochondrion.	Luo et al. (2024)
Receptor-mediated pathway	NIX (also known as BNIP3L), BNIP3, FUNDC1	Facilitates direct interaction with LC3 on the autophagosomal membrane, bypassing ubiquitination	These proteins, embedded in the mitochondrial outer membrane, contain LIR motifs allowing direct binding to LC3, promoting the encapsulation of mitochondria into autophagosomes under conditions like hypoxia or during erythrocyte maturation.	Bi et al. (2024); Liu and Ma (2024); Yamashita et al. (2024)
Cardiolipin-driven pathway	Cardiolipin	Serves as an "eat-me" signal on the outer mitochondrial membrane for autophagic machinery	In response to stress, cardiolipin translocates from the inner to the outer mitochondrial membrane, directly recruiting autophagy-related proteins to encapsulate and degrade the damaged mitochondrion.	Liu and Ma (2024)

MITOPHAGY AND CANCER DRUG RESISTANCE

Cancer drug resistance remains a challenge in oncology and significantly impacts treatment efficacy and patient outcomes. Among the several cellular processes influencing resistance, mitophagy — the selective autophagic degradation of mitochondria — has emerged as a crucial player. This process not only maintains cellular homeostasis by removing damaged mitochondria but also profoundly affects the survival and adaptability of cancer cells under therapeutic stress. This section explains the primary pathway through which mitophagy enhances drug resistance.

Maintenance of Mitochondrial Function and Energy Production

In general, mitochondria are the powerhouses of cells. They are responsible for producing energy in the form of adenosine triphosphate (ATP) through oxidative phosphorylation. However, mitochondria are also the main source of ROS within the cell, and their dysfunction can lead to excessive ROS production. This process is harmful because it can damage DNA, proteins, and lipids, leading to cellular dysfunction and apoptosis (Y. Zhang et al., 2024). Mitophagy is essential for maintaining mitochondrial function because it selectively removes dysfunctional mitochondria. This process is mediated by several key pathways, most notably those involving PTEN-induced putative kinase 1 (PINK1) and E3 ubiquitin mitochondria. PINK1 is stabilized on the outer mitochondrial membrane, where it recruits Parkin. Parkin then ubiquitinates several outer membrane proteins, marking the mitochondrion for engulfment by an autophagosome, which eventually fuses with lysozymes where the contents are degraded. This process ensures optimal mitochondrial function and prevents the accumulation of ROS, which can lead to cellular damage and apoptosis. In cancer therapy, mitophagy can enable cells to sustain ATP production. These findings support survival and continued proliferation despite therapeutic interventions (Zhao et al., 2024).

On the other hand, E3 ubiquitin ligases are crucial components in the regulation of mitophagy, which is a specific process of autophagy focused on the degradation and recycling of damaged or superfluous mitochondria. These enzymes are responsible for catalyzing the transfer of ubiquitin, a small regulatory protein, to specific substrates. In the context of mitochondria, E3 ubiquitin ligases tag dysfunctional or damaged mitochondrial proteins with ubiquitin molecules. This ubiquitination is a key step in the mitophagy pathway because it serves as a signal for identifying mitochondria that need to be degraded (Lee et al., 2024). The ubiquitin tags on mitochondria are recognized by autophagy receptors, such as p62/SQSTM1, NBR1, and optineurin, which link ubiquitinated mitochondria to the autophagic machinery. This connection facilitates the engulfment of the tagged mitochondria into autophagosomes, which then fuse with lysosomes, where the contents are degraded and recycled (Cui et al., 2024). Several E3 ubiquitin ligases, including parkin, Mul1, and SMURF1, are involved in mitophagy. Parkin—perhaps the most well-known E3 ubiquitin ligase involved in mitophagy—is recruited to mitochondria in response to mitochondrial depolarization. Once activated and recruited by PINK1, Parkin ubiquitinates various outer mitochondrial membrane proteins, which signals to the autophagy machinery to initiate the degradation of mitochondria. Mitochondrial E3 ubiquitin protein ligase 1 (Mul1) is another ligase that contributes to mitochondrial homeostasis and can promote the removal of damaged mitochondria through mitophagy. SMURF1 (SMAD specific E3 ubiquitin protein ligase 1) - This E3 ligase has been shown to promote mitophagy through the ubiquitination of mitofusins, which are involved in mitochondrial fusion and maintenance of mitochondrial network integrity (Lv et al., 2024).

Cancer cells have high energy demands due to their rapid growth and proliferation. They often rely on glycolysis for energy production even in the presence of oxygen (a phenomenon known as the Warburg effect). However, mitochondria remain crucial for energy production, particularly under nutrient-stressed conditions or in rapidly dividing cells. In cancer therapy, many anticancer drugs induce mitochondrial damage as a mechanism to kill cancer cells. This effect occurs either directly by targeting mitochondria or indirectly through the induction of ROS. However, by activating mitophagy, cancer cells can selectively remove damaged mitochondria. Thus, it maintains mitochondrial function and sustains ATP production. This enables them to survive and continue proliferating despite the presence of anticancer drugs. Examples from the research are as follows:

1) Thyroid Carcinoma Cells and BRAF Inhibitors

BRAF inhibitors are a class of targeted cancer therapies that specifically inhibit the activity of BRAf protein kinases. The BRAF gene encodes a protein involved in sending signals inside cells, which are crucial for cell growth and division. Mutations in the BRAF gene, particularly the BRAFV600E mutation, can lead to uncontrolled cell growth and are found in various types of cancer, including melanoma, thyroid cancer, and colorectal cancer. In a recent study exploring metabolic dependencies in thyroid carcinoma cells, Díaz-Gago et al. (2024) uncovered significant insights into the role of autophagy in cancer metabolism, particularly in the context of BRAFV600E, the most common mutation associated with aggressive thyroid cancer. The study revealed that the respiration of these cancer cells relies heavily on fatty acid oxidation, which is regulated by macroautophagy. Interestingly, inhibiting autophagy or fatty acid oxidation prompts these cells to increase glycolysis to compensate for the loss of oxidative phosphorylation. This shift is crucial for survival, especially when cells face selective pressure from vemurafenib, a targeted BRAFV600E inhibitor. Furthermore, this study demonstrated that reducing glycolysis can enhance mitochondrial respiration and lead to increased resistance to vemurafenib. These findings suggest that targeting mitochondrial functions alongside BRAF inhibition could enhance therapeutic outcomes in treating BRAFV600E-positive thyroid carcinoma, providing a new avenue for overcoming drug resistance in more advanced tumors.

2) Breast Cancer and Doxorubicin

In breast cancer, a common and often chemoresistant tumor, the interaction between mitophagy and the efficacy of doxorubicin, a widely used anticancer drug, was examined. The study by Naso et al. (2024) specifically targeted the role of mitophagy—a selective autophagic process that degrades damaged mitochondria—in different breast cancer models, including luminal A subtype MCF7 cells and triple-negative subtype MDA-MB-231 cells cultured in both 2D and 3D environments. Microarray analysis revealed a correlation between mitophagy gene expression driven by the canonical PINK1/Parkin pathway and doxorubicin treatment. Furthermore, exogenously expressed miRNA-218-5p, which targets Parkin mRNA, effectively suppressed doxorubicin-induced mitophagy in both cell lines. This suppression increased cell sensitivity to doxorubicin, highlighting a potential strategy to counteract treatment resistance and recurrence in breast cancer by combining mitophagy inhibition with chemotherapy. This novel approach may provide a promising avenue for enhancing therapeutic outcomes in breast cancer treatment.

Regulation of Metabolic Flexibility

Cancer cells are known for their metabolic flexibility, allowing them to adapt to various environmental and intracellular conditions. This flexibility supports their survival, proliferation, and resistance to therapies. Mitophagy, the selective autophagic removal of mitochondria, is central to this adaptation. This ensures that the metabolic machinery of cancer cells operates efficiently, enabling these cells to switch between different metabolic pathways based on the availability of nutrients and energy demands (Masoudi et al., 2024). The role of mitophagy in metabolic regulation is described in detail below.

1) Maintaining Mitochondrial Health and Function

Mitophagy selectively removes damaged or dysfunctional mitochondria, which can compromise cellular function by producing excessive ROS. By clearing these defective mitochondria, mitophagy helps maintain a pool of healthy mitochondria that are essential for optimal cellular respiration and energy production.

2) Facilitating Metabolic Switching

Cancer cells often switch between glycolysis (anaerobic metabolism) and oxidative phosphorylation (OXPHOS, aerobic metabolism). The metabolic switching of cancer cells depends on their growth conditions:

2.1) Under normoxic conditions, where there is adequate oxygen, cancer cells predominantly exhibit the Warburg effect, which favors glycolysis even in the presence of enough oxygen. This metabolic trait allows them to rapidly generate ATP and provides an abundance of glycolytic intermediates required for biosynthesis in proliferating cells. However, cancer cells maintain a flexible metabolic profile and can revert to OXPHOS when necessary. This switch to OXPHOS can occur under several conditions:

2.1.1) Nutrient stress: When nutrients are scarce, particularly glucose, cancer cells may increase their reliance on OXPHOS to efficiently generate ATP from available substrates such as fatty acids and amino acids.

2.1.2) Biosynthetic Demand: During rapid cell proliferation, the demand for biosynthetic precursors increases. OXPHOS plays a crucial role in providing not only ATP but also NADPH and other intermediates essential for the synthesis of nucleotides, amino acids, and lipids.

2.1.3) Therapeutic stress: Some therapies might inhibit specific pathways involved in glycolysis, increasing the reliance of cancer cells on OXPHOS for survival.

2.2) Under hypoxic conditions or when mitochondrial function is compromised (e.g., by mitochondrial toxins), cancer cells enhance glycolysis to compensate for the reduced efficiency of the mitochondria. This metabolic shift is crucial for survival under low oxygen conditions or mitochondrial dysfunction. In this way, mitophagy—the selective degradation of mitochondria via autophagy—plays a vital role:

2.2.1) Protection from ROS: By removing damaged or dysfunctional mitochondria that produce excessive ROS, mitophagy prevents oxidative stress and potential damage to cellular components.

2.2.2) Metabolic reprogramming: Mitophagy facilitates a shift in cellular metabolism from OXPHOS to glycolysis by reducing the mitochondrial mass, thereby allowing the cell to rely more on glycolysis.

2.2.3) Survival under stress: The removal of old and dysfunctional mitochondria helps maintain a pool of healthier mitochondria that are more suited to the challenging environment, promoting cellular survival and adaptation.

A recent study on the regulation of metabolic flexibility in cancer cells focused on the role of pyruvate dehydrogenase kinases (PDKs) and their interaction with the pyruvate dehydrogenase (PDH) complex. This study details how PDKs regulate the PDH complex by phosphorylating it, which in turn inhibits its activity. This regulation is crucial because it determines whether cells utilize glycolysis or OXPHOS for energy production. In cancer cells, the inhibition of PHD by PDK leads to increased glycolysis, even under normoxic conditions where OXPHOS is typically more efficient. This

Metabolic flexibility allows cancer cells to adapt to varying environmental conditions, enhancing their survival and proliferation under different metabolic conditions (Woolbright et al., 2019). By further illustrating the dynamic nature of cancer cell metabolism, another study discussed how cancer cells exhibit metabolic plasticity by adapting their metabolic pathways in response to changes in their microenvironment. For instance, a study revealed differences in metabolic preferences between cancer cells in differently vascularized areas of the same tumor, highlighting how metabolic flexibility supports cancer progression and contributes to the complexity of targeting cancer metabolism therapeutically (Fendt et al., 2020).

Suppression of Apoptosis

Apoptosis, or programmed cell death, is a crucial mechanism targeted by many anticancer therapies. It is designed to eliminate cancer cells by inducing damage that triggers intrinsic cell death pathways. Mitophagy plays a significant role in modulating this process, particularly by influencing the intrinsic (mitochondrial) apoptosis pathway. By selectively removing damaged mitochondria, mitophagy can prevent the release of proapoptotic factors and subsequent cell death, thereby contributing to the resistance of cancer cells to therapeutic interventions (Salehi et al., 2024). The mechanism by which mitophagy suppresses apoptosis is as follows.

1) Removal of Damaged Mitochondria

Mitochondria can incur damage from various sources, including ROS and environmental stresses. Damaged mitochondria are potential sources of apoptosis-inducing factors such as cytochrome c. When released into the cytosol, cytochrome c can activate caspase enzymes that initiate the apoptosis cascade. Mitophagy prevents this cascade by ensuring that damaged mitochondria are sequestered and degraded before they can release these factors (Biswas et al., 2024).

2) Prevention of Mitochondrial Permeabilization

Mitophagy helps maintain the integrity of the mitochondrial network by removing mitochondria that might otherwise undergo permeabilization of their outer membranes, a key event in the activation of intrinsic apoptosis. This includes the control of B-cell lymphoma 2 (BCL-2) family proteins, which regulate the release of proapoptotic factors from mitochondria. The BCL-2 protein plays a crucial role in regulating cell death (apoptosis), particularly by inhibiting this process and thus promoting cell survival. This protein is part of a larger family of BCL-2 family proteins, which include both pro-apoptotic and anti-apoptotic members, playing essential roles in controlling the release of pro-apoptotic factors from mitochondria and the regulation of apoptosis in general (Cauwelier et al., 2024).

The ability of mitophagy to suppress apoptosis has important implications for cancer therapy. This finding suggested that inhibiting mitophagy could be a viable strategy for enhancing the effectiveness of treatments that rely on inducing apoptosis. Targeting mitophagy pathways could sensitize cancer cells to apoptosis, potentially overcoming resistance to therapies that aim to kill cancer cells by damaging their mitochondria.

Modulation of Cellular Signaling Pathways

Mitophagy not only plays a critical role in maintaining mitochondrial integrity but also significantly influences various cellular signaling pathways. This modulation is particularly crucial in cancer, where signaling pathways that regulate cell growth, proliferation, and survival can determine the progression and response to therapy. Mitophagy impacts these pathways either directly by affecting the components involved or indirectly through its role in controlling mitochondrial function and ROS levels.

Key Signaling Pathways Affected by Mitophagy

1) NF-kB Pathway

Nuclear factor kappa-light-chain-enhancer of activated B cells (NF-kB) is a protein complex that controls DNA transcription, cytokine production, and cell survival. NF-κB is activated in response to various stimuli, including oxidative stress and cytokines. Mitophagy directly impacts this pathway by controlling the levels of ROS, which are potent activators of NF-κB. By reducing mitochondrial ROS production through the removal of damaged mitochondria, mitophagy can modulate NF-κB activation, thereby influencing inflammation and survival signals that are crucial for cancer cell resilience and adaptability (Moulana et al., 2024).

2) HIF-1α Pathway

Hypoxia-inducible factor 1-alpha (HIF-1α) is another critical transcription factor that responds to low oxygen conditions in the cellular environment. It promotes the expression of genes involved in angiogenesis, metabolism, and survival under hypoxic conditions. Mitophagy is enhanced under hypoxia to manage increased mitochondrial ROS production, thereby stabilizing HIF-1α. This stabilization supports cancer cell adaptation in hypoxic tumors and contributes to a hypoxia-resistant phenotype (Fu et al., 2024).

The influence of mitophagy on critical signaling pathways such as the NF-kB and HIF-1α pathways highlights its role in cancer biology beyond mere mitochondrial maintenance. By modulating these pathways, mitophagy contributes to the adaptation and survival of cancer cells, especially under therapeutic stress. Therefore, targeting mitophagy represents a potential therapeutic strategy for disrupting these adaptations. Inhibiting mitophagy in conjunction with treatments aimed at inducing oxidative stress or exploiting hypoxic conditions could increase the therapeutic potential of cancer cells.

Contribution to the Cancer Stem Cell Phenotype

Cancer stem cells (CSCs) are a subpopulation of cells within tumors that possess self-renewal and differentiation abilities and are highly implicated in drug resistance and tumor recurrence. Mitophagy, the selective degradation of mitochondria via autophagy, plays a crucial role in regulating the function and survival of these cells under stress, particularly therapeutic stress, which is a key challenge in effective cancer treatment (Masoudi et al., 2024). In CSCs, mitophagy serves several essential functions that contribute to their notorious resilience to mitophagy in cancer stem cells, as described below:

1) Preservation of Mitochondrial Function

CSCs often rely on oxidative phosphorylation for energy rather than glycolysis, which is more common in the bulk of tumor cells. Mitophagy helps maintain efficient mitochondrial function by removing damaged or dysfunctional mitochondria, thereby ensuring optimal ATP production and reducing harmful ROS levels. This energy efficiency is crucial for CSCs because it supports their long-term survival and growth potential (Masoudi et al., 2024).

2) Preservation of Senescence

By removing old and damaged mitochondria, mitophagy helps prevent the onset of senescence in CSCs. Senescence is a state of cell cycle arrest that can be induced by cellular stress or damage, including oxidative stress from dysfunctional mitochondria. Avoiding senescence allows CSCs to maintain their proliferative capabilities, contributing to tumor growth and resistance to treatments that typically induce senescence as a form of cancer therapy (Patra et al., 2024).

3) Supporting Stemness

Mitophagy is linked to the maintenance of 'stemness', the set of characteristics that define stem cells, including self-renewal and differentiation capabilities. By managing mitochondrial quality and function, mitophagy supports metabolic and signaling environments conducive to maintaining these characteristics in CSCs (Masoudi et al., 2024).

Adaptation to Hypoxic Conditions

Hypoxia, or low oxygen conditions, is a hallmark of solid tumors and poses a significant challenge in cancer treatment. It often leads to therapeutic resistance and negatively affects the overall prognosis. Under hypoxic conditions, cells undergo several adaptive responses, including metabolic reprogramming and increased angiogenesis. One of the crucial cellular responses to hypoxia involves the modulation of mitophagy, which helps cells adapt to stress by controlling mitochondrial function and reducing oxidative stress. Under hypoxic conditions, the stabilization of hypoxia-inducible factors (HIFs), particularly HIF-1α, plays a central role. HIF-1α is a transcription factor that mediates the cellular response to low oxygen by activating genes involved in angiogenesis, metabolism, and survival (Liu & Ma, 2024). It also impacts mitophagy both directly and indirectly.

1) Direct Impact

Hypoxia-inducible factor 1-alpha (HIF-1α) plays a pivotal role under hypoxic conditions by influencing the expression of genes such as BCL2/adenovirus E1B 19 kDa interacting protein 3 (BN3) and BNIP3L (NIX). These genes are critical for the induction of mitophagy, a cellular defense mechanism that targets damaged mitochondria for degradation. Both BNIP3 and NIX contribute to this process by disrupting the mitochondrial membrane potential, which is crucial for maintaining mitochondrial integrity. By promoting the removal of damaged mitochondria, they effectively reduce the production of mitochondrial ROS. This action helps to mitigate oxidative stress within the cell, enhancing cellular survival and adaptation in low-oxygen environments (Y.-M. Zhang et al., 2024).

2) Indirect Impact

HIF-1α also influences the metabolic profile of cells under hypoxic conditions, leading to significant changes in mitochondrial dynamics. This metabolic shift, primarily characterized by a transition from oxidative phosphorylation to glycolysis, results in altered mitochondrial function and structure. Such changes can stress the mitochondrial network, necessitating increased mitophagic activity to maintain cellular homeostasis and survival. By enhancing mitophagy, cells can selectively degrade dysfunctional mitochondria, thereby preventing the accumulation of damage and ensuring the maintenance of energy production under oxygen-limited conditions. This adaptive response is crucial for cell survival in varying oxygen environments and underscores the complex role of HIF-1α in cellular metabolism and mitochondrial maintenance (Fu et al., 2024).

A recent study by Yamashita et al. (2024) investigated how mitophagy, the targeted removal of damaged mitochondria, adapts under hypoxic conditions to protect cells from ferroptosis, a form of programmed cell death driven by the accumulation of lipid peroxides. This research highlighted the roles of BNIP3 and NIX, two proteins known to facilitate mitophagy, in modulating this protective mechanism. Under low oxygen conditions, the activation of these proteins enhances mitophagy, which in turn helps reduce mitochondrial ROS levels. This reduction is critical because high levels of ROS can promote ferroptosis by damaging cellular components, including lipids. These findings suggest that by controlling mitochondrial ROS through BNIP3- and NIX-mediated mitophagy, cells can significantly decrease their susceptibility to ferroptosis, especially in hypoxic environments. This insight into the cellular response mechanisms offers potential therapeutic targets for diseases characterized by oxidative stress and hypoxia.

STRATEGIES TO MODULATE MITOPHAGY FOR OVERCOMING DRUG RESISTANCE

The emerging recognition of the role of mitophagy in cancer drug resistance has spurred interest in developing strategies to modulate this process to enhance the efficacy of cancer therapies. Several approaches have been proposed to manipulate mitophagy, either by inhibiting or inducing mitophagy, depending on the context and type of cancer. These strategies aim to disrupt the protective role mitophagy plays in cancer cells, thus sensitizing them to both chemotherapy and targeted therapies.

Inhibition of Mitophagy to Enhance Drug Sensitivity

Mechanisms of Mitophagy Inhibition

Mitophagy is a specific form of autophagy that involves the selective degradation of mitochondria. This process is crucial for cellular health, as it helps remove damaged or dysfunctional mitochondria, thus preventing the buildup of cellular stress and contributing to metabolic homeostasis. In many cancers, however, mitophagy can become a mechanism through which cancer cells evade the cytotoxic effects of therapies. By removing damaged mitochondria, mitophagy helps maintain mitochondrial function and supports the survival and proliferation of cancer cells under therapeutic stress. The strategy of inhibiting mitophagy to enhance drug sensitivity is based on the principle that blocking the removal of damaged mitochondria would increase cellular stress to a level that could synergize with the cytotoxic effects of chemotherapeutic agents. When mitophagy is inhibited, damaged mitochondria accumulate, leading to increased production of ROS. High levels of ROS can cause significant damage to cellular components, including DNA, proteins, and lipids, further sensitizing cancer cells to chemotherapy-induced death (Chen, 2024).

Pharmacological Inhibitors of Mitophagy

1) General Autophagy Inhibitors

Chloroquine and its derivatives, such as hydroxychloroquine, have been extensively studied for their ability to inhibit autophagy, including mitophagy, which is crucial for their use in cancer therapy. These drugs, which are traditionally used for treating malaria, disrupt the final stage of autophagy by blocking the fusion of autophagosomes with lysosomes. This inhibition leads to the accumulation of damaged mitochondria and other cellular debris, which in turn increases ROS production and cellular stress, sensitizing cancer cells to chemotherapy.

Recent studies have demonstrated the effectiveness of chloroquine in combination with various chemotherapeutic agents. For instance, when used with cisplatin, chloroquine can enhance drug cytotoxicity not only in cancer cells but also in other rapidly dividing cells, such as kidney cells, leading to increased DNA damage and cell death. This combination has been shown to induce a more pronounced toxic effect on cancer cells but also highlights the potential for acute kidney injury due to the increased sensitivity of kidney cells to chemotherapy (Liu et al., 2020). Furthermore, in breast cancer therapy, especially for estrogen receptor-positive (ER^+) breast cancer types, chloroquine has been shown to potentiate the responsiveness to antiestrogen drugs. This is achieved by inhibiting the degradation of autophagosomes, leading to their accumulation and increased cellular stress, which increases the susceptibility of cancer cells to treatment (Cook et al., 2014). Moreover, the ability of chloroquine to prevent resistance to PI3K/AKT inhibitors and enhance their antitumor effects in combination with drugs such as paclitaxel has been demonstrated in triple-negative breast cancer models. This suggests the broader application of chloroquine in various cancer treatment regimens, where it can potentiate the effects of multiple anticancer drugs by modulating autophagy (Cocco et al., 2022).

2) PINK1 and Parkin Inhibitors

In addition to general autophagy, targeting specific components of the mitophagy pathway represents a more targeted approach. Key proteins involved in the initiation and progression of mitophagy include PINK1 and Parkin, which are ubiquitin ligases. Under normal conditions, PIK1 accumulates on the outer membrane of damaged mitochondria and recruits Parkin, which then ubiquitinates various mitochondrial proteins to signal the engulfment and degradation of mitochondria by lysosomes. Small molecule inhibitors that specifically target PINK1 or Parkin can inhibit mitophagy. These inhibitors can block the early steps of mitophagy, leading to the accumulation of dysfunctional mitochondria. This targeted inhibition can be effective in cancers where PINK1/Parkin-mediated mitophagy is upregulated and contributes significantly to drug resistance.

PINK1 is a kinase that accumulates on the outer membrane of damaged mitochondria and plays a crucial role in the early stages of mitophagy signaling. By phosphorylating both Parkin and ubiquitin, PINK1 acts as a key signal for the recruitment of Parkin to mitochondria, facilitating its clearance. Small molecule inhibitors of PINK1 can prevent this phosphorylation, thereby preventing the recruitment of Parkin and subsequent mitophagy progression. Currently, one of the notable small molecule inhibitors of PINK1 that has been studied is the MG149 compound. This inhibitor affects the early steps of the PINK1-dependent mitophagy process. MG149 functions by impairing the autophosphorylation and activation of PINK1, which is crucial for the subsequent phosphorylation of Parkin and ubiquitin, key steps required for the recruitment and activation of Parkin on damaged mitochondria. This inhibition blocks the initiation of PINK1-dependent mitophagy, which can be critical in contexts where preventing mitophagy is desired, as in certain cancer therapies where mitophagy contributes to drug resistance (de Talhouët et al., 2024).

Parkin, an E3 ubiquitin ligase, is recruited to mitochondria by PINK1 to label damaged mitochondria with ubiquitin, which marks them for degradation. Inhibiting Parkin directly can prevent this tagging, halting mitophagy. Small molecule inhibitors that disrupt the ability of Parkin to bind to ubiquitin or to mitochondria can effectively reduce its activity. This leads to a failure in the clearance of damaged mitochondria, promoting apoptosis, especially under conditions where mitochondrial function is compromised. To the best of our knowledge, while specific small molecule inhibitors that directly target Parkin have not been extensively reported in recent research, there has been significant exploration of the mechanisms that can indirectly inhibit Parkin activity during mitophagy, particularly through the modulation of other proteins that interact with Parkin. One of the proteins investigated in this context is USP30, a deubiquitinase that opposes the function of Parkin by removing ubiquitin from mitochondria, thereby preventing its degradation through mitophagy.

This finding highlighted the role of USP30 in negatively regulating Parkin activity by deubiquitinating mitochondria, which blocks mitophagy under depolarizing conditions. Inhibiting USP30, therefore, enhances Parkin-mediated mitophagy by allowing the ubiquitination and subsequent degradation of damaged mitochondria. This approach has been suggested to be beneficial for treating conditions such as Parkinson's disease and potentially for treating cancers where mitophagy regulation is crucial for cell survival and drug resistance. Inhibiting USP30 or other similar proteins may effectively serve as an indirect method to modulate Parkin activity in cancer therapies, particularly where mitophagy plays a role in drug resistance or cellular survival mechanisms. This strategy highlights the complex interplay of proteins involved in mitophagy and the potential therapeutic benefits of targeting these interactions in cancer treatment (Tang et al., 2024).

Induction of Mitophagy to Remove Dysfunctional Mitochondria

Mechanisms of Mitophagy Induction

In the context of cancer, especially when cells display a high degree of metabolic flexibility that contributes to drug resistance, targeting dysfunctional mitochondria through mitophagy induction is a promising therapeutic strategy. Dysfunctional mitochondria can lead to increased resilience in cancer cells against various stresses, including chemotherapy, by adapting their metabolic processes to circumvent drug effects. In cancer, where cellular metabolism is often reprogrammed for rapid growth and survival under hypoxic conditions or nutrient scarcity, maintaining mitochondrial health via mitophagy can paradoxically both support and hinder cancer progression. Thus, the context determines whether inhibition or induction of mitophagy may be beneficial (Ji et al., 2024).

Therapeutic Agents Inducing Mitophagy

1) Urolithin A

Urolithin A (Figure 4), a metabolite derived from ellagitannins processed by the gut microbiota, significantly promotes mitophagy through mechanisms involving the PINK1 and Parkin proteins, key regulators in the mitophagy pathway. This compound has been shown to activate mitophagy in a variety of cell types, including those from neurodegenerative disease models and muscle cells, suggesting its broad utility in targeting diseases associated with mitochondrial dysfunction. The activation of mitophagy by urolithin A may contribute to the removal of dysfunctional mitochondria, enhancing cellular function and potentially rendering cancer cells more sensitive to chemotherapy by undermining their metabolic resilience. Research has highlighted its potential in modulating cellular health and treating diseases linked to mitochondrial defects, including cancer, where it could help circumvent drug resistance mechanisms inherent in some cancer cells (Shetty et al., 2024).

2) Spermidine

Spermidine (Figure 4), a polyamine that occurs naturally in cells, induces mitophagy by suppressing the acetyltransferase enzyme EP300. This inhibition leads to the deacetylation of several autophagy-related proteins, triggering autophagic and mitophagic processes. The role of spermidine in promoting mitophagy is crucial for the degradation of damaged mitochondria, potentially limiting the survival of cancer cells under treatment conditions. Its ability to enhance mitochondrial turnover suggests a therapeutic role in cancer treatment, possibly in combination with conventional therapies to overcome drug resistance. This dual action of enhancing autophagy and mitophagy underlines its potential as a supportive treatment in cancers where mitochondrial dysfunction plays a role in therapeutic resistance (Nakashima et al., 2024).

Figure 4. Chemical structures of urolithin A and spermidine

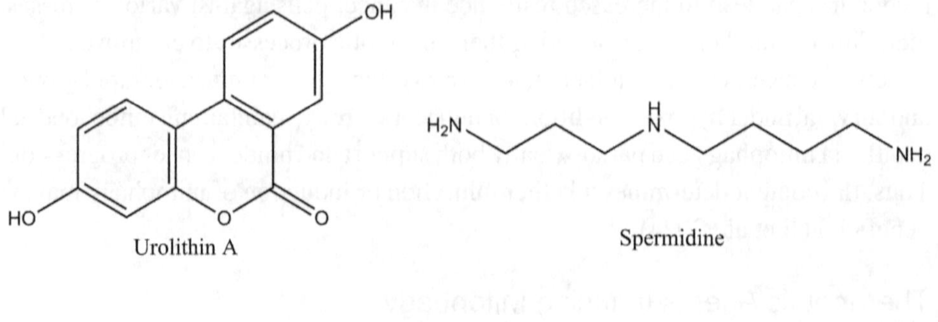

Dual Modulation Strategies

Concept and Rationale

The dual modulation strategy in cancer treatment involves a sophisticated and dynamic approach to manipulate mitophagy—the process by which cells remove damaged mitochondria. This strategy is predicated on the timing and modulation of mitophagy at different phases of cancer therapy to improve therapeutic outcomes. This approach can be particularly useful in managing drug resistance, a major challenge in effective cancer treatment.

Phases of Dual Modulation

1) Inhibition of Mitophagy

The first phase of the dual modulation strategy involves inhibiting mitophagy to sensitize cancer cells to chemotherapy. By temporarily blocking the removal of dysfunctional mitochondria, cells accumulate damaged mitochondria and associated ROS, leading to increased cellular stress and susceptibility to chemotherapeutic agents. This is because the accumulation of damaged mitochondria can disrupt metabolic processes within cancer cells, decreasing their resistance to the cytotoxic effects of chemotherapy.

2) Induction of Mitophagy

Following the initial phase of chemotherapy, the strategy shifts to inducing mitophagy. This phase is aimed at clearing the excessive accumulation of damaged mitochondria after chemotherapy has targeted and killed highly susceptible cancer cells. Inducing mitophagy at this stage helps clean the cellular environment and removes potentially harmful mitochondria that could contribute to cancer recurrence or further resistance.

Table 2 provides a detailed comparative overview of how active versus inhibited mitophagy can affect various mechanisms of drug resistance in cancer cells, highlighting the dual roles of this process in cancer treatment. Mitophagy generally promotes cancer cell survival and adaptation under chemotherapeutic stress by efficiently removing damaged mitochondria that release proapoptotic factors, thereby enhancing resistance to apoptosis. This active removal also leads to reduced levels of ROS, helping cells survive the oxidative stress induced by chemotherapy and supporting a shift in metabolism toward glycolysis, allowing sustained energy production even when mitochondria are dysfunctional. Furthermore, active mitophagy helps cancer cells buffer against therapeutic stress, enabling them to endure and adapt to treatments and enhancing their ability to handle chemical stress through adaptive responses. In terms of genomic stability, active mitophagy contributes to maintaining a healthy cellular environment.

Conversely, inhibiting mitophagy disrupts these adaptive survival mechanisms and can potentially enhance the effectiveness of cancer therapies. Inhibition leads to the accumulation of damaged mitochondria, increasing susceptibility to apoptosis due to the release of cytochrome c and elevated ROS levels, which can enhance oxidative stress and potentially lead to cell death. This buildup also compromises energy production due to mitochondrial dysfunction and decreases the efficiency of metabolic adaptation. Furthermore, the therapeutic efficacy of drugs may increase as the accumulation of dysfunctional mitochondria enhances the cytotoxic effects of these drugs. However, the ability to manage chemical stress is reduced, leading to increased cell mortality under treatment conditions, and there is an increase in genomic instability driven by increased levels of ROS and DNA damage. This comparative analysis underscores the complexity of targeting mitophagy in cancer therapy, where the timing and context of modulating this process are crucial for achieving the desired therapeutic outcome.

Table 2. Comparative overview of drug resistance mechanisms in cancer cells with active vs. inhibited mitophagy

Feature	Active Mitophagy	Inhibited Mitophagy
Apoptosis avoidance	Enhanced resistance to apoptosis due to efficient removal of damaged mitochondria releasing pro-apoptotic factors.	Increased susceptibility to apoptosis due to accumulation of damaged mitochondria and release of cytochrome c.
Reactive oxygen species (ROS) management	Reduced ROS levels due to the removal of dysfunctional mitochondria, helping cells survive oxidative stress induced by chemotherapy.	Elevated ROS levels due to the accumulation of dysfunctional mitochondria, lead to enhanced oxidative stress and potential cell death.
Energy metabolism	Shift toward glycolysis under stress; maintains energy production even with mitochondrial dysfunction.	Compromised energy production due to dysfunctional mitochondria; less efficient metabolic adaptation.
Therapeutic drug efficacy	Reduced, as mitophagy helps to buffer therapeutic stress, allowing cancer cells to endure and adapt to treatment.	Potentially increased, as the buildup of dysfunctional mitochondria can enhance the cytotoxic effects of drugs.
Chemical stress response	Enhanced capability to handle chemical stress through adaptive responses facilitated by mitophagy.	Reduced capability to manage chemical stress, leading to higher cell mortality under treatment conditions.
Genomic stability	Mitophagy can indirectly promote genomic stability by maintaining a healthy cellular environment.	Increased genomic instability due to higher levels of ROS and DNA damage triggered by dysfunctional mitochondria.

Pharmacological Agents

Current research highlights several agents that are being explored for their potential in dual modulation strategies for cancer treatment, particularly through the regulation of mitophagy.

1) Ceramide Analogs

These compounds, such as LCL-461, have been explored for their ability to induce lethal mitophagy. Specifically, in acute myelogenous leukemia patients with FLT3-ITD mutations, ceramide analogs have been shown to be effective at overcoming drug resistance. The induction of mitophagy by these compounds helps in the elimination of dysfunctional mitochondria, potentially leading to cancer cell death (Yan & Li, 2018).

2) Metformin

Known primarily as a diabetes medication, metformin has been found to induce mitophagy via the AMPK-PINK1/Parkin pathway in gastric cancer. This induction is part of the mechanism of action that contributes to resistance to cisplatin, a common chemotherapeutic agent. Although this indicates a challenge in diabetes management for gastric cancer patients, it also opens avenues for using metformin to manipulate mitophagy therapeutically (L. Huang et al., 2024).

3) Salinomycin

This agent induces mitochondrial dysfunction and mitophagy. When combined with mitophagy inhibition strategies, such as ATG5 knockout, the toxicity of salinomycin toward cancer cells is enhanced, suggesting its potential use in combination therapies to target cancer cells more effectively (Patra et al., 2024).

Genetic and Molecular Approaches

The use of genetic manipulation, particularly small interfering RNA (siRNA) and CRISPR/Cas9 gene-editing systems, represents a powerful approach for controlling and studying mitophagy in cancer. These technologies allow scientists to silence or knock out specific genes involved in mitophagy. For example, targeting key proteins such as PINK1 or Parkin, which are crucial for the initiation and progression of mitophagy, can help in understanding their roles in cancer progression and resistance. Researchers can observe how changes in mitophagy affect the survival, proliferation, and drug resistance of cancer cells by manipulating these genes, thereby identifying new therapeutic targets.

Genetic Manipulation Techniques

1) siRNA

This method involves short, double-stranded RNA molecules that interfere with the expression of specific genes. By designing siRNAs that target the mRNA sequences of mitophagy-related genes, researchers can effectively reduce or inhibit the production of proteins that are crucial for mitophagy.

2) CRISPR/Cas9

This more recent and revolutionary gene-editing technology allows for precise cuts and edits in the DNA sequence of a genome. By targeting the DNA sequences of genes involved in mitophagy, CRISPR/Cas9 can be used to generate knockout cells in which specific mitophagy genes are completely inactivated. This helps in studying the direct impact of these genes on cancer cell behavior and therapeutic response.

Molecular Approaches

Modulation of signaling pathways that regulate mitophagy also provides strategic control over this process. Two key pathways often targeted are the AMP-activated protein kinase (AMPK) pathway and the mechanistic target of rapamycin (mTOR) pathway, both of which play critical roles in cellular metabolism and have been linked to mitophagy regulation.

1) AMPK Activation

AMPK is a sensor of cellular energy status and can initiate mitophagy by phosphorylating various substrates that affect mitochondrial dynamics and turnover. Drugs or molecules that can modulate AMPK activity can therefore be used to either promote or inhibit mitophagy depending on the desired therapeutic outcome. For example, metformin, commonly used as a diabetes medication, activates AMPK and has been shown to induce mitophagy, which can affect cancer cell survival and drug resistance.

2) mTOR Inhibition

mTOR acts as a major negative regulator of autophagy and mitophagy. Inhibitors of mTOR, such as rapamycin and its analogs, can induce mitophagy by relieving the inhibition of the ULK1 complex, an essential initiator of autophagy. This pathway is particularly of interest in cancers where suppression of mitophagy contributes to therapy resistance or tumor survival under stress conditions.

Combination Therapies

Combining mitophagy modulation with existing cancer therapies represents a promising strategy for enhancing the overall efficacy of cancer treatments. This approach involves the integration of agents that modulate mitophagy—either by inducing or inhibiting mitophagy—with standard therapeutic modalities such as chemotherapy, immunotherapy, or targeted therapies. The rationale behind this strategy is to target multiple pathways involved in cancer cell survival and resistance, potentially leading to synergistic effects that could reduce tumor growth more effectively and improve patient survival rates (Naso et al., 2024).

Combining Mitophagy Modulators with Immunotherapy

One promising area of combination therapy involves pairing mitophagy modulators with immunotherapies. For example, inhibiting mitophagy in tumor cells can lead to the accumulation of damaged mitochondria, which often results in increased production of reactive oxygen species (ROS) and the release of mitochondrial DNA (mtDNA). These molecules can act as damage-associated molecular patterns (DAMPs) that are recognized by the immune system, potentially enhancing the visibility of cancer cells to immune cells. Examples of immunotherapy combinations are as follows:

1) Checkpoint Inhibitors and Mitophagy Inhibition

Immune checkpoint inhibitors, such as PD-1/PD-L1 or CTLA-4 antagonists, function by stimulating the immune system to attack cancer cells. When combined with mitophagy inhibitors, the increased accumulation of DAMPs from dysfunctional mitochondria can increase the immunogenicity of tumor cells. This potentially increases the efficacy of checkpoint inhibitors by increasing the susceptibility of cancer cells to immune cell-mediated killing.

2) Cancer Vaccines and Mitophagy Modulation

Cancer vaccines aim to initiate an immune response against tumor-specific antigens. Enhancing this strategy with mitophagy inducers could lead to better antigen presentation by dying tumor cells, which are then prompted to undergo regulated cell death through mitophagy. This could improve the overall immunogenicity of the vaccine.

Combining Mitophagy Modulators with Targeted Drugs

Another strategy involves the use of mitophagy modulators combined with targeted therapies that act on specific cancer-driving genes or pathways. For instance, targeted drugs that inhibit specific growth factors or signaling pathways in cancer cells can be combined with mitophagy inducers to enhance cell death in cancer cells that have adapted to survive drug treatment through metabolic flexibility. This approach aims to cut off the protective benefits that mitophagy provides to stressed cancer cells, increasing their susceptibility to targeted therapies. The mechanisms and potential benefits are as follows:

1) Enhanced Efficacy of Targeted Drugs

Many targeted therapies, such as the HER2 receptor in breast cancer or the BCR-ABL tyrosine kinase in chronic myeloid leukemia, inhibit specific growth factors or signaling pathways critical for cancer cell survival and proliferation. When combined with mitophagy inducers, these therapies can be more effective. Mechanistically, mitophagy induction leads to the removal of dysfunctional mitochondria, which are often crucial for cancer cell survival under stress induced by targeted drugs. This can lead to increased cell death and a reduced likelihood of resistance development.

2) Overcoming Drug Resistance

Cancer cells often develop resistance to targeted therapies through various mechanisms, including alterations in drug targets, activation of alternative survival pathways, and enhanced stress response capabilities such as autophagy and mitophagy. By combining targeted therapies with mitophagy inhibitors, it is possible to prevent cancer cells from using mitophagy as a survival tool, potentially increasing their susceptibility to the cytotoxic effects of targeted therapies.

Examples of combination approaches are as follows:

1) BRAF Inhibitors and Mitophagy Modulators in Melanoma

BRAF inhibitors, which are used in melanoma harboring BRAF mutations, can bind to mitophagy modulators to prevent melanoma cells from compensating for the metabolic stress induced by BRAF inhibition. This could prevent cells from escaping drug effects through the management of mitochondrial dysfunction.

2) EGFR Inhibitors in Non-Small Cell Lung Cancer (NSCLC) Patients

For NSCLC patients with specific EGFR mutations, EGFR inhibitors are a standard treatment. Combining these inhibitors with mitophagy inducers could enhance the removal of damaged mitochondria, leading to increased apoptosis in cancer cells stressed by EGFR pathway inhibition.

Overall, the exploration of various therapeutic strategies targeting mitophagy in cancer treatment encompasses a spectrum of innovative approaches. Each is designed to manipulate this critical cellular process to combat cancer more effectively. As shown in Table 3, these strategies range from inhibiting mitophagy, which allows damaged mitochondria to accumulate and promotes cancer cell death, to promoting mitophagy, which enhances the clearance of dysfunctional mitochondria to induce metabolic crises in cancer cells. Moreover, dual modulation approaches dynamically adjust mitophagy activity based on specific needs within the tumor environment, potentially optimizing treatment responses. Genetic and molecular tactics involve precise interventions such as CRISPR/Cas9 or siRNA to specifically alter the expression of genes that regulate mitophagy, aiming to tailor therapies to individual patient tumor profiles. Additionally, combination therapies integrate mitophagy modulation with conventional treatments such as chemotherapy or targeted therapies to increase mitophagy effectiveness and overcome resistance mechanisms. Each strategy reflects a deeper understanding of the role of mitophagy in cancer, providing multiple avenues for potentially enhancing therapeutic outcomes and personalizing cancer treatment.

Table 3. Current therapeutic strategies targeting mitophagy in cancer

Strategy	Mechanism of Action	Examples of Therapeutic Agents	Status/Usage
Inhibition of mitophagy	Block mitophagy to promote the accumulation of damaged mitochondria, leading to cell death.	Mitophagy inhibitors targeting PINK1 or Parkin	Early-stage research and preclinical trials; are not yet widely used in clinical settings.
Promotion of mitophagy	Enhance mitophagy to force the depletion of mitochondria, inducing metabolic crisis in cancer cells.	Drugs that activate PINK1 or Parkin, or small molecules mimicking mitochondrial damage	Investigational; some are in early clinical trials aiming to establish efficacy and safety.
Dual modulation approaches	Using agents that can either inhibit or promote mitophagy depending on the cancer cell context.	Context-dependent modulators of mitochondrial dynamics	Theoretical and experimental; requires further development and understanding of context-specific effects.

continued on following page

Table 3. Continued

Strategy	Mechanism of Action	Examples of Therapeutic Agents	Status/Usage
Genetic and molecular approaches	Manipulate gene expression or signaling pathways influencing mitophagy to control cancer cell survival and death.	siRNA, CRISPR/Cas9 targeting mitophagy-related genes; small molecule regulators of AMPK or mTOR pathways	Advanced research is increasingly utilized in preclinical studies and some early clinical trials.
Combination therapies	Combining mitophagy modulators with conventional cancer therapies to enhance overall efficacy.	Combinations of mitophagy modulators with chemotherapy or targeted therapy agents	Under investigation in clinical trials, aims to overcome resistance to standard therapies.

CHALLENGES AND FUTURE PERSPECTIVES

Challenges in Targeting Mitophagy in Cancer Therapy

Targeting mitophagy in cancer therapy presents a unique set of challenges that stem from the intricate nature of this cellular process. As shown in Table 4, one major hurdle is the specificity of targeting. Mitophagy occurs in both cancerous and normal cells as a fundamental process to manage cellular stress and remove damaged mitochondria. The challenge lies in developing strategies that can selectively inhibit or activate mitophagy in cancer cells without adversely affecting normal cells. This specificity is crucial because unintended effects on normal cells could lead to detrimental impacts on overall cellular health and organ functions. This issue of specificity not only complicates the development of effective therapeutic agents but also raises concerns about potential side effects that could diminish the quality of life for patients.

Moreover, mitophagy regulation involves multiple complex and overlapping pathways that are not yet fully understood. This complexity poses significant challenges in designing drugs that can precisely modulate this process without causing off-target effects. Additionally, the role of mitophagy in cancer varies across different types of cancers, adding another layer of complexity to the development of universal therapeutic strategies. Each type of cancer might utilize mitophagy differently depending on its origin, mutation profile, and microenvironment, necessitating personalized treatment approaches tailored to the specific mitophagy dynamics of each tumor. Furthermore, as with many cancer therapies, there is an ever-present risk that cancer cells might develop resistance to therapies targeting mitophagy, potentially leading to reduced efficacy over time. Due to the lack of reliable biomarkers for dynamically measuring mitophagy in vivo, these challenges make it difficult to assess therapeutic efficacy, monitor treatment responses, and adjust strategies promptly. This complexity affects not only the development phase of mitophagy-targeting therapies but also their implementation in clinical settings, where balancing efficacy with safety becomes a critical concern (Bajinka et al., 2024; Mishra et al., 2024).

Table 4. Challenges in targeting mitophagy for cancer therapy

Challenge	Description	Implications for Therapy
Specificity of targeting	Difficulty in selectively targeting mitophagy in cancer cells without affecting normal cells.	Risk of unintended effects on normal cell functions and overall cellular health.
Complex regulatory mechanisms	Mitophagy is regulated by complex and overlapping pathways that are not fully understood.	Challenges in designing drugs that can precisely modulate mitophagy without off-target effects.
Variability among cancer types	Different cancers may utilize mitophagy in various ways, complicating the application of a one-size-fits-all approach.	Need for personalized treatment strategies based on specific mitophagy profiles of different tumors.
Resistance development	Cancer cells might develop resistance to therapies targeting mitophagy, similar to other cancer therapies.	Potential for reduced long-term efficacy of mitophagy-targeting therapies.
Measurement and monitoring	The lack of reliable biomarkers to measure mitophagy dynamically in vivo complicates the assessment of therapeutic efficacy.	Difficulty in monitoring treatment response and adjusting therapeutic strategies in real-time.
Interactions with other pathways	Mitophagy interacts with various cellular processes like apoptosis and metabolism, which could lead to complex side effects when targeted.	Risk of disrupting other cellular processes that are crucial for normal cell function and survival.

Future Research Directions

Given the challenges and critical role of mitophagy in cancer biology, future research needs to focus on several key areas. As summarized in Table 5, first, a deeper understanding of the molecular regulation of mitophagy in different types of cancer is essential. This includes identifying specific mitophagy triggers, mediators, and inhibitors that are unique to cancer cells. Such knowledge could help in designing drugs that are more selective and less likely to cause harm to normal cells. Second, developing reliable biomarkers for mitophagy is crucial for tracking the process in real time in clinical settings, facilitating better monitoring of treatment responses and adjustments of therapeutic strategies (Cuervo et al., 2024). Another important research direction is the exploration of combination therapies that include mitophagy modulators. Understanding how mitophagy interacts with other cell death and survival pathways could reveal synergistic combinations that are more effective and have fewer side effects (Liu et al., 2024). Moreover, investigating nonpharmacological methods to modulate mitophagy, such as dietary interventions and exercise, could offer low-cost, accessible adjunct therapies (Shorter et al., 2024). Finally, the development of patient-derived xenograft models and organoids that more accurately reflect the patient's tumor microenvironment could improve the preclinical assessment of mitophagy-targeted therapies.

Table 5. Future research directions and potential targets in mitophagy-related cancer therapy

Research Direction	Potential Targets	Description and Impact
Enhancing understanding of mitophagy mechanisms	PINK1, Parkin, BNIP3, NIX, FUNDC1	Further study the molecular details and regulation pathways to identify new therapeutic targets.
Developing specific inhibitors and activators	Mitophagy receptors and regulators	Create drugs that can specifically inhibit or activate mitophagy without affecting other autophagy pathways.
Personalized mitophagy modulation	Patient-specific mitophagy profiles	Tailor mitophagy modulation treatments based on individual genetic and metabolic profiles to enhance efficacy and reduce side effects.
Combination therapies	Combinations of mitophagy modulators with chemotherapeutics or immunotherapies	Investigate how mitophagy modulation can synergize with existing cancer treatments to overcome resistance.
Nonpharmacological approaches	Lifestyle and dietary interventions	Explore how changes in diet or physical activity could naturally modulate mitophagy and complement traditional treatments.
Mitophagy and the immune system interplay	cGAS-STING pathway	Study how mitophagy influences immune responses in tumors to develop strategies that enhance immunogenic cell death.
Biomarker development for mitophagy	Mitophagy-related biomarkers	Identify and validate biomarkers that can accurately measure mitophagy activity in clinical settings for better treatment monitoring.
Addressing Tumor Heterogeneity	Specific subpopulations of cancer cells	Understand mitophagy's role in different tumor microenvironments and subpopulations to design more effective, targeted interventions.

Potential of Mitophagy Modulators in Clinical Practices

The potential of mitophagy modulators in clinical practice is vast and promising. By specifically targeting mitophagy, these modulators can potentially overcome drug resistance, a major obstacle in effective cancer treatment. For example, mitophagy inhibitors could be used to prevent cancer cells from removing damaged mitochondria, thus enhancing the efficacy of chemotherapeutics that induce mitochondrial damage. Conversely, mitophagy inducers might be used in cancers where mitochondrial dysfunction is beneficial, helping to push cancer cells toward metabolic failure and death (Ke et al., 2024). Additionally, increased fine-tuning of mitophagy could facilitate the implementation of a personalized medical strategy. This technique could in turn enable treatments that are more effective and less toxic by tailoring mitophagy-targeted therapies to an individual patient's tumor and its specific mitophagy profile, the researchers say. In addition, combining mitophagy modulators with current treatment regimens may be an effective method for reducing tumor inhibition at multiple time points, suggesting superior clinical results (Ma et al., 2024). Now that progress is starting to be made, the adoption of mitophagy modulators in clinical practice can revolutionize cancer therapy, opening a window of opportunity not only for patients with otherwise intractable diseases but also for much-needed new therapies to be rationalized toward the right patients in clinical trials. Nevertheless, translation of these findings to the clinic will require a robust clinical trial process to assess safety and efficacy, and further research in this evolving field of cancer therapy is needed.

CONCLUSION

Throughout this chapter, the authors have explored the role of mitophagy in cancer, particularly focusing on its contribution to the development of drug resistance in cancer therapy. Key findings have established that mitophagy has dual functions in cancer progression and therapy resistance. It acts as a survival mechanism for cancer cells under therapeutic stress by removing damaged mitochondria and preventing the activation of apoptotic pathways. This capability allows cancer cells to adapt to metabolic changes and endure the cytotoxic effects of both chemotherapy and targeted therapies. Additionally, mitophagy has been shown to interact with various cellular pathways, modulating crucial processes such as apoptosis and metabolic reprogramming and further complicating the landscape of cancer resistance. The mechanisms governing mitophagy in cancer cells, including the roles of key proteins such as PINK1 and Parkin, have been described in detail, providing insights into how this process can potentially be targeted for therapeutic purposes. The ability of mitophagy to influence treatment outcomes by enabling cancer cells to circumvent drug-induced stress highlights its significance as a therapeutic target. These findings underscore the complexity of targeting mitophagy due to its essential functions in both normal and cancer cells, presenting a challenging yet promising frontier in cancer therapy.

The investigation of mitophagy opens up numerous possibilities for novel cancer treatments, offering a promising pathway to overcome drug resistance—a prevalent and challenging issue in oncology. The modulation of mitophagy, whether through inhibition to prevent cancer cells from evading drug effects or induction to promote cellular stress and death in tumor cells, represents a frontier in the design of cancer therapies. The potential for developing mitophagy-targeted drugs, such as inhibitors of the mitophagy pathway or agents that induce excessive mitophagy, offers a strategy to enhance the effectiveness of existing therapies and to treat tumors refractory to current treatments. Future cancer treatments may increasingly rely on a precise understanding of mitophagy dynamics within tumor cells to tailor therapies that can effectively disrupt the survival advantages conferred by mitophagy. Furthermore, the integration of mitophagy modulators with other therapeutic modalities, such as immunotherapy and precision medicine, could yield synergistic effects, maximizing treatment efficacy while minimizing adverse effects. This approach aligns with the ongoing shift toward personalized medicine, where treatments are customized based on the genetic, molecular, and metabolic profiles of individual tumors. Ongoing research and development in this area are expected to lead to clinical trials testing the viability of mitophagy modulation in cancer therapy. Success in these endeavors could pave the way for the inclusion of mitophagy-targeting strategies in standard cancer treatment protocols, offering hope for improved outcomes in patients facing drug-resistant cancers. In conclusion, the exploration of mitophagy in the context of cancer therapy not only sheds light on fundamental cancer biology but also provides insight into innovative and more effective therapeutic strategies.

ABBREVIATION

ATP Adenosine triphosphate
BCL-2 B-cell lymphoma 2
CSCs Cancer stem cells
HIF-1α Hypoxia-inducible factor 1-alpha
HIFs Hypoxia-inducible factors
NF-kB Nuclear factor kappa-light-chain-enhancer of activated B cells
OXPHOS Oxidative phosphorylation
Parkin Parkin RBR E3 ubiquitin protein ligase

PDH Pyruvate dehydrogenase
PDKs Pyruvate dehydrogenase kinases
PINK1 PTEN-induced putative kinase 1
ROS Reactive oxygen species
TKIs Tyrosine kinase inhibitors

REFERENCES

Bajinka, O., Ouedraogo, S. Y., Golubnitschaja, O., Li, N., & Zhan, X. (2024). Energy metabolism as the hub of advanced non-small cell lung cancer management: A comprehensive view in the framework of predictive, preventive, and personalized medicine. *The EPMA Journal, 15*(2), 289–319. DOI: 10.1007/s13167-024-00357-5 PMID: 38841622

Bi, Y., Liu, S., Qin, X., Abudureyimu, M., Wang, L., Zou, R., Ajoolabady, A., Zhang, W., Peng, H., Ren, J., & Zhang, Y. (2024). FUNDC1 interacts with GPx4 to govern hepatic ferroptosis and fibrotic injury through a mitophagy-dependent manner. *Journal of Advanced Research, 55*, 45–60. DOI: 10.1016/j.jare.2023.02.012 PMID: 36828120

Biswas, U., Roy, R., Ghosh, S., & Chakrabarti, G. (2024). The interplay between autophagy and apoptosis: Its implication in lung cancer and therapeutics. *Cancer Letters, 585*, 216662. DOI: 10.1016/j.canlet.2024.216662 PMID: 38309614

Bray, F., Laversanne, M., Sung, H., Ferlay, J., Siegel, R. L., Soerjomataram, I., & Jemal, A. (2024). Global cancer statistics 2022: GLOBOCAN estimates of incidence and mortality worldwide for 36 cancers in 185 countries. *CA: a Cancer Journal for Clinicians, 74*(3), 229–263. DOI: 10.3322/caac.21834 PMID: 38572751

Cauwelier, C., de Ridder, I., & Bultynck, G. (2024). Recent advances in canonical versus noncanonical Ca2+-signaling-related anti-apoptotic Bcl-2 functions and prospects for cancer treatment. *Biochimica et Biophysica Acta (BBA) -. Molecular Cell Research, 1871*(5), 119713. DOI: 10.1016/j.bbamcr.2024.119713 PMID: 38521468

Chen, F. (2024). Inhibiting Pink1/Parkin-mediated mitophagy enhances the anticancer effects of quercetin in hepatocellular carcinomaf. *Biochemical and Biophysical Research Communications, 712–713*, 149899. DOI: 10.1016/j.bbrc.2024.149899 PMID: 38653003

Cocco, S., Leone, A., Roca, M. S., Lombardi, R., Piezzo, M., Caputo, R., Ciardiello, C., Costantini, S., Bruzzese, F., Sisalli, M. J., Budillon, A., & De Laurentiis, M. (2022). Inhibition of autophagy by chloroquine prevents resistance to PI3K/AKT inhibitors and potentiates their antitumor effect in combination with paclitaxel in triple negative breast cancer models. *Journal of Translational Medicine, 20*(1), 290. DOI: 10.1186/s12967-022-03462-z PMID: 35761360

Cook, K. L., Wärri, A., Soto-Pantoja, D. R., Clarke, P. A. G., Cruz, M. I., Zwart, A., & Clarke, R. (2014). Hydroxychloroquine inhibits autophagy to potentiate antiestrogen responsiveness in ER+ breast cancer. *Clinical Cancer Research*, *20*(12), 3222–3232. DOI: 10.1158/1078-0432.CCR-13-3227 PMID: 24928945

Cuervo, A. M., Elazar, Z., Evans, C., Ge, L., Hansen, M., Jäättelä, M., Liang, J. R., Loos, B., Mizushima, N., Simon, A. K., Tooze, S., Yoshimori, T., & Nakamura, S. (2024). Next questions in autophagy. *Nature Cell Biology*, *26*(5), 661–666. DOI: 10.1038/s41556-024-01404-z PMID: 38641661

Cui, Z., Cong, M., Yin, S., Li, Y., Ye, Y., Liu, X., & Tang, J. (2024). Role of protein degradation systems in colorectal cancer. *Cell Death Discovery*, *10*(1), 141. DOI: 10.1038/s41420-023-01781-8 PMID: 38485957

D'Arcy, M. S. (2024). Mitophagy in health and disease. Molecular mechanisms, regulatory pathways, and therapeutic implications. *Apoptosis*, *xx*(x), xxx–xxx. DOI: 10.1007/s10495-024-01977-y PMID: 38758472

de Talhouët, C., Esteras Gallego, N., Soutar, M., O'Callaghan, B., & Plun-Favreau, H. (2024). KAT8 compound inhibition inhibits the initial steps of PINK1-dependant mitophagy. *bioRxiv*, 2023.2008.2003.551835. DOI: 10.1101/2023.08.03.551835

Díaz-Gago, S., Vicente-Gutiérrez, J., Ruiz-Rodríguez, J. M., Calafell, J., Álvarez-Álvarez, A., Lasa, M., Chiloeches, A., & Baquero, P. (2024). Autophagy sustains mitochondrial respiration and determines resistance to BRAFV600E inhibition in thyroid carcinoma cells. *Autophagy*, *20*(6), 1383–1397. DOI: 10.1080/15548627.2024.2312790 PMID: 38436206

Fendt, S. M., Frezza, C., & Erez, A. (2020). Targeting metabolic plasticity and flexibility dynamics for cancer therapy. *Cancer Discovery*, *10*(12), 1797–1807. DOI: 10.1158/2159-8290.CD-20-0844 PMID: 33139243

Fu, J., Lin, J., Dai, Z., Lin, B., & Zhang, J. (2024). Hypoxia-associated autophagy flux dysregulation in human cancers. *Cancer Letters*, *590*, 216823. DOI: 10.1016/j.canlet.2024.216823 PMID: 38521197

Huang, L., Woods, C. M., Dharmawardana, N., Michael, M. Z., & Ooi, E. H. (2024). The mechanisms of action of metformin on head and neck cancer in the preclinical setting: A scoping review. *Frontiers in Oncology*, *14*, 1358854. DOI: 10.3389/fonc.2024.1358854 PMID: 38454932

Huang, X.-Q., Wu, R.-C., Liang, J.-M., Zhou, Z., Qin, Q.-P., & Liang, H. (2024). Anticancer activity of 8-hydroxyquinoline-triphenylphosphine rhodium(III) complexes targeting mitophagy pathways. *European Journal of Medicinal Chemistry*, *272*, 116478. DOI: 10.1016/j.ejmech.2024.116478 PMID: 38718624

International Agency for Research on Cancer, World Health Organization. *New report on global cancer burden in 2022 by world region and human development level.* (2024). Retrieved 16 April 2014 from https://www.iarc.who.int/news-events/new-report-on-global-cancer-burden-in-2022-by-world-region-and-human-development-level/

Jan, S., Fatima, K., Malik, F., Wani, A., & Khan, S. U. (2024). Introduction to Drug Resistance in Cancer. In Khan, S. U., & Malik, F. (Eds.), *Drug Resistance in Cancer: Mechanisms and Strategies* (pp. 1–30). Springer Nature Singapore., DOI: 10.1007/978-981-97-1666-1_1

Ji, M., Sun, L., Zhang, M., Liu, Y., Zhang, Z., & Wang, P. (2024). RN0D, a galactoglucan from Panax notoginseng flower induces cancer cell death via PINK1/Parkin mitophagy. *Carbohydrate Polymers*, *332*, 121889. DOI: 10.1016/j.carbpol.2024.121889 PMID: 38431406

Ke, Q., Wang, Y., Deng, Y., Wang, J., Yuan, M., Liang, A., Wang, J., & Gong, Q. (2024). Identification and validation of mitophagy-related signatures as a novel prognostic model for colorectal cancer. *Translational Cancer Research*, *13*(2), 782–797. DOI: 10.21037/tcr-23-785 PMID: 38482399

Lee, C., Park, S.-H., & Yoon, S. K. (2024). The E3 ligase HUWE1 increases the sensitivity of CRC to oxaliplatin through TOMM20 degradation. *Oncogene*, *43*(9), 636–649. DOI: 10.1038/s41388-023-02928-8 PMID: 38184713

Li, J., Ma, Y., Qiu, T., Wang, J., Zhang, J., Sun, X., Jiang, L., Li, Q., & Yao, X. (2024). Autophagy-dependent lysosomal calcium overload and the ATP5B-regulated lysosomes-mitochondria calcium transmission induce liver insulin resistance under perfluorooctane sulfonate exposure. *Ecotoxicology and Environmental Safety*, *276*, 116318. DOI: 10.1016/j.ecoenv.2024.116318 PMID: 38626609

Ling, Z., Pan, J., Zhang, Z., Chen, G., Geng, J., Lin, Q., Zhang, T., Cao, S., Chen, C., Lin, J., Yuan, H., Ding, W., Xiao, F., Xu, X., Li, F., Wang, G., Zhang, Y., & Li, J. (2024). Small-molecule Molephantin induces apoptosis and mitophagy flux blockage through ROS production in glioblastoma. *Cancer Letters*, *592*, 216927. DOI: 10.1016/j.canlet.2024.216927 PMID: 38697460

Liu, T., Zhang, J., Li, K., Deng, L., & Wang, H. (2020). Combination of an autophagy inducer and an autophagy inhibitor: A smarter strategy emerging in cancer therapy. *Frontiers in Pharmacology, 11*, 48, 408. PMID: 32322202DOI: 10.3389/fphar.2020.00408

Liu, Y., & Ma, Z. (2024). Leukemia and mitophagy: A novel perspective for understanding oncogenesis and resistance. *Annals of Hematology*, *xx*(x), xxx–xxx. DOI: 10.1007/s00277-024-05635-w PMID: 38282059

Liu, Y., Wang, Y., Zhang, J., Peng, Q., Wang, X., Xiao, X., & Shi, K. (2024). Nanotherapeutics targeting autophagy regulation for improved cancer therapy. *Acta Pharmaceutica Sinica. B*, *xx*(x), xxx–xxx. DOI: 10.1016/j.apsb.2024.03.019 PMID: 38828133

Luo, P., An, Y., He, J., Xing, X., Zhang, Q., Liu, X., Chen, Y., Yuan, H., Chen, J., Wong, Y.-K., Huang, J., Gong, Z., Du, Q., Xiao, W., & Wang, J. (2024). Icaritin with autophagy/mitophagy inhibitors synergistically enhances anticancer efficacy and apoptotic effects through PINK1/Parkin-mediated mitophagy in hepatocellular carcinoma. *Cancer Letters*, *587*, 216621. DOI: 10.1016/j.canlet.2024.216621 PMID: 38242198

Lv, S., Zhang, G., Lu, Y., Zhong, X., Huang, Y., Ma, Y., Yan, W., Teng, J., & Wei, S. (2024). Pharmacological mechanism of natural antidepressants: The role of mitochondrial quality control. *Phytomedicine*, *129*, 155669. DOI: 10.1016/j.phymed.2024.155669 PMID: 38696923

Ma, W., Lu, Y., Jin, X., Lin, N., Zhang, L., & Song, Y. (2024). Targeting selective autophagy and beyond: From underlying mechanisms to potential therapies. *Journal of Advanced Research*, *x*(x), xxx–xxx. DOI: 10.1016/j.jare.2024.05.009 PMID: 38750694

Masoudi, M., Moti, D., Masoudi, R., Auwal, A., Hossain, M. M., Pronoy, T. U. H., Rashel, K. M., Gopalan, V., & Islam, F. (2024). Metabolic adaptations in cancer stem cells: A key to therapy resistance. *Biochimica et Biophysica Acta (BBA) -. Biochimica et Biophysica Acta. Molecular Basis of Disease*, *1870*(5), 167164. DOI: 10.1016/j.bbadis.2024.167164 PMID: 38599259

Mishra, S. R., Behera, B. P., Singh, V. K., Mahapatra, K. K., Mundkinajeddu, D., Bhat, D., Minz, A. M., Sethi, G., Efferth, T., Das, S., & Bhutia, S. K. (2024). Anticancer activity of Bacopa monnieri through apoptosis induction and mitophagy-dependent NLRP3 inflammasome inhibition in oral squamous cell carcinoma. *Phytomedicine*, *123*, 155157. DOI: 10.1016/j.phymed.2023.155157 PMID: 37951147

Moulana, M. S., Haiaty, S., Bazmani, A., Shabkhizan, R., Moslehian, M. S., Sadeghsoltani, F., Mostafazadeh, M., Asadi, M. R., Talebi, M., Jafari, Z., Morovati, M. R., Farzaei, M. H., & Rahbarghazi, R. (2024). Tumoricidal properties of thymoquinone on human colorectal adenocarcinoma cells via the modulation of autophagy. *BMC Complementary Medicine and Therapies*, *24*(1), 132. DOI: 10.1186/s12906-024-04432-2 PMID: 38532470

Nakashima, M., Suga, N., & Matsuda, S. (2024). Nutraceuticals modulating mitophagy may combat the mitochondrial dysfunction and redox stress in several cardiac disorders. *Kinases and Phosphatases*, *2*, 166–178. DOI: 10.3390/kinases-phosphatases2020010

Naso, F. D., Bruqi, K., Manzini, V., Chiurchiù, V., D'Onofrio, M., Arisi, I., & Strappazzon, F. (2024). miR-218-5p and doxorubicin combination enhances anticancer activity in breast cancer cells through Parkin-dependent mitophagy inhibition. *Cell Death Discovery*, *10*(1), 149. DOI: 10.1038/s41420-024-01914-7 PMID: 38514650

Patra, S., Naik, P. P., Mahapatra, K. K., Alotaibi, M. R., Patil, S., Patro, B. S., Sethi, G., Efferth, T., & Bhutia, S. K. (2024). Recent advancement of autophagy in polyploid giant cancer cells and its interconnection with senescence and stemness for therapeutic opportunities. *Cancer Letters*, *590*, 216843. DOI: 10.1016/j.canlet.2024.216843 PMID: 38579893

Salehi, M., Kamali, M. J., Arab, D., Safaeian, N., Ashuori, Z., Maddahi, M., Latifi, N., & Jahromi, A. M. (2024). Exosomal microRNAs in regulation of tumor cells resistance to apoptosis. *Biochemistry and Biophysics Reports*, *37*, 101644. DOI: 10.1016/j.bbrep.2024.101644 PMID: 38298209

Shetty, S. S., Shetty, S., & Kumari, N. S. (2024). Therapeutic efficacy of gut microbiota-derived polyphenol metabolite urolithin A. *Beni-Suef University Journal of Basic and Applied Sciences*, *13*(1), 31. DOI: 10.1186/s43088-024-00492-y

Shorter, E., Engman, V., & Lanner, J. T. (2024). Cancer-associated muscle weakness - From triggers to molecular mechanisms. *Molecular Aspects of Medicine*, *97*, 101260. DOI: 10.1016/j.mam.2024.101260 PMID: 38457901

Sun, L., Li, Y., Zhao, R., Fan, Q., Liu, F., Zhu, Y., Han, J., Liu, Y., Jin, N., Li, X., & Li, Y. (2024). Platycodin D2 enhances P21/CyclinA2-mediated senescence of HCC cells by regulating NIX-induced mitophagy. *Cancer Cell International*, *24*(1), 79. DOI: 10.1186/s12935-024-03263-y PMID: 38374035

Tang, G. L. Q., Lai, J. X. H., & Pervaiz, S. (2024). Ubiquitin–proteasome pathway-mediated regulation of the Bcl-2 family: Effects and therapeutic approaches. *Haematologica*, *109*(1), 33–43. DOI: 10.3324/haematol.2023.283730 PMID: 37584295

Wang, L., Wang, X., Zhu, X., Zhong, L., Jiang, Q., Wang, Y., Tang, Q., Li, Q., Zhang, C., Wang, H., & Zou, D. (2024). Drug resistance in ovarian cancer: From mechanism to clinical trial. *Molecular Cancer, 23*(1), 66. DOI: 10.1186/s12943-024-01967-3 PMID: 38539161

Woolbright, B. L., Rajendran, G., Harris, R. A., & Taylor, J. A.III. (2019). Metabolic flexibility in cancer: Targeting the pyruvate dehydrogenase kinase: Pyruvate dehydrogenase axis. *Molecular Cancer Therapeutics, 18*(10), 1673–1681. DOI: 10.1158/1535-7163.MCT-19-0079 PMID: 31511353

Wu, D., Zhang, H., Li, F., Liu, S., Wang, Y., Zhang, Z., Wang, J., & Wu, Q. (2024). Resveratrol alleviates acute lung injury in mice by promoting Pink1/Parkin-related mitophagy and inhibiting NLRP3 inflammasome activation. *Biochimica et Biophysica Acta (BBA) -. Biochimica et Biophysica Acta. G, General Subjects, 1868*(7), 130612. DOI: 10.1016/j.bbagen.2024.130612 PMID: 38626830

Yamashita, S.-i., Sugiura, Y., Matsuoka, Y., Maeda, R., Inoue, K., Furukawa, K., Fukuda, T., Chan, D. C., & Kanki, T. (2024). Mitophagy mediated by BNIP3 and NIX protects against ferroptosis by downregulating mitochondrial reactive oxygen species. *Cell Death and Differentiation, 31*(5), 651–661. DOI: 10.1038/s41418-024-01280-y PMID: 38519771

Yan, C., & Li, T. S. (2018). Dual role of mitophagy in cancer drug resistance. *Anticancer Research, 38*(2), 617–621. DOI: 10.21873/anticanres.12266 PMID: 29374684

Zhang, R., Jiang, W., Wang, G., Zhang, Y., Liu, W., Li, M., Yu, J., Yan, X., Zhou, F., Du, W., Qian, K., Xiao, Y., Liu, T., Ju, L., & Wang, X. (2024). Parkin inhibits proliferation and migration of bladder cancer via ubiquitinating catalase. *Communications Biology, 7*(1), 245. DOI: 10.1038/s42003-024-05935-x PMID: 38424181

Zhang, Y., Yan, H., Wei, Y., & Wei, X. (2024). Decoding mitochondria's role in immunity and cancer therapy. *Biochimica et Biophysica Acta (BBA) -. Revisiones en Cáncer, 1879*(4), 189107. DOI: 10.1016/j.bbcan.2024.189107 PMID: 38734035

Zhang, Y.-M., Miao, Z.-M., Chen, Y.-P., Song, Z.-B., Li, Y.-Y., Liu, Z.-W., Zhou, G.-C., Li, J., Shi, L.-L., Chen, Y., Zhang, S.-Z., Xu, X., He, J.-P., Wang, J.-F., Zhang, L.-Y., & Liu, Y.-Q. (2024). Ononin promotes radiosensitivity in lung cancer by inhibiting HIF-1α/VEGF pathway. *Phytomedicine, 125*, 155290. DOI: 10.1016/j.phymed.2023.155290 PMID: 38308918

Zhao, Y., Han, J., Hu, W., Dai, Y., Wu, X., Liao, X., Zhou, H., & Nie, K. (2024). Xiao-Ban-Xia decoction mitigates cisplatin-induced emesis via restoring PINK1/Parkin mediated mitophagy deficiency in a rat pica model. *Journal of Ethnopharmacology, 318*, 116882. DOI: 10.1016/j.jep.2023.116882 PMID: 37422100

Zheng, J., Jiang, S., Lin, X., Wang, H., Liu, L., Cai, X., & Sun, Y. (2024). Comprehensive analyses of mitophagy-related genes and mitophagy-related lncRNAs for patients with ovarian cancer. *BMC Women's Health*, *24*(1), 37. DOI: 10.1186/s12905-023-02864-5 PMID: 38218807

Zimmermann, A., Madeo, F., Diwan, A., Sadoshima, J., Sedej, S., Kroemer, G., & Abdellatif, M. (2024). Metabolic control of mitophagy. *European Journal of Clinical Investigation*, *54*(4), e14138. DOI: 10.1111/eci.14138 PMID: 38041247

Chapter 12
Natural Products Modulating Mitophagy:
Implications for Cancer Therapy

Odangowei Inetiminebi Ogidi
https://orcid.org/0000-0002-9961-893X
Bayelsa Medical University, Yenagoa, Nigeria

ABSTRACT

Cancer is recognized as the second most significant contributor to death and its occurrence continues to escalate globally, resulting in a mounting burden on global health. Chemotherapy, while being the predominant approach for cancer treatment, is constrained by drug resistance and the occurrence of significant side effects, which restrict its efficacy. Mitophagy is the degradation process that damaged mitochondria go through via autophagy and the lysosome pathway in order to preserve mitochondrial equilibrium. Recent data suggests that mitophagy plays vital roles in the development of tumors, especially in cancer treatment. Several natural substances have been discovered that influence the process of cancer cell death and exhibit anti-cancer characteristics by regulating mitophagy. This chapter discuss the uncertainties and concerns that currently encircle the investigations into the potential of natural compounds as cancer treatments based on mitophagy. Potentially, novel interventional strategies for the treatment of cancer could advance if these restrictions were eliminated.

DOI: 10.4018/979-8-3693-3836-0.ch012

INTRODUCTION

In numerous nations characterised by a high Human Development Index, cancer ranks as the primary cause of mortality among the youth, surpassing cardiovascular disease (Lu et al., 2021). Based on the most recent data provided by the World Health Organisation (WHO) in 2020, a significant global mortality rate of 9.95 million individuals was attributed to cancer. Lung cancer constitutes the primary contributor to cancer-associated fatalities, accounting for 18.0% of the total. Breast cancer is 6.9%, followed by colorectal (8.3%), liver (8.3%), and stomach (7.7%) malignancies (Wang et al., 2020). With all the progress that cancer science has achieved over the years, the field of anticancer medicine still encounters substantial obstacles. Consequently, significant attention has been directed into investigating innovative molecular pathways and creating fresh therapeutic approaches or medications for the treatment of cancer (Ogidi et al., 2025a,b; Ogidi & Tawariowei, 2023).

Autophagy is a catabolic process that has been conserved throughout evolution, serving to breakdown intracellular components via the lysosome. In the past, the autophagy process was initially noticed by Thomas Ashford and Keith Porter, who observed that cells engaged in self-destruction (Pickrell & Youle, 2015). Subsequently, de Duve introduced the word 'autophagy' to describe the role of lysosomes following glucagon therapy (Akabane et al., 2023). Microautophagy, macroautophagy, and chaperone-mediated autophagy (CMA) are the three types of autophagy that are now known to be present in mammalian cells (Wang et al., 2020). Although there are numerous other types of autophagy, macroautophagy has been the subject of the majority of research. An increasing body of research is emphasising the critical role that autophagy plays in numerous physiological processes, including cell fate and stress responses. It has also been discovered that autophagy contributes to the development of disease in humans, such as neurological disorders, cancer, metabolic dysfunctions, and the ageing process (Wang et al., 2020).

Understanding of the mechanisms underlying autophagy has increased significantly over the past few decades. Additional classifications of autophagy include nonselective and selective autophagy. When considering overarching pressures such as starvation, non-selective autophagy is commonly defined as the phagophore's indiscriminate uptake of cargoes. Selective autophagy has the ability to selectively target cargos in a manner that is depending on the unique circumstances. Numerous distinct manifestations of autophagy have been documented thus far, encompassing mitophagy (pertaining to mitochondria), ER-phagy (pertaining to the endoplasmic reticulum, ER), lysophagy (pertaining to lysosomes), aggrephagy (pertaining to protein aggregates), ribophagy (pertaining to ribosomes), and xenophagy (pertaining to bacteria) (Zhang et al., 2008). A notable form of selective autophagy is mitophagy, which destroys damaged or unnecessary mitochondria by means of the autophagy/

lysosome pathway (Zhu et al., 2013). Essential to this process are mitochondria, which generate energy within the cell. In addition, mitochondria play a crucial role in controlling cell proliferation, apoptosis, cell specialisation, and the cell cycle. Therefore, the maintenance of mitochondrial homeostasis is of utmost importance for nearly all cellular processes throughout the lifespan, and mitophagy serves as the primary mechanism for ensuring the integrity of the mitochondrial network (Simpson et al., 2021).

There is considerable interest within the biomedical community regarding the potential health advantages associated with natural products sourced from diverse organic origins. The investigation of potential applications of diverse natural compounds in the prevention and treatment of cancer has witnessed a substantial surge in focus in recent times (Ogidi et al., 2024a,b,c). More recent research has improved our understanding of the crucial role of naturally occurring chemicals in cancer prevention. Notwithstanding the comprehensive examination of the functions of natural compounds in regulating autophagy in prior scholarly works, the applicability of these compounds as mitophagy regulators in the context of anticancer therapy remains unclear (Chen et al., 2014; Tay et al., 2010). Gaining insight into the interaction between natural products and mitophagy is crucial for the advancement of effective therapeutic approaches in anticancer treatment. This chapter presents an overview of the existing knowledge regarding mitophagy in the context of cancer progression. Additionally, it offers a thorough overview of specific natural compounds that have been utilised in cancer treatment, along with their ability to regulate mitophagy. These findings hold significant potential for the advancement of effective therapeutic approaches in the field of anticancer therapy.

BACKGROUND

An Overview of Mitophagy

Mitophagy refers to the process of selectively breaking down mitochondria by the use of autophagic mechanisms, resulting in their transport to the lysosome or vacuole. Researchers and medical professionals have taken a keen interest in the links and pathways that dysfunctional mitophagy and its types of variants (Figure 1) can cause in a variety of physiological processes, including development, ageing, and certain diseases like cancer, neurodegeneration, and immunity (Ding & Yin, 2012; Jin et al., 2013; Taylor & Goldman, 2011). Bhatia-Kišáová & Camougrand (2012), Jin et al. (2013), Ashrafi & Schwarz (2012), and Goldman et al. (2010) are some of the studies that have contributed to our understanding of mitophagy's mechanism, regulation, and specificity. These studies also involve cultured mammalian cells.

Autophagosome formation, also known as macroautophagy or macromitophagy, is the principal mechanism by which mitochondria are ingested, according to these findings.

Yeast contain the ability to engulf their own mitochondria through a mechanism called microautophagy or micromitophagy. The mitochondrion must interact directly with the vacuolar membrane for this process to occur. Autophagosomes are not required for the execution of this procedure. Developmental abnormalities, stress-induced situations, and baseline conditions are the three most common types of circumstances in which mitophagy has been observed. According to the first set of research, mitophagy is involved in a number of cellular activities, such as RBC maturation, stem cell maintenance and specialisation, and paternal mitochondria removal (Vazquez-Martin et al., 2012; Novak & Dikic, 2011; Sato & Sato, 2011). The second group includes common physiological situations where mitophagy helps keep the body's balance and cells working, according to studies by Bhatia-Kičáová & Camougrand (2012) and Goldman et al. (2010), and it does not matter how many cells an organism has. The third category comprises mitophagic events that occur due to compromised or malfunctioning mitochondria, significant alterations in the cellular metabolic milieu (e.g., carbon supply fluctuations or nutrient deficiency), or yeast-specific circumstances. Multiple studies (Bhatia-Kišáová & Camougrand, 2012; Ding & Yin, 2012; Jin et al., 2013; Taylor & Goldman, 2011) have reported that these modifications induce selective engulfment and subsequent degradation of these mitochondria.

Figure 1. Variants of mitophagy

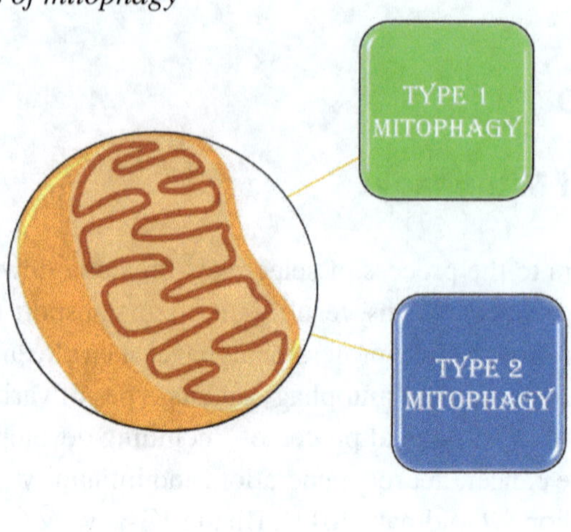

MITOPHAGY MECHANISMS

It is essential to safeguard mitochondria in order to maintain their functionality, which is vital for adaptive metabolism and cell survival under duress. Mitochondrial catalase and additional anti-oxidants collaborate to remediate the unfolded protein response (WPP) and increased concentrations of reactive oxygen species (ROS) within the mitochondria. It is also possible that mitochondrial fusion improves mitochondrial health by decreasing and dispersing defective mitochondrial DNA, proteins, or lipids throughout the broader mitochondrial reticulum. Motility-preserving cellular regulation is profoundly influenced by mitophagy, a specialised form of macroautophagy. While the autophagosome facilitates mitochondrial degradation via various mitophage receptors (Figure 2), NIX-dependent and BNIP3- mitophagy (Choursia et al., 2015) and PINK1/Parkin-induced mitophagy are the most widely recognized (Pickrell & Youle, 2015).

As a consequence of mitochondrial depolarization, PINK1 (PTEN-induced putative kinase 1) serine/threonine kinase accumulates at the outer mitochondrial membrane (OMM). The buildup of ubiquitin phosphorylates mitochondrial proteins, which in turn attracts autophagy cargo adaptors such OPTN and NDP52. LC3 within the autophagosome is the specific site where these adaptors bind to induce the destruction of mitochondria within autophagolysosomes (Pickrell & Youle, 2015). The outer membrane membrane (OMM) ubiquitination of substrates including VDAC, Miro, and Mitofusin-2 can occur via PINK1-induced activation of the E3 ubiquitin ligase Parkin. PINK1 activity initiates a signalling pathway that is augmented by this mechanism (Pickrell & Youle, 2015). Other mitochondrial E3 ubiquitin ligases also exhibit restricted expression patterns, in addition to Parkin. For instance, in skeletal muscle, Mul1 is known to facilitate mitophagy. Mitophagy serves as an adaptive mechanism whereby the quantity of mitochondria is diminished in reaction to various stimuli, including hypoxia, food scarcity, developmental indicators, or defective mitochondria. One possible explanation for stress-responsive mitophagy is that important mitophagy adaptors' expression and activity are controlled by known stress response pathways. As an example of this, consider the transcriptional targeting of BNIP3 by HIF-1, PPARγ, Rb/E2F, FoxO3, active Ras, and p53. Also, NIX (BNIP3L) is controlled by p53 and FUNDC1 is an HIF-1 target. Tissue specification is evident in two proteins that have undergone evolutionary descent from the same family, BNIP3 and NIX. Principal sites of BNIP3 expression are the liver, heart, and muscles; haematological tissues are where NIX is expressed. As RBCs mature into mature adults, NIX is indispensable for facilitating mitochondrial clearance in these tissues (Pickrell & Youle, 2015).

Their mitophagy mechanism is different from the Parkin/PINK1 route because BNIP3 and NIX target the autophagosome via direct adaptors. Induced BNIP3 and NIX (BNIP3L) are typically able to integrate into the OMM through the transmembrane domains found at the C-terminus. Through conserved LC3-interacting region (LIR) motifs, the proteins interact with newly produced phagophores in the cytosol. The proteins' amino termini expand as a result of these interactions. Additional post-translational mechanisms that regulate stress-induced mitophagy are suggested by the fact that phosphorylation of critical serine/threonine residues modulates the interaction between LC3 and BNIP3 (Wu et al., 2014). It is remarkable that BNIP3 and NIX were identified as pro-apoptotic proteins composed exclusively of BH3 residues. It is noteworthy to mention that the BH3 domains exhibit functional redundancy and only moderate conservation. Furthermore, it is worth noting that BNIP3 and NIX predominantly participate in mitophagy rather than cell death, as evidenced by their elevated expression levels in liver, heart, and RBCs in the absence of cell death. FUNDC1, similar to BNIP3 and NIX, functions as a mitochondrial adaptor by directly binding to LC3 via an LIR motif in response to decreased oxygen levels. ULK1 kinase, a critical constituent of the autophagy preinitiation complex, undergoes translocation to the mitochondria in the presence of hypoxia. It facilitates mitophagy by phosphorylating FUNDC1 in mitochondria, thereby strengthening the link between FUNDC1 and LC3 (Wu et al., 2014).

Figure 2. Types of mitophage receptors

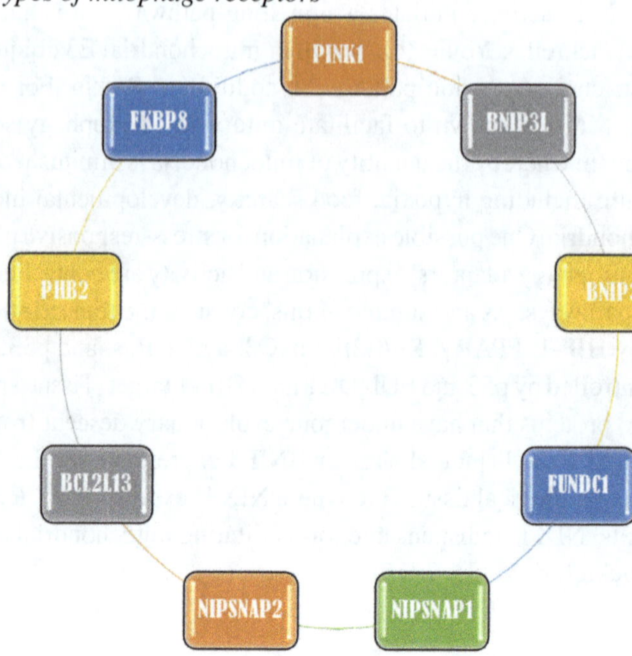

CANCER OVERVIEW

According to Taylor & Goldman (2011), the ability for autophagy to take place decreases with age, which could result in the buildup of damaged cells and the emergence of cancer. The idea was supported by the discovery made by Qu et al. (2003), who found that rats with autophagy malfunction (Beclin 1Ω/Ω) often had spontaneous tumour growth. A chromosomal 17q21 deletion of the Beclin 1 monoallele is also linked to 40–70% of human ovarian, breast, and prostate cancers (Taylor & Goldman, 2011). Mice with this genetic variation have been found to exhibit a variety of cancers, including lymphoma, hepatocellular carcinoma, lung adenocarcinoma, mammary hyperplasia, and allelic deletion of Beclin 1. The role of genes encoding key autophagy proteins as tumour growth suppressors is central to this model of the association between autophagy and cancer. Steatohepatitis, adenocarcinoma, and liver damage owing to the buildup of faulty mitochondria were detected in rats lacking the Atg7 or Atg5 protein primarily in the liver, according to Ding & Yin's (2012) study.

Recent research has indicated that cancer cells lacking the ability to undertake autophagy accumulate reactive oxygen species (ROS), protein aggregates, and damaged mitochondria. It is possible that these variables contribute to the formation and advancement of malignancies (Ogidi, 2024). There is probably a correlation between diminished autophagic and mitophagic capabilities, specifically, and an elevated susceptibility to the development of cancer. Nevertheless, the precise mechanisms by which autophagy mitigates the detrimental effects linked to the proliferation of tumours remain largely unexplored (Taylor & Goldman, 2011). Incorporating information from human malignancies and cancer cell lines has contributed to the expanding corpus of knowledge that establishes a connection between specific somatic mitochondrial DNA mutations and tumour proliferation. Furthermore, it has been observed that cancer cell lines exhibit a diverse array of mtDNA alterations. This suggests that the presence of impaired mitophagy and damaged mitochondria are factors that contribute to the advancement of cancer. Taylor & Goldman (2011) posit that the cumulative results of these studies suggest the potential for mitophagy to eradicate impaired mitochondria, thereby contributing to the reduction of tumours. Mitophagy can provide assistance to tumour tissues that are undergoing metabolic duress as a result of insufficient food or oxygen (Ding & Yin, 2012). In order to enhance comprehension of the role of mitophagy in the progression of tumours, additional research is required.

NATURAL COMPOUNDS AS MITOPHAGIC MODULATORS IN CANCER

The present focus of research and development in the field of autophagy regulatory medications mostly revolves around autophagy inducers and autophagy inhibitors, which are derived from the dual nature of autophagy in tumour cells. This section specifically examines several natural bioactive substances, such as polyphenolic, terpenoid, saponin, alkaloid and quinonoid compounds as shown in Table 1 and Figure 3.

Table 1. Natural compounds as mitophagic modulators in cancer

Compound	Source	Cancer Type	Mitophagy Mechanism	Effect on Cancer	References
Resveratrol	Grapes, red wine	Breast, colon	Induces PINK1/Parkin-mediated mitophagy	Promotes apoptosis, inhibits proliferation	Zou et al. (2020)
Curcumin	Turmeric (Curcuma longa)	Colon, breast	Upregulates BNIP3/NIX-dependent mitophagy	Induces autophagy and mitochondrial dysfunction	Liu et al. (2018)
Berberine	Berberis species	Liver	Enhances AMPK activation, promotes mitophagic flux	Suppresses tumor growth	Zhang et al. (2019)
Quercetin	Onions, apples	Lung, prostate	Activates PINK1/Parkin pathway	Inhibits progression via mitophagy	Wang et al. (2021)
EGCG	Green tea	Breast, prostate	SIRT1/FOXO3a-mediated mitophagy	Induces mitochondrial clearance	Zhang & Liu (2020)
Piperlongumine	Long pepper	Colon, breast	Inhibits mTOR, induces PINK1-mediated mitophagy	Reduces tumor proliferation	Liu et al. (2022)
Ginsenosides	Ginseng	Gastric, lung	ROS-induced AMPK activation	Sensitizes to chemotherapy	Kim et al. (2020)
Withaferin A	Ashwagandha	Pancreatic, breast	Modulates PINK1-Parkin axis	Triggers mitophagy-related apoptosis	Dutta et al. (2019)
Baicalein	Scutellaria baicalensis	Lung, liver	Enhances mitophagy via Beclin1/PINK1	Suppresses cancer cell growth	Cheng et al. (2017)
Honokiol	Magnolia bark	Breast, colon	Induces Parkin-mediated mitophagy	Inhibits metastasis, promotes cell death	Arora et al. (2020)

Compound	Source	Cancer Type	Mitophagy Mechanism	Effect on Cancer	References
Celastrol	Tripterygium wilfordii	Prostate, leukemia	Activates HIF-1α and PINK1 expression	Enhances mitophagy-mediated tumor suppression	Jiang et al. (2021)
Sulforaphane	Broccoli, cruciferous vegetables	Breast, prostate	NRF2 activation leads to mitophagy stimulation	Promotes cytotoxicity via mitophagic flux	Li et al. (2020)
Diosgenin	Fenugreek, yam	Ovarian, colon	Stimulates mitophagy via PINK1/Parkin and ROS	Reduces mitochondrial membrane potential	Gao et al. (2018)

Figure 3. Natural compounds as mitophagic modulators in cancer

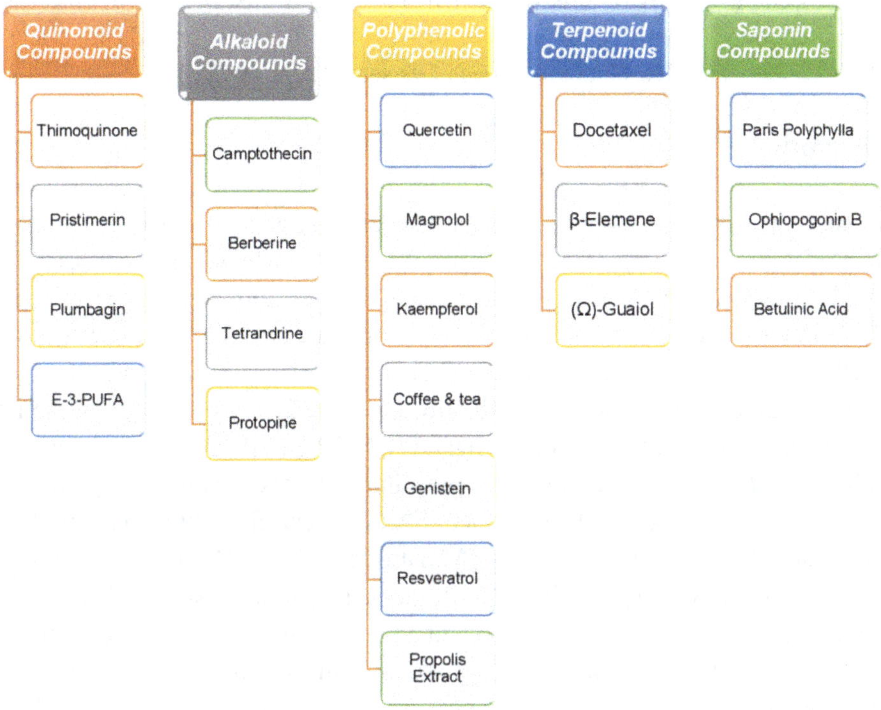

Polyphenolic Compounds

Polyphenolic chemicals, found in fruits, vegetables, seeds, and other plants, are the predominant bioactive secondary metabolites (Ogidi & Emaikwu, 2024). Many diseases, including cancer, can be treated or prevented with these substances (Yessenkyzy et al., 2020). The antioxidant activity of polyphenols has been ascribed to several positive effects (Ogidi & Ajoko, 2024; Messeha et al., 2021). Moreover, polyphenols have the ability to influence several cellular targets that have the potential to regulate mitophage activity, hence disrupting the symptoms and potential etiological factors of cancer (Messeha et al., 2021). Currently, there is a widespread consensus regarding the significant anticancer properties of dietary flavonoids (Ogidi & Felagha, 2024). The anti-inflammatory, proapoptotic, anti-genotoxic, antimetastatic, and antiinvasive actions are only a few of the many recognised activities exhibited by flavonoids such quercetin, kaempferol, apigenin, luteolin, green tea catechins, and genistein. Extensive experimental research using in vitro cell cultures and animal models, namely rodents, has proven that these compounds are effective in fighting cancer (Messeha et al., 2021; Ghasemi et al., 2021).

Quercetin

One of the most well-known antioxidant flavonoids, quercetin, also has anticancer effects (Ogidi & Joshua, 2024; Liu et al., 2021). By influencing the AKTmTOR signalling pathway, quercetin has been found to trigger autophagy in several cancer cells (Almatroodi et al., 2021). Autophagy is stimulated by quercetin's activation of AMPK and the accumulation of HIF-1γ. This process also inhibits mTOR signalling and triggers the synthesis of (Almatroodi et al., 2021) Bcl2/adenovirus E1B 19 kDa protein-interacting protein 3/ligand (BNIP3/BNIP3L), which disrupts the Beclin1/Bcl-2 (Bcl-xL) complex. Scientists have discovered that nanoparticles of quercetin containing poly (DL-lactide-co-glycolide) can cause human neuroglioma cells to die off by inducing autophagy (Almatroodi et al., 2021). Through activating the transcription axis 3 (p-STAT3)/Bcl-2 and causing endoplasmic reticulum (ER) stress, quercetin induces apoptosis and protective autophagy in ovarian cancer cells, according to researchers. Quercetin has a major impact on the control of chemotherapeutic drug sensitivity as a chemopreventive agent (Almatroodi et al., 2021). By modulating pathways linked to autophagy and apoptosis, quercetin increases the sensitivity of human pancreatic cancer cells to the chemotherapy gemcitabine. To achieve this, the receptor involved in the process of advanced glycation end products (RAGE)/PI3K/AKT/mTOR axis is managed. In uterine sarcoma MES-SA cells, quercetin inhibits drug efflux via P-glycoprotein (P-gp) transport proteins, increases

Table 1. Continued

the efficacy of anti-cancer drugs, and suppresses the development of multidrug resistance protein 1 (MDR1) (Almatroodi et al., 2021). Scientists have discovered that quercetin can protect gastric cancer cells from late apoptosis by inducing early autophagy (Wang et al., 2011). Rutin, a compound derived from the Meliaceae plant Toona sinensis Roem, is an antioxidant and anti-inflammatory with promising therapeutic applications (Enogieru et al., 2018). The medicinal herb Gentiana macrophylla contains luteoloside, which, like quercetin, has oncosuppressive effects in humans (Shao et al., 2018).

Magnolol

The magnolia officinalis root yields the botanical chemical magnolol, which finds widespread use in traditional Chinese and Japanese medicine. Many people know that magnolol helps with inflammation, diabetes, bacteria, nerve damage, and depression. Recent research has shown that neuroblastoma cancer cells treated with magnolol undergo mitophagy and ultimately die out. This has been confirmed in both in vitro and in vivo tests. Notably, magnolol's anti-cancer activity is significantly enhanced by inhibiting mitophagy. These findings suggest that fighting chemoresistance and improving the efficacy of cancer treatments may be possible through targeting mitophagy (Tang et al., 2021).

Kaempferol

Grapes and tomatoes are two examples of foods and vegetables that contain the monophenolic flavonoid kaempferol. For the purpose of protecting cells against malfunction, kaempferol influences autophagy in noncancerous cells. Further, it enhances autophagy in gastric cancer cells by upregulating p-AMP-activated kinase protein, LC3-II, and Beclin1, this in turn, accelerates cell death (Ashrafizadeh et al., 2020).

Coffee and Tea

The countries that manufacture the beverages containing EGCG, Catechin, and Epicatechin get a significant boost to their economies because of the large number of people who consume them. The genus Coffea is home to a wide variety of coffee plants, from which coffee is extracted through seed. The consumption of tea derived from the foliage of the Camellia sinensis plant is widely favoured (Landais et al., 2018). A comprehensive investigation demonstrated that caffeine, which is the primary component found in coffee beans and tea leaves, exhibits a strong ability to stimulate the flow of autophagy in the liver. The process of autophagy produced by caffeine involves the suppression of mTOR signalling and changes in the levels of amino acids and sphingolipids in the liver. Caffeine further stimulates AMPK-dependent autophagy in skeletal muscle cells via calcium-mediated mechanisms (Liu et al., 2019). One of the many health benefits of coffee which can include anywhere from 70 to 350 milligrammes of caffeine per cup is a reduced risk of cancer, including breast cancer (Saeed et al., 2019).

However, other cancers, including colorectal cancer (CRC) (Buldak et al., 2018) and bladder cancer (Park et al., 2018), have been associated with coffee use. Mice fed with either natural or decaffeinated coffee increased their autophagic flow in the liver, muscles, and hearts after one to four hours of ingestion, according to research by Pietrocola et al. (2014). By blocking mTORC1 enzyme activity, this result is produced. Their findings do not prove, however, that caffeine is the only element leading to increased autophagy. There may be a larger effect on autophagy activation and protein acetylation reduction from the polyphenols found in coffee and tea, including chlorogenic acid (CGA), epigallocatechin (EGC), catechin, and (Ω)-epicatechin. CGAs have the ability to activate autophagy pathways that are dependent on AMPK. These medications have shown promise in treating a wide range of human diseases, including cancer (Fujiki et al., 2018).

Genistein

Genistein, an isoflavone polyphenol derived from natural sources, has been documented to possess various advantageous impacts on human well-being. This effect's anticancer properties target a wide variety of cancer cells, including human breast MCF-7 cells and ovarian cancer cells (Prietsch et al., 2014). Among the many pathways that lead to these outcomes is an increase in autophagic cell death (Suzuki et al., 2014). Genistein modulates the autophagic-apoptotic pathway, which multiple studies have shown to boost the antitumor characteristics of chemotherapy medicines such gemcitabine, cisplatin, oxaliplatin, and 5-FU. Two key molecules, Bcl-2 and Beclin1, are involved in the control of autophagy, and when 5-FU and genistein are administered together, they cause cancer cells to undergo autophagic cell death (Suzuki et al., 2014). One mechanism by which genistein inhibits cancer growth is via blocking PI3K-AKT signalling (Suzuki et al., 2014). An essential step in the activation of the oncogenic survival pathway in NSCLC is nuclear receptor co-repressor (N-CoR) misfolding, which genistein suppresses, according to Ali et al. (2011).

Also, they discovered that genistein is associated with the autophagy-related molecular chaperone HSC70, which stands at 70 kDa. Genistein promotes autophagy protein expression and, surprisingly, causes an overproduction of TFEB, an important regulator of lysosomal formation (Moskot et al., 2014). In addition, genistein increases dephosphorylation and TFEB nuclear translocation as a result of its suppression of mTOR. This process is linked to a notable augmentation in both the quantity and functionality of lysosomes in both malignant and non-cancerous cells that have been treated. Therefore, it may be inferred that genistein exhibits promising potential as a therapeutic intervention for lysosomal storage disorders and malignancies (Arguello et al., 2021).

Resveratrol

Resveratrol has the capacity to impede the progression of several age-related disorders (ARDs), including cancer. An potential advantage of resveratrol is its ability to stimulate AMPK, a signalling pathway that could potentially enhance glucose tolerance and facilitate the regulation of mitochondrial quality (Suzuki et al., 2014). Numerous studies have shown that resveratrol can inhibit cell development effectively; these studies have focused on HCC, breast cancer, gastric cancer, and leukaemia as well. Resveratrol effectively suppresses the proliferation of breast cancer stem cells via its induction of autophagy and inhibition of the Wnt/β-catenin signalling pathway. Resveratrol activates AMPK, upregulates p62 by JNK, and activates the Beclin1-independent pathway, among many others, when administered to cancer cells, causing them to undergo autophagic cell death (Wang et al., 2016). Rumour has it that resveratrol inhibits p70S6K, a direct substrate of mTOR, which in turn reduces AKT phosphorylation and mTOR signalling. The endoplasmic reticulum (ER) stores and enters calcium ions less efficiently when treated with resveratrol (Zhang et al., 2012).

There is some evidence that resveratrol, due to its effects on apoptosis, could be helpful in the chemotherapeutic treatment of cancers such as leukaemia and hepatocellular carcinoma (HCC) (Zhang et al., 2012). The combination of rapamycin and resveratrol effectively suppresses the proliferation of oestrogen receptor-positive and oestrogen receptor-negative breast cancer cells. This inhibition is achieved by the prevention of AKT pathway activation, autophagy, and the stimulation of apoptosis (Deng et al., 2019). In a separate investigation, the co-administration of resveratrol and carfilzomib proteasome inhibitor at low concentrations was found to exhibit a synergistic effect on enhancing apoptosis in myeloma cells by concurrently stimulating autophagy. Additionally, the chemical has the potential to increase chemotherapy sensitivity in melanoma, prostate, and non-small cell lung cancer (NSCLC) (Sameiyan et al., 2019). Resveratrol was found to reduce autophagy in lung cells affected by cytotoxic stress generated by cigarette smoke. This effect was achieved by activating SIRT1, a powerful autophagy inducer (Deng et al., 2019). Pterostilbene, a resveratrol derivative, has been found to promote autophagy-induced cell death in cisplatin-resistant oral cancer cells in humans. The activation of SIRT1 mediates this action (Cuanalo-Contreras & Moreno-Gonzalez, 2019).

Propolis Extract

A honeybee-produced resinous chemical known as Chrysin Propolis possesses several advantageous pharmacological properties, including the ability to inhibit the proliferation of cancer cells. A compelling contender for cancer therapy is Brazilian green propolis extract, which comprises the active component artepillin C, which is derived from cinnamic acid (Endo et al., 2018). In addition, research has shown that green propolis ethanol extracts from Brazil and China can increase LC3-II expression in CWR22Rv1 cells, a kind of prostate cancer cell, and therefore promote autophagy (Endo et al., 2018). When artepillin C is administered alongside autophagy inhibitors like CQ, the induction of apoptosis is amplified (Endo et al., 2018). Several investigations have verified the biological characteristics of chrysin, such as its ability to reduce inflammation and inhibit tumour growth. The efficacy of chysin as a sensitising agent for temozolomide (TMZ) in human glioblastoma cells (GBM8901) has been demonstrated. By suppressing O6-methylguanine-methyltransferase (MGMT) DNA expression and downregulating the expression levels of LC3-II, ATG7, and Beclin1, the chemical impedes the autophagy process induced by TMZ. The emergence of TMZ chemoresistance may be influenced by this process (Sameiyan et al., 2019).

Terpenoid Compounds

Docetaxel

Docetaxel, a semisynthetic counterpart of paclitaxel, has been widely used as antineoplastic medication for the previous several decades. Ovarian, breast, and non-small cell lung cancer (NSCLC) are among the many malignancies that have benefited from these medicines since their 1992 FDA approval. Paclitaxel is commonly prescribed either as a standalone therapy or in conjunction with cisplatin. The anticancer efficacy of this medication is ascribed to its distinctive mode of operation, specifically inducing mitotic arrest in cancer cells, resulting in death by impeding microtubule depolymerization (Mukhtar et al., 2014). The development of resistance to paclitaxel has emerged as a significant constraint on the achievement of therapeutic success (Mosca et al., 2021). The precise chemical or fundamental mechanism responsible for paclitaxel resistance in malignancies is still unknown, however one possible explanation is that paclitaxel regulates autophagy. Paclitaxel has been discovered to trigger autophagy in a number of cancer cell types, including

BUC, ovarian, cervical, lung, and gastric cancer cells (BGC823 and SiHa, respectively) (Mukhtar et al., 2014).

β- Elemene

Based on studies, β-elemene initiates autophagy and cell death by blocking the PI3K/AKT/mTOR/p70S6K1 pathway in human renal-cell carcinoma 786-0 cells and human non-small cell lung cancer A549 cells (Deng et al., 2019). The treatment cells are protected by autophagy induction since β-elemene's anticancer effects are considerably enhanced when autophagy is inhibited by CQ (Deng et al., 2019). It has been proven that γ-elemene has the ability to reverse chemotherapeutic drug resistance. In p53 wild-type colorectal cancer (CRC) cells, this manifests as an increase in 5-fluorouracil sensitivity, and in non-small cell lung cancer (NSCLC), it reverses resistance to gefitinib (Liu et al., 2020).

(Ω)-Guaiol

The fact that (Ω)-Guaiol is antimicrobial has been acknowledged by many people (Yang et al., 2018). Through the induction of autophagy, which is accomplished by selectively targeting the phosphorylation of mTOR at serine 2481, (Ω)-Guaiol inhibits the growth of NSCLC cells (Yang et al., 2018).

Saponin Compounds

Paris Polyphylla

The growth, invasion, and EMT of cancer cells in lung, ovarian, and breast tissues were all halted by the Paris polyphylla extract (Lin et al., 2019). The ethanolic extract of P. polyphylla (EEPP) contains active components such as pengenin 3-O-beta-chacotrioside and polyphyllin VI. By increasing levels of autophagy markers LC3-II and Beclin1, these compounds induce cell death in DLD-1 human colorectal cancer cells. Moreover, studies have shown that the combination of EEPP treatment and Dox enhances cytotoxicity in these cancer cells (Lin et al., 2019). Research has shown that Diosgenin-enriched P. polyphylla rhizome extract (DPPE) can kill breast cancer cells and prevent their growth (Gupta et al., 2021).

Ophiopogonin B

Ophiopogonin B has been found to decrease cell proliferation in multiple NSCLC cell lines. Several cell types, including adenocarcinoma A549, H157, and H460, can be stimulated to undergo autophagy by ophiopogonin B, according to research. To accomplish this, as mentioned in reference, the treated cells' LC3-I to LC3-II conversion and ATG3 and ATG5-ATG12 expression levels are enhanced (Chen et al., 2016).

Betulinic Acid

Among its several biological roles, betulinic acid (BA) displays anticancer properties. Inhibiting autophagy-mediated apoptosis through the mitochondrial pathway, namely by activating MMP, mitigates the substance's anticancer effects (Zhang et al., 2016). The growth-inhibiting and cell-death-inducing effects of BA have been demonstrated in HepG2, SMMC-7721 hepatocellular carcinoma, and prostate cancer cells (Liu et al., 2019). By inhibiting the AKT/mTOR signalling pathway, BA therapy induces autophagy. Reducing both proliferation and death in colorectal cancer cells with BA is made even more effective by blocking autophagy. One protein that BA targets to limit breast cancer metastasis is GRP78, a major endoplasmic reticulum (ER) chaperone that is often abundantly expressed in most solid cancers. Metastatic traits, including as apoptosis resistance and medication resistance, are influenced by the GRP78 chaperone (Zheng et al., 2019). One of the many pharmacological effects of botulin, a decreased congener of BA, is that it may have anti-cancer capabilities. Betulin activates the AMPK and PI3K/AKT/mTOR signalling pathways, which in turn halts the cell cycle and causes cancer cells to breakdown, so preventing colorectal cancer from spreading. In addition, betulin has been found to reduce MAPK signalling pathway activity in metastatic colorectal cancer (CRC) cells, which leads to caspase-dependent death (Han et al., 2019).

Alkaloid Compounds

Camptothecin

Camptothecin (CPT) is an effective topoisomerase I inhibitor that exhibits oncosuppressive effects against many solid tumour systems, human colon cancer, and leukaemia (Hua et al., 2017). Cancer cells are more effectively targeted by CPT when two powerful autophagy regulators, miR-15a and miR-16, work together synergistically (Hua et al., 2017). After Ca2-mediated AMPK and the JNK/activator protein 1 (AP-1) pathway are activated, autophagy is induced, and CPT enhances the negative effects of c-Myc on endoplasmic reticulum stress and ROS production (Jayasooriya et al., 2018). In esophageal cancer, the production of reactive oxygen species (ROS) by CPT changes the AMPK/mTOR/ULK1 axis, which helps promote protective autophagy (Heng et al., 2021). Pulsatilla saponin D, a powerful autophagy inhibitor, and CPT work together to produce a synergistic effect on breast cancer. Proteins regulated by ubiquitous p62 are more likely to aggregate when this combination is present, as it interferes with autophagic-lysosomal activity (Wang et al., 2020). Belotecan and methylenebis are CPT compounds that promote autophagy as well, although they do it in different ways. While methylenedes have no effect on p62 expression but do boost LC3-II expression, belotecan promotes autophagy by decreasing p62 expression. Note that by inducing cancer cell death, the combination of methylenebis with belotecan enhances the combined antitumoral efficiency (Jang et al., 2017).

Berberine

The capacity to modify cancer is one of the pharmacological properties linked with berberine (BBR) (Zhang et al., 2020). Studies have demonstrated that several human cancer cell types, including as gastric cancer, glioblastoma multiforme (GBM), breast cancer, and hepatoma cells, are able to undergo autophagic cell death and apoptosis. This is achieved by activating Beclin1 and inhibiting the mTOR signalling pathway via BBR (Zhang et al., 2020; Lopes et al., 2020). It is feasible to cause autophagy and cell death in renal cancer cells by combining BBR with photodynamic therapy (Lopes et al., 2020). Beyond that, other studies have demonstrated that BBR can enhance the binding affinity of GRP78 in cancer cells, leading to an increase in autophagic cell death (Zhang et al., 2020; Lopes et al., 2020). By preventing senescence-inducing autophagy and cell-cycle arrest, BBR makes human hepatocellular carcinoma (HCC) more sensitive to ionising radiation (Ramesh et al., 2020).

Tetrandrine

Tetrandrine (TET) shows promise as a treatment for several different kinds of cancer due to its varied pharmacological properties (Luan et al., 2020). The anticancer effects of TET have been associated with its capacity to enhance radiation sensitization, reverse multidrug resistance (MDR), and induce apoptosis and autophagy, and other mechanisms (Luan et al., 2020). Numerous cell lines, including those representing human hepatocellular carcinoma (HCC), nasopharyngeal carcinoma, and triple-negative breast cancer cells, have shown that TET is an effective broad-spectrum autophagy agonist. The PI3K/AKT/mTOR signalling pathways are inhibited to produce these effects (Guo & Pei, 2019). Human PML-RAR[2]positive acute promyelocytic leukaemia (APL) cells are inhibited in their growth and autophagy is initiated by TET through increased ROS production and Notch1 signalling (Liu et al., 2015). TET causes pituitary adenoma (PA) cells to undergo dosage-dependent autophagy and ultimately die. At modest concentrations (1.25 μM), TET causes autophagy in these cells via blocking the MAPK/STAT3 pathway. Pituitary adenoma (PA) cells, however, experience partial apoptosis mediated by caspase when subjected to a higher concentration (5.0 μM) of TET (Lyu et al., 2021). In contrast to an autophagy enhancer, TET demonstrates strong lysosomal inhibitory characteristics, as demonstrated by Qiu et al. (2014). This means that it effectively hinders the autophagic process during lysosomal breakdown in cancer cells. Multiple cancer cells have been found to respond better to gefitinib, cisplatin, and tamoxifen after receiving TET (Ye et al., 2017).

Protopine

Protopine demonstrates various pharmacological characteristics, such as its ability to combat cancer. Protopine exerts a suppressive effect on the growth of cells in colon cancer, hinders the attachment of cells in breast cancer, and triggers the death of damaged cells in prostate cancer (Son et al., 2019). Protopine has the ability to stimulate the transcriptional activity mediated by p53 and enhance the stability of the p53 protein. The induction of autophagy by protopine is achieved by the enhancement of LC3-II turnover, as well as the reduction of p62 levels in human colon cancer cells (Son et al., 2019).

Quinonoid Compounds

The involvement of quinonoid chemicals in various biological oxidative systems is facilitated through their role as crucial components in the electron transport chains of metabolic pathways. The inherent cytotoxicity of quinonoids can be attributed to this redox property (Son et al., 2019).

Thimoquinone

In vitro and in vivo studies have shown that thymoquinone (TQ) has anticancer effects, demonstrating its exceptional pharmacological potency. Multiple myeloma, myeloblastic leukaemia, glioblastoma, and osteosarcoma are among the many cancers that the chemical TQ shows strong anticancer efficacy against (Mostofa et al., 2017). Other cancers that it targets include cervical, breast, colon, ovarian, larynx, ovary, and prostate cancers. Intricate and contradicting molecular processes have been uncovered by studying the influence of TQ on different forms of cancer. Multiple targets, including carcinogen metabolising enzymes and transcription factors, are involved in carcinogenesis and treatment resistance development, which adds complexity (Almajali et al., 2021).

Pristimerin

The many anticancer effects of Pristimerin have been shown to be caused by its ability to trigger autophagy, which is a process that involves the production of reactive oxygen species (ROS) and the activation of the JNK signalling pathway (Li et al., 2019).

Plumbagin

Among plumbabin's many pharmacological effects is its ability to inhibit the growth of many human cancer cell types (Yin et al., 2020). Growing data suggests that plumbagin's anticancer benefits stem from its ability to activate the AMPK pathway, inhibit the PI3K/AKT/mTOR pathway, and produce reactive oxygen species (ROS)—all of which play a role in cell death and autophagy (Lin et al., 2019; Xue et al., 2020).

Omega-3 Polyunsaturated Fatty Acids

Epicosapentaenoic acid (EPA) and docosahexaenoic acid (DHA) are the primary ingredients of β3-PUFAs. Various forms of cancer have shown evidence of the anticancer effects and action mechanism of γ3-PUFAs. But the main ways that DHA-induced cytotoxicity affects these cancer cells are through autophagic and apoptotic cell death. Results from studies using both wild-type and mutant p53 in human cancer cells and prostate cancer cells have demonstrated that DHA administration promotes autophagy and apoptosis, respectively (Jing et al., 2011; Kim et al., 2015). This is facilitated by the signalling cascade that comprises p53, AMPK, and mTOR (Kim et al., 2015). In glioblastoma multiforme (GBM) cell lines, 3-purified fatty acids (PUFAs) like high-dose docosahexaenoic acid (DHA) enhance apoptotic and autophagic cell death by increasing p62 expression, inducing PARP cleavage, and activating the AMPK/mTOR chain (Kim et al., 2018; Tan et al., 2018).

There is growing evidence that β3-PUFAs have anti-melanoma capabilities. When DHA-rich algal oil is given to patients with pulmonary melanoma, it triggers autophagy via activating the JNK pathway and inactivating mTOR, which significantly reduces cell proliferation (Tan et al., 2018). DHA blocks the STAT3 pathway, which triggers immunogenic death in human multiple myeloma cells, without harming dendritic cells (DCs) or peripheral blood mononuclear cells (PBMCs). Also, it may act as immunological enhancers by stimulating autophagy in PBMCs and DCs (D'Eliseo et al., 2017). By transforming them into ethanolamine derivatives, EPA and DHA have demonstrated anticancer effects in breast carcinomas. Various signalling pathways and receptors bind and activate to bring about this process (Giordano et al., 2020).

FUTURE PROSPECTS

Manipulating autophagy can be a preventative or therapeutic strategy for several human tumour types, since autophagy anomalies are associated with a wide range of human disorders. Researchers have found that autophagy promotes tumour growth as well as suppresses tumours in cancer. The microenvironment, the tissues impacted, and the stage of carcinogenesis determine the specific consequences. While autophagy may help with cancer prevention by removing oncogenic components, it can also encourage the spread of cancer to other parts of the body in tumours that have already grown. By blocking autophagy, which results in an overabundance and unchecked production of autophagosomes and auyolysosomes, chemoresistant cancer cells can undergo cell death. Cell death defined by autophagy can be induced by this buildup of autophagosomes and auyolysosomes. We now have a much better understanding of the molecular pathways that drive autophagy because to the discovery of natural compounds that act as modulators (Tan et al., 2018).

In order to study autophagy dynamics and find natural modulators, several labs have built cutting-edge methods, including as high-powered scanning microscopy and high-throughput, image-based screens. Quantitative study of autophagic machinery is now possible because to these developments. Several natural chemicals have anticancer effects due to their capacity to regulate autophagy, either by inhibiting or stimulating it, as stated earlier in this research. Autophagy modulators have the potential to be directly applied in therapeutic settings, however there are several hurdles associated with experimental grounds and clinical trials that have so far precluded this. Many of these issues should be resolved with the advent of more accurate markers of the autophagy apparatus, more animal models of autophagy deficit in vivo, and the creation of more specific autophagy modulators. The consequences of autophagy in tumours in the real world depend on many factors, such as the type of tumour, its developmental stage, its location, and the tumor's genetic, epigenetic, and metabolic background. Understanding the specific function of autophagy in tumorigenesis and progression is crucial for the design of new anticancer therapies aiming at cancer cure. Many questions remain unresolved regarding cancer treatment. Radiation and chemotherapy, the gold standard for cancer treatment, are extremely hazardous to both normal and cancer cells, limiting their efficacy. Therefore, it is crucial to prioritise research into novel therapy agents that are both efficacious and gentle on healthy cells (Giordano et al., 2020).

CONCLUSION

Autophagy has so far been well recognised as having a dual role in carcinogenesis. Within this framework, cytoprotective autophagy helps cancer cells avoid stresses like hypoxia and starvation, which in turn assists cancer cell growth, while defective autophagy is thought to facilitate cancer formation. A growing amount of research has shown that several natural substances can modulate many autophagy-related signalling pathways. So far, several chemicals have shown promise as potential treatments for various cancers. Natural chemicals offer promising new avenues for cancer treatment since they are less toxic, have various targets, and are naturally occurring. A brief summary of the molecular pathways for autophagy control is given in this article, which focuses on five substances ursolic acid, curcumin, paclitaxel, bufalin, and resveratrol that have been examined extensively. Most studies on these natural chemicals have concentrated on their anti-cancer effects in the lab, but there is a lack of data from in vivo trials. However, these obstacles can be efficiently overcome through further study into the validation of animal models and other approaches, which will greatly advance our understanding of the pharmacological actions of natural compounds. Keep in mind that most of these natural compounds can control apoptosis and autophagy. This makes them exceptional prospects for the vibrant and ever-changing Regulated Cell Death (RCD) network. In addition, they have the ability to modulate autophagy, which makes them a great asset in improving standard chemotherapeutic therapies and combating drug resistance. In addition, using a mix of natural substances has the potential to decrease effective dosage while increasing efficacy, which bodes well for future studies along this line. In conclusion, our research on natural chemicals that target autophagy in cancer treatment has the potential to shed new insight on the use of more natural compounds and offer suggestions for new anti-cancer drugs.

REFERENCES

Akabane, S., Watanabe, K., Kosako, H., Yamashita, S. I., Nishino, K., Kato, M., Sekine, S., Kanki, T., Matsuda, N., Endo, T., & Oka, T. (2023). TIM23 facilitates PINK1 activation by safeguarding against OMA1-mediated degradation in damaged mitochondria. *Cell Reports*, *42*(5), 112454. DOI: 10.1016/j.celrep.2023.112454 PMID: 37160114

Ali, A. B., Nin, D. S., Tam, J., & Khan, M. (2011). Role of chaperone mediated autophagy (CMA) in the degradation of misfolded N-CoR protein in non-small cell lung cancer (NSCLC) cells. *PLoS One*, *6*(9), e25268. DOI: 10.1371/journal.pone.0025268 PMID: 21966475

Almajali, B., Al-Jamal, H. A. N., Taib, W. R. W., Ismail, I., Johan, M. F., Doolaanea, A. A., & Ibrahim, W. N. (2021). Thymoquinone, as a Novel Therapeutic Candidate of Cancers. *Pharmaceuticals (Basel, Switzerland)*, *2021*(14), 369. DOI: 10.3390/ph14040369 PMID: 33923474

Almatroodi, S. A., Alsahli, M. A., Almatroudi, A., Verma, A. K., Aloliqi, A., Allemailem, K. S., Khan, A. A., & Rahmani, A. H. (2021). Potential Therapeutic Targets of Quercetin, a Plant Flavonol, and Its Role in the Therapy of Various Types of Cancer through the Modulation of Various Cell Signaling Pathways. *Molecules (Basel, Switzerland)*, *26*(5), 1315. DOI: 10.3390/molecules26051315 PMID: 33804548

Argüello, G., Balboa, E., Tapia, P. J., Castro, J., Yañez, M. J., Mattar, P., Pulgar, R., & Zanlungo, S. (2021). Genistein Activates Transcription Factor EB and Corrects Niemann-Pick C Phenotype. *International Journal of Molecular Sciences*, *22*(8), 4220. DOI: 10.3390/ijms22084220 PMID: 33921734

Arora, S., Singh, S., & Sharma, S. (2020). Honokiol regulates mitochondrial quality control in cancer cells. *Phytotherapy Research*, *34*(3), 470–478. DOI: 10.1002/ptr.6558

Ashrafi, G., & Schwarz, T. L. (2012). The pathways of mitophagy for quality control and clearance of mitochondria. *Cell Death and Differentiation*, *20*(1), 31–42. DOI: 10.1038/cdd.2012.81 PMID: 22743996

Ashrafizadeh, M., Tavakol, S., Ahmadi, Z., Roomiani, S., Mohammadinejad, R., & Samarghandian, S. (2020). Therapeutic effects of kaempferol affecting autophagy and endoplasmic reticulum stress. *Phytotherapy Research*, *34*(5), 911–923. DOI: 10.1002/ptr.6577 PMID: 31829475

Bhatia-Kiššová, I., & Camougrand, N. (2012). Mitophagy: A process that adapts to the cell physiology. *The International Journal of Biochemistry & Cell Biology*, *45*(1), 30–33. DOI: 10.1016/j.biocel.2012.07.006 PMID: 22801005

Buldak, R. J., Hejmo, T., Osowski, M., Buldak, L., Kukla, M., Polaniak, R., & Birkner, E. (2018). The Impact of Coffee and Its Selected Bioactive Compounds on the Development and Progression of Colorectal Cancer In Vivo and In Vitro. *Molecules (Basel, Switzerland)*, *23*(12), 3309. DOI: 10.3390/molecules23123309 PMID: 30551667

Chen, G., Han, Z., Feng, D., Chen, Y., Chen, L., Wu, H., Huang, L., Zhou, C., Cai, X., Fu, C., Duan, L., Wang, X., Liu, L., Liu, X., Shen, Y., Zhu, Y., & Chen, Q. (2014). A regulatory signaling loop comprising the PGAM5 phosphatase and CK2 controls receptor-mediated mitophagy. *Molecular Cell*, *54*(3), 362–377. DOI: 10.1016/j.molcel.2014.02.034 PMID: 24746696

Chen, M., Guo, Y., Zhao, R., Wang, X., Jiang, M., Fu, H., & Zhang, X. (2016). Ophiopogonin B induces apoptosis, mitotic catastrophe and autophagy in A549 cells. *International Journal of Oncology*, *2016*(49), 316–324. DOI: 10.3892/ijo.2016.3514 PMID: 27175570

Cheng, C., Yang, Y., & Liu, X. (2017). Baicalein enhances mitophagy and induces cancer cell apoptosis. *International Journal of Molecular Sciences*, *18*(3), 563. DOI: 10.3390/ijms18030563 PMID: 28273875

Chourasia, A. H., Boland, M. L., & Macleod, K. F. (2015). Macleod KF. Mitophagy & Cancer. *Cancer & Metabolism*, *3*(1), 1–11. DOI: 10.1186/s40170-015-0130-8

Cuanalo-Contreras, K., & Moreno-Gonzalez, I. (2019). Natural Products as Modulators of the Proteostasis Machinery: Implications in Neurodegenerative Diseases. *International Journal of Molecular Sciences*, *20*(19), 4666. DOI: 10.3390/ijms20194666 PMID: 31547084

D'Eliseo, D., Di Renzo, L., Santoni, A., & Velotti, F. (2017). Docosahexaenoic acid (DHA) promotes immunogenic apoptosis in human multiple myeloma cells, induces autophagy and inhibits STAT3 in both tumor and dendritic cells. *Genes & Cancer*, *8*(1-2), 426–437. DOI: 10.18632/genesandcancer.131 PMID: 28435516

Deng, S., Shanmugam, M. K., Kumar, A. P., Yap, C. T., Sethi, G., & Bishayee, A. (2019). Targeting autophagy using natural compounds for cancer prevention and therapy. *Cancer*, *125*(8), 1228–1246. DOI: 10.1002/cncr.31978 PMID: 30748003

Ding, W. X., & Yin, X. M. (2012). Mitophagy: Mechanisms, pathophysiological roles, and analysis. *Biological Chemistry*, *393*(7), 547–564. DOI: 10.1515/hsz-2012-0119 PMID: 22944659

Dutta, R., Khalil, R., & Roy, S. (2019). Withaferin A triggers mitophagy-dependent apoptosis in cancer cells. *Phytotherapy Research*, *33*(7), 1725–1736. DOI: 10.1002/ptr.6403

Endo, S., Hoshi, M., Matsunaga, T., Inoue, T., Ichihara, K., & Ikari, A. (2018). Autophagy inhibition enhances anticancer efficacy of artepillin C, a cinnamic acid derivative in Brazilian green propolis. *Biochemical and Biophysical Research Communications*, *497*(1), 437–443. DOI: 10.1016/j.bbrc.2018.02.105 PMID: 29452093

Enogieru, A. B., Haylett, W., Hiss, D. C., Bardien, S., & Ekpo, O. E. (2018). Rutin as a Potent Antioxidant: Implications for Neurodegenerative Disorders. *Oxidative Medicine and Cellular Longevity*, *2018*(1), 6241017. DOI: 10.1155/2018/6241017 PMID: 30050657

Fujiki, H., Watanabe, T., Sueoka, E., Rawangkan, A., & Suganuma, M. (2018). Cancer Prevention with Green Tea and Its Principal Constituent, EGCG: From Early Investigations to Current Focus on Human Cancer Stem Cells. *Molecules and Cells*, *41*, 73–82. PMID: 29429153

Gao, Y., Liu, X., & Zhao, Y. (2018). Diosgenin modulates ROS-mediated mitophagy in ovarian cancer. *Phytomedicine*, *42*, 203–209. DOI: 10.1016/j.phymed.2018.03.014

Ghasemi, S., Xu, S., Nabavi, S. M., Amirkhani, M. A., Sureda, A., Tejada, S., & Lorigooini, Z. (2021). Epigenetic targeting of cancer stem cells by polyphenols (cancer stem cells targeting). *Phytotherapy Research*, *35*(7), 3649–3664. DOI: 10.1002/ptr.7059 PMID: 33619811

Giordano, C., Plastina, P., Barone, I., Catalano, S., & Bonofiglio, D. (2020). n-3 Polyunsaturated Fatty Acid Amides: New Avenues in the Prevention and Treatment of Breast Cancer. *International Journal of Molecular Sciences*, *21*(7), 2279. DOI: 10.3390/ijms21072279 PMID: 32224850

Goldman, S. J., Taylor, R., Zhang, Y., & Jin, S. (2010). Autophagy and the degradation of mitochondria. *Mitochondrion*, *10*(4), 309–315. DOI: 10.1016/j.mito.2010.01.005 PMID: 20083234

Guo, Y., & Pei, X. (2019). Tetrandrine-Induced Autophagy in MDA-MB-231 Triple-Negative Breast Cancer Cell through the Inhibition of PI3K/AKT/mTOR Signaling. *Evidence-Based Complementary and Alternative Medicine : eCAM*, *2019*, 7517431. DOI: 10.1155/2019/7517431 PMID: 30713576

Gupta, D. D., Mishra, S., Verma, S. S., Shekher, A., Rai, V., Awasthee, N., Das, T. J., Paul, D., Das, S. K., Tag, H., Chandra Gupta, S., & Hui, P. K. (2021). Evaluation of antioxidant, anti-inflammatory and anticancer activities of diosgenin enriched Paris polyphylla rhizome extract of Indian Himalayan landraces. *Journal of Ethnopharmacology*, *270*, 113842. DOI: 10.1016/j.jep.2021.113842 PMID: 33460752

Han, Y. H., Mun, J. G., Jeon, H. D., Kee, J. Y., & Hong, S. H. (2019). Betulin Inhibits Lung Metastasis by Inducing Cell Cycle Arrest, Autophagy, and Apoptosis of Metastatic Colorectal Cancer Cells. *Nutrients*, *12*(1), 66. DOI: 10.3390/nu12010066 PMID: 31887988

Hua, F., Shang, S., & Hu, Z. W. (2017). Seeking new anti-cancer agents from autophagy-regulating natural products. *Journal of Asian Natural Products Research*, *19*(4), 305–313. DOI: 10.1080/10286020.2017.1304385 PMID: 28347180

Jang, M., Kim, H., Park, R., Jo, D., Lee, E. J., Oh, W. K., & Park, J. (2017). 2,2′-Methylenebis (6-tert-butyl 4-methylphenol) enhances the antitumor efficacy of belotecan, a derivative of camptothecin, by inducing autophagy. *Oncotarget*, *8*(70), 115068–115078. DOI: 10.18632/oncotarget.22858 PMID: 29383142

Jayasooriya, R., Dilshara, M. G., Karunarathne, W., Molagoda, I. M. N., Choi, Y. H., & Kim, G. Y. (2018). Camptothecin enhances c-Mycmediated endoplasmic reticulum stress and leads to autophagy by activating Ca2+-mediated AMPK. *Food and Chemical Toxicology*, *121*, 648–656. DOI: 10.1016/j.fct.2018.09.057 PMID: 30266318

Jiang, H., Huang, Q., & Fan, Y. (2021). Celastrol activates HIF-1α-PINK1 axis to trigger mitophagy in cancer suppression. *Frontiers in Pharmacology*, *12*, 654371. DOI: 10.3389/fphar.2021.654371

Jin, M., Liu, X., & Klionsky, D. J. (2013). Snapshot: Selective autophagy. *Cell*, *152*(1-2), 368–368. DOI: 10.1016/j.cell.2013.01.004 PMID: 23332767

Jing, K., Song, K. S., Shin, S., Kim, N., Jeong, S., Oh, H. R., Park, J. H., Seo, K. S., Heo, J. Y., Han, J., Park, J. I., Han, C., Wu, T., Kweon, G. R., Park, S. K., Yoon, W. H., Hwang, B. D., & Lim, K. (2011). Docosahexaenoic acid induces autophagy through p53/AMPK/mTOR signaling and promotes apoptosis in human cancer cells harboring wild-type p53. *Autophagy*, *7*(11), 1348–1358. DOI: 10.4161/auto.7.11.16658 PMID: 21811093

Kim, J., Hwang, J., & Kim, M. (2020). Ginsenosides regulate mitophagy and suppress cancer progression. *Journal of Ginseng Research*, *44*(1), 45–52. DOI: 10.1016/j.jgr.2019.06.002

Kim, N., Jeong, S., Jing, K., Shin, S., Kim, S., Heo, J. Y., Kweon, G. R., Park, S. K., Wu, T., Park, J. I., & Lim, K. (2015). Docosahexaenoic Acid Induces Cell Death in Human Non-Small Cell Lung Cancer Cells by Repressing mTOR via AMPK Activation and PI3K/Akt Inhibition. *BioMed Research International, 239764*, 1–14. Advance online publication. DOI: 10.1155/2015/239764 PMID: 26339598

Kim, S., Jing, K., Shin, S., Jeong, S., Han, S. H., Oh, H., Yoo, Y. S., Han, J., Jeon, Y. J., Heo, J. Y., Kweon, G. R., Park, S. K., Park, J. I., Wu, T., & Lim, K. (2018). ω3-polyunsaturated fatty acids induce cell death through apoptosis and autophagy in glioblastoma cells: In vitro and in vivo. *Oncology Reports, 39*(1), 239–246. DOI: 10.3892/or.2017.6101 PMID: 29192322

Landais, E., Moskal, A., Mullee, A., Nicolas, G., Gunter, M. J., Huybrechts, I., Overvad, K., Roswall, N., Affret, A., Fagherazzi, G., Mahamat-Saleh, Y., Katzke, V., Kühn, T., La Vecchia, C., Trichopoulou, A., Valanou, E., Saieva, C., Santucci de Magistris, M., Sieri, S., & Freisling, H. (2018). Coffee and Tea Consumption and the Contribution of Their Added Ingredients to Total Energy and Nutrient Intakes in 10 European Countries: Benchmark Data from the Late 1990s. *Nutrients, 10*(6), 725. DOI: 10.3390/nu10060725 PMID: 29874819

Li, J., Yang, Y., & Lin, W. (2020). Sulforaphane-induced mitophagy promotes apoptosis in prostate cancer. *Cancer Letters, 482*, 23–34. DOI: 10.1016/j.canlet.2020.05.010

Li, J. J., Yan, Y. Y., Sun, H. M., Liu, Y., Su, C. Y., Chen, H. B., & Zhang, J. Y. (2019). Anti-Cancer Effects of Pristimerin and the Mechanisms: A Critical Review. *Frontiers in Pharmacology, 2019*(10), 746. DOI: 10.3389/fphar.2019.00746 PMID: 31354475

Li, L., Zhang, W., Jiang, Y., Wang, S., & Jia, L. (2021). Camptothecin Inhibits Neddylation to Activate the Protective Autophagy Through NF-kappaB/AMPK/mTOR/ULK1 Axis in Human Esophageal Cancer Cells. *Frontiers in Oncology, 11*, 671180. DOI: 10.3389/fonc.2021.671180 PMID: 33898327

Lin, L. T., Uen, W. C., Choong, C. Y., Shi, Y. C., Lee, B. H., Tai, C. J., & Tai, C. J. (2019). Paris Polyphylla Inhibits Colorectal Cancer Cells via Inducing Autophagy and Enhancing the Efficacy of Chemotherapeutic Drug Doxorubicin. *Molecules (Basel, Switzerland), 24*(11), 2102. DOI: 10.3390/molecules24112102 PMID: 31163662

Lin, Y., Chen, Y., Wang, S., Ma, J., Peng, Y., Yuan, X., Lv, B., Chen, W., & Wei, Y. (2019). Plumbagin induces autophagy and apoptosis of SMMC-7721 cells in vitro and in vivo. *Journal of Cellular Biochemistry, 120*(6), 9820–9830. DOI: 10.1002/jcb.28262 PMID: 30536473

Liu, H., Song, J., Zhou, Y., Cao, L., Gong, Y., Wei, Y., Yang, H., & Tang, L. (2019). Methylxanthine derivatives promote autophagy in gastric cancer cells targeting PTEN. *Anti-Cancer Drugs*, *30*(4), 347–355. DOI: 10.1097/CAD.0000000000000724 PMID: 30875347

Liu, L., Wang, Y., & Ren, J. (2018). Curcumin-induced mitophagy regulates cell fate in cancer therapy. *Autophagy*, *14*(5), 870–886. DOI: 10.1080/15548627.2018.1439431 PMID: 29433359

Liu, Q., Sun, Y., & Liu, Z. (2022). Piperlongumine enhances mitophagy and suppresses colorectal cancer cell growth. *Cellular Physiology and Biochemistry*, *56*(3), 349–360. DOI: 10.33594/000000001

Liu, S., Li, Q., Li, G., Zhang, Q., Zhuo, L., Han, X., Zhang, M., Chen, X., Pan, T., Yan, L., Jin, T., Wang, J., Lv, Q., Sui, X., & Xie, T. (2020). The mechanism of m^6A methyltransferase METTL3-mediated autophagy in reversing gefitinib resistance in NSCLC cells by β-elemene. *Cell Death & Disease*, *11*(11), 969. DOI: 10.1038/s41419-020-03148-8 PMID: 33177491

Liu, T., Men, Q., Wu, G., Yu, C., Huang, Z., Liu, X., & Li, W. (2015). Tetrandrine induces autophagy and differentiation by activating ROS and Notch1 signaling in leukemia cells. *Oncotarget*, *6*(10), 7992–8006. DOI: 10.18632/oncotarget.3505 PMID: 25797266

Liu, Y., Li, C. L., Xu, Q. Q., Cheng, D., Liu, K. D., & Sun, Z. Q. (2021). Quercetin inhibits invasion and angiogenesis of esophageal cancer cells. *Pathology, Research and Practice*, *222*, 153455. DOI: 10.1016/j.prp.2021.153455 PMID: 33962176

Lopes, T. Z., de Moraes, F. R., Tedesco, A. C., Arni, R. K., Rahal, P., & Calmon, M. F. (2020). Berberine associated photodynamic therapy promotes autophagy and apoptosis via ROS generation in renal carcinoma cells. *Biomedicine and Pharmacotherapy*, *123*, 109794. DOI: 10.1016/j.biopha.2019.109794 PMID: 31874443

Lu, G., Wang, L., Zhou, J., Liu, W., & Shen, H. M. (2021). A Destiny for Degradation: Interplay between Cullin-RING E3 Ligases and Autophagy. *Trends in Cell Biology*, *31*(6), 432–444. DOI: 10.1016/j.tcb.2021.01.005 PMID: 33573849

Luan, F., He, X., & Zeng, N. (2020). Tetrandrine: A review of its anticancer potentials, clinical settings, pharmacokinetics and drug delivery systems. *The Journal of Pharmacy and Pharmacology*, *72*(11), 1491–1512. DOI: 10.1111/jphp.13339 PMID: 32696989

Luo, Y., Chen, R., Wei, S., Yang, X., & Wang, Q. (2019). Betulinic acid induces autophagy-mediated apoptosis through suppression of the PI3K/AKT/mTOR signaling pathway and inhibits hepatocellular carcinoma. *American Journal of Translational Research, 11*, 6952–6964. PMID: 31814899

Lyu, L., Hu, Y., Yin, S., Wang, L., Ye, F., Wang, M., Zhou, Y., Ma, W., Chen, C., Jiang, Y., Wang, Z., Jiang, S., Zhou, P., & Wang, X. (2021). Autophagy inhibition enhances anti-pituitary adenoma effect of tetrandrine. *Phytotherapy Research, 35*(7), 4007–4021. DOI: 10.1002/ptr.7117 PMID: 34038010

Messeha, S. S., Zarmouh, N. O., & Soliman, K. F. A. (2021). Polyphenols Modulating Effects of PD-L1/PD-1 Checkpoint and EMT-Mediated PD-L1 Overexpression in Breast Cancer. *Nutrients, 13*(5), 1718. DOI: 10.3390/nu13051718 PMID: 34069461

Mosca, L., Ilari, A., Fazi, F., Assaraf, Y. G., & Colotti, G. (2021). Taxanes in cancer treatment: Activity, chemoresistance and its overcoming. *Drug Resistance Updates, 54*, 100742. DOI: 10.1016/j.drup.2020.100742 PMID: 33429249

Moskot, M., Montefusco, S., Jakobkiewicz-Banecka, J., Mozolewski, P., Wegrzyn, A., Di Bernardo, D., Wegrzyn, G., Medina, D. L., Ballabio, A., & Gabig-Ciminska, M. (2014). The phytoestrogen genistein modulates lysosomal metabolism and transcription factor EB (TFEB) activation. *The Journal of Biological Chemistry, 289*(24), 17054–17069. DOI: 10.1074/jbc.M114.555300 PMID: 24770416

Mostofa, A. G. M., Hossain, M. K., Basak, D., & Bin Sayeed, M. S. (2017). Thymoquinone as a Potential Adjuvant Therapy for Cancer Treatment: Evidence from Preclinical Studies. *Frontiers in Pharmacology, 8*, 295. DOI: 10.3389/fphar.2017.00295 PMID: 28659794

Mukhtar, E., Adhami, V. M., & Mukhtar, H. (2014). Targeting microtubules by natural agents for cancer therapy. *Molecular Cancer Therapeutics, 2014*(13), 275–284. DOI: 10.1158/1535-7163.MCT-13-0791 PMID: 24435445

Novak, I., & Dikic, I. (2011). Autophagy receptors in developmental clearance of mitochondria. *Autophagy, 7*(3), 301–303. DOI: 10.4161/auto.7.3.14509 PMID: 21206218

Ogidi, O. I. (2024). Phytochemical Screening and Bioinformatics Approaches for Anticancer Activity from Potential Plants. In: Computational Approaches in Biomaterials, Bioinformatics and Biomedical Engineering Applications. *CRC Press, Taylor and Francis Group, Florida, USA.*

Ogidi, O. I., & Ajoko, I. (2024). Neuroprotective Potentials of Phytochemicals. In: M.S. Rajput, T. Sarachana, P.D. Sarkar, M. Raval (eds) NeuroPhytomedicine. Published by *CRC Press, Routledge Taylor and Francis Group.*

Ogidi, O. I., Ajoko, I. T., & Chukwudi, P. (2024b). Natural Antioxidant Compounds for Skin Care. In *Eco-Friendly Skin Solutions for Natural Cosmeceuticals.* IGI Global., DOI: 10.4018/979-8-3693-5473-5.ch008

Ogidi, O. I., Barwant, M. M., & Okara, E. (2024a). Biomarker Discovery: Protein Phosphorylation State. In *Spatially Variable Genes in Cancer: Development, Progression, and Treatment Response.* IGI Global., DOI: 10.4018/979-8-3693-7728-4.ch005

Ogidi, O. I., & Emaikwu, N. G. (2024). Plant Phenolic compound isolation and its Bioinformatics Approaches of Molecular Mechanisms in Antimicrobial activities and Resistance. In: Computational Approaches in Biomaterials, Bioinformatics and Biomedical Engineering Applications. *CRC Press, Taylor and Francis Group, Florida, USA.* DOI: 10.1201/9781003354437-8

Ogidi, O. I., Erho, S. A., & Omu, O. (2025a). Reactive Oxygen Species in Cancer. In Prabhakar, P. (Ed.), *The Role of Reactive Oxygen Species in Human Health and Disease* (pp. 339–376). IGI Global Scientific Publishing., DOI: 10.4018/979-8-3693-7919-6.ch010

Ogidi, O. I., & Felagha, I. (2024). Gut Microbiome and Diet Interaction. In *Nutrition Controversies and Advances in Autoimmune Disease. Publisher.* IGI Global. DOI: 10.4018/979-8-3693-5528-2.ch012

Ogidi, O. I., Ijere, N. D., & Sogoi, P. B. (2025b). Neural and Endocrine Regulation of Immunity. In Reddy, K. (Ed.), *Research Methodologies and Practical Applications in Psychoneuroimmunology* (pp. 17–42). IGI Global Scientific Publishing., DOI: 10.4018/979-8-3693-7432-0.ch002

Ogidi, O. I., & Joshua, M. T. (2024). Invitro antioxidant and anti-inflammatory activities of selected polyherbal formulations sold in Nigeria. *Future Natural Products.*, *9*(2), 63–68. DOI: 10.34172/fnp.2307-1252

Ogidi, O. I., Ogoun, T. R., Alex, E. I., Edward, R. B., Joshua, M. T., & Bunu, E. M. (2024c). Radiogenomics and Genetic Diversity of Glioblastoma Characterization. In: Radiomics and Radiogenomics in Neuro-Oncology: An Artificial Intelligence Paradigm- volume 2: Genetics and clinical applications. *Elsevier.* https://doi.org/ DOI: 10.1016/B978-0-443-18509-0.00002-5

Ogidi, O. I., & Tawariowei, A. M. (2023). Endocrine Disrupting Chemicals and their Role in Cancer-A review. *Molecular Sciences And Applications.*, *3*, 5–14. DOI: 10.37394/232023.2023.3.2

Park, S. Y., Freedman, N. D., Haiman, C. A., Le Marchand, L., Wilkens, L. R., & Setiawan, V. W. (2018). Prospective Study of Coffee Consumption and Cancer Incidence in Non-White Populations. *Cancer Epidemiology, Biomarkers & Prevention*, *27*(8), 928–935. DOI: 10.1158/1055-9965.EPI-18-0093 PMID: 29777049

Pickrell, A. M., & Youle, R. J. (2015). The roles of PINK1, parkin, and mitochondrial fidelity in Parkinson's disease. *Neuron*, *85*(2), 257–273. DOI: 10.1016/j.neuron.2014.12.007 PMID: 25611507

Pickrell, A. M., & Youle, R. J. (2015). The roles of PINK1, parkin, and mitochondrial fidelity in Parkinson's disease. *Neuron*, *85*(2), 257–273. DOI: 10.1016/j.neuron.2014.12.007 PMID: 25611507

Pietrocola, F., Malik, S. A., Marino, G., Vacchelli, E., Senovilla, L., Chaba, K., Niso-Santano, M., Maiuri, M. C., Madeo, F., & Kroemer, G. (2014). Coffee induces autophagy in vivo. *Cell Cycle (Georgetown, Tex.)*, *13*(12), 1987–1994. DOI: 10.4161/cc.28929 PMID: 24769862

Prietsch, R. F., Monte, L. G., da Silva, F. A., Beira, F. T., Del Pino, F. A., Campos, V. F., Collares, T., Pinto, L. S., Spanevello, R. M., Gamaro, G. D., & Braganhol, E. (2014). Genistein induces apoptosis and autophagy in human breast MCF-7 cells by modulating the expression of proapoptotic factors and oxidative stress enzymes. *Molecular and Cellular Biochemistry*, *390*(1-2), 235–242. DOI: 10.1007/s11010-014-1974-x PMID: 24573886

Qiu, W., Su, M., Xie, F., Ai, J., Ren, Y., Zhang, J., Guan, R., He, W., Gong, Y., & Guo, Y. (2014). Tetrandrine blocks autophagic flux and induces apoptosis via energetic impairment in cancer cells. *Cell Death & Disease*, *2014*(5), e1123. DOI: 10.1038/cddis.2014.84 PMID: 24625982

Ramesh, G., Das, S., & Bola Sadashiva, S. R. (2020). Berberine, a natural alkaloid sensitizes human hepatocarcinoma to ionizing radiation by blocking autophagy and cell cycle arrest resulting in senescence. *The Journal of Pharmacy and Pharmacology*, *72*(12), 1893–1908. DOI: 10.1111/jphp.13354 PMID: 32815562

Saeed, M., Naveed, M., BiBi, J., Ali Kamboh, A., Phil, L., & Chao, S. (2019). Potential nutraceutical and food additive properties and risks of coffee: A comprehensive overview. *Critical Reviews in Food Science and Nutrition*, *59*(20), 3293–3319. DOI: 10.1080/10408398.2018.1489368 PMID: 30614268

Sameiyan, E., Hayes, A. W., & Karimi, G. (2019). The effect of medicinal plants on multiple drug resistance through autophagy: A review of in vitro studies. *European Journal of Pharmacology*, *852*, 244–253. DOI: 10.1016/j.ejphar.2019.04.001 PMID: 30965056

Sato, M., & Sato, K. (2011). Degradation of paternal mitochondria by fertilization-triggered autophagy in C. elegans embryos. *Science*, *334*(6059), 1141–1144. DOI: 10.1126/science.1210333 PMID: 21998252

Shao, J., Wang, C., Li, L., Liang, H., Dai, J., Ling, X., & Tang, H. (2018). Luteoloside Inhibits Proliferation and Promotes Intrinsic and Extrinsic Pathway-Mediated Apoptosis Involving MAPK and mTOR Signaling Pathways in Human Cervical Cancer Cells. *International Journal of Molecular Sciences*, *19*(6), 1664. DOI: 10.3390/ijms19061664 PMID: 29874795

Simpson, C. L., Tokito, M. K., Uppala, R., Sarkar, M. K., Gudjonsson, J. E., & Holzbaur, E. L. F. (2021). NIX initiates mitochondrial fragmentation via DRP1 to drive epidermal differentiation. *Cell Reports*, *34*(5), 108689. DOI: 10.1016/j.celrep.2021.108689 PMID: 33535046

Son, Y., An, Y., Jung, J., Shin, S., Park, I., Gwak, J., Ju, B. G., Chung, Y. H., Na, M., & Oh, S. (2019). Protopine isolated from Nandina domestica induces apoptosis and autophagy in colon cancer cells by stabilizing p53. *Phytotherapy Research*, *33*(6), 1689–1696. DOI: 10.1002/ptr.6357 PMID: 30932278

Suzuki, R., Kang, Y., Li, X., Roife, D., Zhang, R., & Fleming, J. B. (2014). Genistein potentiates the antitumor effect of 5-Fluorouracil by inducing apoptosis and autophagy in human pancreatic cancer cells. *Anticancer Research*, *34*, 4685–4692. PMID: 25202045

Tan, R. H., Wang, F., Fan, C. L., Zhang, X. H., Zhao, J. S., Zhang, J. J., Yang, Y., Xi, Y., Zou, Z. Q., & Bu, S. Z. (2018). Algal oil rich in n-3 polyunsaturated fatty acids suppresses B16F10 melanoma lung metastasis by autophagy induction. *Food & Function*, *9*(12), 6179–6186. DOI: 10.1039/C8FO01617H PMID: 30450498

Tang, Y., Wang, L., Yi, T., Xu, J., Wang, J., Qin, J. J., Chen, Q., Yip, K. M., Pan, Y., Hong, P., Lu, Y., Shen, H. M., & Chen, H. B. (2021). Synergistic effects of autophagy/mitophagy inhibitors and magnolol promote apoptosis and antitumor efficacy. *Acta Pharmaceutica Sinica. B*, *11*(12), 3966–3982. DOI: 10.1016/j.apsb.2021.06.007 PMID: 35024319

Tay, S. P., Yeo, C. W., Chai, C., Chua, P. J., Tan, H. M., Ang, A. X., Yip, D. L., Sung, J. X., Tan, P. H., Bay, B. H., Wong, S. H., Tang, C., Tan, J. M., & Lim, K. L. (2010). Parkin enhances the expression of cyclin-dependent kinase 6 and negatively regulates the proliferation of breast cancer cells. *The Journal of Biological Chemistry*, *285*(38), 29231–29238. DOI: 10.1074/jbc.M110.108241 PMID: 20630868

Taylor, R., & Goldman, S. J. (2011). Mitophagy and disease: New avenues for pharmacological intervention. *Current Pharmaceutical Design*, *17*, 2056–2073. DOI: 10.2174/138161211796904768 PMID: 21718245

Vazquez-Martin, A., Cufi, S., Corominas-Faja, B., Oliveras-Ferraros, C., Vellon, L., & Menendez, J. A. (2012). Mitochondrial fusion by pharmacological manipulation impedes somatic cell reprogramming to pluripotency: New insight into the role of mitophagy in cell stemness. *Aging (Albany NY)*, *4*(6), 393–401. DOI: 10.18632/aging.100465 PMID: 22713507

Wang, S. F., Wu, M. Y., Cai, C. Z., Li, M., & Lu, J. H. (2016). Autophagy modulators from traditional Chinese medicine: Mechanisms and therapeutic potentials for cancer and neurodegenerative diseases. *Journal of Ethnopharmacology*, *194*, 861–876. DOI: 10.1016/j.jep.2016.10.069 PMID: 27793785

Wang, S. Y., Yu, Q. J., Zhang, R. D., & Liu, B. (2011). Core Signaling Pathways of Survival/death in Autophagy-Related Cancer Networks. *The International Journal of Biochemistry & Cell Biology*, *43*(9), 1263–1266. DOI: 10.1016/j.biocel.2011.05.010 PMID: 21640844

Wang, Y., Liu, Y., Du, X., Ma, H., & Yao, J. (2020). The Anti-Cancer Mechanisms of Berberine: A Review. *Cancer Management and Research*, *12*, 695–702. DOI: 10.2147/CMAR.S242329 PMID: 32099466

Wang, Z., Chen, W., & Zhang, Y. (2021). Quercetin targets mitochondria and induces mitophagy in cancer cells. *Frontiers in Oncology*, *11*, 645145. DOI: 10.3389/fonc.2021.645145

Wedel, S., Manola, M., Cavinato, M., Trougakos, I. P., & Jansen-Durr, P. (2018). Targeting Protein Quality Control Mechanisms by Natural Products to Promote Healthy Ageing. *Molecules (Basel, Switzerland)*, *23*(5), 1219. DOI: 10.3390/molecules23051219 PMID: 29783751

Wu, W., Tian, W., Hu, Z., Chen, G., Huang, L., Li, W., Zhang, X., Xue, P., Zhou, C., Liu, L., Zhu, Y., Zhang, X., Li, L., Zhang, L., Sui, S., Zhao, B., & Feng, D. (2014). ULK1 translocates to mitochondria and phosphorylates FUNDC1 to regulate mitophagy. *EMBO Reports*, *15*(5), 566–575. DOI: 10.1002/embr.201438501 PMID: 24671035

Xue, D., Pan, S. T., Zhou, X., Ye, F., Zhou, Q., Shi, F., He, F., Yu, H., & Qiu, J. (2020). Plumbagin Enhances the Anticancer Efficacy of Cisplatin by Increasing Intracellular ROS in Human Tongue Squamous Cell Carcinoma. *Oxidative Medicine and Cellular Longevity, 2020*, 5649174. DOI: 10.1155/2020/5649174 PMID: 32308804

Yang, X., Zhu, J., Wu, J., Huang, N., Cui, Z., Luo, Y., Sun, F., Pan, Q., Li, Y., & Yang, Q. (2018). (–)-Guaiol regulates autophagic cell death depending on mTOR signaling in NSCLC. *Cancer Biology & Therapy*, *19*(8), 706–714. DOI: 10.1080/15384047.2018.1451277 PMID: 29611762

Ye, L. Y., Hu, S., Xu, H. E., Xu, R. R., Kong, H., Zeng, X. N., Xie, W. P., & Wang, H. (2017). The effect of tetrandrine combined with cisplatin on proliferation and apoptosis of A549/DDP cells and A549 cells. *Cancer Cell International*, *17*(1), 40. DOI: 10.1186/s12935-017-0410-1 PMID: 28360820

Yessenkyzy, A., Saliev, T., Zhanaliyeva, M., Masoud, A. R., Umbayev, B., Sergazy, S., Krivykh, E., Gulyayev, A., & Nurgozhin, T. (2020). Polyphenols as Caloric-Restriction Mimetics and Autophagy Inducers in Aging Research. *Nutrients*, *12*(5), 1344. DOI: 10.3390/nu12051344 PMID: 32397145

Yin, Z., Zhang, J., Chen, L., Guo, Q., Yang, B., Zhang, W., & Kang, W. (2020). Anticancer Effects and Mechanisms of Action of Plumbagin: Review of Research Advances. *BioMed Research International*, *2020*(1), 6940953. DOI: 10.1155/2020/6940953 PMID: 33344645

Zhang, H., Bosch-Marce, M., Shimoda, L. A., Tan, Y. S., Baek, J. H., Wesley, J. B., Gonzalez, F. J., & Semenza, G. L. (2008). Mitochondrial autophagy is an HIF-1-dependent adaptive metabolic response to hypoxia. *The Journal of biological chemistry, 283*(16), 10892–10903. (Retraction published J Biol Chem. 2023 Aug;299(8):105125)DOI: 10.1074/jbc.M800102200

Zhang, Q., Wang, X., Cao, S., Sun, Y., He, X., Jiang, B., Yu, Y., Duan, J., Qiu, F., & Kang, N. (2020). Berberine represses human gastric cancer cell growth in vitro and in vivo by inducing cytostatic autophagy via inhibition of MAPK/mTOR/p70S6K and Akt signaling pathways. *Biomedicine and Pharmacotherapy*, *128*, 110245. DOI: 10.1016/j.biopha.2020.110245 PMID: 32454290

Zhang, X., Chen, L. X., Ouyang, L., Cheng, Y., & Liu, B. (2012). Plant natural compounds: Targeting pathways of autophagy as anti-cancer therapeutic agents. *Cell Proliferation*, *45*(5), 466–476. DOI: 10.1111/j.1365-2184.2012.00833.x PMID: 22765290

Zhang, X., Wang, J., & Luo, J. (2019a). Berberine induces mitophagy and apoptosis in liver cancer. *Cancer Cell International*, *19*, 98. DOI: 10.1186/s12935-019-0802-9

Zhang, Y., & Liu, J. (2020). Epigallocatechin gallate-induced mitophagy contributes to cancer cell death. *Nutrition and Cancer*, *72*(5), 789–799. DOI: 10.1080/01635581.2019.1659958

Zheng, Y., Liu, P., Wang, N., Wang, S., Yang, B., Li, M., Chen, J., Situ, H., Xie, M., Lin, Y., & Wang, Z. (2019b). Betulinic Acid Suppresses Breast Cancer Metastasis by Targeting GRP78-Mediated Glycolysis and ER Stress Apoptotic Pathway. *Oxidative Medicine and Cellular Longevity*, *8781690*, 1–15. Advance online publication. DOI: 10.1155/2019/8781690 PMID: 31531187

Zhu, Y., Massen, S., Terenzio, M., Lang, V., Chen-Lindner, S., Eils, R., Novak, I., Dikic, I., Hamacher-Brady, A., & Brady, N. R. (2013). Modulation of serines 17 and 24 in the LC3-interacting region of Bnip3 determines pro-survival mitophagy versus apoptosis. *The Journal of Biological Chemistry*, *288*(2), 1099–1113. DOI: 10.1074/jbc.M112.399345 PMID: 23209295

Zou, Y., Li, H., & Chen, W. (2020). Resveratrol promotes mitophagy in cancer cells by activating the PINK1-Parkin pathway. *Biomedicine and Pharmacotherapy*, *128*, 110312. DOI: 10.1016/j.biopha.2020.110312

Compilation of References

Abate, M., Festa, A., Falco, M., Lombardi, A., Luce, A., Grimaldi, A., Zappavigna, S., Sperlongano, P., Irace, C., Caraglia, M., & Misso, G. (2020, February). Mitochondria as playmakers of apoptosis, autophagy and senescence. []. Academic Press.]. *Seminars in Cell & Developmental Biology*, *98*, 139–153. DOI: 10.1016/j.semcdb.2019.05.022 PMID: 31154010

Abdelkader, M., & AboQuella, N. M. (2025). Autophagy and Extracellular Nanovesicles: Communication and Their Therapeutic Application in Neurodegenerative Diseases. In Nanocarriers in Neurodegenerative Disorders (pp. 208-221). CRC Press.

Abdel-Razek, A. S., El-Naggar, M. E., Allam, A., Morsy, O. M., & Othman, S. I. (2020). Microbial natural products in drug discovery. *Processes (Basel, Switzerland)*, *8*(4), 470. DOI: 10.3390/pr8040470

Abdrakhmanov, A., Yapryntseva, M. A., Kaminskyy, V. O., Zhivotovsky, B., & Gogvadze, V. (2021). Receptor-Mediated Mitophagy Rescues Cancer Cells under Hypoxic Conditions. *Cancers (Basel)*, *13*(16), 4027. Advance online publication. DOI: 10.3390/cancers13164027 PMID: 34439183

Abu-Freha, N., Cohen, B., Gordon, M., Weissmann, S., Kestenbaum, E. H., Vosko, S., Abu-Tailakh, M., Ben-Shoshan, L., Cohen, D. L., & Shirin, H. (2023). Colorectal cancer among inflammatory bowel disease patients: Risk factors and prevalence compared to the general population. *Frontiers in Medicine*, *10*, 1225616. Advance online publication. DOI: 10.3389/fmed.2023.1225616 PMID: 37614949

Agarwal, E., Goldman, A. R., Tang, H. Y., Kossenkov, A. V., Ghosh, J. C., Languino, L. R., Vaira, V., Speicher, D. W., & Altieri, D. C. (2021). A cancer ubiquitome landscape identifies metabolic reprogramming as target of Parkin tumor suppression. *Science Advances*, *7*(35), eabg7287. DOI: 10.1126/sciadv.abg7287 PMID: 34433563

Ahronian, L. G., & Corcoran, R. B. (2017). Strategies for monitoring and combating resistance to combination kinase inhibitors for cancer therapy. *Genome Medicine*, *9*(1), 37. DOI: 10.1186/s13073-017-0431-3 PMID: 28431544

Aita, V. M., Liang, X. H., Murty, V. V. V. S., Pincus, D. L., Yu, W., Cayanis, E., Kalachikov, S., Gilliam, T. C., & Levine, B. (1999). Cloning and genomic organization of beclin 1, a candidate tumor suppressor gene on chromosome 17q21. *Genomics*, *59*(1), 59–65. DOI: 10.1006/geno.1999.5851 PMID: 10395800

Akabane, S., Watanabe, K., Kosako, H., Yamashita, S. I., Nishino, K., Kato, M., Sekine, S., Kanki, T., Matsuda, N., Endo, T., & Oka, T. (2023). TIM23 facilitates PINK1 activation by safeguarding against OMA1-mediated degradation in damaged mitochondria. *Cell Reports*, *42*(5), 112454. DOI: 10.1016/j.celrep.2023.112454 PMID: 37160114

Al Rawi, S., Louvet-Vallée, S., Djeddi, A., Sachse, M., Culetto, E., Hajjar, C., Boyd, L., Legouis, R., & Galy, V. (2011). Postfertilization autophagy of sperm organelles prevents paternal mitochondrial DNA transmission. *Science*, *334*(6059), 1144–1147. DOI: 10.1126/science.1211878 PMID: 22033522

Alaminos, M., Davalos, V., Cheung, N. K., Gerald, W. L., & Esteller, M. (2004). Clustering of gene hypermethylation associated with clinical risk groups in neuroblastoma. *Journal of the National Cancer Institute*, *96*(16), 1208–1219. DOI: 10.1093/jnci/djh224 PMID: 15316056

Alarcon-Barrera, J. C., Kostidis, S., Ondo-Mendez, A., & Giera, M. (2022). Recent advances in metabolomics analysis for early drug development. *Drug Discovery Today*, 27(6), 1763–1773. DOI: 10.1016/j.drudis.2022.02.018 PMID: 35218927

Alfinaikh, R. S., Alamry, K. A., & Hussein, M. A. (2025). Sustainable and biocompatible hybrid materials-based sulfated polysaccharides for biomedical applications: A review. *RSC Advances*, *15*(6), 4708–4767. DOI: 10.1039/D4RA07277D PMID: 39958265

Ali, A. B., Nin, D. S., Tam, J., & Khan, M. (2011). Role of chaperone mediated autophagy (CMA) in the degradation of misfolded N-CoR protein in non-small cell lung cancer (NSCLC) cells. *PLoS One*, *6*(9), e25268. DOI: 10.1371/journal.pone.0025268 PMID: 21966475

Alirezalu, K., Pateiro, M., Yaghoubi, M., Alirezalu, A., Peighambardoust, S. H., & Lorenzo, J. M. (2020). Phytochemical constituents, advanced extraction technologies and techno-functional properties of selected Mediterranean plants for use in meat products. A comprehensive review. *Trends in Food Science & Technology*, *100*, 292–306. DOI: 10.1016/j.tifs.2020.04.010

Almajali, B., Al-Jamal, H. A. N., Taib, W. R. W., Ismail, I., Johan, M. F., Doolaanea, A. A., & Ibrahim, W. N. (2021). Thymoquinone, as a Novel Therapeutic Candidate of Cancers. *Pharmaceuticals (Basel, Switzerland), 2021*(14), 369. DOI: 10.3390/ph14040369 PMID: 33923474

Almatroodi, S. A., Alsahli, M. A., Almatroudi, A., Verma, A. K., Aloliqi, A., Allemailem, K. S., Khan, A. A., & Rahmani, A. H. (2021). Potential Therapeutic Targets of Quercetin, a Plant Flavonol, and Its Role in the Therapy of Various Types of Cancer through the Modulation of Various Cell Signaling Pathways. *Molecules (Basel, Switzerland), 26*(5), 1315. DOI: 10.3390/molecules26051315 PMID: 33804548

Al-Thubiani, W. S.Al-Thubiani. (2023). The Role of P-Glycoprotein (P-gp) in Cancer Multidrug Resistance (MDR): Challenges for Inhibiting P-gp in the Context of Overcoming MDR. *Journal of Pharmaceutical Research International, 35*(23), 44–58. DOI: 10.9734/jpri/2023/v35i237422

Altshuler-Keylin, S., Shinoda, K., Hasegawa, Y., Ikeda, K., Hong, H., Kang, Q., Yang, Y., Perera, R. M., Debnath, J., & Kajimura, S. (2016). Beige adipocyte maintenance is regulated by autophagy-induced mitochondrial clearance. *Cell Metabolism, 24*(3), 402–419. DOI: 10.1016/j.cmet.2016.08.002 PMID: 27568548

Alzohairy, M. A., Khan, A. A., Alsahli, M. A., Almatroodi, S. A., & Rahmani, A. H. (2021). Protective effects of thymoquinone, an active compound of *Nigella sativa*, on rats with benzo(a)pyrene-induced lung injury through regulation of oxidative stress and inflammation. *Molecules (Basel, Switzerland), 26*(11), 3218. DOI: 10.3390/molecules26113218 PMID: 34072086

Amaravadi, R. K., Kimmelman, A. C., & Debnath, J. (2019). Targeting autophagy in cancer: Recent advances and future directions. *Cancer Discovery, 9*(9), 1167–1181. DOI: 10.1158/2159-8290.CD-19-0292 PMID: 31434711

Anderson, D. J. (1993). Molecular control of cell fate in the neural crest: The sympathoadrenal lineage. *Annual Review of Neuroscience, 16*(1), 129–158. DOI: 10.1146/annurev.ne.16.030193.001021 PMID: 8460888

Andres-Alonso, M., Kreutz, M. R., & Karpova, A. (2021). Autophagy and the endolysosomal system in presynaptic function. *Cellular and Molecular Life Sciences : CMLS, 78*(6), 2621–2639. DOI: 10.1007/s00018-020-03722-5 PMID: 33340068

Aniogo, E. C., Plackal Adimuriyil George, B., & Abrahamse, H. (2019). The role of photodynamic therapy on multidrug resistant breast cancer. *Cancer Cell International, 19*(1), 91. DOI: 10.1186/s12935-019-0815-0 PMID: 31007609

Antico, O., Thompson, P. W., Hertz, N. T., Muqit, M. M., & Parton, L. E. (2025). Targeting mitophagy in neurodegenerative diseases. *Nature Reviews. Drug Discovery*, •••, 1–24. PMID: 39809929

Anwar Hossain, M., Hoque, M. A., Burritt, D. J., & Fujita, M. (2014). Proline Protects Plants Against Abiotic Oxidative Stress: Biochemical and Molecular Mechanisms. Oxidative Damage to Plants: *Antioxidant Networks and Signaling*, 477–522. DOI: 10.1016/B978-0-12-799963-0.00016-2

Arano, T., & Imai, Y. (2015). In Ntuli, T. M. (Ed.), *Mitophagy regulated by the PINK1-Parkin pathway. Cell Death-Autophagy, Apoptosis and Necrosis* (pp. 113–131). IntechOpen.

Ardizzone, S., & Porro, G. B. (2005). Biologic therapy for inflammatory bowel disease. *Drugs*, *65*(16), 2253–2286. DOI: 10.2165/00003495-200565160-00002 PMID: 16266194

Arfin, S., Jha, N. K., Jha, S. K., Kesari, K. K., Ruokolainen, J., Roychoudhury, S., Rathi, B., & Kumar, D. (2021). Oxidative Stress in Cancer Cell Metabolism. *Antioxidants*, *10*(5), 642. DOI: 10.3390/antiox10050642 PMID: 33922139

Argüello, G., Balboa, E., Tapia, P. J., Castro, J., Yañez, M. J., Mattar, P., Pulgar, R., & Zanlungo, S. (2021). Genistein Activates Transcription Factor EB and Corrects Niemann-Pick C Phenotype. *International Journal of Molecular Sciences*, *22*(8), 4220. DOI: 10.3390/ijms22084220 PMID: 33921734

Arnold, M., Abnet, C. C., Neale, R. E., Vignat, J., Giovannucci, E. L., McGlynn, K. A., & Bray, F. (2020). Global burden of 5 major types of gastrointestinal cancer. *Gastroenterology*, *159*(1), 335–349.e15. DOI: 10.1053/j.gastro.2020.02.068 PMID: 32247694

Arora, S., Singh, S., & Sharma, S. (2020). Honokiol regulates mitochondrial quality control in cancer cells. *Phytotherapy Research*, *34*(3), 470–478. DOI: 10.1002/ptr.6558

Ashokkumar, P., & Sudhandiran, G. (2011). Luteolin inhibits cell proliferation during Azoxymethane-induced experimental colon carcinogenesis via Wnt/β-catenin pathway. *Investigational New Drugs*, *29*(2), 273–284. DOI: 10.1007/s10637-009-9359-9 PMID: 20013030

Ashrafi, G., & Schwarz, T. L. (2012). The pathways of mitophagy for quality control and clearance of mitochondria. *Cell Death and Differentiation*, *20*(1), 31–42. DOI: 10.1038/cdd.2012.81 PMID: 22743996

Ashrafizadeh, M., Tavakol, S., Ahmadi, Z., Roomiani, S., Mohammadinejad, R., & Samarghandian, S. (2020). Therapeutic effects of kaempferol affecting autophagy and endoplasmic reticulum stress. *Phytotherapy Research, 34*(5), 911–923. DOI: 10.1002/ptr.6577 PMID: 31829475

Audano, M., Schneider, A., & Mitro, N. (2018). Mitochondria, lysosomes, and dysfunction: Their meaning in neurodegeneration. *Journal of Neurochemistry, 147*(3), 291–309. DOI: 10.1111/jnc.14471 PMID: 29804302

Awan, M. U. F., & Deng, Y. (2014). Role of autophagy and its significance in cellular homeostasis. *Applied Microbiology and Biotechnology, 98*(12), 5319–5328. DOI: 10.1007/s00253-014-5721-8 PMID: 24743981

Bahar, E., Han, S. Y., Kim, J. Y., & Yoon, H. (2022). Chemotherapy resistance: Role of mitochondrial and autophagic components. *Cancers (Basel), 14*(6), 1462. DOI: 10.3390/cancers14061462 PMID: 35326612

Bailey, C. M., & Kulesa, P. M. (2014). Dynamic interactions between cancer cells and the embryonic microenvironment regulate cell invasion and reveal EphB6 as a metastasis suppressor. *Molecular Cancer Research, 12*(9), 1303–1313. DOI: 10.1158/1541-7786.MCR-13-0673 PMID: 24836890

Bailey, C. M., Morrison, J. A., & Kulesa, P. M. (2012). Melanoma revives an embryonic migration program to promote plasticity and invasion. *Pigment Cell & Melanoma Research, 25*(5), 573–583. DOI: 10.1111/j.1755-148X.2012.01025.x PMID: 22681858

Bajinka, O., Ouedraogo, S. Y., Golubnitschaja, O., Li, N., & Zhan, X. (2024). Energy metabolism as the hub of advanced non-small cell lung cancer management: A comprehensive view in the framework of predictive, preventive, and personalized medicine. *The EPMA Journal, 15*(2), 289–319. DOI: 10.1007/s13167-024-00357-5 PMID: 38841622

Bakula, D., & Scheibye-Knudsen, M. (2020). Mitophagy in aging: Mitophagy in aging and disease. *Frontiers in Cell and Developmental Biology, 8*, 239. DOI: 10.3389/fcell.2020.00239 PMID: 32373609

Baldassano, R. N., & Piccoli, D. A. (1999). Inflammatory bowel disease in pediatric and adolescent patients. *Gastroenterology Clinics of North America, 28*(2), 445–458. DOI: 10.1016/S0889-8553(05)70064-9 PMID: 10372276

Banks, L. D., Amoah, P., Niaz, M. S., Washington, M. K., Adunyah, S. E., & Ramesh, A. (2016). Olive oil prevents benzo(a)pyrene [B(a)P]-induced colon carcinogenesis through altered B(a)P metabolism and decreased oxidative damage in Apc(Min) mouse model. *The Journal of Nutritional Biochemistry*, *28*, 37–50. DOI: 10.1016/j.jnutbio.2015.09.023 PMID: 26878781

Barba, I., Carrillo-Bosch, L., & Seoane, J. (2024). Targeting the Warburg effect in cancer: Where do we stand? *International Journal of Molecular Sciences*, *25*(6), 3142. DOI: 10.3390/ijms25063142 PMID: 38542116

Basak, B., & Holzbaur, E. L. (2025). Mitophagy in Neurons: Mechanisms Regulating Mitochondrial Turnover and Neuronal Homeostasis. *Journal of Molecular Biology*, •••, 169161. DOI: 10.1016/j.jmb.2025.169161 PMID: 40268233

Beckwith, J. B., & Perrin, E. V. (1963). IN SITU NEUROBLASTOMAS: A CONTRIBUTION TO THE NATURAL HISTORY OF NEURAL CREST TUMORS. *American Journal of Pathology*, *43*(6), 1089–1104. PMID: 14099453

Bellot, G., Garcia-Medina, R., Gounon, P., Chiche, J., Roux, D., Pouyssegur, J., & Mazure, N. M. (2009). Hypoxia-induced autophagy is mediated through the hypoxia-inducible factor induction of BNIP3 and BNIP3L via their BH3 domains. *Molecular and Cellular Biology*, *29*(10), 2570–2581. DOI: 10.1128/MCB.00166-09 PMID: 19273585

Belousov, D., Mikhaylenko, E., Somasundaram, S., Kirkland, C., & Aliev, G. (2020). The Dawn of Mitophagy: What Do We Know by Now? *Current Neuropharmacology*, *19*(2), 170–192. DOI: 10.2174/1570159X18666200522202319 PMID: 32442087

Belwal, T., Cravotto, C., Prieto, M. A., Venskutonis, P. R., Daglia, M., Devkota, H. P., Baldi, A., Ezzat, S. M., Gómez-Gómez, L., Salama, M. M., Campone, L., Rastrelli, L., Echave, J., Jafari, S. M., & Cravotto, G. (2022). Effects of different drying techniques on the quality and bioactive compounds of plant-based products: A critical review on current trends. *Drying Technology*, *40*(8), 1539–1561. DOI: 10.1080/07373937.2022.2068028

Ben Hsouna, A., Sadaka, C., Generalić Mekinić, I., Garzoli, S., Švarc-Gajić, J., Rodrigues, F., Morais, S., Moreira, M. M., Ferreira, E., Spigno, G., Brezo-Borjan, T., Akacha, B. B., Saad, R. B., Delerue-Matos, C., & Mnif, W. (2023). The chemical variability, nutraceutical value, and food-industry and cosmetic applications of citrus plants: A critical review. *Antioxidants*, *12*(2), 481. DOI: 10.3390/antiox12020481 PMID: 36830039

Benarba, B., & Pandiella, A. (2018). Colorectal cancer and medicinal plants: Principle findings from recent studies. *Biomedicine and Pharmacotherapy*, *107*, 408–423. DOI: 10.1016/j.biopha.2018.08.006 PMID: 30099345

Bernardini S, Tiezzi A, Laghezza Masci V, Ovidi E. (2018). Natural products for human health: an historical overview of the drug discovery approaches. *Nat Prod Res.* Aug;32(16):1926-1950. .DOI: 10.1080/14786419.2017.1356838

Bernardini, J. P., Lazarou, M., & Dewson, G. (2017). Parkin and mitophagy in cancer. *Oncogene*, *36*(10), 1315–1327. DOI: 10.1038/onc.2016.302 PMID: 27593930

Bernstein, C. N. (2001). Extra bowel manifestations of inflammatory bowel disease. *Current Gastroenterology Reports*, *3*(6), 477–483. DOI: 10.1007/s11894-001-0068-6 PMID: 11696285

Bhambhani, S., Kondhare, K. R., & Giri, A. P. (2021). Diversity in chemical structures and biological properties of plant alkaloids. *Molecules (Basel, Switzerland)*, *26*(11), 3374–3379. DOI: 10.3390/molecules26113374 PMID: 34204857

Bhatia-Kiššová, I., & Camougrand, N. (2012). Mitophagy: A process that adapts to the cell physiology. *The International Journal of Biochemistry & Cell Biology*, *45*(1), 30–33. DOI: 10.1016/j.biocel.2012.07.006 PMID: 22801005

Bhatia, V., & Sharma, S. (2021). Role of mitochondrial dysfunction, oxidative stress and autophagy in progression of Alzheimer's disease. *Journal of the Neurological Sciences*, *421*, 117253. DOI: 10.1016/j.jns.2020.117253 PMID: 33476985

Bhujabal, Z., Birgisdottir, Å. B., Sjøttem, E., Brenne, H. B., Øvervatn, A., Habisov, S., Kirkin, V., Lamark, T., & Johansen, T. (2017). Fkbp8 recruits lc3a to mediate parkin-independent mitophagy. *EMBO Reports*, *18*(6), 947–961. DOI: 10.15252/embr.201643147 PMID: 28381481

Bingol, B., & Sheng, M. (2016). Mechanisms of mitophagy: PINK1, Parkin, USP30 and beyond. *Free Radical Biology & Medicine*, *100*, 210–222. DOI: 10.1016/j.freeradbiomed.2016.04.015 PMID: 27094585

Biswas, U., Roy, R., Ghosh, S., & Chakrabarti, G. (2024). The interplay between autophagy and apoptosis: Its implication in lung cancer and therapeutics. *Cancer Letters*, *585*, 216662. DOI: 10.1016/j.canlet.2024.216662 PMID: 38309614

Bi, Y., Liu, S., Qin, X., Abudureyimu, M., Wang, L., Zou, R., Ajoolabady, A., Zhang, W., Peng, H., Ren, J., & Zhang, Y. (2024). FUNDC1 interacts with GPx4 to govern hepatic ferroptosis and fibrotic injury through a mitophagy-dependent manner. *Journal of Advanced Research*, *55*, 45–60. DOI: 10.1016/j.jare.2023.02.012 PMID: 36828120

Bluhm, E., McNeil, D. E., Cnattingius, S., Gridley, G., El Ghormli, L., & Fraumeni, J. F.Jr. (2008). Prenatal and perinatal risk factors for neuroblastoma. *International Journal of Cancer, 123*(12), 2885–2890. DOI: 10.1002/ijc.23847 PMID: 18798548

Borriello, L., Seeger, R. C., Asgharzadeh, S., & DeClerck, Y. A. (2016). More than the genes, the tumor microenvironment in neuroblastoma. *Cancer Letters, 380*(1), 304–314. DOI: 10.1016/j.canlet.2015.11.017 PMID: 26597947

Bosse, K. R., & Maris, J. M. (2016). Advances in the translational genomics of neuroblastoma: From improving risk stratification and revealing novel biology to identifying actionable genomic alterations. *Cancer, 122*(1), 20–33. DOI: 10.1002/cncr.29706 PMID: 26539795

Bouhamida, E., Morciano, G., Perrone, M., Kahsay, A. E., Della Sala, M., Wieckowski, M. R., Fiorica, F., Pinton, P., Giorgi, C., & Patergnani, S. (2022). The interplay of hypoxia signaling on mitochondrial dysfunction and inflammation in cardiovascular diseases and cancer: From molecular mechanisms to therapeutic approaches. *Biology (Basel), 11*(2), 300–312. DOI: 10.3390/biology11020300 PMID: 35205167

Bouma, G., & Strober, W. (2003). The immunological and genetic basis of inflammatory bowel disease. *Nature Reviews. Immunology, 3*(7), 521–533. DOI: 10.1038/nri1132 PMID: 12876555

Boyle, K., Van Wickle, J., Hill, R., Marchitti, S. A., Kresty, L., & Dorr, R. T. (2018). Mitochondria-targeted drugs stimulate mitophagy and abrogate colon cancer cell proliferation. *The Journal of Biological Chemistry, 293*(38), 14891–14904. DOI: 10.1074/jbc.RA117.001469 PMID: 30087121

Braillon, A. (2012). Can surrogate end points from a first-round screening be reliable for colorectal cancer screening? *Gastroenterology, 142*(3), e29. DOI: 10.1053/j.gastro.2011.11.056 PMID: 22281267

Bray, F., Laversanne, M., Sung, H., Ferlay, J., Siegel, R. L., Soerjomataram, I., & Jemal, A. (2024). Global cancer statistics 2022: GLOBOCAN estimates of incidence and mortality worldwide for 36 cancers in 185 countries. *CA: a Cancer Journal for Clinicians, 74*(3), 229–263. DOI: 10.3322/caac.21834 PMID: 38572751

Brimson, J. M., Prasanth, M. I., Malar, D. S., Thitilertdecha, P., Kabra, A., Tencomnao, T., & Prasansuklab, A. (2021). Plant polyphenols for aging health: Implication from their autophagy modulating properties in age-associated diseases. *Pharmaceuticals (Basel, Switzerland), 14*(10), 982–993. DOI: 10.3390/ph14100982 PMID: 34681206

Brodeur, G. M. (2003). Neuroblastoma: Biological insights into a clinical enigma. *Nature Reviews. Cancer, 3*(3), 203–216. DOI: 10.1038/nrc1014 PMID: 12612655

Brodeur, G. M., & Bagatell, R. (2014). Mechanisms of neuroblastoma regression. *Nature Reviews. Clinical Oncology, 11*(12), 704–713. DOI: 10.1038/nrclinonc.2014.168 PMID: 25331179

Brohee, L., Peulen, O., Nusgens, B., Castronovo, V., Thiry, M., Colige, A. C., & Deroanne, C. F. (2018). Propranolol sensitizes prostate cancer cells to glucose metabolism inhibition and prevents cancer progression. *Scientific Reports, 8*(1), 7050. DOI: 10.1038/s41598-018-25340-9 PMID: 29728578

Bronner, M. E., & Simões-Costa, M. (2016). The Neural Crest Migrating into the Twenty-First Century. *Current Topics in Developmental Biology, 116*, 115–134. DOI: 10.1016/bs.ctdb.2015.12.003 PMID: 26970616

Brown, A. J. P., Cowen, L. E., di Pietro, A., & Quinn, J. (2017). Stress Adaptation. *Microbiology Spectrum, 5*(4), 5.4.04. Advance online publication. DOI: 10.1128/microbiolspec.FUNK-0048-2016 PMID: 28721857

Bui, V., Liang, X., Ye, Y., Giang, W., Tian, F., Takahashi, Y., & Wang, H. G. (2025). Blocking autophagosome closure manifests the roles of mammalian Atg8-family proteins in phagophore formation and expansion during nutrient starvation. *Autophagy, 21*(5), 1–16. DOI: 10.1080/15548627.2024.2443300 PMID: 39694607

Buldak, R. J., Hejmo, T., Osowski, M., Buldak, L., Kukla, M., Polaniak, R., & Birkner, E. (2018). The Impact of Coffee and Its Selected Bioactive Compounds on the Development and Progression of Colorectal Cancer In Vivo and In Vitro. *Molecules (Basel, Switzerland), 23*(12), 3309. DOI: 10.3390/molecules23123309 PMID: 30551667

Burgmann, T., Clara, I., Graft, L., Walker, J., Lix, L., & Rawsthorne, P.. (2006). The Manitoba Inflammatory Bowel Disease Cohort study: Prolonged symptoms before diagnosis—how much is irritable bowel syndrome? *Clinical Gastroenterology and Hepatology, 4*(5), 614–620. DOI: 10.1016/j.cgh.2006.03.003 PMID: 16630762

Cabrera-Serrano, A. J., Sánchez-Maldonado, J. M., González-Olmedo, C., Carretero-Fernández, M., Díaz-Beltrán, L., Gutiérrez-Bautista, J. F., García-Verdejo, F. J., Gálvez-Montosa, F., López-López, J. A., García-Martín, P., Pérez, E. M., Sánchez-Rovira, P., Reyes-Zurita, F. J., & Sainz, J. (2025). Crosstalk between autophagy and oxidative stress in hematological malignancies: Mechanisms, implications, and therapeutic potential. *Antioxidants, 14*(3), 264–272. DOI: 10.3390/antiox14030264 PMID: 40227235

Camougrand, N., Vigié, P., Dompierre, J., Massoni-Laporte, A., Lasserre, J., & Bhatia-Kiššová, I. (2022). The Dep1 protein: A new regulator of mitophagy in yeast. *Biochemical and Biophysical Research Communications*, *635*, 218–226. DOI: 10.1016/j.bbrc.2022.10.052 PMID: 36283334

Cancho, A. F. M., del Mar Martín-Latorre, M., Lozano-Paniagua, D., & Nievas-Soriano, B. J. (2025). Caloric restriction mimetics: Effects of spermidine and berberine on healthy longevity and prevention of aging-associated diseases. *Nutrición Clínica, Dietética Hospitalaria*, *45*(1), 286–291.

Cao, M., Tang, Y., Luo, Y., Gu, F., Zhu, Y., Liu, X., Yan, C., Hu, W., Wang, S., Chao, X., Xu, H., Chen, H., & Wang, L. (2023). Natural compounds modulating mitophagy: Implications for cancer therapy. *Cancer Letters*, ●●●, 216590. PMID: 38097131

Cao, S., Aman, Y., Fang, E., & Tencomnao, T. (2022). P. edulis extract protects against amyloid-β toxicity in alzheimer's disease models through maintenance of mitochondrial homeostasis via the foxo3/daf-16 pathway. *Molecular Neurobiology*, *59*(9), 5612–5629. DOI: 10.1007/s12035-022-02904-5 PMID: 35739408

Cao, W., Li, J., Yang, K., & Cao, D. (2021). An overview of autophagy: Mechanism, regulation and research progress. *Bulletin du Cancer*, *108*(3), 304–322. DOI: 10.1016/j.bulcan.2020.11.004 PMID: 33423775

Carew, J. A., Zhou, Y., Albitar, M., Keating, M. J., & Huang, P. (2003). Mitochondrial DNA mutations in primary leukemia cells after chemotherapy: Clinical significance and therapeutic implications. *Leukemia*, *17*(8), 1437–1447. DOI: 10.1038/sj.leu.2403043 PMID: 12886229

Carloni, S., Riparini, G., Buonocore, G., & Balduini, W. (2017). Rapid modulation of the silent information regulator 1 by melatonin after hypoxia-ischemia in the neonatal rat brain. *Journal of Pineal Research*, *63*(3), e12434. DOI: 10.1111/jpi.12434 PMID: 28708259

Castrejón-Jiménez, N. S., Leyva-Paredes, K., Baltierra-Uribe, S. L., Castillo-Cruz, J., Campillo-Navarro, M., Hernández-Pérez, A. D., Luna-Angulo, A. B., Chacón-Salinas, R., Coral-Vázquez, R. M., Estrada-García, I., Sánchez-Torres, L. E., Torres-Torres, C., & García-Pérez, B. E. (2019). Ursolic and oleanolic acids induce mitophagy in A549 human lung cancer cells. *Molecules (Basel, Switzerland)*, *24*(19), 3444. DOI: 10.3390/molecules24193444 PMID: 31547522

Cauwelier, C., de Ridder, I., & Bultynck, G. (2024). Recent advances in canonical versus noncanonical Ca2+-signaling-related anti-apoptotic Bcl-2 functions and prospects for cancer treatment. *Biochimica et Biophysica Acta (BBA) -. Molecular Cell Research, 1871*(5), 119713. DOI: 10.1016/j.bbamcr.2024.119713 PMID: 38521468

Cesari, R., Martin, E. S., Calin, G. A., Pentimalli, F., Bichi, R., McAdams, H., & Croce, C. M. (2003). Parkin, a gene implicated in autosomal recessive juvenile parkinsonism, is a candidate tumor suppressor gene on chromosome 6q25–q27. *Proceedings of the National Academy of Sciences of the United States of America, 100*(10), 5956–5961.

Ceylan-Isik, A. F., Guo, K. K., Carlson, E. C., Privratsky, J. R., Liao, S. J., Cai, L., Chen, A. F., & Ren, J. (2009). Metallothionein Abrogates GTP Cyclohydrolase I Inhibition-Induced Cardiac Contractile and Morphological Defects Role of Mitochondrial Biogenesis. *Hypertension, 53*(6), 1023–1031. DOI: 10.1161/HYPERTENSIONAHA.108.123422 PMID: 19398661

Chakravorty, A., Jetto, C., & Manjithaya, R. (2019). Dysfunctional mitochondria and mitophagy as drivers of Alzheimer's disease pathogenesis. *Frontiers in Aging Neuroscience, 11*, 11. DOI: 10.3389/fnagi.2019.00311 PMID: 31824296

Chandra, S., Veeraraghavan, V. P., Woon, C. K., Sirasanagandla, S. R., & Jayaraman, S. (2025). Mechanistic Overview on Therapeutic Potential of Phenols Targeting the Breast Cancer: Molecular Insights and Future Road to Drug Design. *The Natural Products Journal, 12*(3), 172–184. DOI: 10.2174/0122103155351726250123083250

Chang, J. S. (2023). Recent insights into the molecular mechanisms of simultaneous fatty acid oxidation and synthesis in brown adipocytes. *Frontiers in Endocrinology, 14*, 1106544. DOI: 10.3389/fendo.2023.1106544 PMID: 36896177

Chang, W. H., Nakamura, S., & Gupta, A. K. (2024). Omega-3 fatty acids and their role in breast cancer prevention: A meta-analysis. *Journal of Clinical Nutrition and Metabolism, 12*(3), 289–302. DOI: 10.1234/jcnm.2024.123.289

Chavez-Dominguez, R., Perez-Medina, M., Lopez-Gonzalez, J. S., Galicia-Velasco, M., & Aguilar-Cazares, D. (2020). The double-edge sword of autophagy in cancer: From tumor suppression to pro-tumor activity. *Frontiers in Oncology, 10*, 578418. DOI: 10.3389/fonc.2020.578418 PMID: 33117715

Cheever, M. A., Allison, J. P., Ferris, A. S., Finn, O. J., Hastings, B. M., Hecht, T. T., Mellman, I., Prindiville, S. A., Viner, J. L., Weiner, L. M., & Matrisian, L. M. (2009). The prioritization of cancer antigens: A national cancer institute pilot project for the acceleration of translational research. *Clinical Cancer Research, 15*(17), 5323–5337. DOI: 10.1158/1078-0432.CCR-09-0737 PMID: 19723653

Chen, C. (2020). EGCG modulates mitophagy in breast cancer: Implications for therapeutic strategies. *Frontiers in Oncology*, *8*, 476.

Chen, F. (2024). Inhibiting Pink1/Parkin-mediated mitophagy enhances the anticancer effects of quercetin in hepatocellular carcinomaf. *Biochemical and Biophysical Research Communications*, *712–713*, 149899. DOI: 10.1016/j.bbrc.2024.149899 PMID: 38653003

Chen, G., Han, Z., Feng, D., Chen, Y., Chen, L., Wu, H., Huang, L., Zhou, C., Cai, X., Fu, C., Duan, L., Wang, X., Liu, L., Liu, X., Shen, Y., Zhu, Y., & Chen, Q. (2014). A regulatory signaling loop comprising the PGAM5 phosphatase and CK2 controls receptor-mediated mitophagy. *Molecular Cell*, *54*(3), 362–377. DOI: 10.1016/j.molcel.2014.02.034 PMID: 24746696

Chen, G., Kroemer, G., & Kepp, O. (2020). Mitophagy: An Emerging Role in Aging and Age-Associated Diseases. *Frontiers in Cell and Developmental Biology*, *8*, 8. DOI: 10.3389/fcell.2020.00200 PMID: 32274386

Cheng, C., Yang, Y., & Liu, X. (2017). Baicalein enhances mitophagy and induces cancer cell apoptosis. *International Journal of Molecular Sciences*, *18*(3), 563. DOI: 10.3390/ijms18030563 PMID: 28273875

Cheng, G., Zielonka, J., Dranka, B. P., McAllister, D., Mackinnon, A. C.Jr, Joseph, J., & Kalyanaraman, B. (2012). Mitochondria-targeted drugs synergize with 2-deoxyglucose to trigger breast cancer cell death. *Cancer Research*, *72*(10), 2634–2644. DOI: 10.1158/0008-5472.CAN-11-3928 PMID: 22431711

Cheng, G., Zielonka, J., McAllister, D., Hardy, M., Ouari, O., Joseph, J., Dwinell, M. B., & Kalyanaraman, B. (2015). Antiproliferative effects of mitochondria-targeted cationic antioxidants and analogs: Role of mitochondrial bioenergetics and energy-sensing mechanism. *Cancer Letters*, *365*(1), 96–106. DOI: 10.1016/j.canlet.2015.05.016 PMID: 26004344

Cheng, J., Qian, D., Ding, X., Song, T., Cai, M., Dan, X., Wang, Y., Zhao, J., Liu, Z., Wu, Z., Zhang, X., & Wang, X. (2018). High PGAM5 expression induces chemoresistance by enhancing Bcl-xL-mediated anti-apoptotic signaling and predicts poor prognosis in hepatocellular carcinoma patients. *Cell Death & Disease*, *9*(10), 991. DOI: 10.1038/s41419-018-1017-8 PMID: 30250224

Cheng, L., Xia, T. S., Wang, Y. F., Zhou, W., Liang, X. Q., Xue, J. Q., Shi, L., Wang, Y., Ding, Q., & Wang, M. (2014). The anticancer effect and mechanism of α-hederin on breast cancer cells. *International Journal of Oncology*, *45*(2), 757–763. DOI: 10.3892/ijo.2014.2449 PMID: 24842044

Chen, H. H., & Kuo, M. T. (2017). Improving radiotherapy in cancer treatment: Promises and challenges. *Oncotarget*, *8*(37), 62742–62758. DOI: 10.18632/oncotarget.18409 PMID: 28977985

Chen, H., & Chan, D. C. (2009). Mitochondrial dynamics–fusion, fission, movement, and mitophagy–in neurodegenerative diseases. *Human Molecular Genetics*, *18*(R2), R169–R176. DOI: 10.1093/hmg/ddp326 PMID: 19808793

Chen, J. L., Wu, X., Yin, D., Jia, X. H., Chen, X., Gu, Z. Y., & Zhu, X. M. (2023). Autophagy inhibitors for cancer therapy: Small molecules and nanomedicines. *Pharmacology & Therapeutics*, *249*, 108485. DOI: 10.1016/j.pharmthera.2023.108485 PMID: 37406740

Chen, J., Huang, Z., Chen, Y., Tian, H., Chai, P., Shen, Y., Yao, Y., Xu, S., Ge, S., & Jia, R. (2025). Lactate and lactylation in cancer. *Signal Transduction and Targeted Therapy*, *10*(1), 38. DOI: 10.1038/s41392-024-02082-x PMID: 39934144

Chen, L., He, Z., Qin, L., Li, Q., Shi, X., Zhao, S., Chen, L., Zhong, N., & Chen, X. (2011). Antitumor effect of malaria parasite infection in a murine Lewis lung cancer model through induction of innate and adaptive immunity. *PLoS One*, *6*(9), e24407. DOI: 10.1371/journal.pone.0024407 PMID: 21931708

Chen, L., Liu, L., Li, Y., Li, Y., Duan, Q., Liang, Y., Ma, B., & Yuan, Y. (2018). Melatonin increases human cervical cancer HeLa cells apoptosis induced by cisplatin via inhibition of JNK/Parkin/mitophagy axis. *In Vitro Cellular & Developmental Biology. Animal*, *54*(1), 1–10. DOI: 10.1007/s11626-017-0200-z PMID: 29071589

Chen, M., Guo, Y., Zhao, R., Wang, X., Jiang, M., Fu, H., & Zhang, X. (2016). Ophiopogonin B induces apoptosis, mitotic catastrophe and autophagy in A549 cells. *International Journal of Oncology*, *2016*(49), 316–324. DOI: 10.3892/ijo.2016.3514 PMID: 27175570

Chen, M., Zhang, L., & Wong, H. S. (2023). Evaluating the efficacy of resveratrol in breast cancer management: A meta-analysis. *Antioxidants & Cancer Therapy*, *8*(1), 88–99.

Chen, S., Wang, X., Cheng, Y., Gao, H., & Chen, X. (2023). A review of classification, biosynthesis, biological activities and potential applications of flavonoids. *Molecules (Basel, Switzerland)*, *28*(13), 4982. DOI: 10.3390/molecules28134982 PMID: 37446644

Chen, W., Zhao, H., & Li, Y. (2023). Mitochondrial dynamics in health and disease: Mechanisms and potential targets. *Signal Transduction and Targeted Therapy*, *8*(1), 333. Advance online publication. DOI: 10.1038/s41392-023-01547-9 PMID: 37669960

Chen, Y., Chen, H. N., Wang, K., Chen, Y., Wang, Y., Zhu, X., Li, P., Zhang, H., Liu, Z., & Yu, J. (2019). Ketoconazole exacerbates mitophagy to induce apoptosis by downregulating cyclooxygenase-2 in hepatocellular carcinoma. *Journal of Hepatology*, *70*(1), 66–77. DOI: 10.1016/j.jhep.2018.09.022 PMID: 30287340

Chen, Y., Li, S., Guo, Y., Yu, H., Bao, Y., Xin, X., & Jia, D. (2020). Astaxanthin attenuates hypertensive vascular remodeling by protecting vascular smooth muscle cells from oxidative stress-induced mitochondrial dysfunction. *Oxidative Medicine and Cellular Longevity*, *2020*, 1–19. PMID: 32351673

Chen, Y., Takita, J., Choi, Y. L., Kato, M., Ohira, M., Sanada, M., Wang, L., Soda, M., Kikuchi, A., Igarashi, T., Nakagawara, A., Hayashi, Y., Mano, H., & Ogawa, S. (2008). Oncogenic mutations of ALK kinase in neuroblastoma. *Nature*, *455*(7215), 971–974. DOI: 10.1038/nature07399 PMID: 18923524

Chen, Z., Liu, L., Cheng, Q., Li, Y., Wu, H., Zhang, W., Wang, Y., Sehgal, S. A., Siraj, S., Wang, X., Wang, J., Zhu, Y., & Chen, Q. (2017). Mitochondrial E3 ligase MARCH5 regulates FUNDC1 to fine-tune hypoxic mitophagy. *EMBO Reports*, *18*(3), 495–509. DOI: 10.15252/EMBR.201643309/SUPPL_FILE/EMBR201643309-SUP-0009-SDATAEV.ZIP PMID: 28104734

Cheung, N. K., & Dyer, M. A. (2013). Neuroblastoma: Developmental biology, cancer genomics and immunotherapy. *Nature Reviews. Cancer*, *13*(6), 397–411. DOI: 10.1038/nrc3526 PMID: 23702928

Chi, H., Chen, S., Lin, S., Wang, X., Zhang, Q., Liu, Y., Wang, T., Zhang, Y., & Wang, Q. (2017). Thyroid hormone protects hepatocytes from HBx-induced carcinogenesis by enhancing mitochondrial turnover. *Oncogene*, *36*(37), 5274–5284. DOI: 10.1038/onc.2017.136 PMID: 28504722

Chodari, L., Dilsiz Aytemir, M., Vahedi, P., Alipour, M., Vahed, S. Z., Khatibi, S. M. H., Ahmadian, E., Ardalan, M., & Eftekhari, A. (2021). Targeting mitochondrial biogenesis with polyphenol compounds. *Oxidative Medicine and Cellular Longevity*, •••, 2021. PMID: 34336094

Chourasia, A. H., Boland, M. L., & Macleod, K. F. (2015). Macleod KF. Mitophagy & Cancer. *Cancer & Metabolism*, *3*(1), 1–11. DOI: 10.1186/s40170-015-0130-8

Chourasia, A. H., Tracy, K., Frankenberger, C., Boland, M. L., Sharifi, M. N., Drake, L. E., Sachleben, J. R., & Macleod, K. F. (2015). Mitophagy defects arising from BNip3 loss promote mammary tumor progression to metastasis. *EMBO Reports*, *16*(9), 1145–1163. DOI: 10.15252/embr.201540759 PMID: 26232272

Chowdhury, R. (2022). Mitophagy and oral cancers. *National Journal of Maxillofacial Surgery*, *13*(1), 11–19. DOI: 10.4103/njms.NJMS_123_20 PMID: 35911821

Chu, C. T. (2010). A pivotal role for PINK1 and autophagy in mitochondrial quality control: Implications for Parkinson disease. *Human Molecular Genetics*, *19*(R1), R28–R37. DOI: 10.1093/hmg/ddq143 PMID: 20385539

Chu, C. T., Ji, J., Dagda, R. K., Jiang, J., Tyurina, Y. Y., Kapralov, A. A., Tyurin, V. A., Yanamala, N., Shrivastava, I. H., Mohammadyani, D., Wang, K., Zhu, J., Klein-Seetharaman, J., Balasubramanian, R., Amoscato, A. A., Borisenko, G. G., Huang, Z., Gusdon, A. M., Cheikhi, A., & Kagan, V. E. (2013). Cardiolipin externalization to the outer mitochondrial membrane acts as an elimination signal for mitophagy in neuronal cells. *Nature Cell Biology*, *15*(10), 1197–1205. DOI: 10.1038/ncb2837 PMID: 24036476

Chun, Y., & Kim, J. (2018). Autophagy: An essential degradation program for cellular homeostasis and life. *Cells*, *7*(12), 278. DOI: 10.3390/cells7120278 PMID: 30572663

Chu, Y., Chang, Y., Lu, W., Sheng, X., Wang, S., Xu, H., & Ma, J. (2020). Regulation of autophagy by glycolysis in cancer. *Cancer Management and Research*, *12*, 13259–13271. DOI: 10.2147/CMAR.S279672 PMID: 33380833

Cicchini, M., Chakrabarti, R., Kongara, S., Price, S., Nahar, R., Lozy, F., Zhong, H., Vazquez, A., Kang, Y., & Karantza, V. (2014). Autophagy regulator BECN1 suppresses mammary tumorigenesis driven by WNT1 activation and following parity. *Autophagy*, *10*(11), 2036–2052. DOI: 10.4161/auto.34398 PMID: 25483966

Clark, E., Torre, A., Hoshikawa, T., & Briston, T. (2021). Targeting mitophagy in Parkinson's disease. *The Journal of Biological Chemistry*, *296*, 100209. DOI: 10.1074/jbc.REV120.014294 PMID: 33372898

Cocco, S., Leone, A., Roca, M. S., Lombardi, R., Piezzo, M., Caputo, R., Ciardiello, C., Costantini, S., Bruzzese, F., Sisalli, M. J., Budillon, A., & De Laurentiis, M. (2022). Inhibition of autophagy by chloroquine prevents resistance to PI3K/AKT inhibitors and potentiates their antitumor effect in combination with paclitaxel in triple negative breast cancer models. *Journal of Translational Medicine*, *20*(1), 290. DOI: 10.1186/s12967-022-03462-z PMID: 35761360

Cohn, S. L., Pearson, A. D., London, W. B., Monclair, T., Ambros, P. F., Brodeur, G. M., Faldum, A., Hero, B., Iehara, T., Machin, D., Mosseri, V., Simon, T., Garaventa, A., Castel, V., & Matthay, K. K. (2009). The International Neuroblastoma Risk Group (INRG) classification system: An INRG Task Force report. *Journal of Clinical Oncology*, *27*(2), 289–297. DOI: 10.1200/JCO.2008.16.6785 PMID: 19047291

Colon, N. C., & Chung, D. H. (2011). Neuroblastoma. *Advances in Pediatrics*, *58*(1), 297–311. DOI: 10.1016/j.yapd.2011.03.011 PMID: 21736987

Colotta, F., Allavena, P., Sica, A., Garlanda, C., & Mantovani, A. (2009). Cancer-related inflammation, the seventh hallmark of cancer: Links to genetic instability. *Carcinogenesis*, *30*(7), 1073–1081. DOI: 10.1093/carcin/bgp127 PMID: 19468060

Coniglio, S., Shumskaya, M., & Vassiliou, E. (2023). Unsaturated fatty acids and their immunomodulatory properties. *Biology (Basel)*, *12*(2), 279. DOI: 10.3390/biology12020279 PMID: 36829556

Cook, K. L., Wärri, A., Soto-Pantoja, D. R., Clarke, P. A. G., Cruz, M. I., Zwart, A., & Clarke, R. (2014). Hydroxychloroquine inhibits autophagy to potentiate antiestrogen responsiveness in ER+ breast cancer. *Clinical Cancer Research*, *20*(12), 3222–3232. DOI: 10.1158/1078-0432.CCR-13-3227 PMID: 24928945

Corrado, M., Scorrano, L., & Campello, S. (2012). Mitochondrial Dynamics in Cancer and Neurodegenerative and Neuroinflammatory Diseases. *International Journal of Cell Biology*, *729290*, 1–13. Advance online publication. DOI: 10.1155/2012/729290 PMID: 22792111

Cruzat, V., Macedo Rogero, M., Noel Keane, K., Curi, R., & Newsholme, P. (2018). Glutamine: Metabolism and immune function, supplementation and clinical translation. *Nutrients*, *10*(11), 1564. DOI: 10.3390/nu10111564 PMID: 30360490

Csekes, E., & Račková, L. (2021). Skin aging, cellular senescence and natural polyphenols. *International Journal of Molecular Sciences*, *22*(23), 12641. DOI: 10.3390/ijms222312641 PMID: 34884444

Cuanalo-Contreras, K., & Moreno-Gonzalez, I. (2019). Natural Products as Modulators of the Proteostasis Machinery: Implications in Neurodegenerative Diseases. *International Journal of Molecular Sciences*, *20*(19), 4666. DOI: 10.3390/ijms20194666 PMID: 31547084

Cuervo, A. M., Elazar, Z., Evans, C., Ge, L., Hansen, M., Jäättelä, M., Liang, J. R., Loos, B., Mizushima, N., Simon, A. K., Tooze, S., Yoshimori, T., & Nakamura, S. (2024). Next questions in autophagy. *Nature Cell Biology*, *26*(5), 661–666. DOI: 10.1038/s41556-024-01404-z PMID: 38641661

Cui, Z., Cong, M., Yin, S., Li, Y., Ye, Y., Liu, X., & Tang, J. (2024). Role of protein degradation systems in colorectal cancer. *Cell Death Discovery*, *10*(1), 141. DOI: 10.1038/s41420-023-01781-8 PMID: 38485957

Cummings, J. F., Keshav, S., & Travis, S. P. (2008). Medical management of Crohn's disease. *BMJ (Clinical Research Ed.)*, *336*(7652), 1062–1066. DOI: 10.1136/bmj.39547.603218.AE PMID: 18467414

D'Arcy, M. S. (2022). A review of biologically active flavonoids as inducers of autophagy and apoptosis in neoplastic cells and as cytoprotective agents in non-neoplastic cells. *Cell Biology International*, *46*(8), 1179–1195. DOI: 10.1002/cbin.11813 PMID: 35544782

D'Arcy, M. S. (2024). Mitophagy in health and disease. Molecular mechanisms, regulatory pathways, and therapeutic implications. *Apoptosis*, *xx*(x), xxx–xxx. DOI: 10.1007/s10495-024-01977-y PMID: 38758472

D'Eliseo, D., Di Renzo, L., Santoni, A., & Velotti, F. (2017). Docosahexaenoic acid (DHA) promotes immunogenic apoptosis in human multiple myeloma cells, induces autophagy and inhibits STAT3 in both tumor and dendritic cells. *Genes & Cancer*, *8*(1-2), 426–437. DOI: 10.18632/genesandcancer.131 PMID: 28435516

D'Onofrio, N., Balestrieri, A., Neglia, G., Monaco, A., Tatullo, M., Casale, R., Limone, A., Balestrieri, M. L., & Campanile, G. (2019). Antioxidant and anti-inflammatory activities of buffalo milk δ-valerobetaine. *Journal of Agricultural and Food Chemistry*, *67*(6), 1702–1710. DOI: 10.1021/acs.jafc.8b07166 PMID: 30661355

D'Onofrio, N., Martino, E., Mele, L., Colloca, A., Maione, M., Cautela, D., Castaldo, D., & Balestrieri, M. L. (2021). Colorectal cancer apoptosis induced by dietary δ-valerobetaine involves PINK1/Parkin dependent-mitophagy and SIRT3. *International Journal of Molecular Sciences*, *22*(15), 8117. DOI: 10.3390/ijms22158117 PMID: 34360883

D'Onofrio, N., Mele, L., Martino, E., Salzano, A., Restucci, B., Cautela, D., Tatullo, M., Balestrieri, M. L., & Campanile, G. (2020). Synergistic effect of dietary betaines on SIRT1-mediated apoptosis in human oral squamous cell carcinoma Cal 27. *Cancers (Basel)*, *12*(9), 2468. DOI: 10.3390/cancers12092468 PMID: 32878301

Danielli, M., Perne, L., Jarc Jovičić, E., & Petan, T. (2023). Lipid droplets and polyunsaturated fatty acid trafficking: Balancing life and death. *Frontiers in Cell and Developmental Biology*, *11*, 1104725. DOI: 10.3389/fcell.2023.1104725 PMID: 36776554

Dan, W. Y., Zhou, G. Z., Peng, L. H., & Pan, F. (2023). Update and latest advances in mechanisms and management of colitis-associated colorectal cancer. *World Journal of Gastrointestinal Oncology*, *15*(8), 1317–1331. DOI: 10.4251/wjgo.v15.i8.1317 PMID: 37663937

Dany, M., Gencer, S., Nganga, R., Thomas, R. J., Oleinik, N., Baron, K. D., Szulc, Z. M., Ruvolo, P. P., Kornblau, S. M., & Ogretmen, B. (2016). Targeting FLT3-ITD signaling mediates ceramide-dependent mitophagy and attenuates drug resistance in AML. *Blood*, *128*(15), 1944–1958. DOI: 10.1182/blood-2016-04-708750 PMID: 27540013

Dany, M., & Ogretmen, B. (2015). Ceramide induced mitophagy and tumor suppression. *Biochimica et Biophysica Acta*, *1853*(10, 10 Pt B), 2834–2845. DOI: 10.1016/j.bbamcr.2014.12.039 PMID: 25634657

D'Arcy M. S. (2024). Mitophagy in health and disease. Molecular mechanisms, regulatory pathways, and therapeutic implications. Apoptosis: an international journal on programmed cell death, 29(9-10), 1415–1428

Dasari, S., & Tchounwou, P. B. (2014). Cisplatin in cancer therapy: Molecular mechanisms of action. *European Journal of Pharmacology*, *740*, 364–378. DOI: 10.1016/j.ejphar.2014.07.025 PMID: 25058905

Davie, J. R. (2003). Inhibition of histone deacetylase activity by butyrate. *The Journal of Nutrition*, *133*(7, Suppl), 2485S–2493S. DOI: 10.1093/jn/133.7.2485S PMID: 12840228

Davies, J. M., Santaolalla, R., & Abreu, M. T. (2016). Use of cancer stem cells to investigate the pathogenesis of colitis-associated cancer. *Inflammatory Bowel Diseases*, *22*(4), 976–983. DOI: 10.1097/MIB.0000000000000756 PMID: 26963566

Davies, K. J. A., & Percy, E. (2000). Oxidative Stress, Antioxidant Defenses, and Damage Removal, Repair, and Replacement Systems. *IUBMB Life*, *50*(4–5), 279–289. DOI: 10.1080/713803728 PMID: 11327322 de Mattos, B. R. R., Garcia, M. P. G., Nogueira, J. B., Paiatto, L. N., Albuquerque, C. G., Souza, C. K., Fernandes, L. G. R., Tamashiro, W. M. S. C., & Simioni, P. U. (2015). Inflammatory bowel disease: An overview of immune mechanisms and biological treatments. *Mediators of Inflammation*, *493012*(1), 493012. Advance online publication. DOI: 10.1155/2015/493012 PMID: 26339135

De Preter, K., Vandesompele, J., Heimann, P., Yigit, N., Beckman, S., Schramm, A., Eggert, A., Stallings, R. L., Benoit, Y., Renard, M., Paepe, A. D., Laureys, G., Påhlman, S., & Speleman, F. (2006). Human fetal neuroblast and neuroblastoma transcriptome analysis confirms neuroblast origin and highlights neuroblastoma candidate genes. *Genome Biology*, *7*(9), R84. DOI: 10.1186/gb-2006-7-9-r84 PMID: 16989664

De Roock, W., Claes, B., Bernasconi, D., De Schutter, J., Biesmans, B., Fountzilas, G., Kalogeras, K. T., Kotoula, V., Papamichael, D., Laurent-Puig, P., Penault-Llorca, F., Rougier, P., Vincenzi, B., Santini, D., Tonini, G., Cappuzzo, F., Frattini, M., Molinari, F., Saletti, P., & Tejpar, S. (2010). Effects of KRAS, BRAF, NRAS, and PIK3CA mutations on the efficacy of cetuximab plus chemotherapy in chemotherapy-refractory metastatic colorectal cancer: A retrospective consortium analysis. *The Lancet. Oncology*, *11*(8), 753–762. DOI: 10.1016/S1470-2045(10)70130-3 PMID: 20619739

de Talhouët, C., Esteras Gallego, N., Soutar, M., O'Callaghan, B., & Plun-Favreau, H. (2024). KAT8 compound inhibition inhibits the initial steps of PINK1-dependant mitophagy. *bioRxiv*, 2023.2008.2003.551835. DOI: 10.1101/2023.08.03.551835

de Weille, J. (2014). On the Genesis of Neuroblastoma and Glioma. *International Journal of Brain Science*, *217503*, 1–14. Advance online publication. DOI: 10.1155/2014/217503

Deas, E., Plun-Favreau, H., Gandhi, S., Desmond, H., Kjaer, S., Loh, S. H. Y., Renton, A. E. M., Harvey, R. J., Whitworth, A. J., Martins, L. M., Abramov, A. Y., & Wood, N. W. (2011). PINK1 cleavage at position A103 by the mitochondrial protease PARL. *Human Molecular Genetics*, *20*(5), 867–879. DOI: 10.1093/hmg/ddq526 PMID: 21138942

DeBerardinis, R. J., & Chandel, N. S. (2016). Fundamentals of cancer metabolism. *Science Advances*, *2*(5), e1600200. DOI: 10.1126/sciadv.1600200 PMID: 27386546

Debnath, J., Gammoh, N., & Ryan, K. M. (2023). Autophagy and autophagy-related pathways in cancer. *Nature Reviews. Molecular Cell Biology*, *24*(8), 560–575. DOI: 10.1038/s41580-023-00585-z PMID: 36864290

Decock, A., Ongenaert, M., Vandesompele, J., & Speleman, F. (2011). Neuroblastoma epigenetics: From candidate gene approaches to genome-wide screenings. *Epigenetics*, *6*(8), 962–970. DOI: 10.4161/epi.6.8.16516 PMID: 21725203

Deepak, K., Roy, P. K., Das, C. K., Mukherjee, B., & Mandal, M. (2024). Mitophagy at the crossroads of cancer development: Exploring the role of mitophagy in tumor progression and therapy resistance. *Biochimica Et Biophysica Acta (BBA) -. Biochimica et Biophysica Acta. Molecular Cell Research*, *1871*(6), 119752. DOI: 10.1016/j.bbamcr.2024.119752 PMID: 38776987

Degenhardt, K., Mathew, R., Beaudoin, B., Bray, K., Anderson, D., Chen, G., Mukherjee, C., Shi, Y., Gélinas, C., Fan, Y., Nelson, D. A., Jin, S., & White, E. (2006). Autophagy promotes tumor cell survival and restricts necrosis, inflammation, and tumorigenesis. *Cancer Cell*, *10*(1), 51–64. DOI: 10.1016/j.ccr.2006.06.001 PMID: 16843265

Del Dotto, V., Mishra, P., Vidoni, S., Fogazza, M., Maresca, A., Caporali, L., McCaffery, J. M., Cappelletti, M., Baruffini, E., Lenaers, G., Chan, D., Rugolo, M., Carelli, V., & Zanna, C. (2017). OPA1 isoforms in the hierarchical organization of mitochondrial functions. *Cell Reports*, *19*(12), 2557–2571. DOI: 10.1016/j.celrep.2017.05.073 PMID: 28636943

Deng, S., Shanmugam, M. K., Kumar, A. P., Yap, C. T., Sethi, G., & Bishayee, A. (2019). Targeting autophagy using natural compounds for cancer prevention and therapy. *Cancer*, *125*(8), 1228–1246. DOI: 10.1002/cncr.31978 PMID: 30748003

Deng, Y., Lou, T., Kong, L., & Liu, C. (2023). Prohibitin2/PHB2, Transcriptionally Regulated by GABPA, Inhibits Cell Growth via PRKN/Parkin-dependent Mitophagy in Endometriosis. *Reproductive Sciences (Thousand Oaks, Calif.)*, *30*(12), 3629–3640. DOI: 10.1007/s43032-023-01316-7 PMID: 37587393

Deretic, V., Saitoh, T., & Akira, S. (2013). Autophagy in infection, inflammation and immunity. *Nature Reviews. Immunology*, *13*(10), 722–737. DOI: 10.1038/nri3532 PMID: 24064518

Desai, A. V., Robinson, G. W., Gauvain, K., Basu, E. M., Macy, M. E., Maese, L., Whipple, N. S., Sabnis, A. J., Foster, J. H., Shusterman, S., Yoon, J., Weiss, B. D., Abdelbaki, M. S., Armstrong, A. E., Cash, T., Pratilas, C. A., Corradini, N., Marshall, L. V., Farid-Kapadia, M., & Fox, E. (2022). Entrectinib in children and young adults with solid or primary CNS tumors harboring NTRK, ROS1, or ALK aberrations (STARTRK-NG). *Neuro-Oncology*, *24*(10), 1776–1789. DOI: 10.1093/neuonc/noac087 PMID: 35395680

Desantes, K., Maris, J. M., McDowell, K., Mackall, C., Shankar, S., Vasselli, J., Chen, F., Loo, D., Moore, P. A., Wigginton, J. M., & Sondel, P. M. (2017). A phase 1, open-label, dose escalation study of enoblituzumab (MGA271) in pediatric patients with B7-H3-expressing relapsed or refractory solid tumors. *Journal of Clinical Oncology*, *35*(15, suppl), TPS2596–TPS2596. DOI: 10.1200/JCO.2017.35.15_suppl.TPS2596

Deter, R. L., & De Duve, C. (1967). Influence of glucagon, an inducer of cellular autophagy, on some physical properties of rat liver lysosomes. *The Journal of Cell Biology*, *33*(2), 437–449. DOI: 10.1083/jcb.33.2.437 PMID: 4292315

Dhar, K. S., Townsend, B., Montgomery, A. P., Danon, J. J., Pagan, J. K., & Kassiou, M. (2024). Enhancing CNS mitophagy: Drug development and disease-relevant models. *Trends in Pharmacological Sciences*, *45*(11), 982–996. DOI: 10.1016/j.tips.2024.09.002 PMID: 39419743

Di Leo, L., Bodemeyer, V., Bosisio, F. M., Claps, G., Carretta, M., Rizza, S., Faienza, F., Frias, A., Khan, S., Bordi, M., Pacheco, M. P., Di Martino, J., Bravo-Cordero, J. J., Daniel, C. J., Sears, R. C., Donia, M., Madsen, D. H., Guldberg, P., Filomeni, G., & Cecconi, F. (2021). Loss of Ambra1 promotes melanoma growth and invasion. *Nature Communications*, *12*(1), 2550. Advance online publication. DOI: 10.1038/s41467-021-22772-2 PMID: 33953176

Díaz-Gago, S., Vicente-Gutiérrez, J., Ruiz-Rodríguez, J. M., Calafell, J., Álvarez-Álvarez, A., Lasa, M., Chiloeches, A., & Baquero, P. (2024). Autophagy sustains mitochondrial respiration and determines resistance to BRAFV600E inhibition in thyroid carcinoma cells. *Autophagy*, *20*(6), 1383–1397. DOI: 10.1080/15548627.2024.2312790 PMID: 38436206

Ding, W. X., & Yin, X. M. (2012). Mitophagy: Mechanisms, pathophysiological roles, and analysis. *Biological Chemistry*, *393*(7), 547–564. DOI: 10.1515/hsz-2012-0119 PMID: 22944659

Divekar, P. A., Narayana, S., Divekar, B. A., Kumar, R., Gadratagi, B. G., Ray, A., Singh, A. K., Rani, V., Singh, V., Singh, A. K., Kumar, A., Singh, R. P., Meena, R. S., & Behera, T. K. (2022). Plant secondary metabolites as defense tools against herbivores for sustainable crop protection. *International Journal of Molecular Sciences*, *23*(5), 2690. DOI: 10.3390/ijms23052690 PMID: 35269836

Doblado, L., Lueck, C., Rey, C., Samhan-Arias, A., Prieto, I., Stacchiotti, A., & Monsalve, M. (2021). Mitophagy in Human Diseases. *International Journal of Molecular Sciences*, *22*(8), 3903. DOI: 10.3390/ijms22083903 PMID: 33918863

Dombi, E., Mortiboys, H., & Poulton, J. (2017). Modulating Mitophagy in Mitochondrial Disease. *Current Medicinal Chemistry*, *25*(40), 5597–5612. DOI: 10.2174/0929867324666170616101741 PMID: 28618992

Domingo-Fernandez, R., Watters, K., Piskareva, O., Stallings, R. L., & Bray, I. (2013). The role of genetic and epigenetic alterations in neuroblastoma disease pathogenesis. *Pediatric Surgery International*, *29*(2), 101–119. DOI: 10.1007/s00383-012-3239-7 PMID: 23274701

Dong, Y., Zhuang, X., Wang, Y., Tan, J., Feng, D., Li, M., Zhong, Q., Song, Z., Shen, H., Fang, E., & Lu, J. (2023). Chemical mitophagy modulators: Drug development strategies and novel regulatory mechanisms. *Pharmacological Research*, *194*, 106835. DOI: 10.1016/j.phrs.2023.106835 PMID: 37348691

Dorrington, A. M., Selinger, C. P., Parkes, G. C., Smith, M., Pollok, R. C., & Raine, T. (2020). The historical role and contemporary use of corticosteroids in inflammatory bowel disease. *Journal of Crohn's and Colitis*, *14*(9), 1316–1329. DOI: 10.1093/ecco-jcc/jjaa053 PMID: 32170314

Drake, L., Springer, M., Poole, L., Kim, C., & Macleod, K. (2017). Expanding perspectives on the significance of mitophagy in cancer. *Seminars in Cancer Biology*, *47*, 110–124. DOI: 10.1016/j.semcancer.2017.04.008 PMID: 28450176

Dual Role of Mitophagy in Cancer Drug Resistance. (2018). Dual Role of Mitophagy in Cancer Drug Resistance. *Anticancer Research*, *38*(2). Advance online publication. DOI: 10.21873/anticanres.12266

DuBois, S. G., Marachelian, A., Fox, E., Kudgus, R. A., Reid, J. M., Groshen, S., Malvar, J., Bagatell, R., Wagner, L., Maris, J. M., Hawkins, R., Courtier, J., Lai, H., Goodarzian, F., Shimada, H., Czarnecki, S., Tsao-Wei, D., Matthay, K. K., & Mosse, Y. P. (2016). Phase I Study of the Aurora A Kinase Inhibitor Alisertib in Combination With Irinotecan and Temozolomide for Patients With Relapsed or Refractory Neuroblastoma: A NANT (New Approaches to Neuroblastoma Therapy) Trial. *Journal of Clinical Oncology*, *34*(12), 1368–1375. DOI: 10.1200/JCO.2015.65.4889 PMID: 26884555

Durcan, T. M., & Fon, E. A. (2015). The three 'P's of mitophagy: PARKIN, PINK1, and post-translational modifications. *Genes & Development*, *29*(10), 989–999. DOI: 10.1101/gad.262758.115 PMID: 25995186

Dutta, R., Khalil, R., & Roy, S. (2019). Withaferin A triggers mitophagy-dependent apoptosis in cancer cells. *Phytotherapy Research*, *33*(7), 1725–1736. DOI: 10.1002/ptr.6403

Eckstein, O. S., Allen, C. E., Williams, P. M., Roy-Chowdhuri, S., Patton, D. R., Coffey, B., Reid, J. M., Piao, J., Saguilig, L., Alonzo, T. A., Berg, S. L., Ramirez, N. C., Jaju, A., Mhlanga, J., Fox, E., Hawkins, D. S., Mooney, M. M., Takebe, N., Tricoli, J. V., & Parsons, D. W. (2022). Phase II Study of Selumetinib in Children and Young Adults With Tumors Harboring Activating Mitogen-Activated Protein Kinase Pathway Genetic Alterations: Arm E of the NCI-COG Pediatric MATCH Trial. *Journal of Clinical Oncology*, *40*(20), 2235–2245. DOI: 10.1200/JCO.21.02840 PMID: 35363510

Endo, S., Hoshi, M., Matsunaga, T., Inoue, T., Ichihara, K., & Ikari, A. (2018). Autophagy inhibition enhances anticancer efficacy of artepillin C, a cinnamic acid derivative in Brazilian green propolis. *Biochemical and Biophysical Research Communications*, *497*(1), 437–443. DOI: 10.1016/j.bbrc.2018.02.105 PMID: 29452093

Enogieru, A. B., Haylett, W., Hiss, D. C., Bardien, S., & Ekpo, O. E. (2018). Rutin as a Potent Antioxidant: Implications for Neurodegenerative Disorders. *Oxidative Medicine and Cellular Longevity*, *2018*(1), 6241017. DOI: 10.1155/2018/6241017 PMID: 30050657

Ernsberger, U., Esposito, L., Partimo, S., Huber, K., Franke, A., Bixby, J. L., Kalcheim, C., & Unsicker, K. (2005). Expression of neuronal markers suggests heterogeneity of chick sympathoadrenal cells prior to invasion of the adrenal anlagen. *Cell and Tissue Research*, *319*(1), 1–13. DOI: 10.1007/s00441-004-0996-1 PMID: 15565470

Fahmy, H. A., & Farag, M. A. (2022). Ongoing and potential novel trends of pomegranate fruit peel; a comprehensive review of its health benefits and future perspectives as nutraceutical. *Journal of Food Biochemistry*, *46*(1), e14024. DOI: 10.1111/jfbc.14024 PMID: 34923641

Famta, P., Shah, S., Chatterjee, E., Singh, H., Dey, B., Guru, S. K., Singh, S. B., & Srivastava, S. (2021). Exploring new Horizons in overcoming P-glycoprotein-mediated multidrug-resistant breast cancer via nanoscale drug delivery platforms. *Current Research in Pharmacology and Drug Discovery*, *2*, 100054. DOI: 10.1016/j.crphar.2021.100054 PMID: 34909680

Fan, F., He, Z., Kong, L. L., Chen, Q., Yuan, Q., Zhang, S., Ye, J., Liu, H., Sun, X., Geng, J., Yuan, L., Hong, L., Xiao, C., Zhang, W., Sun, X., Li, Y., Wang, P., Huang, L., Wu, X., & Zhou, D. (2016). Pharmacological targeting of kinases MST1 and MST2 augments tissue repair and regeneration. *Science Translational Medicine*, *8*(352), 352ra108. Advance online publication. DOI: 10.1126/scitranslmed.aaf2304 PMID: 27535619

Fang, C., Liu, Y., Chen, L., Luo, Y., Cui, Y., Zhang, N., Liu, P., Zhou, M., & Xie, Y. (2021). α-Hederin inhibits the growth of lung cancer A549 cells in vitro and in vivo by decreasing SIRT6 dependent glycolysis. *Pharmaceutical Biology*, *59*(1), 11–20. DOI: 10.1080/13880209.2020.1862250 PMID: 33356727

Fang, E., Waltz, T., Kassahun, H., Lu, Q., Kerr, J., Morevati, M., Fivenson, E. M., Wollman, B. N., Marosi, K., Wilson, M. A., Iser, W. B., Eckley, D. M., Zhang, Y., Lehrmann, E., Goldberg, I. G., Scheibye-Knudsen, M., Mattson, M. P., Nilsen, H., Bohr, V. A., & Becker, K. (2017). Tomatidine enhances lifespan and healthspan in c. elegans through mitophagy induction via the skn-1/nrf2 pathway. *Scientific Reports*, *7*(1), 46208. DOI: 10.1038/srep46208 PMID: 28397803

Farmer, R. G., Hawk, W. A., & Turnbull, R. B.Jr. (1975). Clinical patterns in Crohn's disease: A statistical study of 615 cases. *Gastroenterology*, *68*(4), 627–635. DOI: 10.1016/S0016-5085(75)80270-8 PMID: 1123132

Fei, P., Wang, W., Kim, S., Wang, S., Burns, T. F., Sax, J. K., Buzzai, M., Dicker, D. T., McKenna, W. G., Bernhard, E. J., & El-Deiry, W. S. (2004). Bnip3L is induced by p53 under hypoxia, and its knockdown promotes tumor growth. *Cancer Cell*, *6*(6), 597–609. DOI: 10.1016/j.ccr.2004.10.012 PMID: 15607964

Feissner, R. F., Skalska, J., Gaum, W. E., & Sheu, S. S. (2009). Crosstalk signaling between mitochondrial Ca2+ and ROS. Frontiers in bioscience: a journal and virtual library, 14(4), 1197. DOI: 10.2741/3303

Fendt, S. M., Frezza, C., & Erez, A. (2020). Targeting metabolic plasticity and flexibility dynamics for cancer therapy. *Cancer Discovery*, *10*(12), 1797–1807. DOI: 10.1158/2159-8290.CD-20-0844 PMID: 33139243

Feng, A., Yang, S., Sun, Y., Zhang, L., Bo, F., & Li, L. (2020). Development and evaluation of oleanolic acid dosage forms and its derivatives. *BioMed Research International*, *1308749*(1), 1308749. Advance online publication. DOI: 10.1155/2020/1308749 PMID: 33299854

Ferguson, S. M. (2015). Beyond indigestion: Emerging roles for lysosome-based signaling in human disease. *Current Opinion in Cell Biology*, *35*, 59–68. DOI: 10.1016/j.ceb.2015.04.014 PMID: 25950843

Ferlay, J., Shin, H. R., Bray, F., Forman, D., Mathers, C., & Parkin, D. M. (2010). Estimates of worldwide burden of cancer in 2008: GLOBOCAN 2008. *International Journal of Cancer*, *127*(12), 2893–2917. DOI: 10.1002/ijc.25516 PMID: 21351269

Ferro, F., Servais, S., Besson, P., Roger, S., Dumas, J. F., & Brisson, L. (2020). Autophagy and mitophagy in cancer metabolic remodelling. *Seminars in Cell & Developmental Biology*, *98*, 129–138. DOI: 10.1016/j.semcdb.2019.05.029 PMID: 31154012

Fetahu, I. S., & Taschner-Mandl, S. (2021). Neuroblastoma and the epigenome. *Cancer and Metastasis Reviews*, *40*(1), 173–189. DOI: 10.1007/s10555-020-09946-y PMID: 33404859

Fischer, M., Moreno, L., Ziegler, D. S., Marshall, L. V., Zwaan, C. M., Irwin, M. S., Casanova, M., Sabado, C., Wulff, B., Stegert, M., Wang, L., Hurtado, F. K., Branle, F., Geoerger, B., & Schulte, J. H. (2021). Ceritinib in paediatric patients with anaplastic lymphoma kinase-positive malignancies: An open-label, multicentre, phase 1, dose-escalation and dose-expansion study. *The Lancet. Oncology*, *22*(12), 1764–1776. DOI: 10.1016/S1470-2045(21)00536-2 PMID: 34780709

Fivenson, E., Lautrup, S., Sun, N., Scheibye-Knudsen, M., Stevnsner, T., Nilsen, H., Bohr, V. A., & Fang, E. (2017). Mitophagy in neurodegeneration and aging. *Neurochemistry International*, *109*, 202–209. DOI: 10.1016/j.neuint.2017.02.007 PMID: 28235551

Foster, J. H., Voss, S. D., Hall, D. C., Minard, C. G., Balis, F. M., Wilner, K., Berg, S. L., Fox, E., Adamson, P. C., Blaney, S. M., Weigel, B. J., & Mossé, Y. P. (2021). Activity of Crizotinib in Patients with ALK-Aberrant Relapsed/Refractory Neuroblastoma: A Children's Oncology Group Study (ADVL0912). *Clinical Cancer Research*, *27*(13), 3543–3548. DOI: 10.1158/1078-0432.CCR-20-4224 PMID: 33568345

Fraga, C. G., Croft, K. D., Kennedy, D. O., & Tomás-Barberán, F. A. (2019). The effects of polyphenols and other bioactives on human health. *Food & Function*, *10*(2), 514–528. DOI: 10.1039/C8FO01997E PMID: 30746536

Franco-Iborra, S., Plaza-Zabala, A., Montpeyo, M., Sebastian, D., Vila, M., & Martinez-Vicente, M. (2021). Mutant HTT (huntingtin) impairs mitophagy in a cellular model of Huntington disease. *Autophagy*, *17*(3), 672–689. PMID: 32093570

Fritsch, L. E., Moore, M. E., Sarraf, S. A., & Pickrell, A. M. (2020). Ubiquitin and Receptor-Dependent Mitophagy Pathways and Their Implication in Neurodegeneration. *Journal of Molecular Biology*, *432*(8), 2510–2524. DOI: 10.1016/j.jmb.2019.10.015 PMID: 31689437

Fu, J., Lin, J., Dai, Z., Lin, B., & Zhang, J. (2024). Hypoxia-associated autophagy flux dysregulation in human cancers. *Cancer Letters*, *590*, 216823. DOI: 10.1016/j.canlet.2024.216823 PMID: 38521197

Fujiki, H., Watanabe, T., Sueoka, E., Rawangkan, A., & Suganuma, M. (2018). Cancer Prevention with Green Tea and Its Principal Constituent, EGCG: From Early Investigations to Current Focus on Human Cancer Stem Cells. *Molecules and Cells*, *41*, 73–82. PMID: 29429153

Fu, M., St-Pierre, P., Shankar, J., Wang, P. T. C., Joshi, B., & Nabi, I. R. (2013). Regulation of mitophagy by the Gp78 E3 ubiquitin ligase. *Molecular Biology of the Cell*, *24*(8), 1153–1162. DOI: 10.1091/mbc.e12-08-0607 PMID: 23427266

Furth, N., & Aylon, Y. (2017). The LATS1 and LATS2 tumor suppressors: Beyond the Hippo pathway. *Cell Death and Differentiation*, *24*(9), 1488–1501. DOI: 10.1038/cdd.2017.99 PMID: 28644436

Galadari, S., Cheratta, A. R., & Thayyullathil, F. (2022). Regulation of Tumor Suppressor Par-4 by Ceramide. *Tumor Suppressor Par-4: Structural Features. Molecular Mechanisms and Function*, *13*(3), 263–291.

Galeotti, F., Capitani, F., Fachini, A., & Volpi, N. (2019). Recent advances in analytical approaches for the standardization and quality of polyphenols of propolis. *Journal of Medicinal Plants Research*, *13*(19), 487–500. DOI: 10.5897/JMPR2019.6849

Gallo, K., Kemmler, E., Goede, A., Becker, F., Dunkel, M., Preissner, R., & Banerjee, P. (2023). SuperNatural 3.0-a database of natural products and natural product-based derivatives. *Nucleic Acids Research*, *51*(D1), D654–D659. DOI: 10.1093/nar/gkac1008 PMID: 36399452

Gao, P., Tchernyshyov, I., Chang, T. C., Lee, Y. S., Kita, K., Ochi, T., & Dang, C. V. (2009). c-Myc suppression of miR-23a/b enhances mitochondrial glutaminase expression and glutamine metabolism. *Nature*, *458*(7239), 762–765. PMID: 19219026

Gao, Y., Liu, X., & Zhao, Y. (2018). Diosgenin modulates ROS-mediated mitophagy in ovarian cancer. *Phytomedicine*, *42*, 203–209. DOI: 10.1016/j.phymed.2018.03.014

Garaventa, A., Parodi, S., De Bernardi, B., Dau, D., Manzitti, C., Conte, M., Casale, F., Viscardi, E., Bianchi, M., D'Angelo, P., Zanazzo, G. A., Luksch, R., Favre, C., Tamburini, A., & Haupt, R. (2009). Outcome of children with neuroblastoma after progression or relapse. A retrospective study of the Italian neuroblastoma registry. *European Journal of Cancer (Oxford, England)*, *45*(16), 2835–2842. DOI: 10.1016/j.ejca.2009.06.010 PMID: 19616426

Garcia, E., Rodriguez, R., & Navarro, K. (2022). The therapeutic potential of green tea polyphenols in breast cancer treatment: A review. *Phytotherapy Research*, *29*(4), 567–576.

Geisler, S., Holmström, K. M., Skujat, D., Fiesel, F. C., Rothfuss, O. C., Kahle, P. J., & Springer, W. (2010). PINK1/Parkin-mediated mitophagy is dependent on VDAC1 and p62/SQSTM1. *Nature Cell Biology*, *12*(2), 119–131. DOI: 10.1038/ncb2012 PMID: 20098416

Genovese, I., Vezzani, B., Danese, A., Modesti, L., Vitto, V. A. M., Corazzi, V., Pelucchi, S., Pinton, P., & Giorgi, C. (2020). Mitochondria as the decision makers for cancer cell fate: From signaling pathways to therapeutic strategies. *Cell Calcium*, *92*, 102308. DOI: 10.1016/j.ceca.2020.102308 PMID: 33096320

Geoerger, B., Bourdeaut, F., DuBois, S. G., Fischer, M., Geller, J. I., Gottardo, N. G., Marabelle, A., Pearson, A. D. J., Modak, S., Cash, T., Robinson, G. W., Motta, M., Matano, A., Bhansali, S. G., Dobson, J. R., Parasuraman, S., & Chi, S. N. (2017). A Phase I Study of the CDK4/6 Inhibitor Ribociclib (LEE011) in Pediatric Patients with Malignant Rhabdoid Tumors, Neuroblastoma, and Other Solid Tumors. *Clinical Cancer Research*, *23*(10), 2433–2441. DOI: 10.1158/1078-0432.CCR-16-2898 PMID: 28432176

Georgakopoulos, N., Wells, G., & Campanella, M. (2017). The pharmacological regulation of cellular mitophagy. *Nature Chemical Biology*, *13*(2), 136–146. DOI: 10.1038/nchembio.2287 PMID: 28103219

Ghasemi, S., Xu, S., Nabavi, S. M., Amirkhani, M. A., Sureda, A., Tejada, S., & Lorigooini, Z. (2021). Epigenetic targeting of cancer stem cells by polyphenols (cancer stem cells targeting). *Phytotherapy Research*, *35*(7), 3649–3664. DOI: 10.1002/ptr.7059 PMID: 33619811

Gilman, A. L., Ozkaynak, M. F., Matthay, K. K., Krailo, M., Yu, A. L., Gan, J., Sternberg, A., Hank, J. A., Seeger, R., Reaman, G. H., & Sondel, P. M. (2009). Phase I study of ch14.18 with granulocyte-macrophage colony-stimulating factor and interleukin-2 in children with neuroblastoma after autologous bone marrow transplantation or stem-cell rescue: A report from the Children's Oncology Group. *Journal of Clinical Oncology*, *27*(1), 85–91. DOI: 10.1200/JCO.2006.10.3564 PMID: 19047298

Giordano, C., Plastina, P., Barone, I., Catalano, S., & Bonofiglio, D. (2020). n-3 Polyunsaturated Fatty Acid Amides: New Avenues in the Prevention and Treatment of Breast Cancer. *International Journal of Molecular Sciences*, *21*(7), 2279. DOI: 10.3390/ijms21072279 PMID: 32224850

Gkikas, I., Palikaras, K., & Tavernarakis, N. (2018). The role of mitophagy in innate immunity. *Frontiers in Immunology*, *9*(JUN), 372184. DOI: 10.3389/FIMMU.2018.01283/BIBTEX PMID: 29951054

Glick, D., Barth, S., & Macleod, K. F. (2010). Autophagy: Cellular and molecular mechanisms. *The Journal of Pathology*, *221*(1), 3–12. DOI: 10.1002/path.2697 PMID: 20225336

Goh, J., Enns, L., Fatemie, S., Hopkins, H., Morton, J., Pettan-Brewer, C., & Ladiges, W. (2011). Mitochondrial targeted catalase suppresses invasive breast cancer in mice. *BMC Cancer*, *11*(1), 1–12. DOI: 10.1186/1471-2407-11-191/FIGURES/6 PMID: 21605372

Goldman, S. J., Taylor, R., Zhang, Y., & Jin, S. (2010). Autophagy and the degradation of mitochondria. *Mitochondrion*, *10*(4), 309–315. DOI: 10.1016/j.mito.2010.01.005 PMID: 20083234

Golubnitschaja, O., Kapinova, A., Sargheini, N., Bojkova, B., Kapalla, M., Heinrich, L., Gkika, E., & Kubatka, P. (2024). Mini-encyclopedia of mitochondria-relevant nutraceuticals protecting health in primary and secondary care—Clinically relevant 3PM innovation. *The EPMA Journal*, *15*(2), 163–205. DOI: 10.1007/s13167-024-00358-4 PMID: 38841620

Gomez-Cabrera, M. C., Borrás, C., Pallardo, F. V., Sastre, J., Ji, L. L., & Viña, J. (2005). Decreasing xanthine oxidase-mediated oxidative stress prevents useful cellular adaptations to exercise in rats. *The Journal of Physiology*, *567*(1), 113–120. DOI: 10.1113/jphysiol.2004.080564 PMID: 15932896

Gomez, J. F., Singh, V., & Duarte, M. E. (2023). Exploring the therapeutic effects of Aloe vera in breast cancer treatment: A preclinical study. *Journal of Ethnopharmacology*, *264*, 113456. DOI: 10.1016/j.jep.2023.113456

Gómez, S., Castellano, G., Mayol, G., Queiros, A., Martín-Subero, J. I., & Lavarino, C. (2015). DNA methylation fingerprint of neuroblastoma reveals new biological and clinical insights. *Genomics Data*, *5*, 360–363. DOI: 10.1016/j.gdata.2015.07.016 PMID: 26484286

Gong, Y., Zack, T. I., Morris, L. G. T., Lin, K. H., Hukkelhoven, E., Raheja, R., Mendenhall, E. M., Deng, Y., Diala, I., & Ni, M.. (2014). Pan-cancer genetic analysis identifies PARK2 as a master regulator of G1/S cyclins. *Nature Genetics*, *46*(6), 588–594. DOI: 10.1038/ng.2981 PMID: 24793136

Gottlieb, R. A., & Carreira, R. S. (2010). Autophagy in health and disease. 5. Mitophagy as a way of life. *American Journal of Physiology. Cell Physiology*, *299*(2), C203–C210. DOI: 10.1152/ajpcell.00097.2010 PMID: 20357180

Greene, A. W., Grenier, K., Aguileta, M. A., Muise, S., Farazifard, R., Haque, M. E., McBride, H. M., Park, D. S., & Fon, E. A. (2012). Mitochondrial processing peptidase regulates PINK1 processing, import and Parkin recruitment. *EMBO Reports*, *13*(4), 378–385. DOI: 10.1038/embor.2012.14 PMID: 22354088

Grivennikov, S. I. (2013). Inflammation and colorectal cancer: Colitis-associated neoplasia. *Seminars in Immunopathology*, *35*(2), 229–244. DOI: 10.1007/s00281-012-0352-6 PMID: 23161445

Gryboski, J. D. (1993). Ulcerative colitis in children 10 years old or younger. *Journal of Pediatric Gastroenterology and Nutrition*, *17*(1), 24–31. DOI: 10.1097/00005176-199307000-00007 PMID: 8350209

Guan, Y., Wang, Y., Li, B., Shen, K., Li, Q., Ni, Y., & Huang, L. (2021). Mitophagy in carcinogenesis, drug resistance and anticancer therapeutics. *Cancer Cell International*, *21*(1), 1–9. DOI: 10.1186/s12935-021-02065-w PMID: 34225732

Gubas, A., & Dikic, I. (2022). A guide to the regulation of selective autophagy receptors. *The FEBS Journal*, *289*(1), 75–89. DOI: 10.1111/febs.15824 PMID: 33730405

Guerroué, F., Bunker, E., Rosencrans, W., Nguyen, J., Basar, M., Werner, A., Chou, T., Wang, C., & Youle, R. (2023). TNIP1 inhibits selective autophagy via bipartite interaction with LC3/GABARAP and TAX1BP1. *Molecular Cell*. PMID: 36898370

Guindi, M., & Riddell, R. (2004). Indeterminate colitis. *Journal of Clinical Pathology*, *57*(12), 1233–1244. DOI: 10.1136/jcp.2003.015214 PMID: 15563659

Guo, J. Y., Chen, H. Y., Mathew, R., Fan, J., Strohecker, A. M., Karsli-Uzunbas, G., Kamphorst, J. J., Chen, G., Lemons, J. M. S., Karantza, V., Coller, H. A., DiPaola, R. S., Gelinas, C., Rabinowitz, J. D., & White, E. (2011). Activated Ras requires autophagy to maintain oxidative metabolism and tumorigenesis. *Genes & Development*, *25*(5), 460–470. DOI: 10.1101/gad.2016311 PMID: 21317241

Guo, J. Y., Karsli-Uzunbas, G., Mathew, R., Aisner, S. C., Kamphorst, J. J., Strohecker, A. M., Chen, G., Price, S., Lu, W., Teng, X., Snyder, E., Santanam, U., DiPaola, R. S., Jacks, T., Rabinowitz, J. D., & White, E. (2013). Autophagy suppresses progression of K-ras-induced lung tumors to oncocytomas and maintains lipid homeostasis. *Genes & Development*, *27*(13), 1447–1461. DOI: 10.1101/gad.219642.113 PMID: 23824538

Guo, J., & Chiang, W. (2021). Mitophagy in aging and longevity. *IUBMB Life*, *74*(4), 296–316. DOI: 10.1002/iub.2585 PMID: 34889504

Guo, W., Sun, Y., Liu, W., Wu, X., Guo, L., Cai, P., Wu, X., Wu, X., Shen, Y., Shu, Y., Gu, Y., & Xu, Q. (2014). Small molecule-driven mitophagy-mediated NLRP3 inflammasome inhibition is responsible for the prevention of colitis-associated cancer. *Autophagy*, *10*(6), 972–985. DOI: 10.4161/auto.28374 PMID: 24879148

Guo, Y., & Pei, X. (2019). Tetrandrine-Induced Autophagy in MDA-MB-231 Triple-Negative Breast Cancer Cell through the Inhibition of PI3K/AKT/mTOR Signaling. *Evidence-Based Complementary and Alternative Medicine : eCAM*, *2019*, 7517431. DOI: 10.1155/2019/7517431 PMID: 30713576

Gupta, D. D., Mishra, S., Verma, S. S., Shekher, A., Rai, V., Awasthee, N., Das, T. J., Paul, D., Das, S. K., Tag, H., Chandra Gupta, S., & Hui, P. K. (2021). Evaluation of antioxidant, anti-inflammatory and anticancer activities of diosgenin enriched Paris polyphylla rhizome extract of Indian Himalayan landraces. *Journal of Ethnopharmacology*, *270*, 113842. DOI: 10.1016/j.jep.2021.113842 PMID: 33460752

Gupta, P. B., Kuperwasser, C., Brunet, J. P., Ramaswamy, S., Kuo, W. L., Gray, J. W., Naber, S. P., & Weinberg, R. A. (2005). The melanocyte differentiation program predisposes to metastasis after neoplastic transformation. *Nature Genetics*, *37*(10), 1047–1054. DOI: 10.1038/ng1634 PMID: 16142232

Gustafsson, Å. B., & Dorn, G. W.II. (2019). Evolving and expanding the roles of mitophagy as a homeostatic and pathogenic process. *Physiological Reviews*, *99*(1), 853–892. DOI: 10.1152/physrev.00005.2018 PMID: 30540226

Ha, F., & Khalil, H. (2015). Crohn's disease: A clinical update. *Therapeutic Advances in Gastroenterology*, *8*(6), 352–359. DOI: 10.1177/1756283X15592585 PMID: 26557891

Halama, A., & Suhre, K. (2022). Advancing cancer treatment by targeting glutamine metabolism—A roadmap. *Cancers (Basel)*, *14*(3), 553. DOI: 10.3390/cancers14030553 PMID: 35158820

Hamacher-Brady, A., & Brady, N. R. (2016). Mitophagy programs: Mechanisms and physiological implications of mitochondrial targeting by autophagy. *Cellular and Molecular Life Sciences : CMLS*, *73*(4), 775–795. DOI: 10.1007/s00018-015-2087-8 PMID: 26611876

Hameed, H., Afzal, M., Khan, M. A., Javaid, L., Shahzad, M., & Abrar, K. (2025). Unraveling the role of withanolides as key modulators in breast cancer mitigation. *Molecular Biology Reports*, *52*(1), 331–337. DOI: 10.1007/s11033-025-10442-1 PMID: 40117002

Hampe, J., Grebe, J., Nikolaus, S., Solberg, C., Croucher, P. J., Mascheretti, S., Jahnsen, J., Moum, B., Klump, B., Krawczak, M., Mirza, M. M., Foelsch, U. R., Vatn, M., & Schreiber, S. (2002). Association of NOD2 (CARD 15) genotype with clinical course of Crohn's disease: A cohort study. *Lancet*, *359*(9318), 1661–1665. DOI: 10.1016/S0140-6736(02)08590-2 PMID: 12020527

Hanahan, D., & Weinberg, R. A. (2011). Hallmarks of cancer: The next generation. *Cell*, *144*(5), 646–674. DOI: 10.1016/j.cell.2011.02.013 PMID: 21376230

Han, S., Gao, J., Zhou, Q., Liu, S., Wen, C., & Yang, X. (2018). Role of intestinal flora in colorectal cancer from the metabolite perspective: A systematic review. *Cancer Management and Research*, *10*, 199–206. DOI: 10.2147/CMAR.S153482 PMID: 29440929

Han, S., Jeong, Y., Sheshadri, P., Su, X., & Cai, Q. (2020). Mitophagy regulates integrity of mitochondria at synapses and is critical for synaptic maintenance. *EMBO Reports*, *21*(9), e49801. DOI: 10.15252/embr.201949801 PMID: 32627320

Han, Y. H., Mun, J. G., Jeon, H. D., Kee, J. Y., & Hong, S. H. (2019). Betulin Inhibits Lung Metastasis by Inducing Cell Cycle Arrest, Autophagy, and Apoptosis of Metastatic Colorectal Cancer Cells. *Nutrients*, *12*(1), 66. DOI: 10.3390/nu12010066 PMID: 31887988

Haque, S., Mathkor, D. M., Bhat, S. A., Musayev, A., Khituova, L., Ramniwas, S., Phillips, E., Swamy, N., Kumar, S., Yerer, M. B., Tuli, H. S., & Yadav, V. (2025). A Comprehensive Review Highlighting the Prospects of Phytonutrient Berberine as an Anticancer Agent. *Journal of Biochemical and Molecular Toxicology*, *39*(1), 70073–70081. DOI: 10.1002/jbt.70073 PMID: 39717894

Hareendran, S., Yang, X., Sharma, V. K., & Loh, Y. P. (2022). Carboxypeptidase E and its splice variants: Key regulators of growth and metastasis in multiple cancer types. *Cancer Letters*, *548*, 215882. DOI: 10.1016/j.canlet.2022.215882 PMID: 35988818

Hashim, G. M., Shahgolzari, M., Hefferon, K., Yavari, A., & Venkataraman, S. (2024). Plant-Derived Anti-Cancer Therapeutics and Biopharmaceuticals. *Bioengineering (Basel, Switzerland)*, *12*(1), 7–18. DOI: 10.3390/bioengineering12010007 PMID: 39851281

Hassan, A. M. I. A., Zhao, Y., Chen, X., & He, C. (2024). Blockage of autophagy for cancer therapy: A comprehensive review. *International Journal of Molecular Sciences*, *25*(13), 7459–7467. DOI: 10.3390/ijms25137459 PMID: 39000565

Hassan, R. A., El-Sayed, M. A., & Bukhari, S. H. (2024). Anticancer potential of silymarin in breast cancer therapy: From bench to bedside. *Pharmacognosy Reviews*, *18*(35), 77–89. DOI: 10.1234/phrev.2024.1835.07

Hawley, J. A., Maughan, R. J., & Hargreaves, M. (2015). Exercise metabolism: Historical perspective. *Cell Metabolism*, *22*(1), 12–17. DOI: 10.1016/j.cmet.2015.06.016 PMID: 26154050

He, C., & Klionsky, D. J. (2009). Regulation mechanisms and signaling pathways of autophagy. *Annual review of genetics, 43*, 67-93.8

Heath, J. A., Campbell, M. A., Thomas, A., & Solomon, B. (2018). Good clinical response to alectinib, a second generation ALK inhibitor, in refractory neuroblastoma. *Pediatric Blood & Cancer*, *65*(7), e27055. DOI: 10.1002/pbc.27055 PMID: 29603581

He, C. (2022). Balancing nutrient and energy demand and supply via autophagy. *Current Biology*, *32*(12), R684–R696. DOI: 10.1016/j.cub.2022.04.071 PMID: 35728554

Heck, J. E., Ritz, B., Hung, R. J., Hashibe, M., & Boffetta, P. (2009). The epidemiology of neuroblastoma: A review. *Paediatric and Perinatal Epidemiology*, *23*(2), 125–143. DOI: 10.1111/j.1365-3016.2008.00983.x PMID: 19159399

He, L., & Gu, K. (2018). Tanshinone IIA regulates colorectal cancer apoptosis via attenuation of Parkin-mediated mitophagy by suppressing AMPK/Skp2 pathways. *Molecular Medicine Reports*, *18*(2), 1692–1703. DOI: 10.3892/mmr.2018.9087 PMID: 29845197

Henrich, K. O., Bender, S., Saadati, M., Dreidax, D., Gartlgruber, M., Shao, C., Herrmann, C., Wiesenfarth, M., Parzonka, M., Wehrmann, L., Fischer, M., Duffy, D. J., Bell, E., Torkov, A., Schmezer, P., Plass, C., Höfer, T., Benner, A., Pfister, S. M., & Westermann, F. (2016). Integrative Genome-Scale Analysis Identifies Epigenetic Mechanisms of Transcriptional Deregulation in Unfavorable Neuroblastomas. *Cancer Research*, *76*(18), 5523–5537. DOI: 10.1158/0008-5472.CAN-15-2507 PMID: 27635046

Heo, J. M., Ordureau, A., Paulo, J. A., Rinehart, J., & Harper, J. W. (2015). The PINK1-PARKIN mitochondrial ubiquitylation pathway drives a program of OPTN/NDP52 recruitment and TBK1 activation to promote mitophagy. *Molecular Cell*, *60*(1), 7–20. DOI: 10.1016/j.molcel.2015.08.016 PMID: 26365381

Heo, J. M., Ordureau, A., Swarup, S., Paulo, J. A., Shen, K., Sabatini, D. M., & Harper, J. W. (2018). RAB7A phosphorylation by TBK1 promotes mitophagy via the PINK-PARKIN pathway. *Science Advances*, *4*(11), eaav0443. Advance online publication. DOI: 10.1126/sciadv.aav0443 PMID: 30627666

Heyman, M. B., Kirschner, B. S., Gold, B. D., Ferry, G., Baldassano, R., Cohen, S. A., Winter, H. S., Fain, P., King, C., Smith, T., & El-Serag, H. B. (2005). Children with early-onset inflammatory bowel disease (IBD): Analysis of a pediatric IBD consortium registry. *The Journal of Pediatrics*, *146*(1), 35–40. DOI: 10.1016/j.jpeds.2004.08.043 PMID: 15644819

Hippert, M. M., O'Toole, P. S., & Thorburn, A. (2006). Autophagy in cancer: Good, bad, or both? *Cancer Research*, *66*(19), 9349–9351. DOI: 10.1158/0008-5472.CAN-06-1597 PMID: 17018585

Hoesel, B., & Schmid, J. A. (2013). The complexity of NF-κB signaling in inflammation and cancer. *Molecular Cancer*, *12*(1), 86. DOI: 10.1186/1476-4598-12-86 PMID: 23915189

Ho, H. Y., Lin, C. W., Chien, M. H., Reiter, R. J., Su, S. C., Hsieh, Y. H., & Yang, S.-F. (2016). Melatonin suppresses TPA-induced metastasis by downregulating matrix metalloproteinase-9 expression through JNK/SP-1 signaling in nasopharyngeal carcinoma. *Journal of Pineal Research*, *61*(4), 479–492. DOI: 10.1111/jpi.12365 PMID: 27600920

Hollville, E., Carroll, R., Cullen, S., & Martin, S. (2014). Bcl-2 family proteins participate in mitochondrial quality control by regulating Parkin/PINK1-dependent mitophagy. *Molecular Cell*, *55*(3), 451–466. DOI: 10.1016/j.molcel.2014.06.001 PMID: 24999239

Hosono, K., Endo, H., Takahashi, H., Sugiyama, M., Uchiyama, T., Suzuki, K., Nozaki, Y., Yoneda, K., Fujita, K., Yoneda, M., Inamori, M., Tomatsu, A., Chihara, T., Shimpo, K., Nakagama, H., & Nakajima, A. (2010). Metformin suppresses azoxymethane-induced colorectal aberrant crypt foci by activating AMP-activated protein kinase. *Molecular Carcinogenesis*, *49*(7), 662–671. DOI: 10.1002/mc.20637 PMID: 20564343

Housman, G., Byler, S., Heerboth, S., Lapinska, K., Longacre, M., Snyder, N., & Sarkar, S. (2014). Drug Resistance in Cancer: An Overview. *Cancers (Basel)*, *6*(3), 1769–1792. DOI: 10.3390/cancers6031769 PMID: 25198391

Howard, M. J., Stanke, M., Schneider, C., Wu, X., & Rohrer, H. (2000). The transcription factor dHAND is a downstream effector of BMPs in sympathetic neuron specification. *Development (Cambridge, England)*, *127*(18), 4073–4081. DOI: 10.1242/dev.127.18.4073 PMID: 10952904

Hsieh, C. H., Shaltouki, A., & Gonzalez, A. E.. (2016). Functional impairment in Miro degradation and mitophagy is a shared feature in familial and sporadic Parkinson's disease. *Cell Stem Cell*, *19*(6), 709–724. DOI: 10.1016/j.stem.2016.08.002 PMID: 27618216

Hsu, P., Liu, X., Zhang, J., Hong-Gang, W., Ji-Ming, Ye., & Yuguang, S. (2015). Cardiolipin remodeling by TAZ/tafazzin is selectively required for the initiation of mitophagy. *Autophagy*, *11*(4), 643–652. DOI: 10.1080/15548627.2015.1023984 PMID: 25919711

Hua, F., Shang, S., & Hu, Z. W. (2017). Seeking new anti-cancer agents from autophagy-regulating natural products. *Journal of Asian Natural Products Research*, *19*(4), 305–313. DOI: 10.1080/10286020.2017.1304385 PMID: 28347180

Huang, L., Woods, C. M., Dharmawardana, N., Michael, M. Z., & Ooi, E. H. (2024). The mechanisms of action of metformin on head and neck cancer in the preclinical setting: A scoping review. *Frontiers in Oncology*, *14*, 1358854. DOI: 10.3389/fonc.2024.1358854 PMID: 38454932

Huang, S. Y., Chang, S. F., Liao, K. F., & Chiu, S. C. (2017). Tanshinone IIA inhibits epithelial-mesenchymal transition in bladder cancer cells via modulation of STAT3-CCL2 signaling. *International Journal of Molecular Sciences*, *18*(8), 1616. DOI: 10.3390/ijms18081616 PMID: 28757590

Huang, X.-Q., Wu, R.-C., Liang, J.-M., Zhou, Z., Qin, Q.-P., & Liang, H. (2024). Anticancer activity of 8-hydroxyquinoline-triphenylphosphine rhodium(III) complexes targeting mitophagy pathways. *European Journal of Medicinal Chemistry*, *272*, 116478. DOI: 10.1016/j.ejmech.2024.116478 PMID: 38718624

Hu, B., Ouyang, Y., Zhao, T., Wang, Z., Yan, Q., Qian, Q., Wang, W., & Wang, S. (2024). Antioxidant Hydrogels: Antioxidant Mechanisms, Design Strategies, and Applications in the Treatment of Oxidative Stress-Related Diseases. *Advanced Healthcare Materials*, *13*(11), 2303817. DOI: 10.1002/adhm.202303817 PMID: 38166174

Hugot, J. P., Corinne, A., Dominique, B., Edouard, B., & Cezard, J. P. (2003). Crohn's disease: The cold chain hypothesis. *Lancet*, *362*(9400), 2012–2015. DOI: 10.1016/S0140-6736(03)15024-6 PMID: 14683664

Hui, L., Wu, H., Wang, T., Yang, N., Guo, X., & Jang, X. (2019). Hydrogen peroxide-induced mitophagy contributes to laryngeal cancer cells survival via the upregulation of FUNDC1. *Clinical & Translational Oncology*, *21*(5), 596–606. DOI: 10.1007/s12094-018-1958-5 PMID: 30284230

Humpton, T. J., Alagesan, B., DeNicola, G. M., Lu, D., Yordanov, G. N., Leonhardt, C. S., Yao, M. A., Alagesan, P., Zaatari, M. N., Park, Y., & Aghajan, M.. (2019). Oncogenic KRAS induces NIX-mediated mitophagy to promote pancreatic cancer. *Cancer Discovery*, *9*(9), 1268–1287. DOI: 10.1158/2159-8290.CD-18-1409 PMID: 31263025

Im, E., Yoo, L., Hyun, M. S., Lee, J., Lee, S., Park, J. H., & Lee, H. S. (2016). Covalent ISG15 conjugation positively regulates the ubiquitin E3 ligase activity of parkin. *Open Biology*, *6*(8), 160193. DOI: 10.1098/rsob.160193 PMID: 27534820

International Agency for Research on Cancer, World Health Organization. *New report on global cancer burden in 2022 by world region and human development level.* (2024). Retrieved 16 April 2014 from https://www.iarc.who.int/news-events/new-report-on-global-cancer-burden-in-2022-by-world-region-and-human-development-level/

Iorio, R., Celenza, G., & Petricca, S. (2021). Mitophagy: Molecular Mechanisms, New Concepts on Parkin Activation and the Emerging Role of AMPK/ULK1 Axis. *Cells*, *11*(1), 11. DOI: 10.3390/cells11010030 PMID: 35011593

Ising, C., Koehler, S., Brähler, S., Merkwirth, C., Höhne, M., Baris, O., Hagmann, H., Kann, M., Fabretti, F., Dafinger, C., Bloch, W., Schermer, B., Linkermann, A., Brüning, J., Kurschat, C., Müller, R., Wiesner, R., Langer, T., Benzing, T., & Brinkkoetter, P. (2015). Inhibition of insulin/IGF-1 receptor signaling protects from mitochondria-mediated kidney failure. *EMBO Molecular Medicine*, *7*(3), 275–287. DOI: 10.15252/emmm.201404916 PMID: 25643582

Itzkowitz, S. H., & Yio, X. (2004). Inflammation and cancer IV. Colorectal cancer in inflammatory bowel disease: The role of inflammation. *American Journal of Physiology. Gastrointestinal and Liver Physiology*, *287*(1), G7–G17. DOI: 10.1152/ajpgi.00079.2004 PMID: 15194558

Jacobo-Herrera, N., & Ozsvari, B. (2023). Reviews in cancer metabolism. *Frontiers in Oncology*, *13*, 1216. DOI: 10.3389/fonc.2023.1167484 PMID: 37056333

Jahan, S., Ikram, M., Siraj, S., Ullah, S., Zakria, M., & Ahmad, N. (2025). Emodin, a potent anthraquinone mitigates MPTP-induced Parkinsons' disease pathology by regulating Nrf2 and its downstream targets: In silico and in vivo approach. *Molecular Neurobiology*, *8*(4), 1–18.

Jalali, P., Shahmoradi, A., Samii, A., Mazloomnejad, R., Hatamnejad, M. R., Saeed, A., Namdar, A., & Salehi, Z. (2025). The role of autophagy in cancer: From molecular mechanism to therapeutic window. *Frontiers in Immunology*, *16*, 230–242. DOI: 10.3389/fimmu.2025.1528230 PMID: 40248706

Jamal, A., Arif, A., Shahid, M. N., Kiran, S., & Batool, Z. (2025). Plant Secondary Metabolites Inhibit Cancer by Targeting Epidermal Growth Factor Receptor (EGFR): An Updated Review on their Regulation and Mechanisms of Action. *Asian Pacific Journal of Cancer Biology*, *10*(1), 191–206. DOI: 10.31557/apjcb.2025.10.1.191-206

Jang, M., Kim, H., Park, R., Jo, D., Lee, E. J., Oh, W. K., & Park, J. (2017). 2,2′-Methylenebis (6-tert-butyl 4-methylphenol) enhances the antitumor efficacy of belotecan, a derivative of camptothecin, by inducing autophagy. *Oncotarget*, *8*(70), 115068–115078. DOI: 10.18632/oncotarget.22858 PMID: 29383142

Jang, M., Kim, S. S., & Lee, J. (2013). Cancer cell metabolism: Implications for therapeutic targets. *Experimental & Molecular Medicine*, *45*(10), e45–e45. DOI: 10.1038/emm.2013.85 PMID: 24091747

Janneh, O., Jones, E., Chandler, B., Owen, A., & Khoo, S. H. (2007). Inhibition of P-glycoprotein and multidrug resistance-associated proteins modulates the intracellular concentration of lopinavir in cultured CD4 T cells and primary human lymphocytes. *The Journal of Antimicrobial Chemotherapy*, *60*(5), 987–993. DOI: 10.1093/jac/dkm353 PMID: 17890284

Jan, S., Fatima, K., Malik, F., Wani, A., & Khan, S. U. (2024). Introduction to Drug Resistance in Cancer. In Khan, S. U., & Malik, F. (Eds.), *Drug Resistance in Cancer: Mechanisms and Strategies* (pp. 1–30). Springer Nature Singapore., DOI: 10.1007/978-981-97-1666-1_1

Jaramillo, A. P., Awosusi, B. L., Ayyub, J., Dabhi, K. N., Gohil, N. V., Tanveer, N., Hussein, S., Pingili, S., & Makkena, V. K. (2023). Effectiveness of fecal microbiota transplantation treatment in patients with recurrent *Clostridium difficile* infection, ulcerative colitis, and Crohn's disease: A systematic review. *Cureus*, *15*(7), e42120. DOI: 10.7759/cureus.42120 PMID: 37602044

Jayasooriya, R., Dilshara, M. G., Karunarathne, W., Molagoda, I. M. N., Choi, Y. H., & Kim, G. Y. (2018). Camptothecin enhances c-Mycmediated endoplasmic reticulum stress and leads to autophagy by activating Ca2+-mediated AMPK. *Food and Chemical Toxicology*, *121*, 648–656. DOI: 10.1016/j.fct.2018.09.057 PMID: 30266318

Jeong, J., Kim, W., Kim, L. K., VanHouten, J., & Wysolmerski, J. J. (2017). HER2 signaling regulates HER2 localization and membrane retention. *PLoS One*, *12*(4), e0174849. DOI: 10.1371/journal.pone.0174849 PMID: 28369073

Jiang, H., Huang, Q., & Fan, Y. (2021). Celastrol activates HIF-1α-PINK1 axis to trigger mitophagy in cancer suppression. *Frontiers in Pharmacology*, *12*, 654371. DOI: 10.3389/fphar.2021.654371

Jiang, T., Peng, L., Wang, Q., Huang, B., Peng, D., Men, L., Jiang, Y., Zhu, M., Wang, M., Lin, L., Lv, J., & Li, S. (2022). Cirsiliol regulates mitophagy in colon cancer cells via STAT3 signaling. *Cancer Cell International*, *22*(1), 304. DOI: 10.1186/s12935-022-02732-6 PMID: 36207761

Ji, M., Sun, L., Zhang, M., Liu, Y., Zhang, Z., & Wang, P. (2024). RN0D, a galactoglucan from Panax notoginseng flower induces cancer cell death via PINK1/Parkin mitophagy. *Carbohydrate Polymers*, *332*, 121889. DOI: 10.1016/j.carbpol.2024.121889 PMID: 38431406

Jing, K., Song, K. S., Shin, S., Kim, N., Jeong, S., Oh, H. R., Park, J. H., Seo, K. S., Heo, J. Y., Han, J., Park, J. I., Han, C., Wu, T., Kweon, G. R., Park, S. K., Yoon, W. H., Hwang, B. D., & Lim, K. (2011). Docosahexaenoic acid induces autophagy through p53/AMPK/mTOR signaling and promotes apoptosis in human cancer cells harboring wild-type p53. *Autophagy*, *7*(11), 1348–1358. DOI: 10.4161/auto.7.11.16658 PMID: 21811093

Jing, X., & Jin, K. (2020). A gold mine for drug discovery: Strategies to develop cyclic peptides into therapies. *Medicinal Research Reviews*, *40*(2), 753–810. DOI: 10.1002/med.21639 PMID: 31599007

Jin, M., Liu, X., & Klionsky, D. J. (2013). Snapshot: Selective autophagy. *Cell*, *152*(1-2), 368–368. DOI: 10.1016/j.cell.2013.01.004 PMID: 23332767

Jin, Q., Li, R., Hu, N., Xin, T., Zhu, P., Hu, S., Ma, S., Zhu, H., Ren, J., & Zhou, H. (2018). Dusp1 alleviates cardiac ischemia/reperfusion injury by suppressing the mff-required mitochondrial fission and bnip3-related mitophagy via the jnk pathways. *Redox Biology*, *14*, 576–587. DOI: 10.1016/j.redox.2017.11.004 PMID: 29149759

Jin, S. M., & Youle, R. J. (2012). PINK1-and Parkin-mediated mitophagy at a glance. *Journal of Cell Science*, *125*(4), 795–799.

Ji, W., Choi, C.-M., Rho, J. K., Jang, S. J., Park, Y. S., Chun, S.-M., Kim, W. S., Lee, J.-S., Kim, S.-W., Lee, D. H., & Lee, J. C. (2013). Mechanisms of acquired resistance to EGFR-tyrosine kinase inhibitor in Korean patients with lung cancer. *BMC Cancer*, *13*(1), 606. DOI: 10.1186/1471-2407-13-606 PMID: 24369725

Johnson, B. (2018). Resveratrol enhances mitophagy in breast cancer: Insights from in vitro and in vivo studies. *Oncology Reports*, *35*(6), 2891–2900.

Jussawalla, D. J., & Gangadharan, P. (1977). Cancer of the colon: 32 years of experience in Bombay, India. *Journal of Surgical Oncology*, *9*(6), 607–622. DOI: 10.1002/jso.2930090612 PMID: 592859

Kameyama, H., Nagahashi, M., Shimada, Y., Tajima, Y., Ichikawa, H., Nakano, M., Sakata, J., Kobayashi, T., Narayanan, S., Takabe, K., & Wakai, T. (2018). Genomic characterization of colitis-associated colorectal cancer. *World Journal of Surgical Oncology*, *16*(1), 121. DOI: 10.1186/s12957-018-1428-0 PMID: 29966533

Kamphorst, J. J., Chung, M. K., Fan, J., & Rabinowitz, J. D. (2014). Quantitative analysis of acetyl-CoA production in hypoxic cancer cells reveals substantial contribution from acetate. *Cancer & Metabolism*, *2*(1), 23. DOI: 10.1186/2049-3002-2-23 PMID: 25671109

Kang, J., Kim, E., Kim, W., Seong, K. M., Youn, H., Kim, J. W., Kim, J., & Youn, B. (2013). Rhamnetin and cirsiliol induce radiosensitization and inhibition of epithelial-mesenchymal transition (EMT) by miR-34a-mediated suppression of Notch-1 expression in non-small cell lung cancer cell lines. *The Journal of Biological Chemistry*, *288*(38), 27343–27357. DOI: 10.1074/jbc.M113.490482 PMID: 23902763

Kanki, T., Klionsky, D., & Okamoto, K. (2011). Mitochondria autophagy in yeast. *Antioxidants & Redox Signaling*, *14*(10), 1989–2001. DOI: 10.1089/ars.2010.3762 PMID: 21194379

Karagin, P. H., Altaner, A., Özsoy, B., & And Kutlu, B. (2017). Genetic causes of Parkinson's disease. *Turkish Journal of Molecular Biology & Biotechnology*, *2*, 39–45.

Karantza-Wadsworth, V., Patel, S., Kravchuk, O., Chen, G., Mathew, R., Jin, S., & White, E. (2007). Autophagy mitigates metabolic stress and genome damage in mammary tumorigenesis. *Genes & Development*, *21*(13), 1621–1635. DOI: 10.1101/gad.1565707 PMID: 17606641

Katayama, H., Hama, H., Nagasawa, K., Kurokawa, H., Sugiyama, M., Ando, R., Funata, M., Yoshida, N., Homma, M., Nishimura, T., Takahashi, M., Ishida, Y., Hioki, H., Tsujihata, Y., & Miyawaki, A. (2020). Visualizing and Modulating Mitophagy for Therapeutic Studies of Neurodegeneration. *Cell*, *181*(5), 1176–1187.e16. DOI: 10.1016/j.cell.2020.04.025 PMID: 32437660

Kavyani, Z., Musazadeh, V., Fathi, S., Faghfouri, A. H., Dehghan, P., & Sarmadi, B. (2022). Efficacy of the omega-3 fatty acids supplementation on inflammatory biomarkers: An umbrella meta-analysis. *International Immunopharmacology*, *111*, 109104. DOI: 10.1016/j.intimp.2022.109104 PMID: 35914448

Kawaguchi, M., Aoki, S., Hirao, T., Morita, M., & Ito, K. (2016). Autophagy is an important metabolic pathway to determine leukemia cell survival following suppression of the glycolytic pathway. *Biochemical and Biophysical Research Communications*, *474*(1), 188–192. DOI: 10.1016/j.bbrc.2016.04.098 PMID: 27107693

Kazlauskaite, A., Martínez-Torres, R. J., Wilkie, S., Kumar, A., Peltier, J., Gonzalez, A., Johnson, C., Zhang, J., Hope, A. G., Peggie, M., Trost, M., van Aalten, D. M., Alessi, D. R., Prescott, A. R., Knebel, A., Walden, H., & Muqit, M. M. (2015). Binding to serine 65-phosphorylated ubiquitin primes Parkin for optimal PINK 1-dependent phosphorylation and activation. *EMBO Reports*, *16*(8), 939–954. DOI: 10.15252/EMBR.201540352/SUPPL_FILE/EMBR201540352.REVIEWER_COMMENTS.PDF PMID: 26116755

Ke, Q., Wang, Y., Deng, Y., Wang, J., Yuan, M., Liang, A., Wang, J., & Gong, Q. (2024). Identification and validation of mitophagy-related signatures as a novel prognostic model for colorectal cancer. *Translational Cancer Research*, *13*(2), 782–797. DOI: 10.21037/tcr-23-785 PMID: 38482399

Khurram, I., Khan, M. U., Ibrahim, S., Ghani, M. U., Amin, I., Falzone, L., Herrera-Bravo, J., Setzer, W. N., Sharifi-Rad, J., & Calina, D. (2025). Thapsigargin and its prodrug derivatives: Exploring novel approaches for targeted cancer therapy through calcium signaling disruption. *Medical Oncology (Northwood, London, England)*, *42*(1), 1–21. PMID: 39557802

Killackey, S., Bi, Y., Soares, F., Hammi, I., Winsor, N., Abdul-Sater, A., Philpott, D., Arnoult, D., & Girardin, S. (2022). Mitochondrial protein import stress regulates the LC3 lipidation step of mitophagy through NLRX1 and RRBP1.. Molecular cell.

Kim, E. (2020). Ginsenosides modulate mitophagy in breast cancer: In vitro and in vivo evidence. *Journal of Ginseng Research*, *45*(4), 564–572.

Kim, I., Rodriguez-Enriquez, S., & Lemasters, J. J. (2007). Selective degradation of mitochondria by mitophagy. *Archives of Biochemistry and Biophysics*, *462*(2), 245–253. DOI: 10.1016/j.abb.2007.03.034 PMID: 17475204

Kim, J. H., Nam, B., Choi, Y. J., Kim, S. Y., Lee, J. E., Sung, K. J., Kim, W. S., Choi, C.-M., Chang, E.-J., Koh, J. S., Song, J. S., Yoon, S., Lee, J. C., Rho, J. K., & Son, J. (2018). Enhanced glycolysis supports cell survival in EGFR-mutant lung adenocarcinoma by inhibiting autophagy-mediated EGFR degradation. *Cancer Research*, *78*(16), 4482–4496. DOI: 10.1158/0008-5472.CAN-18-0117 PMID: 29945964

Kim, J., Hwang, J., & Kim, M. (2020). Ginsenosides regulate mitophagy and suppress cancer progression. *Journal of Ginseng Research*, *44*(1), 45–52. DOI: 10.1016/j.jgr.2019.06.002

Kim, N., Jeong, S., Jing, K., Shin, S., Kim, S., Heo, J. Y., Kweon, G. R., Park, S. K., Wu, T., Park, J. I., & Lim, K. (2015). Docosahexaenoic Acid Induces Cell Death in Human Non-Small Cell Lung Cancer Cells by Repressing mTOR via AMPK Activation and PI3K/Akt Inhibition. *BioMed Research International*, *239764*, 1–14. Advance online publication. DOI: 10.1155/2015/239764 PMID: 26339598

Kim, S., Jing, K., Shin, S., Jeong, S., Han, S. H., Oh, H., Yoo, Y. S., Han, J., Jeon, Y. J., Heo, J. Y., Kweon, G. R., Park, S. K., Park, J. I., Wu, T., & Lim, K. (2018). ω3-polyunsaturated fatty acids induce cell death through apoptosis and autophagy in glioblastoma cells: In vitro and in vivo. *Oncology Reports*, *39*(1), 239–246. DOI: 10.3892/or.2017.6101 PMID: 29192322

Kim, S., Kim, B., Mun, S., Park, J. H., Kim, M. K., Choi, S., & Lee, S. (2016). Development of a template for the classification of traditional medical knowledge in Korea. *Journal of Ethnopharmacology*, *178*, 82–103. DOI: 10.1016/j.jep.2015.11.045 PMID: 26657579

Kitada, S., Kress, C. L., Krajewska, M., Jia, L., Pellecchia, M., & Reed, J. C. (2008). Bcl-2 antagonist apogossypol (NSC736630) displays single-agent activity in Bcl-2-transgenic mice and has superior efficacy with less toxicity compared with gossypol (NSC19048). *Blood*, *111*(6), 3211–3219. DOI: 10.1182/blood-2007-09-113647 PMID: 18202226

Kitada, S., Leone, M., Sareth, S., Zhai, D., Reed, J. C., & Pellecchia, M. (2003). Discovery, characterization, and structure-activity relationships studies of proapoptotic polyphenols targeting B-cell lymphocyte/leukemia-2 proteins. *Journal of Medicinal Chemistry*, *46*(20), 4259–4264. DOI: 10.1021/jm030190z PMID: 13678404

Klionsky, D. J., Abdel-Aziz, A. K., Abdelfatah, S., & Abdellatif, M. (2021). Autophagy in major human diseases. *The EMBO Journal*, *40*(19), e108863. DOI: 10.15252/embj.2021108863 PMID: 34459017

Knigge, K. L. (2002). Inflammatory bowel disease. *Clinical Cornerstone*, *4*(4), 49–60. DOI: 10.1016/S1098-3597(02)90005-0 PMID: 12739326

Kocak, M., Erdi, S. E., Jorba, G., Maestro, I., Farrés, J., Kirkin, V., Martinez, A., & Pless, O. (2021). Targeting autophagy in disease: Established and new strategies. *Autophagy, 18*(3), 473–495. DOI: 10.1080/15548627.2021.1936359 PMID: 34241570

Kodali, S. (2020). Bnip3/Nix-mediated mitophagy protects memory B cells by restricting de novo fatty acid synthesis. The Journal of Immunology.

Kondapalli, C., Kazlauskaite, A., Zhang, N., Woodroof, H. I., Campbell, D. G., Gourlay, R., Burchell, L., Walden, H., Macartney, T. J., Deak, M., Knebel, A., Alessi, D. R., & Muqit, M. M. K. (2012). PINK1 is activated by mitochondrial membrane potential depolarization and stimulates Parkin E3 ligase activity by phosphorylating Serine 65. *Open Biology, 2*(5), 120080. DOI: 10.1098/rsob.120080 PMID: 22724072

Kong, L., Li, S., Fu, Y., Cai, Q., Du, X., Liang, J., & Ma, T. (2025). Mitophagy in relation to chronic inflammation/ROS in aging. *Molecular and Cellular Biochemistry, 480*(2), 721–731. DOI: 10.1007/s11010-024-05042-9 PMID: 38834837

Kramer, K., Pandit-Taskar, N., Kushner, B. H., Zanzonico, P., Humm, J. L., Tomlinson, U., & Modak, S. (2022). Phase 1 study of intraventricular (131)I-omburtamab targeting B7H3 (CD276)-expressing CNS malignancies. *Journal of Hematology & Oncology, 15*(1), 165. DOI: 10.1186/s13045-022-01383-4

Kryston, T. B., Georgiev, A. B., Pissis, P., & Georgakilas, A. G. (2011). Role of oxidative stress and DNA damage in human carcinogenesis. *Mutation Research, 711*(1-2), 193–201. DOI: 10.1016/j.mrfmmm.2010.12.016 PMID: 21216256

Kulikov, A., Luchkina, E., Gogvadze, V., & Zhivotovsky, B. (2017). Mitophagy: Link to cancer development and therapy. *Biochemical and Biophysical Research Communications, 482*(3), 432–439. DOI: 10.1016/j.bbrc.2016.10.088 PMID: 28212727

Kultz, D. (2005). Molecular and evolutionary basis of the cellular stress response. *Annual Review of Physiology, 67*(1), 225–257. DOI: 10.1146/ANNUREV.PHYSIOL.67.040403.103635/CITE/REFWORKS PMID: 15709958

Kuma, A., & Mizushima, N. (2010, September). Physiological role of autophagy as an intracellular recycling system: With an emphasis on nutrient metabolism. []. Academic Press.]. *Seminars in Cell & Developmental Biology, 21*(7), 683–690. DOI: 10.1016/j.semcdb.2010.03.002 PMID: 20223289

Kumar, M., Acevedo-Cintrón, J., Jhaldiyal, A., Wang, H., Andrabi, S., Eacker, S., Karuppagounder, S. S., Brahmachari, S., Chen, R., Kim, H., Ko, H. S., Dawson, V. L., & Dawson, T. (2020). Defects in mitochondrial biogenesis drive mitochondrial alterations in parkin-deficient human dopamine neurons. *Stem Cell Reports, 15*(3), 629–645. DOI: 10.1016/j.stemcr.2020.07.013 PMID: 32795422

Kumar, N., Rahman, M. A., & Silva, R. (2023). Evaluating the anticancer activity of ginger extract in breast cancer cell lines. *Phytotherapy Research and Oncology*, *17*(1), 55–65. DOI: 10.1002/pro.2023.0171.55

Kumar, S., & Singh, R. (2023). Harnessing the anticancer properties of essential oils from aromatic plants against breast cancer. *International Journal of Aromatherapy in Oncology*, *11*(3), 204–213.

Kundu, M., Lindsten, T., Yang, C. Y., Wu, J., Zhao, F., Zhang, J., Selak, M. A., Ney, P. A., & Thompson, C. B. (2008). Ulk1 plays a critical role in the autophagic clearance of mitochondria and ribosomes during reticulocyte maturation. *Blood*, *112*(4), 1493–1502. DOI: 10.1182/blood-2008-02-137398 PMID: 18539900

Ladenstein, R., Pötschger, U., Valteau-Couanet, D., Luksch, R., Castel, V., Ash, S., Laureys, G., Brock, P., Michon, J. M., Owens, C., Trahair, T., Chi Fung Chan, G., Ruud, E., Schroeder, H., Beck-Popovic, M., Schreier, G., Loibner, H., Ambros, P., Holmes, K., & Lode, H. N. (2020). Investigation of the Role of Dinutuximab Beta-Based Immunotherapy in the SIOPEN High-Risk Neuroblastoma 1 Trial (HR-NBL1). *Cancers (Basel)*, *12*(2), 309. Advance online publication. DOI: 10.3390/cancers12020309 PMID: 32013055

Lakatos, P. L., & Lakatos, L. (2008). Risk for colorectal cancer in ulcerative colitis: Changes, causes and management strategies. *World Journal of Gastroenterology*, *14*(25), 3937–3947. DOI: 10.3748/wjg.14.3937 PMID: 18609676

Lambert, J. D., Hong, J., Yang, G. Y., Liao, J., & Yang, C. S. (2005). Inhibition of carcinogenesis by polyphenols: Evidence from laboratory investigations. *The American Journal of Clinical Nutrition*, *81*(1, Suppl), 284S–291S. DOI: 10.1093/ajcn/81.1.284S PMID: 15640492

Lampert, M., Orogo, A., Najor, R., Hammerling, B., Leon, L., Wang, B., Kim, T., Sussman, M., & Gustafsson, Å. (2019). BNIP3L/NIX and FUNDC1-mediated mitophagy is required for mitochondrial network remodeling during cardiac progenitor cell differentiation. *Autophagy*, *15*(7), 1182–1198. DOI: 10.1080/15548627.2019.1580095 PMID: 30741592

Landais, E., Moskal, A., Mullee, A., Nicolas, G., Gunter, M. J., Huybrechts, I., Overvad, K., Roswall, N., Affret, A., Fagherazzi, G., Mahamat-Saleh, Y., Katzke, V., Kühn, T., La Vecchia, C., Trichopoulou, A., Valanou, E., Saieva, C., Santucci de Magistris, M., Sieri, S., & Freisling, H. (2018). Coffee and Tea Consumption and the Contribution of Their Added Ingredients to Total Energy and Nutrient Intakes in 10 European Countries: Benchmark Data from the Late 1990s. *Nutrients*, *10*(6), 725. DOI: 10.3390/nu10060725 PMID: 29874819

Lauzier, A., Normandeau-Guimond, J., Vaillancourt-Lavigueur, V., Boivin, V., Charbonneau, M., Rivard, N., Scott, M. S., Dubois, C. M., & Jean, S. (2019). Colorectal cancer cells respond differentially to autophagy inhibition in vivo. *Scientific Reports*, *9*(1), 11316. Advance online publication. DOI: 10.1038/s41598-019-47659-7 PMID: 31383875

Lazarou, M., Sliter, D. A., Kane, L. A., Sarraf, S. A., Wang, C., Burman, J. L., Sideris, D. P., Fogel, A. I., & Youle, R. J. (2015). The ubiquitin kinase PINK1 recruits' autophagy receptors to induce mitophagy. Nature 2015 524:7565, 524(7565), 309–314. DOI: 10.1038/nature14893

Lazova, R., Camp, R. L., Klump, V., Siddiqui, S. F., Amaravadi, R. K., & Pawelek, J. M. (2012). Punctate LC3B expression is a common feature of solid tumors and associated with proliferation, metastasis, and poor outcome. *Clinical Cancer Research*, *18*(2), 370–379. DOI: 10.1158/1078-0432.CCR-11-1282 PMID: 22080440

Lee, C., Park, S.-H., & Yoon, S. K. (2024). The E3 ligase HUWE1 increases the sensitivity of CRC to oxaliplatin through TOMM20 degradation. *Oncogene*, *43*(9), 636–649. DOI: 10.1038/s41388-023-02928-8 PMID: 38184713

Lee, H. (2023). Integrative analysis of herbal medicine's efficacy in breast cancer treatment. *Frontiers in Pharmacology and Herbal Medicine*, *14*(5), 1122–1138.

Lee, I. H., Kawai, Y., Fergusson, M. M., Rovira, I. I., Bishop, A. J. R., Motoyama, N., Cao, L., & Finkel, T. (2012). Atg7 modulates p53 activity to regulate cell cycle and survival during metabolic stress. *Science*, *336*(6078), 225–228. DOI: 10.1126/science.1218395 PMID: 22499945

Lee, J. (2019). Epicatechin enhances mitophagy in breast cancer: Mechanistic insights. *Food and Chemical Toxicology*, *128*, 35–44.

Lee, J. Y., Nagano, Y., Taylor, J. P., Lim, K. L., & Yao, T. P. (2010). Disease-causing mutations in parkin impair mitochondrial ubiquitination, aggregation, and HDAC6-dependent mitophagy. *The Journal of Cell Biology*, *189*(4), 671–679. DOI: 10.1083/jcb.201001039 PMID: 20457763

Lee, K., & Yun, J. (2022). Mitophagy stimulation as a novel strategy for the treatment of mitochondrial diseases. *Journal of Genetic Medicine*, *19*(2), 49–56. DOI: 10.5734/JGM.2022.19.2.49

Lee, S., Son, J. Y., Lee, J., & Cheong, H. (2023). Unraveling the Intricacies of Autophagy and Mitophagy: Implications in Cancer Biology. *Cells*, *12*(23), 2742. DOI: 10.3390/cells12232742 PMID: 38067169

Lee, Y. H., Martin-Orozco, N., Zheng, P., Li, J., Zhang, P., Tan, H., Park, H. J., Jeong, M., Chang, S. H., Kim, B.-S., Xiong, W., Zang, W., Guo, L., Liu, Y., Dong, Z., Overwijk, W. W., Hwu, P., Yi, Q., Kwak, L., & Dong, C. (2017). Inhibition of the B7-H3 immune checkpoint limits tumor growth by enhancing cytotoxic lymphocyte function. *Cell Research*, *27*(8), 1034–1045. DOI: 10.1038/cr.2017.90 PMID: 28685773

Lei, Y., Gan, M., Qiu, Y., Chen, Q., Wang, X., Liao, T., Zhao, M., Chen, L., Zhang, S., Zhao, Y., Niu, L., Wang, Y., Zhu, L., & Shen, L. (2024). The role of mitochondrial dynamics and mitophagy in skeletal muscle atrophy: From molecular mechanisms to therapeutic insights. *Cellular & Molecular Biology Letters*, *29*(1), 59. DOI: 10.1186/s11658-024-00572-y PMID: 38654156

Lemasters, J. J. (2005). Selective mitochondrial autophagy, or mitophagy, as a targeted defense against oxidative stress, mitochondrial dysfunction, and aging. *Rejuvenation Research*, *8*(1), 3–5. DOI: 10.1089/rej.2005.8.3 PMID: 15798367

Levine, B., & Kroemer, G. (2019). Biological functions of autophagy genes: A disease perspective. *Cell*, *176*(1–2), 11–42. DOI: 10.1016/j.cell.2018.09.048 PMID: 30633901

Levy, J. M. M., Towers, C. G., & Thorburn, A. (2017). Targeting autophagy in cancer. *Nature Reviews. Cancer*, *17*(9), 528–542. DOI: 10.1038/nrc.2017.53 PMID: 28751651

Liang, C., Feng, P., Ku, B., Dotan, I., Canaani, D., Oh, B. H., & Jung, J. U. (2006). Autophagic and tumour suppressor activity of a novel Beclin1-binding protein UVRAG. *Nature Cell Biology*, *8*(7), 688–698. DOI: 10.1038/ncb1426 PMID: 16799551

Liang, H., Ma, Z., Zhong, W., Liu, J., Sugimoto, K., & Chen, H. (2024). Regulation of mitophagy and mitochondrial function: Natural compounds as potential therapeutic strategies for Parkinson's disease. *Phytotherapy Research*, *38*(4), 1838–1862. DOI: 10.1002/ptr.8156 PMID: 38356178

Liang, J., Wang, X. S., Zhen, H. S., Zhong, Z. G., Zhang, W. Y., Zhang, W. W., & Li, W. L. (2007). [Study on anti-tumor effect of extractions from roots of *Actinidia deliciosa*]. *Zhong Yao Cai*, *30*(10), 1279–1282. PMID: 18300504

Liang, K., Zhou, G., Zhang, Q., Li, J., & Zhang, C. (2014). Expression of Hippo pathway in colorectal cancer. *Saudi Journal of Gastroenterology : Official Journal of the Saudi Gastroenterology Association*, *20*(3), 188–194. DOI: 10.4103/1319-3767.133025 PMID: 24976283

Liang, W., He, X., Bi, J., Hu, T., & Sun, Y. (2021). Role of reactive oxygen species in tumors based on the 'seed and soil'theory: A complex interaction. *Oncology Reports*, *46*(3), 1–15. DOI: 10.3892/or.2021.8159 PMID: 34328200

Liang, X. H., Jackson, S., Seaman, M., Brown, K., Kempkes, B., Hibshoosh, H., & Levine, B. (1999). Induction of autophagy and inhibition of tumorigenesis by beclin 1. *Nature*, *402*(6762), 672–676. DOI: 10.1038/45257 PMID: 10604474

Liao, J., Li, Q., Hu, Z., Yu, W., Zhang, K., Ma, F., Han, Q., Zhang, H., Guo, J., Hu, L., Pan, J., Li, Y., & Tang, Z. (2021). Mitochondrial miR-1285 regulates copper-induced mitochondrial dysfunction and mitophagy by impairing IDH2 in pig jejunal epithelial cells. *Journal of Hazardous Materials*, *422*, 126899. DOI: 10.1016/j.jhazmat.2021.126899 PMID: 34418838

Li, C., Zhang, Y., Cheng, X., Yuan, H., Zhu, S., Liu, J., Wen, Q., Wang, X., Zhang, Y., & Kang, R. (2018). PINK1 and PARK2 suppress pancreatic tumorigenesis through control of mitochondrial iron-mediated immunometabolism. *Developmental Cell*, *46*(4), 441–455. DOI: 10.1016/j.devcel.2018.07.012 PMID: 30100261

Li, J. J., Yan, Y. Y., Sun, H. M., Liu, Y., Su, C. Y., Chen, H. B., & Zhang, J. Y. (2019). Anti-Cancer Effects of Pristimerin and the Mechanisms: A Critical Review. *Frontiers in Pharmacology*, *2019*(10), 746. DOI: 10.3389/fphar.2019.00746 PMID: 31354475

Li, J., Ji, Y., Chen, N., Dai, L., & Deng, H. (2023). Colitis-associated carcinogenesis: Crosstalk between tumors, immune cells and gut microbiota. *Cell & Bioscience*, *13*(1), 194. DOI: 10.1186/s13578-023-01139-8 PMID: 37875976

Li, J., Ma, Y., Qiu, T., Wang, J., Zhang, J., Sun, X., Jiang, L., Li, Q., & Yao, X. (2024). Autophagy-dependent lysosomal calcium overload and the ATP5B-regulated lysosomes-mitochondria calcium transmission induce liver insulin resistance under perfluorooctane sulfonate exposure. *Ecotoxicology and Environmental Safety*, *276*, 116318. DOI: 10.1016/j.ecoenv.2024.116318 PMID: 38626609

Li, J., Wu, J., Zhou, X., Lü, Y., Ge, Y., & Zhang, X. (2023). Targeting neuronal mitophagy in ischemic stroke: An update. *Burns and Trauma*, *11*, 11. DOI: 10.1093/burnst/tkad018 PMID: 37274155

Li, J., Yang, D., Li, Z., Zhao, M., Wang, D., Sun, Z., Wen, P., Dai, Y., Gou, F., Ji, Y., Zhao, D., & Yang, L. (2022). PINK1/Parkin-mediated mitophagy in neurodegenerative diseases. *Ageing Research Reviews*, •••, 84. PMID: 36503124

Li, J., Yang, Y., & Lin, W. (2020). Sulforaphane-induced mitophagy promotes apoptosis in prostate cancer. *Cancer Letters*, *482*, 23–34. DOI: 10.1016/j.canlet.2020.05.010

Li, K., & Lai, H. (2017). Tanshinone IIA enhances the chemosensitivity of breast cancer cells to doxorubicin through down-regulating the expression of MDR-related ABC transporters. *Biomedicine and Pharmacotherapy*, *96*, 371–377. DOI: 10.1016/j.biopha.2017.10.016 PMID: 29028589

Li, L., & Moore, P. K. (2007). An overview of the biological significance of endogenous gases: New roles for old molecules. *Biochemical Society Transactions*, *35*(5), 1138–1141. DOI: 10.1042/BST0351138 PMID: 17956296

Li, L., Zhang, W., Jiang, Y., Wang, S., & Jia, L. (2021). Camptothecin Inhibits Neddylation to Activate the Protective Autophagy Through NF-kappaB/AMPK/mTOR/ULK1 Axis in Human Esophageal Cancer Cells. *Frontiers in Oncology*, *11*, 671180. DOI: 10.3389/fonc.2021.671180 PMID: 33898327

Li, M., Ding, L., Cao, L., Zhang, Z., Li, X., Li, Z., Xia, Q., Yin, K., Song, S., Wang, Z., & Du, H. (2025). Natural products targeting AMPK signaling pathway therapy, diabetes mellitus and its complications. *Frontiers in Pharmacology*, *16*, 4634–4644.

Li, N., Ragheb, K., Lawler, G., Sturgis, J., Rajwa, B., Melendez, J. A., & Robinson, J. P. (2003). Mitochondrial complex I inhibitor rotenone induces apoptosis through enhancing mitochondrial reactive oxygen species production. *The Journal of Biological Chemistry*, *278*(10), 8516–8525. DOI: 10.1074/jbc.M210432200 PMID: 12496265

Ling, Z., Pan, J., Zhang, Z., Chen, G., Geng, J., Lin, Q., Zhang, T., Cao, S., Chen, C., Lin, J., Yuan, H., Ding, W., Xiao, F., Xu, X., Li, F., Wang, G., Zhang, Y., & Li, J. (2024). Small-molecule Molephantin induces apoptosis and mitophagy flux blockage through ROS production in glioblastoma. *Cancer Letters*, *592*, 216927. DOI: 10.1016/j.canlet.2024.216927 PMID: 38697460

Lin, L. T., Uen, W. C., Choong, C. Y., Shi, Y. C., Lee, B. H., Tai, C. J., & Tai, C. J. (2019). Paris Polyphylla Inhibits Colorectal Cancer Cells via Inducing Autophagy and Enhancing the Efficacy of Chemotherapeutic Drug Doxorubicin. *Molecules (Basel, Switzerland)*, *24*(11), 2102. DOI: 10.3390/molecules24112102 PMID: 31163662

Lin, X., Liu, W., Hu, X., Liu, Z., Wang, F., & Wang, J. (2024). The Role of Polyphenols in Modulating Mitophagy: Implications for Therapeutic Interventions. *Pharmacological Research*, *207*, 107324. DOI: 10.1016/j.phrs.2024.107324 PMID: 39059613

Lin, Y., Chen, Y., Wang, S., Ma, J., Peng, Y., Yuan, X., Lv, B., Chen, W., & Wei, Y. (2019). Plumbagin induces autophagy and apoptosis of SMMC-7721 cells in vitro and in vivo. *Journal of Cellular Biochemistry*, *120*(6), 9820–9830. DOI: 10.1002/jcb.28262 PMID: 30536473

Li, Q., Qi, F., Meng, X., Zhu, C., & Gao, Y. (2018). Mst1 regulates colorectal cancer stress response via inhibiting Bnip3-related mitophagy by activation of JNK/p53 pathway. *Cell Biology and Toxicology*, *34*(4), 263–277. DOI: 10.1007/s10565-017-9417-6 PMID: 29063978

Liu, T., Zhang, J., Li, K., Deng, L., & Wang, H. (2020). Combination of an autophagy inducer and an autophagy inhibitor: A smarter strategy emerging in cancer therapy. *Frontiers in Pharmacology, 11*, 48, 408. PMID: 32322202DOI: 10.3389/fphar.2020.00408

Liu, C., Wang, J., Yang, Y., Liu, X., Zhu, Y., Zou, J., Peng, S., Le, T. H., Chen, Y., Zhao, S., He, B., Mi, Q., Zhang, X., & Du, Q. (2018). Ginsenoside Rd ameliorates colitis by inducing p62-driven mitophagy-mediated NLRP3 inflammasome inactivation in mice. *Biochemical Pharmacology*, *155*, 366–379. DOI: 10.1016/j.bcp.2018.07.010 PMID: 30012462

Liu, H., Song, J., Zhou, Y., Cao, L., Gong, Y., Wei, Y., Yang, H., & Tang, L. (2019). Methylxanthine derivatives promote autophagy in gastric cancer cells targeting PTEN. *Anti-Cancer Drugs*, *30*(4), 347–355. DOI: 10.1097/CAD.0000000000000724 PMID: 30875347

Liu, H., Song, Y., Wang, H., Zhou, Y., Xu, M., & Xian, J. (2025). Deciphering the Power of Resveratrol in Mitophagy: From Molecular Mechanisms to Therapeutic Applications. *Phytotherapy Research*, *39*(3), 1319–1343. DOI: 10.1002/ptr.8433 PMID: 39754508

Liu, J., Liu, W., Li, R., & Yang, H. (2019). Mitophagy in Parkinson's disease: From pathogenesis to treatment. *Cells*, *8*(7), 712. DOI: 10.3390/cells8070712 PMID: 31336937

Liu, J., Ma, H., Wu, Z., Ji, Y., & Liang, Y. (2024). The Knowns and Unknowns of Membrane Features and Changes During Autophagosome–Lysosome/Vacuole Fusion. *International Journal of Molecular Sciences*, *25*(20), 11160. DOI: 10.3390/ijms252011160 PMID: 39456939

Liu, L., Feng, D., Chen, G., Chen, M., Zheng, Q., Song, P., Ma, Q., Zhu, C., Wang, R., Qi, W., Huang, L., Xue, P., Li, B., Wang, X., Jin, H., Wang, J., Yang, F., Liu, Y., & Chen, Q. (2012). Mitochondrial outer-membrane protein FUNDC1 mediates hypoxia-induced mitophagy in mammalian cells. *Nature Cell Biology*, *14*(2), 177–185. DOI: 10.1038/ncb2422 PMID: 22267086

Liu, L., Wang, Y., & Ren, J. (2018). Curcumin-induced mitophagy regulates cell fate in cancer therapy. *Autophagy*, *14*(5), 870–886. DOI: 10.1080/15548627.2018.1439431 PMID: 29433359

Liu, Q., Sun, Y., & Liu, Z. (2022). Piperlongumine enhances mitophagy and suppresses colorectal cancer cell growth. *Cellular Physiology and Biochemistry*, *56*(3), 349–360. DOI: 10.33594/000000001

Liu, Q., Yang, Y., Tan, X., Tao, Z., Adah, D., Yu, S., Lu, J., Zhao, S., Qin, L., Qin, L., & Chen, X. (2017). Plasmodium parasite as an effective hepatocellular carcinoma antigen glypican-3 delivery vector. *Oncotarget*, *8*(15), 24785–24796. DOI: 10.18632/oncotarget.15806 PMID: 28445973

Liu, S., Li, Q., Li, G., Zhang, Q., Zhuo, L., Han, X., Zhang, M., Chen, X., Pan, T., Yan, L., Jin, T., Wang, J., Lv, Q., Sui, X., & Xie, T. (2020). The mechanism of m^6A methyltransferase METTL3-mediated autophagy in reversing gefitinib resistance in NSCLC cells by β-elemene. *Cell Death & Disease*, *11*(11), 969. DOI: 10.1038/s41419-020-03148-8 PMID: 33177491

Liu, S., Yao, S., Yang, H., Liu, S., & Wang, Y. (2023). Autophagy: Regulator of cell death. *Cell Death & Disease*, *14*(10), 648. Advance online publication. DOI: 10.1038/s41419-023-06154-8 PMID: 37794028

Liu, T., Men, Q., Wu, G., Yu, C., Huang, Z., Liu, X., & Li, W. (2015). Tetrandrine induces autophagy and differentiation by activating ROS and Notch1 signaling in leukemia cells. *Oncotarget*, *6*(10), 7992–8006. DOI: 10.18632/oncotarget.3505 PMID: 25797266

Liu, Y., Fu, Y., Hu, X., Wang, Y., Zhou, Y., Zhang, L., & Wang, L. (2020). Caveolin-1 knockdown increases the therapeutic sensitivity of lung cancer to cisplatin-induced apoptosis by repressing Parkin-related mitophagy and activating the ROCK1 pathway. *Journal of Cellular Physiology*, *235*(2), 1197–1208. DOI: 10.1002/jcp.29033 PMID: 31270811

Liu, Y., Li, C. L., Xu, Q. Q., Cheng, D., Liu, K. D., & Sun, Z. Q. (2021). Quercetin inhibits invasion and angiogenesis of esophageal cancer cells. *Pathology, Research and Practice*, *222*, 153455. DOI: 10.1016/j.prp.2021.153455 PMID: 33962176

Liu, Y., & Ma, Z. (2024). Leukemia and mitophagy: A novel perspective for understanding oncogenesis and resistance. *Annals of Hematology*, *xx*(x), xxx–xxx. DOI: 10.1007/s00277-024-05635-w PMID: 38282059

Liu, Y., Wang, Y., Zhang, J., Peng, Q., Wang, X., Xiao, X., & Shi, K. (2024). Nanotherapeutics targeting autophagy regulation for improved cancer therapy. *Acta Pharmaceutica Sinica. B*, *xx*(x), xxx–xxx. DOI: 10.1016/j.apsb.2024.03.019 PMID: 38828133

Liu, Z., Sun, Q., Zhang, C., Yuan, H., & He, W. (2021). Activity-based fluorescent molecular logic gate probe for dynamic tracking of mitophagy induced by oxidative stress. *Analytical Chemistry*, *93*(7), 3502–3509. DOI: 10.1021/acs.analchem.0c04854 PMID: 33544570

Li, W., Li, Y., Siraj, S., Jin, H., Fan, Y., Yang, X., & Chen, Q. (2019). FUN14 Domain-containing 1–mediated mitophagy suppresses hepatocarcinogenesis by inhibition of inflammasome activation in mice. *Hepatology (Baltimore, Md.)*, *69*(2), 604–621. DOI: 10.1002/hep.30191/suppinfo PMID: 30053328

Li, W., Tanikawa, T., Kryczek, I., Xia, H., Li, G., Wu, K. E., Wei, S., Zhao, L., Vatan, L., Wen, B., Shu, P., Sun, D., Kleer, C., Wicha, M., Sabel, M., Tao, K., Wang, G., & Zou, W. (2018). Aerobic glycolysis controls myeloid-derived suppressor cells and tumor immunity via a specific CEBPB isoform in triple-negative breast cancer. *Cell Metabolism*, *28*(1), 87–103. DOI: 10.1016/j.cmet.2018.04.022 PMID: 29805099

Li, W., & Xu, X. (2023). Advances in mitophagy and mitochondrial apoptosis pathway-related drugs in glioblastoma treatment. *Frontiers in Pharmacology*, *14*, 1719–1725. DOI: 10.3389/fphar.2023.1211719 PMID: 37456742

Li, X., He, S., & Ma, B. (2020). Autophagy and autophagy-related proteins in cancer. *Molecular Cancer*, *19*(1), 12. DOI: 10.1186/s12943-020-1138-4 PMID: 31969156

Li, Y., Zhang, X., Yang, J., Zhang, Y., Zhu, D., Zhang, L., Zhu, Y., Li, D., & Zhou, J. (2017). Methylation of BNIP3 in pancreatic cancer inhibits the induction of mitochondrial-mediated tumor cell apoptosis. *Oncotarget*, *8*(38), 63208–63222. DOI: 10.18632/oncotarget.18736 PMID: 28968982

Li, Y., Zheng, W., Lu, Y., Zheng, Y., Pan, L., Wu, X., Yuan, Y., Shen, Z., Ma, S., Zhang, X., Wu, J., Chen, Z., & Zhang, X. (2021). BNIP3L/NIX-mediated mitophagy: Molecular mechanisms and implications for human disease. *Cell Death & Disease*, *13*(1), 14. DOI: 10.1038/s41419-021-04469-y PMID: 34930907

Li, Z., Wang, Y., Wu, L., Wang, C., Wang, P., Ma, Q., & Zhang, L. (2019). Apurinic endonuclease 1 promotes the cisplatin resistance of lung cancer cells by inducing Parkin-mediated mitophagy. *Oncology Reports*, *42*(6), 2245–2254. DOI: 10.3892/or.2019.7345 PMID: 31578585

Lock, R., Roy, S., Kenific, C. M., Su, J. S., Salas, E., Ronen, S. M., & Debnath, J. (2011). Autophagy facilitates glycolysis during Ras-mediated oncogenic transformation. *Molecular Biology of the Cell*, *22*(2), 165–178. DOI: 10.1091/mbc.e10-06-0500 PMID: 21119005

London, W. B., Bagatell, R., Weigel, B. J., Fox, E., Guo, D., Van Ryn, C., Naranjo, A., & Park, J. R. (2017). Historical time to disease progression and progression-free survival in patients with recurrent/refractory neuroblastoma treated in the modern era on Children's Oncology Group early-phase trials. *Cancer*, *123*(24), 4914–4923. DOI: 10.1002/cncr.30934 PMID: 28885700

Longo, M., Paolini, E., Meroni, M., & Dongiovanni, P. (2021). Remodeling of Mitochondrial Plasticity: The Key Switch from NAFLD/NASH to HCC. *International Journal of Molecular Sciences*, *22*(8), 4173. DOI: 10.3390/ijms22084173 PMID: 33920670

Loos, M., Hedderich, D. M., Friess, H., & Kleeff, J. (2010). B7-h3 and its role in antitumor immunity. *Clinical & Developmental Immunology*, *683875*(1), 683875. Advance online publication. DOI: 10.1155/2010/683875 PMID: 21127709

Lopes, T. Z., de Moraes, F. R., Tedesco, A. C., Arni, R. K., Rahal, P., & Calmon, M. F. (2020). Berberine associated photodynamic therapy promotes autophagy and apoptosis via ROS generation in renal carcinoma cells. *Biomedicine and Pharmacotherapy*, *123*, 109794. DOI: 10.1016/j.biopha.2019.109794 PMID: 31874443

Lorent, J. H., Léonard, C., Abouzi, M., Akabi, F., Quetin-Leclercq, J., & Mingeot-Leclercq, M. P. (2016). α-Hederin induces apoptosis, membrane permeabilization and morphologic changes in two cancer cell lines through a cholesterol-dependent mechanism. *Planta Medica*, *82*(18), 1532–1539. DOI: 10.1055/s-0042-114780 PMID: 27574896

Lou, G., Palikaras, K., Lautrup, S., Scheibye-Knudsen, M., Tavernarakis, N., & Fang, E. (2020). Mitophagy and neuroprotection. *Trends in Molecular Medicine*, *26*(1), 8–20. DOI: 10.1016/j.molmed.2019.07.002 PMID: 31375365

Luan, F., He, X., & Zeng, N. (2020). Tetrandrine: A review of its anticancer potentials, clinical settings, pharmacokinetics and drug delivery systems. *The Journal of Pharmacy and Pharmacology*, *72*(11), 1491–1512. DOI: 10.1111/jphp.13339 PMID: 32696989

Luan, Y., Jiang, L., Luan, Y., Xie, Y., Yang, Y., & Ren, K. (2023). Mitophagy and traumatic brain injury: Regulatory mechanisms and therapeutic potentials. *Oxidative Medicine and Cellular Longevity*, *2023*, 1–15. DOI: 10.1155/2023/1649842 PMID: 36846712

Lu, G., Wang, L., Zhou, J., Liu, W., & Shen, H. M. (2021). A Destiny for Degradation: Interplay between Cullin-RING E3 Ligases and Autophagy. *Trends in Cell Biology*, *31*(6), 432–444. DOI: 10.1016/j.tcb.2021.01.005 PMID: 33573849

Lu, J., Chew, E. L., & Holmgren, A. (2007). Targeting thioredoxin reductase is a basis for cancer therapy by arsenic trioxide. *Proceedings of the National Academy of Sciences of the United States of America*, *104*(30), 12288–12293. DOI: 10.1073/pnas.0701549104 PMID: 17640917

Lu, J., Guan, S., Zhao, Y., Yu, Y., Woodfield, S. E., Zhang, H., Yang, K. L., Bieerkehazhi, S., Qi, L., Li, X., Gu, J., Xu, X., Jin, J., Muscal, J. A., Yang, T., Xu, G.-T., & Yang, J. (2017). The second-generation ALK inhibitor alectinib effectively induces apoptosis in human neuroblastoma cells and inhibits tumor growth in a TH-MYCN transgenic neuroblastoma mouse model. *Cancer Letters*, *400*, 61–68. DOI: 10.1016/j.canlet.2017.04.022 PMID: 28455243

Luo, P., An, Y., He, J., Xing, X., Zhang, Q., Liu, X., Chen, Y., Yuan, H., Chen, J., Wong, Y.-K., Huang, J., Gong, Z., Du, Q., Xiao, W., & Wang, J. (2024). Icaritin with autophagy/mitophagy inhibitors synergistically enhances anticancer efficacy and apoptotic effects through PINK1/Parkin-mediated mitophagy in hepatocellular carcinoma. *Cancer Letters*, *587*, 216621. DOI: 10.1016/j.canlet.2024.216621 PMID: 38242198

Luo, Y., Chen, R., Wei, S., Yang, X., & Wang, Q. (2019). Betulinic acid induces autophagy-mediated apoptosis through suppression of the PI3K/AKT/mTOR signaling pathway and inhibits hepatocellular carcinoma. *American Journal of Translational Research*, *11*, 6952–6964. PMID: 31814899

Lushchak, V. I. (2011). Adaptive response to oxidative stress: Bacteria, fungi, plants, and animals. *Comparative Biochemistry and Physiology. Toxicology & Pharmacology : CBP*, *153*(2), 175–190. DOI: 10.1016/j.cbpc.2010.10.004 PMID: 20959147

Lu, X., Altshuler-Keylin, S., Wang, Q., Chen, Y. C., Sponton, C. H., & Kajimura, S. (2018). Mitophagy controls beige adipocyte maintenance through a Parkin-dependent and UCP1-independent mechanism. *Science Signaling*, *11*(527), eaap8526. Advance online publication. DOI: 10.1126/scisignal.aap8526 PMID: 29692364

Lu, X., Liu, Q., Zhang, J., Zhou, D., Yang, G., Li, M., Qiu, Y., Chen, Q., Zheng, H., & Dai, J. (2020). PINK1 overexpression promotes cell migration and proliferation via regulation of autophagy and predicts a poor prognosis in lung cancer cases. *Cancer Management and Research*, *12*, 7703–7714. DOI: 10.2147/CMAR.S262466 PMID: 32904694

L , Y., Li, Z., Zhang, S., Zhang, T., Liu, Y., & Zhang, L. (2023). Cellular mitophagy: Mechanism, roles in diseases and small molecule pharmacological regulation. *Theranostics*, *13*(2), 736–766. DOI: 10.7150/thno.79876 PMID: 36632220

Lv, S., Zhang, G., Lu, Y., Zhong, X., Huang, Y., Ma, Y., Yan, W., Teng, J., & Wei, S. (2024). Pharmacological mechanism of natural antidepressants: The role of mitochondrial quality control. *Phytomedicine*, *129*, 155669. DOI: 10.1016/j.phymed.2024.155669 PMID: 38696923

Lystad, A. H., & Simonsen, A. (2019). Mechanisms and pathophysiological roles of the ATG8 conjugation machinery. *Cells*, *8*(9), 973. DOI: 10.3390/cells8090973 PMID: 31450711

Lyu, L., Hu, Y., Yin, S., Wang, L., Ye, F., Wang, M., Zhou, Y., Ma, W., Chen, C., Jiang, Y., Wang, Z., Jiang, S., Zhou, P., & Wang, X. (2021). Autophagy inhibition enhances anti-pituitary adenoma effect of tetrandrine. *Phytotherapy Research*, *35*(7), 4007–4021. DOI: 10.1002/ptr.7117 PMID: 34038010

MacKeigan, J. P., Murphy, L. O., & Blenis, J. (2005). Sensitized RNAi screen of human kinases and phosphatases identifies new regulators of apoptosis and chemoresistance. *Nature Cell Biology*, *7*(6), 591–600. DOI: 10.1038/ncb1258 PMID: 15864305

Macleod, K. F. (2020). Mitophagy and Mitochondrial Dysfunction in Cancer. *4*(Volume 4, 2020), 41-60. doi:https://doi.org/DOI: 10.1146/annurev-cancerbio-030419-033405

Maestro, I., de la Ballina, L. R., Porras, G., Corrochano, S., De Lago, E., Simonsen, A., Boya, P., & Martinez, A. (2022). Discovery of Mitophagy Inhibitors with Therapeutic Potential in Different Familial Amyotrophic Lateral Sclerosis Mutations. *International Journal of Molecular Sciences*, *23*(20), 12676. DOI: 10.3390/ijms232012676 PMID: 36293534

Magistretti, P. J., & Allaman, I. (2015). A cellular perspective on brain energy metabolism and functional imaging. *Neuron*, *86*(4), 883–901. DOI: 10.1016/j.neuron.2015.03.035 PMID: 25996133

Maiti, P., Scott, J., Sengupta, D., Al-Gharaibeh, A., & Dunbar, G. (2019). Curcumin and Solid Lipid Curcumin Particles Induce Autophagy, but Inhibit Mitophagy and the PI3K-Akt/mTOR Pathway in Cultured Glioblastoma Cells. *International Journal of Molecular Sciences*, *20*(2), 20. DOI: 10.3390/ijms20020399 PMID: 30669284

Ma, K., Chen, G., Li, W., Kepp, O., Zhu, Y., & Chen, Q. (2020). Mitophagy, Mitochondrial Homeostasis, and Cell Fate. *Frontiers in Cell and Developmental Biology*, •••, 8. PMID: 32671064

Ma, K., Chen, G., Li, W., Kepp, O., Zhu, Y., & Chen, Q. (2020). Mitophagy, mitochondrial homeostasis, and cell fate. *Frontiers in Cell and Developmental Biology*, *8*, 467. DOI: 10.3389/fcell.2020.00467 PMID: 32671064

Malpartida, A. B., Williamson, M., Narendra, D. P., Wade-Martins, R., & Ryan, B. J. (2021). Mitochondrial dysfunction and mitophagy in Parkinson's disease: From mechanism to therapy. *Trends in Biochemical Sciences*, *46*(4), 329–343. DOI: 10.1016/j.tibs.2020.11.007 PMID: 33323315

Manczak, M., Kandimalla, R., Yin, X., & Reddy, P. H. (2018). Hippocampal mutant APP and amyloid beta-induced cognitive decline, dendritic spine loss, defective autophagy, mitophagy and mitochondrial abnormalities in a mouse model of Alzheimer's disease. *Human Molecular Genetics*, *27*(8), 1332–1342. DOI: 10.1093/hmg/ddy042 PMID: 29408999

Manganelli, V., Salvatori, I., Costanzo, M., Capozzi, A., Caissutti, D., Caterino, M., Valle, C., Ferri, A., Sorice, M., Ruoppolo, M., Garofalo, T., & Misasi, R. (2021). Overexpression of Neuroglobin Promotes Energy Metabolism and Autophagy Induction in Human Neuroblastoma SH-SY5Y Cells. *Cells*, *10*(12), 3394. Advance online publication. DOI: 10.3390/cells10123394 PMID: 34943907

Mansoori, B., Mohammadi, A., Davudian, S., Shirjang, S., & Baradaran, B. (2017a). The Different Mechanisms of Cancer Drug Resistance: A Brief Review. *Advanced Pharmaceutical Bulletin*, *7*(3), 339–348. DOI: 10.15171/apb.2017.041 PMID: 29071215

Mantovani, A. (2010). The growing diversity and spectrum of action of myeloid-derived suppressor cells. *European Journal of Immunology*, *40*(12), 3317–3320. DOI: 10.1002/eji.201041170 PMID: 21110315

Mao, K., Wang, K., Liu, X., & Klionsky, D. (2013). The scaffold protein atg11 recruits fission machinery to drive selective mitochondria degradation by autophagy. *Developmental Cell*, *26*(1), 9–18. DOI: 10.1016/j.devcel.2013.05.024 PMID: 23810512

Marinković, M., & Novak, I. (2021). A brief overview of BNIP3L/NIX receptor-mediated mitophagy. *FEBS Open Bio*, *11*(12), 3230–3236. DOI: 10.1002/2211-5463.13307 PMID: 34597467

Maris, J. M. (2010). Recent advances in neuroblastoma. *The New England Journal of Medicine*, *362*(23), 2202–2211. DOI: 10.1056/NEJMra0804577 PMID: 20558371

Maris, J. M., Morton, C. L., Gorlick, R., Kolb, E. A., Lock, R., Carol, H., Keir, S. T., Reynolds, C. P., Kang, M. H., Wu, J., Smith, M. A., & Houghton, P. J. (2010). Initial testing of the aurora kinase A inhibitor MLN8237 by the Pediatric Preclinical Testing Program (PPTP). *Pediatric Blood & Cancer*, *55*(1), 26–34. DOI: 10.1002/pbc.22430 PMID: 20108338

Martínez Reyes, I., & Chandel, N. S. (2020). Mitochondrial TCA cycle metabolites control physiology and disease. *Nature Communications*, *11*(1), 102. DOI: 10.1038/s41467-019-13668-3 PMID: 31900386

Martinez-Lopez, N., Garcia-Macia, M., Sahu, S., Athonvarangkul, D., Liebling, E., Merlo, P., Cecconi, F., Schwartz, G. J., & Singh, R. (2016). Autophagy in the CNS and periphery coordinate lipophagy and lipolysis in the brown adipose tissue and liver. *Cell Metabolism*, *23*(1), 113–127. DOI: 10.1016/j.cmet.2015.10.008 PMID: 26698918

Martínez-Reyes, I., & Chandel, N. S. (2021). Cancer metabolism: Looking forward. *Nature Reviews. Cancer*, *21*(10), 669–680. DOI: 10.1038/s41568-021-00378-6 PMID: 34272515

Masoudi, M., Moti, D., Masoudi, R., Auwal, A., Hossain, M. M., Pronoy, T. U. H., Rashel, K. M., Gopalan, V., & Islam, F. (2024). Metabolic adaptations in cancer stem cells: A key to therapy resistance. *Biochimica et Biophysica Acta (BBA) -. Biochimica et Biophysica Acta. Molecular Basis of Disease*, *1870*(5), 167164. DOI: 10.1016/j.bbadis.2024.167164 PMID: 38599259

Mathew, R., Karp, C. M., Beaudoin, B., Vuong, N., Chen, G., Chen, H. Y., Bray, K., Reddy, A., Bhanot, G., Gelinas, C., DiPaola, R. S., Karantza-Wadsworth, V., & White, E. (2009). Autophagy suppresses tumorigenesis through elimination of p62. *Cell*, *137*(6), 1062–1075. DOI: 10.1016/j.cell.2009.03.048 PMID: 19524509

Mathew, R., Khor, S., Hackett, S. R., Rabinowitz, J. D., Perlman, D. H., & White, E. (2014). Functional role of autophagy-mediated proteome remodeling in cell survival signaling and innate immunity. *Molecular Cell*, *55*(6), 916–930. DOI: 10.1016/j.molcel.2014.07.019 PMID: 25175026

Mathew, R., Kongara, S., Beaudoin, B., Karp, C. M., Bray, K., Degenhardt, K., Chen, G., Jin, S., & White, E. (2007). Autophagy suppresses tumor progression by limiting chromosomal instability. *Genes & Development*, *21*(11), 1367–1381. DOI: 10.1101/gad.1545107 PMID: 17510285

Mathiassen, S. G., De Zio, D., & Cecconi, F. (2017). Autophagy and the cell cycle: A complex landscape. *Frontiers in Oncology*, *7*, 51. Advance online publication. DOI: 10.3389/fonc.2017.00051 PMID: 28409123

Matsuyama, S., Llopis, J., Deveraux, Q. L., Tsien, R. Y., & Reed, J. C. (2000). Changes in intramitochondrial and cytosolic pH: Early events that modulate caspase activation during apoptosis. *Nature Cell Biology*, *2*(6), 318–325. DOI: 10.1038/35014006 PMID: 10854321

Matthay, K. K., Maris, J. M., Schleiermacher, G., Nakagawara, A., Mackall, C. L., Diller, L., & Weiss, W. A. (2016). Neuroblastoma. *Nature Reviews. Disease Primers*, *2*(1), 16078. DOI: 10.1038/nrdp.2016.78 PMID: 27830764

Mattio, L. M., Catinella, G., Dallavalle, S., & Pinto, A. (2020). Stilbenoids: A natural arsenal against bacterial pathogens. *Antibiotics (Basel, Switzerland)*, *9*(6), 336. DOI: 10.3390/antibiotics9060336 PMID: 32570824

Ma, W., Lu, Y., Jin, X., Lin, N., Zhang, L., & Song, Y. (2024). Targeting selective autophagy and beyond: From underlying mechanisms to potential therapies. *Journal of Advanced Research*, *x*(x), xxx–xxx. DOI: 10.1016/j.jare.2024.05.009 PMID: 38750694

Ma, X. H., Piao, S., Wang, D., Mcafee, Q. W., Nathanson, K. L., Lum, J. J., Li, L. Z., & Amaravadi, R. K. (2011). Measurements of tumor cell autophagy predict invasiveness, resistance to chemotherapy, and survival in melanoma. *Clinical Cancer Research*, *17*(10), 3478–3489. DOI: 10.1158/1078-0432.CCR-10-2372 PMID: 21325076

McLelland, G. L., Soubannier, V., Chen, C. X., McBride, H. M., & Fon, E. A. (2014). Parkin and PINK1 function in a vesicular trafficking pathway regulating mitochondrial quality control. *The EMBO Journal*, *33*(4), 282–295. DOI: 10.1002/embj.201385902 PMID: 24446486

McWilliams, T. G., & Muqit, M. M. (2017). PINK1 and Parkin: Emerging themes in mitochondrial homeostasis. *Current Opinion in Cell Biology*, *45*, 83–91. DOI: 10.1016/j.ceb.2017.03.013 PMID: 28437683

Mehdizadeh, S., Chen, G., Enayati, P. J., Cheng, D. W., Han, N. J., Shaye, O. A., Ippoliti, A., Vasiliauskas, E., Lo, S., & Papadakis, K. (2008). Diagnostic yield of capsule endoscopy in ulcerative colitis and inflammatory bowel disease of unclassified type (IBDU). *Endoscopy*, *40*(1), 30–35. DOI: 10.1055/s-2007-995359 PMID: 18058654

Mella-Raipán, J., Romero-Parra, J., & Recabarren-Gajardo, G. (2020). DARK classics in chemical neuroscience: Heroin and desomorphine. *ACS Chemical Neuroscience*, *11*(23), 3905–3927. DOI: 10.1021/acschemneuro.0c00262 PMID: 32568519

Meng, T., Wen, Z., Cheng, X., Li, C., Zhang, P., Xiao, D., & Xu, Y. (2025). Unlocking Gut Health: The Potent Role of Stilbenoids in Intestinal Homeostasis. *Animals (Basel), 15*(3), 417–426. DOI: 10.3390/ani15030417 PMID: 39943187

Messeha, S. S., Zarmouh, N. O., & Soliman, K. F. A. (2021). Polyphenols Modulating Effects of PD-L1/PD-1 Checkpoint and EMT-Mediated PD-L1 Overexpression in Breast Cancer. *Nutrients, 13*(5), 1718. DOI: 10.3390/nu13051718 PMID: 34069461

Miceli, C., Leri, M., Stefani, M., & Bucciantini, M. (2023). Autophagy-related proteins: Potential diagnostic and prognostic biomarkers of aging-related diseases. *Ageing Research Reviews, 89*, 101967. DOI: 10.1016/j.arr.2023.101967 PMID: 37270146

Misale, S., Di Nicolantonio, F., Sartore-Bianchi, A., Siena, S., & Bardelli, A. (2014). Resistance to Anti-EGFR Therapy in Colorectal Cancer: From Heterogeneity to Convergent Evolution. *Cancer Discovery, 4*(11), 1269–1280. DOI: 10.1158/2159-8290.CD-14-0462 PMID: 25293556

Mishra, S. R., Behera, B. P., Singh, V. K., Mahapatra, K. K., Mundkinajeddu, D., Bhat, D., Minz, A. M., Sethi, G., Efferth, T., Das, S., & Bhutia, S. K. (2024). Anticancer activity of Bacopa monnieri through apoptosis induction and mitophagy-dependent NLRP3 inflammasome inhibition in oral squamous cell carcinoma. *Phytomedicine, 123*, 155157. DOI: 10.1016/j.phymed.2023.155157 PMID: 37951147

Mishra, T., Singh, S., & Singh, T. G. (2024). Therapeutic Implications and Regulations of Protein Post-translational Modifications in Parkinsons Disease. *Cellular and Molecular Neurobiology, 44*(1), 53. DOI: 10.1007/s10571-024-01471-8 PMID: 38960968

Mizushima, N., & Levine, B. (2020). Autophagy in human diseases. *The New England Journal of Medicine, 383*(16), 1564–1576. DOI: 10.1056/NEJMra2022774 PMID: 33053285

Mlakar, V., Morel, E., Mlakar, S. J., Ansari, M., & Gumy-Pause, F. (2021). A review of the biological and clinical implications of RAS-MAPK pathway alterations in neuroblastoma. *Journal of Experimental & Clinical Cancer Research : CR, 40*(1), 189. DOI: 10.1186/s13046-021-01967-x PMID: 34103089

Mody, R., Naranjo, A., Van Ryn, C., Yu, A. L., London, W. B., Shulkin, B. L., Parisi, M. T., Servaes, S.-E.-N., Diccianni, M. B., Sondel, P. M., Bender, J. G., Maris, J. M., Park, J. R., & Bagatell, R. (2017). Irinotecan-temozolomide with temsirolimus or dinutuximab in children with refractory or relapsed neuroblastoma (COG ANBL1221): An open-label, randomised, phase 2 trial. *The Lancet. Oncology, 18*(7), 946–957. DOI: 10.1016/S1470-2045(17)30355-8 PMID: 28549783

Mohandas, K. M. (2011). Colorectal cancer in India: Controversies, enigmas and primary prevention. *Indian Journal of Gastroenterology*, *30*(1), 3–6. DOI: 10.1007/s12664-010-0076-2 PMID: 21222189

Mohebali, N., Pandurangan, A. K., Mustafa, M. R., Anandasadagopan, S. K., & Alagumuthu, T. (2020). Vernodalin induces apoptosis through ROS/JNK pathway activation in human colon cancer cells. *Journal of Biochemical and Molecular Toxicology*, *34*(12), e22577. DOI: 10.1002/jbt.22587 PMID: 32726518

Mohsen, S., Sobash, P. T., Algwaiz, G. F., Nasef, N., Al-Zeidaneen, S. A., & Karim, N. A. (2022). Autophagy Agents in Clinical Trials for Cancer Therapy: A Brief Review. *Current Oncology (Toronto, Ont.)*, *29*(3), 1695–1708. DOI: 10.3390/curroncol29030141 PMID: 35323341

Moindjie, H., Rodrigues-Ferreira, S., & Nahmias, C. (2021). Mitochondrial Metabolism in Carcinogenesis and Cancer Therapy. *Cancers (Basel)*, *13*(13), 3311. DOI: 10.3390/cancers13133311 PMID: 34282749

Molodecky, N. A., Soon, I. S., Rabi, D. M., Ghali, W. A., Ferris, M., Chernoff, G., Benchimol, E. I., Panaccione, R., Ghosh, S., Barkema, H. W., & Kaplan, G. G. (2012). Increasing incidence and prevalence of inflammatory bowel diseases with time, based on systematic review. *Gastroenterology*, *142*(1), 46–54.e42. DOI: 10.1053/j.gastro.2011.10.001 PMID: 22001864

Montemorano, L., Lightfoot, M. D., & Bixel, K. (2019). Role of Olaparib as Maintenance Treatment for Ovarian Cancer: The Evidence to Date. *OncoTargets and Therapy*, *12*, 11497–11506. DOI: 10.2147/OTT.S195552 PMID: 31920338

Mora, J., Chan, G. C.-F., Morgenstern, D. A., Nysom, K., Bear, M., Tornøe, K., Sørensen, P. S., & Kushner, B. H. (2022). Naxitamab (NAX) treatment for refractory/relapsed (R/R) high-risk neuroblastoma (HR-NB): Response data and efficacy in patient (pt) subgroups. *Journal of Clinical Oncology*, *40*(16, suppl), e22019–e22019. DOI: 10.1200/JCO.2022.40.16_suppl.e22019

Morales, D. M., Liu, F., & Herrera, N. (2023). Pomegranate extract as a potential adjuvant in breast cancer therapy: Insights into its mechanisms of action. *Cancer Biology & Therapy*, *24*(7), 1024–1037. DOI: 10.1080/15384047.2023.1924738

Morciano, G., Patergnani, S., Bonora, M., Pedriali, G., Tarocco, A., Bouhamida, E., Marchi, S., Ancora, G., Anania, G., Wieckowski, M., Giorgi, C., & Pinton, P. (2020). Mitophagy in Cardiovascular Diseases. *Journal of Clinical Medicine*, •••, 9. PMID: 32214047

Mosadegh, M., Noori Goodarzi, N., & Erfani, Y. (2025). A Comprehensive Insight into Apoptosis: Molecular Mechanisms, Signaling Pathways, and Modulating Therapeutics. *Cancer Investigation*, *7*(3), 1–26. DOI: 10.1080/07357907.2024.2445528 PMID: 39760426

Mosca, L., Ilari, A., Fazi, F., Assaraf, Y. G., & Colotti, G. (2021). Taxanes in cancer treatment: Activity, chemoresistance and its overcoming. *Drug Resistance Updates*, *54*, 100742. DOI: 10.1016/j.drup.2020.100742 PMID: 33429249

Moskot, M., Montefusco, S., Jakobkiewicz-Banecka, J., Mozolewski, P., Wegrzyn, A., Di Bernardo, D., Wegrzyn, G., Medina, D. L., Ballabio, A., & Gabig-Ciminska, M. (2014). The phytoestrogen genistein modulates lysosomal metabolism and transcription factor EB (TFEB) activation. *The Journal of Biological Chemistry*, *289*(24), 17054–17069. DOI: 10.1074/jbc.M114.555300 PMID: 24770416

Mossé, Y. P., Laudenslager, M., Longo, L., Cole, K. A., Wood, A., Attiyeh, E. F., Laquaglia, M. J., Sennett, R., Lynch, J. E., Perri, P., Laureys, G., Speleman, F., Kim, C., Hou, C., Hakonarson, H., Torkamani, A., Schork, N. J., Brodeur, G. M., Tonini, G. P., & Maris, J. M. (2008). Identification of ALK as a major familial neuroblastoma predisposition gene. *Nature*, *455*(7215), 930–935. DOI: 10.1038/nature07261 PMID: 18724359

Mostofa, A. G. M., Hossain, M. K., Basak, D., & Bin Sayeed, M. S. (2017). Thymoquinone as a Potential Adjuvant Therapy for Cancer Treatment: Evidence from Preclinical Studies. *Frontiers in Pharmacology*, *8*, 295. DOI: 10.3389/fphar.2017.00295 PMID: 28659794

Moulana, M. S., Haiaty, S., Bazmani, A., Shabkhizan, R., Moslehian, M. S., Sadeghsoltani, F., Mostafazadeh, M., Asadi, M. R., Talebi, M., Jafari, Z., Morovati, M. R., Farzaei, M. H., & Rahbarghazi, R. (2024). Tumoricidal properties of thymoquinone on human colorectal adenocarcinoma cells via the modulation of autophagy. *BMC Complementary Medicine and Therapies*, *24*(1), 132. DOI: 10.1186/s12906-024-04432-2 PMID: 38532470

Mu, D., Gao, Z., Guo, H., Zhou, G., & Sun, B. (2013). Sodium butyrate induces growth inhibition and apoptosis in human prostate cancer DU145 cells by up-regulation of the expression of annexin A1. *PLoS One*, *8*(9), e74922. DOI: 10.1371/journal.pone.0074922 PMID: 24086397

Mukherjee, S., Bhatti, G. K., Chhabra, R., Reddy, P. H., & Bhatti, J. S. (2023). Targeting mitochondria as a potential therapeutic strategy against chemoresistance in cancer. *Biomedicine and Pharmacotherapy*, *160*, 114398. DOI: 10.1016/j.biopha.2023.114398 PMID: 36773523

Mukhtar, E., Adhami, V. M., & Mukhtar, H. (2014). Targeting microtubules by natural agents for cancer therapy. *Molecular Cancer Therapeutics*, *2014*(13), 275–284. DOI: 10.1158/1535-7163.MCT-13-0791 PMID: 24435445

Mukhtar, Y. M., Adu-Frimpong, M., Xu, X., & Yu, J. (2018). Biochemical significance of limonene and its metabolites: Future prospects for designing and developing highly potent anticancer drugs. *Bioscience Reports*, *38*(6), BSR20181253. DOI: 10.1042/BSR20181253 PMID: 30287506

Murai, M., Toyota, M., Suzuki, H., Satoh, A., Sasaki, Y., Akino, K., Kikuchi, T., Mita, H., Tanaka, N., Itoh, F., & Tokino, T. (2005). Aberrant methylation and silencing of the BNIP3 gene in colorectal and gastric cancer. *Clinical Cancer Research*, *11*(3), 1021–1027. DOI: 10.1158/1078-0432.1021.11.3 PMID: 15709167

Nagdas, S. K., Daniel, F., Nascimento, A. L., Hussain, S. S., Trainor, R. E., Pollock, S. R., Adair, S. J., Michaels, A. D., Sesaki, H. S., & Elizabeth, B.. (2019). Drp1 promotes KRas-driven metabolic changes to drive pancreatic tumor growth. *Cell Reports*, *28*(7), 1845–1859.e5. DOI: 10.1016/j.celrep.2019.07.031 PMID: 31412251

Nah, J., Yuan, J., & Jung, Y. K. (2015). Autophagy in neurodegenerative diseases: From mechanism to therapeutic approach. *Molecules and Cells*, *38*(5), 381–389. DOI: 10.14348/molcells.2015.0034 PMID: 25896254

Nakahira, K., Haspel, J. A., Rathinam, V. A. K., Lee, S. J., Dolinay, T., Lam, H. C., Englert, J. A., Rabinovitch, M., Cernadas, M., Kim, H. P., Fitzgerald, K. A., Ryter, S. W., & Choi, A. M. K. (2011). Autophagy proteins regulate innate immune responses by inhibiting the release of mitochondrial DNA mediated by the NALP3 inflammasome. *Nature Immunology*, *12*(3), 222–230. DOI: 10.1038/ni.1980 PMID: 21151103

Nakashima, M., Suga, N., Ikeda, Y., Yoshikawa, S., & Matsuda, S. (2024). Inspiring tactics with the improvement of mitophagy and redox balance for the development of innovative treatment against polycystic kidney disease. *Biomolecules*, *14*(2), 207. DOI: 10.3390/biom14020207 PMID: 38397444

Nakashima, M., Suga, N., & Matsuda, S. (2024). Nutraceuticals modulating mitophagy may combat the mitochondrial dysfunction and redox stress in several cardiac disorders. *Kinases and Phosphatases*, *2*, 166–178. DOI: 10.3390/kinasesphosphatases2020010

Nakatogawa, H., Suzuki, K., Kamada, Y., & Ohsumi, Y. (2009). Dynamics and diversity in autophagy mechanisms: Lessons from yeast. *Nature Reviews. Molecular Cell Biology*, *10*(7), 458–467. DOI: 10.1038/nrm2708 PMID: 19491929

Nardone, O. M., Zammarchi, I., Santacroce, G., Ghosh, S., & Iacucci, M. (2023). Inflammation-driven colorectal cancer associated with colitis: From pathogenesis to changing therapy. *Cancers (Basel), 15*(8), 2389. DOI: 10.3390/cancers15082389 PMID: 37190315

Narendra, D. P., Jin, S. M., Tanaka, A., Suen, D. F., Gautier, C. A., Shen, J., Cookson, M. R., & Youle, R. J. (2010). PINK1 is selectively stabilized on impaired mitochondria to activate Parkin. *PLoS Biology, 8*(1), e1000298. DOI: 10.1371/journal.pbio.1000298 PMID: 20126261

Narendra, D. P., & Youle, R. J. (2011). Targeting mitochondrial dysfunction: Role for PINK1 and Parkin in mitochondrial quality control. *Antioxidants & Redox Signaling, 14*(10), 1929–1938. DOI: 10.1089/ars.2010.3799 PMID: 21194381

Narendra, D. P., & Youle, R. J. (2024). The role of PINK1–Parkin in mitochondrial quality control. *Nature Cell Biology, 26*(10), 1639–1651. DOI: 10.1038/s41556-024-01513-9 PMID: 39358449

Naso, F. D., Bruqi, K., Manzini, V., Chiurchiù, V., D'Onofrio, M., Arisi, I., & Strappazzon, F. (2024). miR-218-5p and doxorubicin combination enhances anticancer activity in breast cancer cells through Parkin-dependent mitophagy inhibition. *Cell Death Discovery, 10*(1), 149. DOI: 10.1038/s41420-024-01914-7 PMID: 38514650

Nazeam, J. A., El-Hefnawy, H. M., & Singab, A. B. (2020). Structural elucidation of immunomodulators, acetylated heteroglycan and galactosamine, isolated from *Aloe arborescens* leaves. *Journal of Medicinal Food, 23*(8), 895–901. DOI: 10.1089/jmf.2019.0229 PMID: 31976801

Nazha, B., Inal, C., & Owonikoko, T. K. (2020). Disialoganglioside GD2 Expression in Solid Tumors and Role as a Target for Cancer Therapy. *Frontiers in Oncology, 10*, 1000. DOI: 10.3389/fonc.2020.01000 PMID: 32733795

Newsholme, P., Cruzat, V. F., Keane, K. N., Carlessi, R., & De Bittencourt, P. I. H.Jr. (2016). Molecular mechanisms of ROS production and oxidative stress in diabetes. *The Biochemical Journal, 473*(24), 4527–4550. DOI: 10.1042/BCJ20160503C PMID: 27941030

Ney, P. A. (1853). 2015. Mitochondrial autophagy: Origins, significance, and role of BNIP3 and NIX. *Biochimica et Biophysica Acta (BBA)-. Molecular Cell Research*, (10), 2775–2783.

Ney, P. A. (2015). Mitochondrial autophagy: Origins, significance, and role of BNIP3 and NIX. *Biochimica et Biophysica Acta (BBA) -. Biochimica et Biophysica Acta. Molecular Cell Research, 1853*(10), 2775–2783. DOI: 10.1016/j.bbamcr.2015.02.022 PMID: 25753537

Nguyen, D. H., El-Ramady, H., Llanaj, X., Törős, G., Hajdú, P., & Prokisch, J. (2023). Chemical composition and health attributes of agri-foods: A scientific overview on black foods. *Sustainability (Basel), 15*(4), 3852. DOI: 10.3390/su15043852

Nicholson, J. K., Holmes, E., Kinross, J., Burcelin, R., Gibson, G., Jia, W., & Pettersson, S. (2012). Host-gut microbiota metabolic interactions. *Science, 336*(6086), 1262–1267. DOI: 10.1126/science.1223813 PMID: 22674330

Niemi, N. M., & Friedman, J. R. (2024). Coordinating BNIP3/NIX-mediated mitophagy in space and time. *Biochemical Society Transactions, 52*(5), 1969–1979. DOI: 10.1042/BST20221364 PMID: 39377319

Niewiadomski, O., Studd, C., Hair, C., Wilson, J., Ding, N. S., Heerasing, N., Ting, A., McNeill, J., Knight, R., Santamaria, J., Prewett, E., Dabkowski, P., Dowling, D., Alexander, S., Allen, B., Popp, B., Connell, W., Desmond, P., & Bell, S. (2015). Prospective population-based cohort of inflammatory bowel disease in the biologics era: Disease course and predictors of severity. *Journal of Gastroenterology and Hepatology, 30*(9), 1346–1353. DOI: 10.1111/jgh.12967 PMID: 25867770

Nikfardjam, M. S. P., Márk, L., Avar, P., Figler, M., & Ohmacht, R. (2006). Polyphenols, anthocyanins, and trans-resveratrol in red wines from the Hungarian Villány region. *Food Chemistry, 98*(3), 453–462. DOI: 10.1016/j.foodchem.2005.06.014

Niu, X., Fan, T., Li, W., Huang, H., Zhang, Y., & Xing, W. (2013). Protective effect of sanguinarine against acetic acid-induced ulcerative colitis in mice. *Toxicology and Applied Pharmacology, 267*(3), 256–265. DOI: 10.1016/j.taap.2013.01.009 PMID: 23352506

Noshita, N., Sugawara, T., Lewén, A., Hayashi, T., & Chan, P. H. (2003). Copper-zinc superoxide dismutase affects Akt activation after transient focal cerebral ischemia in mice. *Stroke, 34*(6), 1513–1518. DOI: 10.1161/01.STR.0000072986.46924.F4 PMID: 12738898

Novak, I. (2012). Mitophagy: A complex mechanism of mitochondrial removal. *Antioxidants & Redox Signaling, 17*(5), 794–802. DOI: 10.1089/ars.2011.4407 PMID: 22077334

Novak, I., & Dikic, I. (2011). Autophagy receptors in developmental clearance of mitochondria. *Autophagy*, *7*(3), 301–303. DOI: 10.4161/auto.7.3.14509 PMID: 21206218

Novak, I., Kirkin, V., McEwan, D. G., Zhang, J., Wild, P., Rozenknop, A., Rogov, V., Löhr, F., Popovic, D., Occhipinti, A., Reichert, A. S., Terzic, J., Dötsch, V., Ney, P. A., & Dikic, I. (2010). Nix is a selective autophagy receptor for mitochondrial clearance. *EMBO Reports*, *11*(1), 45–51. DOI: 10.1038/embor.2009.256 PMID: 20010802

Ntie-Kang, F., Telukunta, K. K., Döring, K., Simoben, C. V. A., Moumbock, A. F., Malange, Y. I., Njume, L. E., Yong, J. N., Sippl, W., & Günther, S. (2017). NANPDB: A Resource for Natural Products from Northern African Sources. *Journal of Natural Products*, *80*(7), 2067–2076. DOI: 10.1021/acs.jnatprod.7b00283 PMID: 28641017

Nunnari, J., & Suomalainen, A. (2012). Mitochondria: In sickness and in health. *Cell*, *148*(6), 1145–1159. DOI: 10.1016/j.cell.2012.02.035 PMID: 22424226

Ogidi, O. I. (2024). Phytochemical Screening and Bioinformatics Approaches for Anticancer Activity from Potential Plants. In: Computational Approaches in Biomaterials, Bioinformatics and Biomedical Engineering Applications. *CRC Press, Taylor and Francis Group, Florida, USA*.

Ogidi, O. I., & Ajoko, I. (2024). Neuroprotective Potentials of Phytochemicals. In: M.S. Rajput, T. Sarachana, P.D. Sarkar, M. Raval (eds) NeuroPhytomedicine. Published by *CRC Press, Routledge Taylor and Francis Group.*

Ogidi, O. I., & Emaikwu, N. G. (2024). Plant Phenolic compound isolation and its Bioinformatics Approaches of Molecular Mechanisms in Antimicrobial activities and Resistance. In: Computational Approaches in Biomaterials, Bioinformatics and Biomedical Engineering Applications. *CRC Press, Taylor and Francis Group, Florida, USA*. DOI: 10.1201/9781003354437-8

Ogidi, O. I., Ogoun, T. R., Alex, E. I., Edward, R. B., Joshua, M. T., & Bunu, E. M. (2024c). Radiogenomics and Genetic Diversity of Glioblastoma Characterization. In: Radiomics and Radiogenomics in Neuro-Oncology: An Artificial Intelligence Paradigm- volume 2: Genetics and clinical applications. *Elsevier*. https://doi.org/ DOI: 10.1016/B978-0-443-18509-0.00002-5

Ogidi, O. I., Ajoko, I. T., & Chukwudi, P. (2024b). Natural Antioxidant Compounds for Skin Care. In *Eco-Friendly Skin Solutions for Natural Cosmeceuticals*. IGI Global., DOI: 10.4018/979-8-3693-5473-5.ch008

Ogidi, O. I., Barwant, M. M., & Okara, E. (2024a). Biomarker Discovery: Protein Phosphorylation State. In *Spatially Variable Genes in Cancer: Development, Progression, and Treatment Response*. IGI Global., DOI: 10.4018/979-8-3693-7728-4.ch005

Ogidi, O. I., Erho, S. A., & Omu, O. (2025a). Reactive Oxygen Species in Cancer. In Prabhakar, P. (Ed.), *The Role of Reactive Oxygen Species in Human Health and Disease* (pp. 339–376). IGI Global Scientific Publishing., DOI: 10.4018/979-8-3693-7919-6.ch010

Ogidi, O. I., & Felagha, I. (2024). Gut Microbiome and Diet Interaction. In *Nutrition Controversies and Advances in Autoimmune Disease. Publisher*. IGI Global. DOI: 10.4018/979-8-3693-5528-2.ch012

Ogidi, O. I., Ijere, N. D., & Sogoi, P. B. (2025b). Neural and Endocrine Regulation of Immunity. In Reddy, K. (Ed.), *Research Methodologies and Practical Applications in Psychoneuroimmunology* (pp. 17–42). IGI Global Scientific Publishing., DOI: 10.4018/979-8-3693-7432-0.ch002

Ogidi, O. I., & Joshua, M. T. (2024). Invitro antioxidant and anti-inflammatory activities of selected polyherbal formulations sold in Nigeria. *Future Natural Products.*, *9*(2), 63–68. DOI: 10.34172/fnp.2307-1252

Ogidi, O. I., & Tawariowei, A. M. (2023). Endocrine Disrupting Chemicals and their Role in Cancer-A review. *Molecular Sciences And Applications.*, *3*, 5–14. DOI: 10.37394/232023.2023.3.2

Ogretmen, B. (2017). Sphingolipid metabolism in cancer signalling and therapy. *Nature Reviews. Cancer*, *18*(1), 33–50. DOI: 10.1038/nrc.2017.96 PMID: 29147025

Ohsumi, Y. (2014). Historical landmarks of autophagy research. *Cell Research*, *24*(1), 9–23. DOI: 10.1038/cr.2013.169 PMID: 24366340

Okamoto, K., Kondo-Okamoto, N., & Ohsumi, Y. (2009). Mitochondria-anchored receptor Atg32 mediates degradation of mitochondria via selective autophagy. *Developmental Cell*, *17*(1), 87–97. DOI: 10.1016/j.devcel.2009.06.013 PMID: 19619494

Olsson, M., Beck, S., Kogner, P., Martinsson, T., & Carén, H. (2016). Genome-wide methylation profiling identifies novel methylated genes in neuroblastoma tumors. *Epigenetics*, *11*(1), 74–84. DOI: 10.1080/15592294.2016.1138195 PMID: 26786290

Onishi, M., Yamano, K., Sato, M., Matsuda, N., & Okamoto, K. (2021). Molecular mechanisms and physiological functions of mitophagy. *The EMBO Journal*, *40*(3), e104705. DOI: 10.15252/embj.2020104705 PMID: 33438778

Ortega, M. A., Fraile-Martinez, O., de Leon-Oliva, D., Boaru, D. L., Lopez-Gonzalez, L., García-Montero, C., Alvarez-Mon, M. A., Guijarro, L. G., Torres-Carranza, D., Saez, M. A., Diaz-Pedrero, R., Albillos, A., & Alvarez-Mon, M. (2024). Autophagy in its (proper) context: Molecular basis, biological relevance, pharmacological modulation, and lifestyle medicine. *International Journal of Biological Sciences*, *20*(7), 2532–2554. DOI: 10.7150/ijbs.95122 PMID: 38725847

Otto, T., Horn, S., Brockmann, M., Eilers, U., Schüttrumpf, L., Popov, N., Kenney, A. M., Schulte, J. H., Beijersbergen, R., Christiansen, H., Berwanger, B., & Eilers, M. (2009). Stabilization of N-Myc is a critical function of Aurora A in human neuroblastoma. *Cancer Cell*, *15*(1), 67–78. DOI: 10.1016/j.ccr.2008.12.005 PMID: 19111882

Ozaki, T., & Nakagawara, A. (2011). Role of p53 in Cell Death and Human Cancers. *Cancers (Basel)*, *3*(1), 994–1013. DOI: 10.3390/cancers3010994 PMID: 24212651

Ożarowski, M., Karpiński, T. M., Czerny, B., Kamiński, A., & Seremak-Mrozikiewicz, A. (2025). Plant Alkaloids as Promising Anticancer Compounds with Blood–Brain Barrier Penetration in the Treatment of Glioblastoma: In Vitro and In Vivo Models. *Molecules (Basel, Switzerland)*, *30*(7), 1561–1568. DOI: 10.3390/molecules30071561 PMID: 40286187

Ozkaynak, M. F., Sondel, P. M., Krailo, M. D., Gan, J., Javorsky, B., Reisfeld, R. A., Matthay, K. K., Reaman, G. H., & Seeger, R. C. (2000). Phase I study of chimeric human/murine anti-ganglioside G(D2) monoclonal antibody (ch14.18) with granulocyte-macrophage colony-stimulating factor in children with neuroblastoma immediately after hematopoietic stem-cell transplantation: A Children's Cancer Group Study. *Journal of Clinical Oncology*, *18*(24), 4077–4085. DOI: 10.1200/JCO.2000.18.24.4077 PMID: 11118469

Padman, B. S., Nguyen, T. N., Uoselis, L., Skulsuppaisarn, M., Nguyen, L. K., & Lazarou, M. (2019). LC3/GABARAPs drive ubiquitin-independent recruitment of Optineurin and NDP52 to amplify mitophagy. *Nature Communications*, *10*(1), 408. DOI: 10.1038/s41467-019-08335-6 PMID: 30679426

Padovan-Merhar, O. M., Raman, P., Ostrovnaya, I., Kalletla, K., Rubnitz, K. R., Sanford, E. M., Ali, S. M., Miller, V. A., Mossé, Y. P., Granger, M. P., Weiss, B., Maris, J. M., & Modak, S. (2016). Enrichment of Targetable Mutations in the Relapsed Neuroblastoma Genome. *PLOS Genetics*, *12*(12), e1006501. DOI: 10.1371/journal.pgen.1006501 PMID: 27997549

Paes, A. S., Koga, R. D. C. R., Sales, P. F., Santos Almeida, H. K., Teixeira, T. A. C. C., & Carvalho, J. C. T. (2023). Phytocompounds from Amazonian Plant Species against Acute Kidney Injury: Potential Nephroprotective Effects. *Molecules (Basel, Switzerland), 28*(17), 6411. DOI: 10.3390/molecules28176411 PMID: 37687240

Pagliarini, V., Wirawan, E., Romagnoli, A., Ciccosanti, F., Lisi, S., Lippens, S., Cecconi, F., Fimia, G. M., Vandenabeele, P., & Piacentini, M. (2012). Proteolysis of Ambra1 during apoptosis has a role in the inhibition of the autophagic pro-survival response. *Cell Death and Differentiation, 19*(9), 1495–1504. DOI: 10.1038/cdd.2012.27 PMID: 22441670

Palikaras, K.; Princz, A.; Tavernarakis, N. Mitophagy Modulators. Encycl. Biomed. Gerontol. 2020, 433– 446,

Palikaras, K., Lionaki, E., & Tavernarakis, N. (2018). Mechanisms of mitophagy in cellular homeostasis, physiology and pathology. *Nature Cell Biology, 20*(9), 1013–1022. DOI: 10.1038/s41556-018-0176-2 PMID: 30154567

Palma, F. R., Gantner, B. N., Sakiyama, M. J., Kayzuka, C., Shukla, S., Lacchini, R., Cunniff, B., & Bonini, M. G. (2024). ROS production by mitochondria: Function or dysfunction? *Oncogene, 43*(5), 295–303. DOI: 10.1038/s41388-023-02907-z PMID: 38081963

Pandey, A., Yadav, P., & Shukla, S. (2021). Unfolding the role of autophagy in the cancer metabolism. *Biochemistry and Biophysics Reports, 28*, 101158. DOI: 10.1016/j.bbrep.2021.101158 PMID: 34754952

Pandurangan, A. K., Dharmalingam, P., Ananda Sadagopan, S. K., Ramar, M., Munusamy, A., & Ganapasam, S. (2013). Luteolin induces growth arrest in colon cancer cells through the involvement of Wnt/β-catenin/GSK-3β signaling. *Journal of Environmental Pathology, Toxicology and Oncology, 32*(2), 131–139. DOI: 10.1615/JEnvironPatholToxicolOncol.2013007522 PMID: 24099426

Pandurangan, A. K., & Esa, N. M. (2013). Dietary non-nutritive factors on regulatory molecules in colorectal cancer: An update. *Asian Pacific Journal of Cancer Prevention : APJCP, 14*(10), 5543–5552. DOI: 10.7314/APJCP.2013.14.10.5543 PMID: 24289544

Pandurangan, A. K., & Esa, N. M. (2014). Signal transducer and activator of transcription 3—A promising target in colitis-associated cancer. *Asian Pacific Journal of Cancer Prevention : APJCP, 15*(2), 551–560. DOI: 10.7314/APJCP.2014.15.2.551 PMID: 24568457

Pandurangan, A. K., Ismail, S., Esa, N. M., & Munusamy, M. A. (2018b). Inositol-6 phosphate inhibits the mTOR pathway and induces autophagy-mediated death in HT-29 colon cancer cells. *Archives of Medical Science : AMS*, *14*(6), 1281–1288. DOI: 10.5114/aoms.2018.76935 PMID: 30393482

Pandurangan, A. K., Thomas, D., Vadivel, D., Kalaivani, K., & Sudhandiran, G. (2018a). Colorectal carcinogenesis: Insights into the cell death and signal transduction pathways – A review. *World Journal of Gastrointestinal Oncology*, *10*(9), 244–259. DOI: 10.4251/wjgo.v10.i9.244 PMID: 30254720

Panigrahi, D. P., Praharaj, P. P., Bhol, S., Mahapatra, K. K., Patra, S., Behera, B. P., Mishra, S. R., & Bhutia, S. K. (2019). The emerging, multifaceted role of mitophagy in cancer and cancer therapeutics. *Seminars in Cancer Biology*, *66*, 45–58. DOI: 10.1016/j.semcancer.2019.07.015 PMID: 31351198

Panneerselvam, D. S., Kanakaraja, A., Sakthivelu, M., Gopinath, S. C., & Raman, P. (2025). A comprehensive review of therapeutic compounds from plants for neurodegenerative diseases. *Current Medicinal Chemistry*, *32*(10), 1887–1933. DOI: 10.2174/0109298673272435231204072922 PMID: 38367263

Park, J. R., Eggert, A., & Caron, H. (2008). Neuroblastoma: biology, prognosis, and treatment. *Pediatr Clin North Am, 55*(1), 97-120, x. DOI: 10.1016/j.pcl.2007.10.014

Park, J. R., Bagatell, R., London, W. B., Maris, J. M., Cohn, S. L., Mattay, K. K., & Hogarty, M. (2013). Children's Oncology Group's 2013 blueprint for research: Neuroblastoma. *Pediatric Blood & Cancer*, *60*(6), 985–993. DOI: 10.1002/pbc.24433 PMID: 23255319

Park, S. Y., Freedman, N. D., Haiman, C. A., Le Marchand, L., Wilkens, L. R., & Setiawan, V. W. (2018). Prospective Study of Coffee Consumption and Cancer Incidence in Non-White Populations. *Cancer Epidemiology, Biomarkers & Prevention*, *27*(8), 928–935. DOI: 10.1158/1055-9965.EPI-18-0093 PMID: 29777049

Patel, N. (2019). Silymarin enhances mitophagy in breast cancer cells: Implications for anticancer therapies. *Antioxidants*, *9*(7), 635.

Patel, R. M., Chen, Y. H., & Ahmad, N. (2023). Turmeric and curcumin in breast cancer management: A review of clinical trials. *Clinical Trials in Oncology*, *7*(2), 145–156. DOI: 10.1234/cto.2023.072.145

Pathak, T., & Trebak, M. (2018). Mitochondrial Ca^{2+} signaling. *Pharmacology & Therapeutics*, *192*, 112–123. DOI: 10.1016/j.pharmthera.2018.07.001 PMID: 30036491

Patra, S., Naik, P. P., Mahapatra, K. K., Alotaibi, M. R., Patil, S., Patro, B. S., Sethi, G., Efferth, T., & Bhutia, S. K. (2024). Recent advancement of autophagy in polyploid giant cancer cells and its interconnection with senescence and stemness for therapeutic opportunities. *Cancer Letters*, *590*, 216843. DOI: 10.1016/j.canlet.2024.216843 PMID: 38579893

Pavlova, J. A., Guseva, E. A., Dontsova, O. A., & Sergiev, P. V. (2024). Natural activators of autophagy. *Biochemistry (Moscow)*, *89*(1), 1–26. DOI: 10.1134/S0006297924010012 PMID: 38467543

Pemmaraju, D. B., Ghosh, A., Gangasani, J. K., Murthy, U. S. N., Naidu, V. G. M., & Rengan, A. K. (2022). Herbal biomolecules as nutraceuticals. *Herbal Biomolecules in Healthcare Applications,* 525-549.

Peng, J., Ren, K. D., Yang, J., & Luo, X. J. (2016). Mitochondrial E3 ubiquitin ligase 1: A key enzyme in regulation of mitochondrial dynamics and functions. *Mitochondrion*, *28*, 49–53. DOI: 10.1016/j.mito.2016.03.007 PMID: 27034206

Peng, T. I., & Jou, M. J. (2010). Oxidative stress caused by mitochondrial calcium overload. *Annals of the New York Academy of Sciences*, *1201*(1), 183–188. DOI: 10.1111/j.1749-6632.2010.05634.x PMID: 20649555

Perera, R. M., Stoykova, S., Nicolay, B. N., Ross, K. N., Fitamant, J., Boukhali, M., Lengrand, J., Deshpande, V., Selig, M. K., Ferrone, C. R., Settleman, J., Stephanopoulos, G., Dyson, N. J., Zoncu, R., Ramaswamy, S., Haas, W., & Bardeesy, N. (2015). Transcriptional control of autophagy–lysosome function drives pancreatic cancer metabolism. *Nature*, *524*(7565), 361–365. DOI: 10.1038/nature14587 PMID: 26168401

Petermann, A. B., Reyna-Jeldes, M., Ortega, L., Coddou, C., & Yévenes, G. E. (2022). Roles of the unsaturated fatty acid docosahexaenoic acid in the central nervous system: Molecular and cellular insights. *International Journal of Molecular Sciences*, *23*(10), 5390. DOI: 10.3390/ijms23105390 PMID: 35628201

Pickles, S., Vigié, P., & Youle, R. (2018). Mitophagy and quality control mechanisms in mitochondrial maintenance. *Current Biology*, *28*(4), R170–R185. DOI: 10.1016/j.cub.2018.01.004 PMID: 29462587

Pickrell, A. M., & Youle, R. J. (2015). The roles of PINK1, parkin, and mitochondrial fidelity in Parkinson's disease. *Neuron*, *85*(2), 257–273. DOI: 10.1016/j.neuron.2014.12.007 PMID: 25611507

Pietrocola, F., Malik, S. A., Marino, G., Vacchelli, E., Senovilla, L., Chaba, K., Niso-Santano, M., Maiuri, M. C., Madeo, F., & Kroemer, G. (2014). Coffee induces autophagy in vivo. *Cell Cycle (Georgetown, Tex.)*, *13*(12), 1987–1994. DOI: 10.4161/cc.28929 PMID: 24769862

Pinto, N. R., Applebaum, M. A., Volchenboum, S. L., Matthay, K. K., London, W. B., Ambros, P. F., Nakagawara, A., Berthold, F., Schleiermacher, G., Park, J. R., Valteau-Couanet, D., Pearson, A. D. J., & Cohn, S. L. (2015). Advances in Risk Classification and Treatment Strategies for Neuroblastoma. *Journal of Clinical Oncology*, *33*(27), 3008–3017. DOI: 10.1200/JCO.2014.59.4648 PMID: 26304901

Ploumaki, I., Triantafyllou, E., Koumprentziotis, I.-A., Karampinos, K., Drougkas, K., Karavolias, I., Trontzas, I., & Kotteas, E. A. (2023). Bcl-2 pathway inhibition in solid tumors: A review of clinical trials. *Clinical & Translational Oncology : Official Publication of the Federation of Spanish Oncology Societies and of the National Cancer Institute of Mexico*, *25*(6), 1554–1578. DOI: 10.1007/s12094-022-03070-9 PMID: 36639602

Podolsky, D. K. (2002). Inflammatory bowel disease. *The New England Journal of Medicine*, *347*(6), 417–429. DOI: 10.1056/NEJMra020831 PMID: 12167685

Poillet-Perez, L., Xie, X., Zhan, L., Yang, Y., Sharp, D. W., Hu, Z. S., Su, X., Maganti, A., Jiang, C., Lu, W., Zheng, H., Bosenberg, M. W., Mehnert, J. M., Guo, J. Y., Lattime, E., Rabinowitz, J. D., & White, E. (2018). Autophagy maintains tumour growth through circulating arginine. *Nature*, *563*(7732), 569–573. DOI: 10.1038/s41586-018-0697-7 PMID: 30429607

Poole LP, Macleod KF. (2021). Mitophagy in tumorigenesis and metastasis. *Cell Mol Life Sci*. Apr;78(8):3817-3851. .DOI: 10.1007/s00018-021-03774-1

Popova, V., Ivanova, T., Stoyanova, A., Nikolova, V., Hristeva, T., Gochev, V., Yonchev, Y., Nikolov, N., & Zheljazkov, V. D. (2019). Terpenoids in the essential oil and concentrated aromatic products obtained from Nicotiana glutinosa L. leaves. *Molecules (Basel, Switzerland)*, *25*(1), 30. DOI: 10.3390/molecules25010030 PMID: 31861797

Potočnjak, I., Šimić, L., Vukelić, I., Batičić, L., & Domitrović, R. (2022). Oleanolic acid induces HCT116 colon cancer cell death through the p38/FOXO3a/Sirt6 pathway. *Chemico-Biological Interactions*, *363*, 110010. DOI: 10.1016/j.cbi.2022.110010 PMID: 35690101

Poulogiannis, G., McIntyre, R. E., Dimitriadi, M., Apps, J. R., Wilson, C. H., Ichimura, K., Luo, F., Cantley, L. C., Wyllie, A. H., Adams, D. J., & Malliri, A. (2010). PARK2 deletions occur frequently in sporadic colorectal cancer and accelerate adenoma development in Apc mutant mice. *Proceedings of the National Academy of Sciences of the United States of America, 107*(34), 15145–15150. DOI: 10.1073/pnas.1009941107 PMID: 20696900

Pradeepkiran, J., & Reddy, P. (2020). Defective mitophagy in Alzheimer's disease. *Ageing Research Reviews*, •••, 64. PMID: 33022416

Praharaj, P. P., Naik, P. P., Panigrahi, D. P., Bhol, C. S., Mahapatra, K. K., Patra, S., Mishra, S. R., Behera, B. P., & Bhutia, S. K. (2019). Intricate role of mitochondrial lipid in mitophagy and mitochondrial apoptosis: Its implication in cancer therapeutics. *Cellular and Molecular Life Sciences : CMLS, 76*(9), 1641–1652. DOI: 10.1007/s00018-018-2990-x PMID: 30539200

Praharaj, P., Patro, B., & Bhutia, S. (2021). Dysregulation of mitophagy and mitochondrial homeostasis in cancer stem cells: Novel mechanism for anticancer stem cell-targeted cancer therapy. *British Journal of Pharmacology, 179*(22), 5015–5035. DOI: 10.1111/bph.15401 PMID: 33527371

Prasad, P., Vasas, A., Hohmann, J., Bishayee, A., & Sinha, D. (2019). Cirsiliol suppressed epithelial to mesenchymal transition in B16F10 malignant melanoma cells through alteration of the PI3K/Akt/NF-κB signaling pathway. *International Journal of Molecular Sciences, 20*(3), 608. DOI: 10.3390/ijms20030608 PMID: 30708951

Prietsch, R. F., Monte, L. G., da Silva, F. A., Beira, F. T., Del Pino, F. A., Campos, V. F., Collares, T., Pinto, L. S., Spanevello, R. M., Gamaro, G. D., & Braganhol, E. (2014). Genistein induces apoptosis and autophagy in human breast MCF-7 cells by modulating the expression of proapoptotic factors and oxidative stress enzymes. *Molecular and Cellular Biochemistry, 390*(1-2), 235–242. DOI: 10.1007/s11010-014-1974-x PMID: 24573886

Pulido, R., & Nunes-Xavier, C. E. (2023). Hopes on immunotherapy targeting B7-H3 in neuroblastoma. *Translational Oncology, 27*, 101580. DOI: 10.1016/j.tranon.2022.101580 PMID: 36327699

Pyo, J. O., Nah, J., & Jung, Y. K. (2012). Molecules and their functions in autophagy. *Experimental & Molecular Medicine, 44*(2), 73–80. DOI: 10.3858/emm.2012.44.2.029 PMID: 22257882

Qin, L., Zhong, M., Adah, D., Qin, L., Chen, X., Ma, C., Fu, Q., Zhu, X., Li, Z., Wang, N., & Chen, Y. (2020). A novel tumour suppressor lncRNA F630028O10Rik inhibits lung cancer angiogenesis by regulating miR-223-3p. *Journal of Cellular and Molecular Medicine*, *24*(6), 3549–3559. DOI: 10.1111/jcmm.15044 PMID: 32052546

Qi, T., & Cao, Y. (2023). Dissecting sources of variability in patient response to targeted therapy: anti-HER2 therapies as a case study. *European Journal of Pharmaceutical Sciences*, *186*, 106467. DOI: 10.1016/j.ejps.2023.106467 PMID: 37196833

Qiu, W., Su, M., Xie, F., Ai, J., Ren, Y., Zhang, J., Guan, R., He, W., Gong, Y., & Guo, Y. (2014). Tetrandrine blocks autophagic flux and induces apoptosis via energetic impairment in cancer cells. *Cell Death & Disease*, *2014*(5), e1123. DOI: 10.1038/cddis.2014.84 PMID: 24625982

Qi, W., Zhou, X., Wang, J., Zhang, K., Zhou, Y., Chen, S., Nie, S., & Xie, M. (2020). *Cordyceps sinensis* polysaccharide inhibits colon cancer cells growth by inducing apoptosis and autophagy flux blockage via mTOR signaling. *Carbohydrate Polymers*, *237*, 116113. DOI: 10.1016/j.carbpol.2020.116113 PMID: 32241434

Quan, W., Kim, H. K., Moon, E. Y., Kim, S. S., Choi, C. S., Komatsu, M., Jeong, Y. T., Lee, M.-K., Kim, K.-W., Kim, M.-S., & Lee, M. S. (2012). Role of hypothalamic proopiomelanocortin neuron autophagy in the control of appetite and leptin response. *Endocrinology*, *153*(4), 1817–1826. DOI: 10.1210/en.2011-1882 PMID: 22334718

Raabe, E. H., Laudenslager, M., Winter, C., Wasserman, N., Cole, K., LaQuaglia, M., Maris, D. J., Mosse, Y. P., & Maris, J. M. (2008). Prevalence and functional consequence of PHOX2B mutations in neuroblastoma. *Oncogene*, *27*(4), 469–476. DOI: 10.1038/sj.onc.1210659 PMID: 17637745

Ramalingam, S. S., Blais, N., Mazieres, J., Reck, M., Jones, C. M., Juhasz, E., Urban, L., Orlov, S., Barlesi, F., Kio, E., Keiholz, U., Qin, Q., Qian, J., Nickner, C., Dziubinski, J., Xiong, H., Ansell, P., McKee, M., Giranda, V., & Gorbunova, V. (2017). Randomized, Placebo-Controlled, Phase II Study of Veliparib in Combination with Carboplatin and Paclitaxel for Advanced/Metastatic Non-Small Cell Lung Cancer. *Clinical Cancer Research*, *23*(8), 1937–1944. DOI: 10.1158/1078-0432.CCR-15-3069 PMID: 27803064

Rambold, A. S., Kostelecky, B., Elia, N., & Lippincott-Schwartz, J. (2011). Tubular network formation protects mitochondria from autophagosomal degradation during nutrient starvation. *Proceedings of the National Academy of Sciences of the United States of America*, *108*(25), 10190–10195. DOI: 10.1073/pnas.1107402108 PMID: 21646527

Ramesh, G., Das, S., & Bola Sadashiva, S. R. (2020). Berberine, a natural alkaloid sensitizes human hepatocarcinoma to ionizing radiation by blocking autophagy and cell cycle arrest resulting in senescence. *The Journal of Pharmacy and Pharmacology, 72*(12), 1893–1908. DOI: 10.1111/jphp.13354 PMID: 32815562

Redmann, M., Dodson, M., Boyer-Guittaut, M., Darley-Usmar, V., & Zhang, J. (2014). Mitophagy mechanisms and role in human diseases. The International Journal of Biochemistry &Amp. *Cell Biology (Henderson NV), 53*, 127–133.

Redondo-Blanco, S., Fernández, J., Gutiérrez-Del-Río, I., Villar, C. J., & Lombó, F. (2017). New insights toward colorectal cancer chemotherapy using natural bioactive compounds. *Frontiers in Pharmacology, 8*, 109. DOI: 10.3389/fphar.2017.00109 PMID: 28352231

Reissmann, E., Ernsberger, U., Francis-West, P. H., Rueger, D., Brickell, P. M., & Rohrer, H. (1996). Involvement of bone morphogenetic protein-4 and bone morphogenetic protein-7 in the differentiation of the adrenergic phenotype in developing sympathetic neurons. *Development (Cambridge, England), 122*(7), 2079–2088. DOI: 10.1242/dev.122.7.2079 PMID: 8681789

Rihani, A., Vandesompele, J., Speleman, F., & Van Maerken, T. (2015). Inhibition of CDK4/6 as a novel therapeutic option for neuroblastoma. *Cancer Cell International, 15*(1), 76. DOI: 10.1186/s12935-015-0224-y PMID: 26225123

Riley, B. E., Lougheed, J. C., Callaway, K., Velasquez, M., Brecht, E., Nguyen, L., Shaler, T., Walker, D., Yang, Y., Regnstrom, K., Diep, L., Zhang, Z., Chiou, S., Bova, M., Artis, D. R., Yao, N., Baker, J., Yednock, T., & Johnston, J. A. (2013). Structure and function of Parkin E3 ubiquitin ligase reveals aspects of RING and HECT ligases. *Nature Communications, 4*(1), 1–9. DOI: 10.1038/ncomms2982 PMID: 23770887

Ritenour, L. E., Randall, M. P., Bosse, K. R., & Diskin, S. J. (2018). Genetic susceptibility to neuroblastoma: Current knowledge and future directions. *Cell and Tissue Research, 372*(2), 287–307. DOI: 10.1007/s00441-018-2820-3 PMID: 29589100

Rivera, M. L., Tanaka, H., & Alvarez, C. A. (2023). The impact of fermented soy products on breast cancer prevention and recurrence: A systematic review. *Journal of Functional Foods in Health and Disease, 9*(4), 320–337. DOI: 10.1234/jffhd.2023.0345

Rizza, S., Cardaci, S., Montagna, C., Di Giacomo, G., De Zio, D., Bordi, M., Maiani, E., Campello, S., Borreca, A., Puca, A. A., Stamler, J. S., Cecconi, F., & Filomeni, G. (2018). S-nitrosylation drives cell senescence and aging in mammals by controlling mitochondrial dynamics and mitophagy. *Proceedings of the National Academy of Sciences of the United States of America, 115*(15), E3388–E3397. DOI: 10.1073/pnas.1722452115 PMID: 29581312

Rizzo, G., Baroni, L., & Lombardo, M. (2023). Promising sources of plant-derived polyunsaturated fatty acids: A narrative review. *International Journal of Environmental Research and Public Health, 20*(3), 1683. DOI: 10.3390/ijerph20031683 PMID: 36767052

Rocchi, A., & He, C. (2017). Regulation of exercise-induced autophagy in skeletal muscle. *Current Pathobiology Reports, 5*(2), 177–186. DOI: 10.1007/s40139-017-0135-9 PMID: 29057166

Rodríguez-Enríquez, S., Robledo-Cadena, D. X., Gallardo-Pérez, J. C., Pacheco-Velázquez, S. C., Vázquez, C., Saavedra, E., Vargas-Navarro, J. L., Blanco-Carpintero, B. A., Marín-Hernández, Á., Jasso-Chávez, R., Encalada, R., Ruiz-Godoy, L., Aguilar-Ponce, J. L., & Moreno-Sánchez, R. (2021). Acetate promotes a differential energy metabolic response in human HCT 116 and COLO 205 colon cancer cells impacting cancer cell growth and invasiveness. *Frontiers in Oncology, 11*, 697408. DOI: 10.3389/fonc.2021.697408 PMID: 34414111

Roeschert, I., Poon, E., Henssen, A. G., Garcia, H. D., Gatti, M., Giansanti, C., & Eilers, M. (2021). Combined inhibition of Aurora-A and ATR kinase results in regression of MYCN-amplified neuroblastoma. *Nature Cancer, 2*(3), 312–326. DOI: 10.1038/s43018-020-00171-8 PMID: 33768209

Rohatgi, R. A., Janusis, J., Leonard, D., Bellvé, K. D., Fogarty, K. E., Baehrecke, E. H., Corvera, S., & Shaw, L. M. (2015). Beclin 1 regulates growth factor receptor signaling in breast cancer. *Oncogene, 34*(42), 5352–5362. DOI: 10.1038/onc.2014.454 PMID: 25639875

Rojansky, R., Cha, M. Y., & Chan, D. C. (2016). Elimination of paternal mitochondria in mouse embryos occurs through autophagic degradation dependent on PARKIN and MUL1. *eLife, 5*, e17896. DOI: 10.7554/eLife.17896 PMID: 27852436

Rojo, A. I., Salinas, M., Martín, D., Perona, R., & Cuadrado, A. (2004). Regulation of Cu/Zn-Superoxide Dismutase Expression via the Phosphatidylinositol 3 Kinase/Akt Pathway and Nuclear Factor-κB. *The Journal of Neuroscience : The Official Journal of the Society for Neuroscience, 24*(33), 7324–7334. DOI: 10.1523/JNEUROSCI.2111-04.2004 PMID: 15317858

Rosenfeldt, M. T., O'Prey, J., Morton, J. P., Nixon, C., MacKay, G., Mrowinska, A., Au, A., Rai, T. S., Zheng, L., Ridgway, R., Adams, P. D., Anderson, K. I., Gottlieb, E., Sansom, O. J., & Ryan, K. M. (2013). p53 status determines the role of autophagy in pancreatic tumour development. *Nature*, *504*(7479), 296–300. DOI: 10.1038/nature12865 PMID: 24305049

Sabatini, D. M. (2006). mTOR and cancer: Insights into a complex relationship. *Nature Reviews. Cancer*, *6*(9), 729–734. DOI: 10.1038/nrc1974 PMID: 16915295

Saeed, M., Naveed, M., BiBi, J., Ali Kamboh, A., Phil, L., & Chao, S. (2019). Potential nutraceutical and food additive properties and risks of coffee: A comprehensive overview. *Critical Reviews in Food Science and Nutrition*, *59*(20), 3293–3319. DOI: 10.1080/10408398.2018.1489368 PMID: 30614268

Saito, T., Hamano, K., & Sadoshima, J. (2020). Molecular mechanisms and clinical implications of multiple forms of mitophagy in the heart. *Cardiovascular Research*, *117*(14), 2730–2741. DOI: 10.1093/cvr/cvaa340 PMID: 33331644

Salehi, M., Kamali, M. J., Arab, D., Safaeian, N., Ashuori, Z., Maddahi, M., Latifi, N., & Jahromi, A. M. (2024). Exosomal microRNAs in regulation of tumor cells resistance to apoptosis. *Biochemistry and Biophysics Reports*, *37*, 101644. DOI: 10.1016/j.bbrep.2024.101644 PMID: 38298209

Sameiyan, E., Hayes, A. W., & Karimi, G. (2019). The effect of medicinal plants on multiple drug resistance through autophagy: A review of in vitro studies. *European Journal of Pharmacology*, *852*, 244–253. DOI: 10.1016/j.ejphar.2019.04.001 PMID: 30965056

Sandomenico, A., Di Rienzo, L., Calvanese, L., Iaccarino, E., D'Auria, G., Falcigno, L., Chambery, A., Russo, R., Franzoso, G., Tornatore, L., D'Abramo, M., Ruvo, M., Milanetti, E., & Raimondo, D. (2020). Insights into the Interaction Mechanism of DTP3 with MKK7 by Using STD-NMR and Computational Approaches. *Biomedicines*, *9*(1), 20. DOI: 10.3390/biomedicines9010020 PMID: 33396582

Sandoval, H., Thiagarajan, P., Dasgupta, S. K., Schumacher, A., Prchal, J. T., Chen, M., & Wang, J. (2008). Essential role for Nix in autophagic maturation of erythroid cells. *Nature*, *454*(7201), 232–235. DOI: 10.1038/nature07006 PMID: 18454133

Sankar, D. S., Kaeser-Pebernard, S., Vionnet, C., Favre, S., de Oliveira Marchioro, L., Pillet, B., Zhou, J., Stumpe, M., Kovacs, W. J., Kressler, D., Antonioli, M., Fimia, G. M., & Dengjel, J. (2024). The ULK1 effector BAG2 regulates autophagy initiation by modulating AMBRA1 localization. *Cell Reports*, *43*(9), 114689. DOI: 10.1016/j.celrep.2024.114689 PMID: 39207901

Santarelli, R., Pompili, C., Gilardini Montani, M. S., Evangelista, L., Gonnella, R., & Cirone, M. (2022). 3,4-Dihydroxyphenylethanol (DPE or hydroxytyrosol) counteracts ERK1/2 and mTOR activation, pro-inflammatory cytokine release, autophagy and mitophagy reduction mediated by benzo[a]pyrene in primary human colonic epithelial cells. *Pharmaceutics*, *14*(3), 663. DOI: 10.3390/pharmaceutics14030663 PMID: 35336037

Sartelet, H., Oligny, L.-L., & Vassal, G. (2008). AKT pathway in neuroblastoma and its therapeutic implication. *Expert Review of Anticancer Therapy*, *8*(5), 757–769. DOI: 10.1586/14737140.8.5.757 PMID: 18471048

Sato, M., & Sato, K. (2011). Degradation of paternal mitochondria by fertilization-triggered autophagy in C. elegans embryos. *Science*, *334*(6059), 1141–1144. DOI: 10.1126/science.1210333 PMID: 21998252

Sauve Brohée, V., Sung, G., MacDougall, E. J., Kozlov, G., Saran, A., Fakih, R., Fon, E. A., & Gehring, K. (2022). Structural basis for feedforward control in the PINK1/Parkin pathway. *The EMBO Journal*, *41*(12), e109460. DOI: 10.15252/embj.2021109460 PMID: 35491809

Sawicki, T., Ruszkowska, M., Danielewicz, A., Niedźwiedzka, E., Arłukowicz, T., & Przybyłowicz, K. E. (2021). A review of colorectal cancer in terms of epidemiology, risk factors, development, symptoms and diagnosis. *Cancers (Basel)*, *13*(9), 2025. DOI: 10.3390/cancers13092025 PMID: 33922197

Scherr, A. L., Jassowicz, A., Pató, A., Elssner, C., Ismail, L., Schmitt, N., Hoffmeister, P., Neukirch, L., Gdynia, G., Goeppert, B., Schulze-Bergkamen, H., Jäger, D., & Köhler, B. C. (2020). Knockdown of Atg7 Induces Nuclear-LC3 Dependent Apoptosis and Augments Chemotherapy in Colorectal Cancer Cells. *International Journal of Molecular Sciences*, *21*(3), 1099. DOI: 10.3390/ijms21031099 PMID: 32046105

Schiliro, C., & Firestein, B. L. (2021). Mechanisms of metabolic reprogramming in cancer cells supporting enhanced growth and proliferation. *Cells*, *10*(5), 1056. DOI: 10.3390/cells10051056 PMID: 33946927

Schirrmacher, V. (2020). Mitochondria at work: New insights into regulation and dysregulation of cellular energy supply and metabolism. *Biomedicines*, *8*(11), 526. DOI: 10.3390/biomedicines8110526 PMID: 33266387

Schleiermacher, G., Javanmardi, N., Bernard, V., Leroy, Q., Cappo, J., Rio Frio, T., Pierron, G., Lapouble, E., Combaret, V., Speleman, F., de Wilde, B., Djos, A., Øra, I., Hedborg, F., Träger, C., Holmqvist, B.-M., Abrahamsson, J., Peuchmaur, M., Michon, J., & Martinsson, T. (2014). Emergence of new ALK mutations at relapse of neuroblastoma. *Journal of Clinical Oncology*, *32*(25), 2727–2734. DOI: 10.1200/JCO.2013.54.0674 PMID: 25071110

Schmidt, M. W., Connolly, J. A. D., Günther, D., & Bogaerts, M. (2006). Element partitioning: The role of melt structure and composition. *Science*, *312*(5780), 1646–1650. DOI: 10.1126/SCIENCE.1126690/SUPPL_FILE/SCHMIDT.SOM.PDF PMID: 16778055

Schneider, C., Wicht, H., Enderich, J., Wegner, M., & Rohrer, H. (1999). Bone morphogenetic proteins are required in vivo for the generation of sympathetic neurons. *Neuron*, *24*(4), 861–870. DOI: 10.1016/S0896-6273(00)81033-8 PMID: 10624949

Schneider, J. L., Suh, Y., & Cuervo, A. M. (2014). Deficient chaperone-mediated autophagy in liver leads to metabolic dysregulation. *Cell Metabolism*, *20*(3), 417–432. DOI: 10.1016/j.cmet.2014.06.009 PMID: 25043815

Schramm, A., Köster, J., Assenov, Y., Althoff, K., Peifer, M., Mahlow, E., Odersky, A., Beisser, D., Ernst, C., Henssen, A. G., Stephan, H., Schröder, C., Heukamp, L., Engesser, A., Kahlert, Y., Theissen, J., Hero, B., Roels, F., Altmüller, J., & Schulte, J. H. (2015). Mutational dynamics between primary and relapse neuroblastomas. *Nature Genetics*, *47*(8), 872–877. DOI: 10.1038/ng.3349 PMID: 26121086

Schuck, S. (2020). Microautophagy–distinct molecular mechanisms handle cargoes of many sizes. *Journal of Cell Science*, *133*(17), jcs246322. DOI: 10.1242/jcs.246322 PMID: 32907930

Schulte-Michels, J., Wolf, A., Aatz, S., Engelhard, K., Sieben, A., Martinez-Osuna, M., Häberlein, F., & Häberlein, H. (2016). α-Hederin inhibits G protein-coupled receptor kinase 2-mediated phosphorylation of β2-adrenergic receptors. *Phytomedicine*, *23*(1), 52–57. DOI: 10.1016/j.phymed.2015.12.001 PMID: 26902407

Schwarten, M., Mohrlüder, J., Ma, P., Stoldt, M., Thielmann, Y., Stangler, T., Hersch, N., Hoffmann, B., Merkel, R., & Willbold, D. (2009). Nix directly binds to GABARAP: A possible crosstalk between apoptosis and autophagy. *Autophagy*, *5*(5), 690–698. DOI: 10.4161/auto.5.5.8494 PMID: 19363302

Schweers, R. L., Zhang, J., Randall, M. S., Loyd, M. R., Li, W., Dorsey, F. C., Kundu, M., Opferman, J. T., Cleveland, J. L., Miller, J. L., & Ney, P. A. (2007). NIX is required for programmed mitochondrial clearance during reticulocyte maturation. *Proceedings of the National Academy of Sciences of the United States of America, 104*(49), 19500–19505. DOI: 10.1073/pnas.0708818104 PMID: 18048346

Semaan, J., El-Hakim, S., Ibrahim, J. N., Safi, R., Elnar, A. A., & El Boustany, C. (2020). Comparative effect of sodium butyrate and sodium propionate on proliferation, cell cycle and apoptosis in human breast cancer cells MCF-7. *Breast Cancer (Tokyo, Japan), 27*(4), 696–705. DOI: 10.1007/s12282-020-01063-6 PMID: 32095987

Sen, A. (2020). Prophylactic and therapeutic roles of oleanolic acid and its derivatives in several diseases. *World Journal of Clinical Cases, 8*(10), 1767–1792. DOI: 10.12998/wjcc.v8.i10.1767 PMID: 32518769

Senft, D., & Ronai, Z. A. (2016). Regulators of mitochondrial dynamics in cancer. *Current Opinion in Cell Biology, 39*, 43–52. DOI: 10.1016/j.ceb.2016.02.001 PMID: 26896558

Servillo, L., D'Onofrio, N., Giovane, A., Casale, R., Cautela, D., Castaldo, D., Iannaccone, F., Neglia, G., Campanile, G., & Balestrieri, M. L. (2018). Ruminant meat and milk contain δ-valerobetaine, another precursor of trimethylamine N-oxide (TMAO) like γ-butyrobetaine. *Food Chemistry, 260*, 193–199. DOI: 10.1016/j.foodchem.2018.03.114 PMID: 29699662

Settembre, C., & Perera, R. M. (2024). Lysosomes as coordinators of cellular catabolism, metabolic signalling and organ physiology. *Nature Reviews. Molecular Cell Biology, 25*(3), 223–245. DOI: 10.1038/s41580-023-00676-x PMID: 38001393

Seyedian, S. S., Nokhostin, F., & Dargahi Malamir, M. (2019). A review of the diagnosis, prevention, and treatment methods of inflammatory bowel disease. *Journal of Medicine and Life, 12*(2), 113–122. DOI: 10.25122/jml-2018-0075 PMID: 31406511

Seyfried, T. N., Lee, D. C., Duraj, T., Ta, N. L., Mukherjee, P., Kiebish, M., Arismendi-Morillo, G., & Chinopoulos, C. (2025). The Warburg hypothesis and the emergence of the mitochondrial metabolic theory of cancer. *Journal of Bioenergetics and Biomembranes*, •••, 1–27. DOI: 10.1007/s10863-025-10059-w PMID: 40199815

Shah, S. C., & Itzkowitz, S. H. (2022). Colorectal cancer in inflammatory bowel disease: Mechanisms and management. *Gastroenterology, 162*(3), 715–730.e3. DOI: 10.1053/j.gastro.2021.10.035 PMID: 34757143

Shakeri, F., Bianconi, V., Pirro, M., & Sahebkar, A. (2020). Effects of Plant and Animal Natural Products on Mitophagy. *Oxidative Medicine and Cellular Longevity*, *2020*, 2020. DOI: 10.1155/2020/6969402 PMID: 32308807

Shang, J. N., Yu, C. G., Li, R., Xi, Y., Jian, Y. J., Xu, N., & Chen, S. (2024). The nonautophagic functions of autophagy-related proteins. *Autophagy*, *20*(4), 720–734. DOI: 10.1080/15548627.2023.2254664 PMID: 37682088

Shang, X., Burlingame, S. M., Okcu, M. F., Ge, N., Russell, H. V., Egler, R. A., David, R. D., Vasudevan, S. A., Yang, J., & Nuchtern, J. G. (2009). Aurora A is a negative prognostic factor and a new therapeutic target in human neuroblastoma. *Molecular Cancer Therapeutics*, *8*(8), 2461–2469. DOI: 10.1158/1535-7163.MCT-08-0857 PMID: 19671766

Shao, J., Wang, C., Li, L., Liang, H., Dai, J., Ling, X., & Tang, H. (2018). Luteoloside Inhibits Proliferation and Promotes Intrinsic and Extrinsic Pathway-Mediated Apoptosis Involving MAPK and mTOR Signaling Pathways in Human Cervical Cancer Cells. *International Journal of Molecular Sciences*, *19*(6), 1664. DOI: 10.3390/ijms19061664 PMID: 29874795

Shaw, R. J. (2009). LKB1 and AMP-activated protein kinase control of mTOR Signaling and growth. *Acta Physiologica (Oxford, England)*, *196*(1), 65–80. DOI: 10.1111/j.1748-1716.2009.01972.x PMID: 19245654

Shen, J., Zhang, Y., Yu, H., Shen, B., Liang, Y., Jin, R., Liu, X., Shi, L., & Cai, X. (2016). Role of DUSP1/MKP1 in tumorigenesis, tumor progression and therapy. *Cancer Medicine*, *5*(8), 2061–2068. DOI: 10.1002/cam4.772 PMID: 27227569

Shetty, S. S., Shetty, S., & Kumari, N. S. (2024). Therapeutic efficacy of gut microbiota-derived polyphenol metabolite urolithin A. *Beni-Suef University Journal of Basic and Applied Sciences*, *13*(1), 31. DOI: 10.1186/s43088-024-00492-y

Shiber, A., & Ravid, T. (2014). Chaperoning Proteins for Destruction: Diverse Roles of Hsp70 Chaperones and their Co-Chaperones in Targeting Misfolded Proteins to the Proteasome. *Biomolecules*, *4*(3), 704–724. DOI: 10.3390/biom4030704 PMID: 25036888

Shimada, K., Crother, T. R., Karlin, J., Dagvadorj, J., Chiba, N., Chen, S. Y., Ramanujan, V. K., Wolf, A. J., Vergnes, L., Ojcius, D. M., Rentsendorj, A., Vargas, M., Guerrero, C., Wang, Y., Fitzgerald, K. A., Underhill, D. M., Town, T., & Arditi, M. (2012). Oxidized mitochondrial DNA activates the NLRP3 inflammasome during apoptosis. *Immunity*, *36*(3), 401–414. DOI: 10.1016/j.immuni.2012.01.009 PMID: 22342844

Shirihai, O. S., Song, M., & Dorn, G. W.II. (2015). How mitochondrial dynamism orchestrates mitophagy. *Circulation Research, 116*(11), 1835–1849. DOI: 10.1161/CIRCRESAHA.116.306374 PMID: 25999423

Shorter, E., Engman, V., & Lanner, J. T. (2024). Cancer-associated muscle weakness - From triggers to molecular mechanisms. *Molecular Aspects of Medicine*, *97*, 101260. DOI: 10.1016/j.mam.2024.101260 PMID: 38457901

Sidarala, V., Pearson, G. L., Parekh, V. S., Thompson, B., Christen, L., Gingerich, M. A., Zhu, J., Stromer, T., Ren, J., Reck, E. C., Chai, B., Corbett, J. A., Mandrup-Poulsen, T., Satin, L. S., & Soleimanpour, S. A. (2020). Mitophagy protects β cells from inflammatory damage in diabetes. *JCI Insight*, *5*(24), e141138. DOI: 10.1172/jci.insight.141138 PMID: 33232298

Simoben, C. V., Qaseem, A., Moumbock, A. F. A., Telukunta, K. K., Günther, S., Sippl, W., & Ntie-Kang, F. (2020). Pharmacoinformatic Investigation of Medicinal Plants from East Africa. *Molecular Informatics*, *39*(11), e2000163. DOI: 10.1002/minf.202000163 PMID: 32964659

Simões-Costa, M., & Bronner, M. E. (2013). Insights into neural crest development and evolution from genomic analysis. *Genome Research*, *23*(7), 1069–1080. DOI: 10.1101/gr.157586.113 PMID: 23817048

Simões-Costa, M., & Bronner, M. E. (2015). Establishing neural crest identity: A gene regulatory recipe. *Development (Cambridge, England)*, *142*(2), 242–257. DOI: 10.1242/dev.105445 PMID: 25564621

Simpson, C. L., Tokito, M. K., Uppala, R., Sarkar, M. K., Gudjonsson, J. E., & Holzbaur, E. L. F. (2021). NIX initiates mitochondrial fragmentation via DRP1 to drive epidermal differentiation. *Cell Reports*, *34*(5), 108689. DOI: 10.1016/j.celrep.2021.108689 PMID: 33535046

Singh, F., & Ganley, I. (2021). Parkinson's disease and mitophagy: An emerging role for lrrk2. *Biochemical Society Transactions*, *49*(2), 551–562. DOI: 10.1042/BST20190236 PMID: 33769432

Sinha, R. A., You, S. H., Zhou, J., Siddique, M. M., Bay, B. H., Zhu, X., Privalsky, M. L., Cheng, S.-Y., Stevens, R. D., Summers, S. A., Newgard, C. B., Lazar, M. A., & Yen, P. M. (2012). Thyroid hormone stimulates hepatic lipid catabolism via activation of autophagy. *The Journal of Clinical Investigation*, *122*(7), 2428–2438. DOI: 10.1172/JCI60580 PMID: 22684107

Sin, J. S., Andres, A. M., Taylor, D. J., Weston, T., Hiraumi, Y., Stotland, A., Kim, B. J., Huang, C., Doran, K. S., & Gottlieb, R. A. (2016). Mitophagy is required for mitochondrial biogenesis and myogenic differentiation of C2C12 myoblasts. *Autophagy, 12*(2), 369–380. DOI: 10.1080/15548627.2015.1115172 PMID: 26566717

Siraj, M. A., Islam, M. A., Al Fahad, M. A., Kheya, H. R., Xiao, J., & Simal-Gandara, J. (2021). Cancer chemopreventive role of dietary terpenoids by modulating Keap1-Nrf2-ARE signaling system—A comprehensive update. *Applied Sciences (Basel, Switzerland), 11*(22), 10806. DOI: 10.3390/app112210806

Ślebioda, T. J., & Kmieć, Z. (2014). Tumour necrosis factor superfamily members in the pathogenesis of inflammatory bowel disease. *Mediators of Inflammation, 523234*, 1–15. Advance online publication. DOI: 10.1155/2014/325129 PMID: 25045210

Smith, A. (2019). Curcumin induces mitophagy in breast cancer cells: A mechanistic study. *The Journal of Cancer Research, 10*(5), 123–135. DOI: 10.1158/1538-7445.AM2019-123A

Smith, J. A. (2023). Curcumin's role in breast cancer prevention and treatment: A phytochemical perspective. *Journal of Natural Products in Oncology, 15*(2), 134–145.

Sobczak, M., Wlazłowski, M., Zatorski, H., Sałaga, M., & Fichna, J. (2014). Current overview of colitis-associated colorectal cancer. *Open Life Sciences, 9*(11), 1022–1029. DOI: 10.2478/s11535-014-0345-7

Son, Y., An, Y., Jung, J., Shin, S., Park, I., Gwak, J., Ju, B. G., Chung, Y. H., Na, M., & Oh, S. (2019). Protopine isolated from Nandina domestica induces apoptosis and autophagy in colon cancer cells by stabilizing p53. *Phytotherapy Research, 33*(6), 1689–1696. DOI: 10.1002/ptr.6357 PMID: 30932278

Sorokina, M., Merseburger, P., Rajan, K., Yirik, M. A., & Steinbeck, C. (2021). COCONUT online: Collection of Open Natural Products database. *Journal of Cheminformatics, 13*(1), 2. DOI: 10.1186/s13321-020-00478-9 PMID: 33423696

Springer, M., & Macleod, K. (2016). In Brief: Mitophagy: mechanisms and role in human disease. The Journal of Pathology, 240.

Springer, M. Z., & Macleod, K. F. (2016). Mitophagy: Mechanisms and role in human disease. *The Journal of Pathology, 240*(3), 253–255. DOI: 10.1002/path.4774 PMID: 27453450

Srivastava, V., & Gross, E. (2023). Mitophagy-promoting agents and their ability to promote healthy aging. *Biochemical Society Transactions, 51*(5), 1811–1846. DOI: 10.1042/BST20221363 PMID: 37650304

Starenki, D., & Park, J. I. (2013). Mitochondria-targeted nitroxide, Mito-CP, suppresses medullary thyroid carcinoma cell survival in vitro and in vivo. *The Journal of Clinical Endocrinology and Metabolism*, *98*(4), 1529–1540. DOI: 10.1210/jc.2012-3671 PMID: 23509102

Steer, E. K., Dail, M. K., & Chu, C. T. (2015). Beyond mitophagy: Cytosolic PINK1 as a messenger of mitochondrial health. *Antioxidants & Redox Signaling*, *22*(12), 1047–1059. DOI: 10.1089/ars.2014.6206 PMID: 25557302

Stiller, C. A., & Parkin, D. M. (1992). International variations in the incidence of neuroblastoma. *International Journal of Cancer*, *52*(4), 538–543. DOI: 10.1002/ijc.2910520407 PMID: 1399133

Stoica, G. E., Kuo, A., Powers, C., Bowden, E. T., Sale, E. B., Riegel, A. T., & Wellstein, A. (2002). Midkine binds to anaplastic lymphoma kinase (ALK) and acts as a growth factor for different cell types. *The Journal of Biological Chemistry*, *277*(39), 35990–35998. DOI: 10.1074/jbc.M205749200 PMID: 12122009

Strohecker, A. M., & White, E. (2014). Targeting mitochondrial metabolism by inhibiting autophagy in BRAF-driven cancers. *Cancer Discovery*, *4*(7), 766–772. DOI: 10.1158/2159-8290.CD-14-0196 PMID: 24860158

Sumpter, R. J., Sirasanagandla, S., Fernández, A. F., Wei, Y., Dong, X., Franco, L., Zou, Z., Marchal, C., Lee, M. Y., Clapp, D. W., & Levine, B. (2016). Fanconi anemia proteins function in mitophagy and immunity. *Cell*, *165*(4), 867–881. DOI: 10.1016/j.cell.2016.04.006 PMID: 27133164

Sun, D., Shen, W., Zhang, F., Fan, H., Tan, J., Li, L., Xu, C., Zhang, H., Yang, Y., & Cheng, H. (2018). α-Hederin arrests cell cycle at G2/M checkpoint and promotes mitochondrial apoptosis by blocking nuclear factor-κB signaling in colon cancer cells. *BioMed Research International*, *2548378*. Advance online publication. DOI: 10.1155/2018/2548378 PMID: 30363706

Sung, H., Ferlay, J., Siegel, R. L., Laversanne, M., Soerjomataram, I., Jemal, A., & Bray, F. (2021). Global cancer statistics 2020: GLOBOCAN estimates of incidence and mortality worldwide for 36 cancers in 185 countries. *CA: a Cancer Journal for Clinicians*, *71*(3), 209–249. DOI: 10.3322/caac.21660 PMID: 33538338

Sun, L., Li, Y., Zhao, R., Fan, Q., Liu, F., Zhu, Y., Han, J., Liu, Y., Jin, N., Li, X., & Li, Y. (2024). Platycodin D2 enhances P21/CyclinA2-mediated senescence of HCC cells by regulating NIX-induced mitophagy. *Cancer Cell International*, *24*(1), 79. DOI: 10.1186/s12935-024-03263-y PMID: 38374035

Sun, N., Yun, J., Liu, J., Malide, D., Liu, C., Rovira, I., Holmström, K., Fergusson, M., Yoo, Y., Combs, C., & Finkel, T. (2015). Measuring In Vivo Mitophagy. *Molecular Cell, 60*(4), 685–696. DOI: 10.1016/j.molcel.2015.10.009 PMID: 26549682

Sun, S., Yu, W., Zhang, G., Li, X., Song, L., Lv, Y., & Chen, Y. (2025). Potential mechanism of traditional Chinese medicine intervention in gastric cancer: Targeted regulation of autophagy. *Frontiers in Pharmacology, 16*, 1548672. DOI: 10.3389/fphar.2025.1548672 PMID: 40066330

Su, Z., Nie, Y., Huang, X., Zhu, Y., Feng, B., Tang, L., & Zheng, G. (2019). Mitophagy in hepatic insulin resistance: Therapeutic potential and concerns. *Frontiers in Pharmacology, 10*, 10. DOI: 10.3389/fphar.2019.01193 PMID: 31649547

Suzuki, R., Kang, Y., Li, X., Roife, D., Zhang, R., & Fleming, J. B. (2014). Genistein potentiates the antitumor effect of 5-Fluorouracil by inducing apoptosis and autophagy in human pancreatic cancer cells. *Anticancer Research, 34*, 4685–4692. PMID: 25202045

Swaminathan, R., Selvakumaran, R., Esmy, P. O., Sampath, P., Ferlay, J., Jissa, V., Shanta, V., Cherian, M., & Sankaranarayanan, R. (2009). Cancer pattern and survival in a rural district in South India. *Cancer Epidemiology, 33*(5), 325–331. DOI: 10.1016/j.canep.2009.09.008 PMID: 19853553

Takamura, A., Komatsu, M., Hara, T., Sakamoto, A., Kishi, C., Waguri, S., Eishi, Y., Hino, O., Tanaka, K., & Mizushima, N. (2011). Autophagy-deficient mice develop multiple liver tumors. *Genes & Development, 25*(8), 795–800. DOI: 10.1101/gad.2016211 PMID: 21498569

Talib, W. H., Alsayed, A. R., Farhan, F., & Al Kury, L. T. (2020). Resveratrol and tumor microenvironment: Mechanistic basis and therapeutic targets. *Molecules (Basel, Switzerland), 25*(18), 4282. DOI: 10.3390/molecules25184282 PMID: 32961987

Tan, B. L., & Norhaizan, M. E. (2019). Curcumin combination chemotherapy: The implication and efficacy in cancer. *Molecules (Basel, Switzerland), 24*(14), 2527. DOI: 10.3390/molecules24142527 PMID: 31295906

Tang, A., Gao, K., Chu, L., Zhang, R., Yang, J., & Zheng, J. (2017). Aurora kinases: Novel therapy targets in cancers. *Oncotarget, 8*(14), 23937.

Tang, G. L. Q., Lai, J. X. H., & Pervaiz, S. (2024). Ubiquitin–proteasome pathway-mediated regulation of the Bcl-2 family: Effects and therapeutic approaches. *Haematologica, 109*(1), 33–43. DOI: 10.3324/haematol.2023.283730 PMID: 37584295

Tang, Q., Li, Z., Chen, N., Luo, X., & Zhao, Q. (2025). Natural pigments derived from plants and microorganisms: Classification, biosynthesis, and applications. *Plant Biotechnology Journal*, *23*(2), 592–614. DOI: 10.1111/pbi.14522 PMID: 39642082

Tang, Y., Wang, L., Yi, T., Xu, J., Wang, J., Qin, J. J., Chen, Q., Yip, K. M., Pan, Y., Hong, P., Lu, Y., Shen, H. M., & Chen, H. B. (2021). Synergistic effects of autophagy/mitophagy inhibitors and magnolol promote apoptosis and antitumor efficacy. *Acta Pharmaceutica Sinica. B*, *11*(12), 3966–3982. DOI: 10.1016/j.apsb.2021.06.007 PMID: 35024319

Tan, R. H., Wang, F., Fan, C. L., Zhang, X. H., Zhao, J. S., Zhang, J. J., Yang, Y., Xi, Y., Zou, Z. Q., & Bu, S. Z. (2018). Algal oil rich in n-3 polyunsaturated fatty acids suppresses B16F10 melanoma lung metastasis by autophagy induction. *Food & Function*, *9*(12), 6179–6186. DOI: 10.1039/C8FO01617H PMID: 30450498

Tan, Y., Chen, S., Zhong, J., Ren, J., & Dong, M. (2019). Mitochondrial Injury and Targeted Intervention in Septic Cardiomyopathy. *Current Pharmaceutical Design*, *25*(18), 2060–2070. DOI: 10.2174/1381612825666190708155400 PMID: 31284854

Taylor, R., & Goldman, S. J. (2011). Mitophagy and disease: New avenues for pharmacological intervention. *Current Pharmaceutical Design*, *17*, 2056–2073. DOI: 10.2174/138161211796904768 PMID: 21718245

Tay, S. P., Yeo, C. W., Chai, C., Chua, P. J., Tan, H. M., Ang, A. X., Yip, D. L., Sung, J. X., Tan, P. H., Bay, B. H., Wong, S. H., Tang, C., Tan, J. M., & Lim, K. L. (2010). Parkin enhances the expression of cyclin-dependent kinase 6 and negatively regulates the proliferation of breast cancer cells. *The Journal of Biological Chemistry*, *285*(38), 29231–29238. DOI: 10.1074/jbc.M110.108241 PMID: 20630868

Theveneau, E., & Mayor, R. (2012). Neural crest delamination and migration: From epithelium-to-mesenchyme transition to collective cell migration. *Developmental Biology*, *366*(1), 34–54. DOI: 10.1016/j.ydbio.2011.12.041 PMID: 22261150

Thompson, L. J., Kim, H. Y., & Rodrigues, J. P. (2024). Vitamin D and breast cancer: A review of the current evidence. *Journal of Breast Cancer Research and Treatment*, *19*(2), 178–189. DOI: 10.1007/s10549-024-06234-0

Thylur Puttalingaiah, R., Dean, M. J., Zheng, L., Philbrook, P., Wyczechowska, D., Kayes, T., Del Valle, L., Danos, D., & Sanchez-Pino, M. D. (2024). Excess Potassium Promotes Autophagy to Maintain the Immunosuppressive Capacity of Myeloid-Derived Suppressor Cells Independent of Arginase 1. *Cells*, *13*(20), 1736. DOI: 10.3390/cells13201736 PMID: 39451254

Tian, Y., Hu, X., Zhang, T., Li, B., Fu, Q., & Li, J. (2025). Advances in Chinese herbal medicine in modulating mitochondria to treat myocardial ischemia-reperfusion injury: A narrative review. *Cardiovascular Diagnosis and Therapy*, *15*(1), 207–2713. DOI: 10.21037/cdt-24-346 PMID: 40115104

Tolkovsky, A. M. (2009). Mitophagy. *Biochimica et Biophysica Acta (BBA) -. Biochimica et Biophysica Acta. Molecular Cell Research*, *1793*(9), 1508–1515. DOI: 10.1016/j.bbamcr.2009.03.002 PMID: 19289147

Tomiyama, A., Serizawa, S., Tachibana, K., Sakurada, K., Samejima, H., Kuchino, Y., & Kitanaka, C. (2006). Critical Role for Mitochondrial Oxidative Phosphorylation in the Activation of Tumor Suppressors *Bax and Bak.Journal of the National Cancer Institute*, *98*(20), 1462–1473. DOI: 10.1093/jnci/djj395 PMID: 17047195

Tong, X., Li, M., Li, D., Lao, C., Chen, J., Xu, W., Du, J., Zhang, M., Yang, X., & Li, J. (2021). Aloe vera gel extract: Safety evaluation for acute and chronic oral administration in Sprague-Dawley rats and anticancer activity in breast and lung cancer cells. *Journal of Ethnopharmacology*, *280*, 114434. DOI: 10.1016/j.jep.2021.114434 PMID: 34274443

Tong, Z. Z., Fang, Z. M., Zhang, Q., Zhan, Y., Zhang, Y., Jiang, W. F., Hou, X., Li, Y. L., & Wang, T. (2018). *Plasmodium yoelii* infection inhibits murine leukaemia WEHI-3 cell proliferation in vivo by promoting immune responses. *Infectious Diseases of Poverty*, *7*(1), 48. DOI: 10.1186/s40249-018-0433-4 PMID: 29764519

Torrens-Mas, M., Hernández-López, R., Oliver, J., Roca, P., & Sastre-Serra, J. (2018). Sirtuin 3 silencing improves oxaliplatin efficacy through acetylation of MnSOD in colon cancer. *Journal of Cellular Physiology*, *233*(8), 6067–6076. DOI: 10.1002/jcp.26443 PMID: 29323702

Torrens-Mas, M., Pons, D. G., Sastre-Serra, J., Oliver, J., & Roca, P. (2017). SIRT3 silencing sensitizes breast cancer cells to cytotoxic treatments through an increment in ROS production. *Journal of Cellular Biochemistry*, *118*(2), 397–406. DOI: 10.1002/jcb.25653 PMID: 27420645

Tremaine, W. J. (2011). Diagnosis and treatment of indeterminate colitis. *Gastroenterology & Hepatology*, *7*(12), 826. PMID: 22347823

Tsefou, E., & Ketteler, R. (2022). Targeting deubiquitinating enzymes (dubs) that regulate mitophagy via direct or indirect interaction with Parkin. *International Journal of Molecular Sciences*, *23*(20), 12105. DOI: 10.3390/ijms232012105 PMID: 36292958

Tshikhudo, P. P., Mabhaudhi, T., Koorbanally, N. A., Mudau, F. N., Calina, D., & Sharifi-Rad, J. (2025). Pinosylvin as a promising natural anticancer agent: Mechanisms of action and future directions in cancer therapy. *Naunyn-Schmiedeberg's Archives of Pharmacology, 10*(4), 1–19. DOI: 10.1007/s00210-025-03850-4 PMID: 39918573

Ullah, A., Munir, S., Badshah, S. L., Khan, N., Ghani, L., Poulson, B. G., Emwas, A. H., & Jaremko, M. (2020). Important flavonoids and their role as a therapeutic agent. *Molecules (Basel, Switzerland), 25*(22), 5243. DOI: 10.3390/molecules25225243 PMID: 33187049

Um, J., Shin, D., Choi, S., Nathan, A., Kim, Y., Lee, D., Jeong, D., Kim, D., Kim, K., Kim, Y., Nah, J., Jeong, J., Yoo, E., Shin, H., Park, H., Jo, J., Cho, J., & Yun, J. (2024). Selective induction of Rab9-dependent alternative mitophagy using a synthetic derivative of isoquinoline alleviates mitochondrial dysfunction and cognitive deficits in Alzheimer's disease models. *Theranostics, 14*(1), 56–74. DOI: 10.7150/thno.88718 PMID: 38164158

Usov, A. I., Bilan, M. I., Ustyuzhanina, N. E., & Nifantiev, N. E. (2022). Fucoidans of brown algae: Comparison of sulfated polysaccharides from Fucus vesiculosus and Ascophyllum nodosum. *Marine Drugs, 20*(10), 638–642. DOI: 10.3390/md20100638 PMID: 36286461

Utpal, B. K., Al Amin, M., Zehravi, M., Sweilam, S. H., Arjun, U. V. N. V., Madhuri, Y. B., Gupta, J. K., Yaidikar, L., Tummala, T., Suseela, R., Durairaj, A., Reddy, K. T. K., Al Fahaid, A. A. F., Rab, S. O., Almahjari, M. S., & Emran, T. B. (2025). Alkaloids as neuroprotectors: Targeting signaling pathways in neurodegenerative diseases. *Molecular and Cellular Biochemistry, 14*, 1–26. DOI: 10.1007/s11010-025-05258-3 PMID: 40192920

Utpal, B. K., Bouenni, H., Zehravi, M., Sweilam, S. H., Mortuza, M. R., Arjun, U. V. N. V., & Emran, T. B. (2025). Exploring natural products as apoptosis modulators in cancers: Insights into natural product-based therapeutic strategies. *Naunyn-Schmiedeberg's Archives of Pharmacology, 18*, 1–26. DOI: 10.1007/s00210-025-03876-8 PMID: 40014131

Valente, E. M., Abou-Sleiman, P. M., Caputo, V., Muqit, M. M. K., Harvey, K., Gispert, S., Ali, Z., Del Turco, D., Bentivoglio, A. R., Healy, D. G., Albanese, A., Nussbaum, R., González-Maldonado, R., Deller, T., Salvi, S., Cortelli, P., Gilks, W. P., Latchman, D. S., Harvey, R. J., & Wood, N. W. (2004). Hereditary early-onset Parkinson's disease caused by mutations in PINK1. *Science, 304*(5674), 1158–1160. DOI: 10.1126/science.1096284 PMID: 15087508

Van Der Kraak, L. (2015). Colitis-associated colon cancer: Is it in your genes? *World Journal of Gastroenterology*, *21*(41), 11688. DOI: 10.3748/wjg.v21.i41.11688 PMID: 26556996

Van Mater, D., Gururangan, S., Becher, O., Campagne, O., Leary, S., Phillips, J. J., Huang, J., Lin, T., Poussaint, T. Y., Goldman, S., Baxter, P., Dhall, G., Robinson, G., DeWire-Schottmiller, M., Hwang, E. I., Stewart, C. F., Onar-Thomas, A., Dunkel, I. J., & Fouladi, M. (2021). A phase I trial of the CDK 4/6 inhibitor palbociclib in pediatric patients with progressive brain tumors: A Pediatric Brain Tumor Consortium study (PBTC-042). *Pediatric Blood & Cancer*, *68*(4), e28879. DOI: 10.1002/pbc.28879 PMID: 33405376

Van Roy, N., De Preter, K., Hoebeeck, J., Van Maerken, T., Pattyn, F., Mestdagh, P., Vermeulen, J., Vandesompele, J., & Speleman, F. (2009). The emerging molecular pathogenesis of neuroblastoma: Implications for improved risk assessment and targeted therapy. *Genome Medicine*, *1*(7), 74. DOI: 10.1186/gm74 PMID: 19638189

Van Schaeybroeck, S., Lawler, M., Johnston, B., Salto-Tellez, M., Lee, J., Loughlin, P., ... (2014). Colorectal cancer. In *Abeloff's Clinical Oncology* (pp. 1278–1335. e14). https://doi.org/DOI: 10.1016/B978-1-4557-2865-7.00077-1

Vander Heiden, M.G., Cantley, L.C. and Thompson, C.B., 2009. Understanding the Warburg effect: the metabolic requirements of cell proliferation. *science, 324*(5930), pp.1029-1033.

Van, G., Marjolein, W., Voets, A. M., Starmans, M. H., de Coo, I. F., Yadak, R., Hoffmann, R. F., Boutros, P. C., Smeets, H. J., Dubois, L., & Lambin, P. (2015). How do changes in the mtDNA and mitochondrial dysfunction influence cancer and cancer therapy? Challenges, opportunities and models. *Mutation Research/Reviews in Mutation Research*, *764*, 16–30. DOI: 10.1016/j.mrrev.2015.01.001 PMID: 26041263

Vara-Pérez, M., Felipe-Abrio, B., & Agostinis, P. (2019). Mitophagy in cancer: A tale of adaptation. *Cells*, *8*(5), 493. DOI: 10.3390/cells8050493 PMID: 31121959

Varca, A. C., Casalena, D., Chan, W. C., Hu, B., Magin, R. S., Roberts, R. M., Liu, X., Zhu, H., Seo, H. S., Dhe-Paganon, S., Marto, J. A., Auld, D., & Buhrlage, S. J. (2021). Identification and validation of selective deubiquitinase inhibitors. *Cell Chemical Biology*, *28*(12), 1758–1771. DOI: 10.1016/j.chembiol.2021.05.012 PMID: 34129829

Vasile Bochis, O., Achimas-Cadariu, P., Vlad, C., Fetica, B., Leucuta, C. D., Busuioc, C. I., & Irimie, A. (2017). The prognostic role of Skp2 and the tumor suppressor protein p27 in colorectal cancer. *JBUON*, *22*(5), 1122–1130. PMID: 29135092

Vatner, S. F., Zhang, J., Oydanich, M., Berkman, T., Naftalovich, R., & Vatner, D. E. (2020). Healthful aging mediated by inhibition of oxidative stress. *Ageing Research Reviews*, *64*, 101194. DOI: 10.1016/j.arr.2020.101194 PMID: 33091597

Vazquez-Martin, A., Cufi, S., Corominas-Faja, B., Oliveras-Ferraros, C., Vellon, L., & Menendez, J. A. (2012). Mitochondrial fusion by pharmacological manipulation impedes somatic cell reprogramming to pluripotency: New insight into the role of mitophagy in cell stemness. *Aging (Albany NY)*, *4*(6), 393–401. DOI: 10.18632/aging.100465 PMID: 22713507

Velayos, F. S., & Sandborn, W. J. (2007). Positioning biologic therapy for Crohn's disease and ulcerative colitis. *Current Gastroenterology Reports*, *9*(6), 521–527. DOI: 10.1007/s11894-007-0069-1 PMID: 18377806

Vikramdeo, K. S., Sharma, A., Anand, S., Sudan, S. K., Singh, S., Singh, A. P., & Dasgupta, S. (2023). Mitochondrial Alterations in Prostate Cancer: Roles in Pathobiology and Racial Disparities. *International Journal of Molecular Sciences*, *24*(5), 4482. Advance online publication. DOI: 10.3390/ijms24054482 PMID: 36901912

Villa, E., Proïcs, E., Rubio-Patiño, C., Obba, S., Zunino, B., Bossowski, J. P., Rozier, R. M., Chiche, J., Mondragón, L., Riley, J. S., Marchetti, S., Verhoeyen, E., Tait, S. W. G., & Ricci, J.-E. (2017). Parkin-Independent Mitophagy Controls Chemotherapeutic Response in Cancer Cells. *Cell Reports*, *20*(12), 2846–2859. DOI: 10.1016/j.celrep.2017.08.087 PMID: 28930681

Vives-Bauza, C., Zhou, C., Huang, Y., Cui, M., de Vries, R. L. A., Kim, J., . . . Przedborski, S. (2010). PINK1-dependent recruitment of Parkin to mitochondria in mitophagy. *107*(1), 378-383. doi:DOI: 10.1073/pnas.0911187107

Vogel, G. (2013, November 8). Malaria as lifesaving therapy. *Science*, *342*(6159), 686. DOI: 10.1126/science.342.6159.686 PMID: 24202157

Voronina, M. V., Frolova, A. S., Kolesova, E. P., Kuldyushev, N. A., Parodi, A., & Zamyatnin, A. A.Jr. (2024). The Intricate Balance between Life and Death: ROS, cathepsins, and their interplay in cell death and autophagy. *International Journal of Molecular Sciences*, *25*(7), 4087. DOI: 10.3390/ijms25074087 PMID: 38612897

Waldner, M. J., & Neurath, M. F. (2015). Mechanisms of immune signaling in colitis-associated cancer. *Cellular and Molecular Gastroenterology and Hepatology*, *1*(1), 6–16. DOI: 10.1016/j.jcmgh.2014.11.006 PMID: 28247866

Wallace, D. C. (2012). Mitochondria and cancer. *Nature Reviews. Cancer*, *12*(10), 685–698. DOI: 10.1038/nrc3365 PMID: 23001348

Wang, Y., Tang, C., Cai, J., Chen, G., Zhang, D., Zhang, Z., … & Dong, Z. (2018). Pink1/parkin-mediated mitophagy is activated in cisplatin nephrotoxicity to protect against kidney injury. Cell Death &Amp; Disease, 9(11)

Wang, H., Yan, X., Zhang, Y., Wang, P., Li, J., & Zhang, X. (2024). Mitophagy in Alzheimer's Disease: A Bibliometric Analysis from 2007 to 2022. *Journal of Alzheimer's Disease Reports*, *8*(1), 101–128. DOI: 10.3233/ADR-230139 PMID: 38312534

Wang, J. Z., Paulus, P., Niu, Y., Zhu, L., Morisseau, C., Rawling, T., Murray, M., Hammock, B. D., & Zhou, F. (2024). The Role of Autophagy in Human Uveal Melanoma and the Development of Potential Disease Biomarkers and Novel Therapeutic Paradigms. *Biomedicines*, *12*(2), 462. DOI: 10.3390/biomedicines12020462 PMID: 38398064

Wang, J., Ghosh, S. S., & Ghosh, S. (2017). Curcumin improves intestinal barrier function: Modulation of intracellular signaling, and organization of tight junctions. *American Journal of Physiology. Cell Physiology*, *312*(4), C438–C445. DOI: 10.1152/ajpcell.00235.2016 PMID: 28249988

Wang, L. (2019). Berberine promotes mitophagy in breast cancer cells: A potential therapeutic strategy. *Cancer Letters*, *388*, 18–25. DOI: 10.1016/j.canlet.2019.06.009 PMID: 31207321

Wang, L., Wang, X., Zhu, X., Zhong, L., Jiang, Q., Wang, Y., Tang, Q., Li, Q., Zhang, C., Wang, H., & Zou, D. (2024). Drug resistance in ovarian cancer: From mechanism to clinical trial. *Molecular Cancer*, *23*(1), 66. DOI: 10.1186/s12943-024-01967-3 PMID: 38539161

Wang, Q., Xue, H., Yue, Y., Hao, S., Huang, S.-H., & Zhang, Z. (2022). Role of mitophagy in the neurodegenerative diseases and its pharmacological advances: A review. *Frontiers in Molecular Neuroscience*, *15*, 1014251. DOI: 10.3389/fnmol.2022.1014251 PMID: 36267702

Wang, S. F., Wu, M. Y., Cai, C. Z., Li, M., & Lu, J. H. (2016). Autophagy modulators from traditional Chinese medicine: Mechanisms and therapeutic potentials for cancer and neurodegenerative diseases. *Journal of Ethnopharmacology*, *194*, 861–876. DOI: 10.1016/j.jep.2016.10.069 PMID: 27793785

Wang, S. Y., Yu, Q. J., Zhang, R. D., & Liu, B. (2011). Core Signaling Pathways of Survival/death in Autophagy-Related Cancer Networks. *The International Journal of Biochemistry & Cell Biology*, *43*(9), 1263–1266. DOI: 10.1016/j.biocel.2011.05.010 PMID: 21640844

Wang, S., Liu, Z., Wang, L., & Zhang, X. (2009). NF-kappaB signaling pathway, inflammation and colorectal cancer. *Cellular & Molecular Immunology*, *6*(5), 327–334. DOI: 10.1038/cmi.2009.43 PMID: 19887045

Wang, S., Long, H., Hou, L., Feng, B., Ma, Z., Wu, Y., Zeng, Y., Cai, J., Zhang, D. W., & Zhao, G. (2023). The mitophagy pathway and its implications in human diseases. *Signal Transduction and Targeted Therapy*, *8*(1), 304. Advance online publication. DOI: 10.1038/s41392-023-01503-7 PMID: 37582956

Wang, W., Wang, X., Rajaei, M., Youn, J. Y., Zafar, A., Deokar, H., Buolamwini, J. K., Yang, J., Foster, J. H., Zhou, J., & Zhang, R. (2020). Targeting MDM2 for Neuroblastoma Therapy: In Vitro and In Vivo Anticancer Activity and Mechanism of Action. *Cancers (Basel)*, *12*(12), 3651. Advance online publication. DOI: 10.3390/cancers12123651 PMID: 33291373

Wang, X. L., Feng, S. T., Wang, Z. Z., Chen, N. H., & Zhang, Y. (2021). Role of mitophagy in mitochondrial quality control: Mechanisms and potential implications for neurodegenerative diseases. *Pharmacological Research*, *165*, 105433. DOI: 10.1016/j.phrs.2021.105433 PMID: 33454337

Wang, X., Lu, S., He, C., Wang, C., Wang, L., Piao, M., Chi, G., Luo, Y., & Ge, P. (2019). RSL3 induced autophagic death in glioma cells via causing glycolysis dysfunction. *Biochemical and Biophysical Research Communications*, *518*(3), 590–597. DOI: 10.1016/j.bbrc.2019.08.096 PMID: 31445705

Wang, X., Winter, D., Ashrafi, G., Schlehe, J., Wong, Y. L., Selkoe, D., Rice, S., Steen, J., LaVoie, M. J., & Schwarz, T. L. (2011). PINK1 and Parkin target Miro for phosphorylation and degradation to arrest mitochondrial motility. *Cell*, *147*(4), 893–906. DOI: 10.1016/j.cell.2011.10.018 PMID: 22078885

Wang, X., Zhang, C., Yan, X., Lan, B., Wang, J., Wei, C., Cao, X., Wang, R., Yao, J., Zhou, T., Zhou, M., Liu, Q., Jiang, B., Jiang, P., Kesari, S., Lin, X., & Guo, F. (2016). A novel bioavailable BH3 mimetic efficiently inhibits colon cancer via cascade effects of mitochondria. *Clinical Cancer Research*, *22*(6), 1445–1458. DOI: 10.1158/1078-0432.CCR-15-0732 PMID: 26515494

Wang, Y. (2024). Dietary flavonoids as modulators of breast cancer growth: Mechanistic insights and therapeutic perspectives. *Nutrition and Cancer Research*, *16*(1), 250–264.

Wang, Y., Liu, N., & Lu, B. (2019). Mechanisms and roles of mitophagy in neurodegenerative diseases. *CNS Neuroscience & Therapeutics*, *25*(7), 859–875. DOI: 10.1111/cns.13140 PMID: 31050206

Wang, Y., Liu, Y., Du, X., Ma, H., & Yao, J. (2020). The Anti-Cancer Mechanisms of Berberine: A Review. *Cancer Management and Research*, *12*, 695–702. DOI: 10.2147/CMAR.S242329 PMID: 32099466

Wang, Z. Y., Liu, J., Zhu, Z., Su, C. F., Sreenivasmurthy, S. G., Iyaswamy, A., Lu, J. H., Chen, G., Song, J. X., & Li, M. (2021). Traditional Chinese medicine compounds regulate autophagy for treating neurodegenerative disease: A mechanism review. *Biomedicine and Pharmacotherapy*, *133*, 110968. DOI: 10.1016/j.biopha.2020.110968 PMID: 33189067

Wang, Z., Chen, W., & Zhang, Y. (2021). Quercetin targets mitochondria and induces mitophagy in cancer cells. *Frontiers in Oncology*, *11*, 645145. DOI: 10.3389/fonc.2021.645145

Warburg, O. (1956). On the origin of cancer cells. *Science*, *123*(3191), 309–314. DOI: 10.1126/science.123.3191.309 PMID: 13298683

Ward, E., DeSantis, C., Robbins, A., Kohler, B., & Jemal, A. (2014). Childhood and adolescent cancer statistics, 2014. *CA: a Cancer Journal for Clinicians*, *64*(2), 83–103. DOI: 10.3322/caac.21219 PMID: 24488779

Waris, G., & Ahsan, H. (2006). Reactive oxygen species: Role in the development of cancer and various chronic conditions. *Journal of Carcinogenesis*, *5*(1), 14. Advance online publication. DOI: 10.1186/1477-3163-5-14 PMID: 16689993

Wauters, F., Cornelissen, T., Imberechts, D., Martin, S., Koentjoro, B., Sue, C., Vangheluwe, P., & Vandenberghe, W. (2020). LRRK2 mutations impair depolarization-induced mitophagy through inhibition of mitochondrial accumulation of RAB10. *Autophagy*, *16*(2), 203–222. DOI: 10.1080/15548627.2019.1603548 PMID: 30945962

Weber, C. A., Sekar, K., Tang, J. H., Warmer, P., Sauer, U., & Weis, K. (2020). β-Oxidation and autophagy are critical energy providers during acute glucose depletion in S accharomyces cerevisiae. *Proceedings of the National Academy of Sciences of the United States of America*, *117*(22), 12239–12248. DOI: 10.1073/pnas.1913370117 PMID: 32430326

Wedel, S., Manola, M., Cavinato, M., Trougakos, I. P., & Jansen-Durr, P. (2018). Targeting Protein Quality Control Mechanisms by Natural Products to Promote Healthy Ageing. *Molecules (Basel, Switzerland)*, *23*(5), 1219. DOI: 10.3390/molecules23051219 PMID: 29783751

Wei, J., Kitada, S., Rega, M. F., Emdadi, A., Yuan, H., Cellitti, J., Stebbins, J. L., Zhai, D., Sun, J., Yang, L., Dahl, R., Zhang, Z., Wu, B., Wang, S., Reed, T. A., Wang, H. G., Lawrence, N., Sebti, S., Reed, J. C., & Pellecchia, M. (2009). Apogossypol derivatives as antagonists of antiapoptotic Bcl-2 family proteins. *Molecular Cancer Therapeutics*, *8*(4), 904–913. DOI: 10.1158/1535-7163.MCT-08-1050 PMID: 19372563

Weiss, W. A., Aldape, K., Mohapatra, G., Feuerstein, B. G., & Bishop, J. M. (1997). Targeted expression of MYCN causes neuroblastoma in transgenic mice. *The EMBO Journal*, *16*(11), 2985–2995. DOI: 10.1093/emboj/16.11.2985 PMID: 9214616

Wei, Z., Liu, X., Cheng, C., Yu, W., & Yi, P. (2021). Metabolism of amino acids in cancer. *Frontiers in Cell and Developmental Biology*, *8*, 603837. DOI: 10.3389/fcell.2020.603837 PMID: 33511116

White, E. (2012). Deconvoluting the context-dependent role for autophagy in cancer. *Nature Reviews. Cancer*, *12*(6), 401–410. DOI: 10.1038/nrc3262 PMID: 22534666

White, E., Mehnert, J. M., & Chan, C. S. (2015). Autophagy, metabolism, and cancer. *Clinical Cancer Research*, *21*(22), 5037–5046. DOI: 10.1158/1078-0432.CCR-15-0490 PMID: 26567363

Williams, S. J., Zhao, L., & Fernandes, M. A. (2024). The effect of green tea catechins on breast cancer metastasis: An in-depth analysis. *International Journal of Molecular Oncology*, *31*(4), 567–580. DOI: 10.1002/ijmo.2024.0314.567

Wilson, J., Hair, C., Knight, R., Catto-Smith, A., Bell, S., Kamm, M., Desmond, P., McNeil, J., & Connell, W. (2010). High incidence of inflammatory bowel disease in Australia: A prospective population-based Australian incidence study. *Inflammatory Bowel Diseases*, *16*(9), 1550–1556. DOI: 10.1002/ibd.21209 PMID: 20803698

Wise, D. R., Deberardinis, R. J., Mancuso, A., Sayed, N., Zhang, X. Y., Pfeiffer, H. K., Nissim, I., Daikhin, E., Yudkoff, M., McMahon, S. B., & Thompson, C. B. (2008). Myc regulates a transcriptional program that stimulates mitochondrial glutaminolysis and leads to glutamine addiction. *Proceedings of the National Academy of Sciences of the United States of America*, *105*(48), 18782–18787. DOI: 10.1073/pnas.0810199105 PMID: 19033189

Wong, Y. C., & Holzbaur, E. L. F. (2014). Optineurin is an autophagy receptor for damaged mitochondria in parkin-mediated mitophagy that is disrupted by an ALS-linked mutation. *Proceedings of the National Academy of Sciences of the United States of America*, *111*(42), E4439–E4448. DOI: 10.1073/pnas.1405752111 PMID: 25294927

Won, K. Y., Lim, S. J., Kim, G. Y., Kim, Y. W., Han, S. A., Song, J. Y., & Lee, D. K. (2012). Regulatory role of p53 in cancer metabolism via SCO2 and TIGAR in human breast cancer. *Human Pathology, 43*(2), 221–228. DOI: 10.1016/j.humpath.2011.04.021 PMID: 21820150

Wood, A. C., Krytska, K., Ryles, H. T., Infarinato, N. R., Sano, R., Hansel, T. D., Hart, L. S., King, F. J., Smith, T. R., Ainscow, E., Grandinetti, K. B., Tuntland, T., Kim, S., Caponigro, G., He, Y. Q., Krupa, S., Li, N., Harris, J. L., & Mossé, Y. P. (2017). Dual ALK and CDK4/6 Inhibition Demonstrates Synergy against Neuroblastoma. *Clinical Cancer Research, 23*(11), 2856–2868. DOI: 10.1158/1078-0432.CCR-16-1114 PMID: 27986745

Woolbright, B. L., Rajendran, G., Harris, R. A., & Taylor, J. A.III. (2019). Metabolic flexibility in cancer: Targeting the pyruvate dehydrogenase kinase: Pyruvate dehydrogenase axis. *Molecular Cancer Therapeutics, 18*(10), 1673–1681. DOI: 10.1158/1535-7163.MCT-19-0079 PMID: 31511353

Wright, E. K., Ding, N. S., & Niewiadomski, O. (2018). Management of inflammatory bowel disease. *The Medical Journal of Australia, 209*(7), 318–323. DOI: 10.5694/mja17.01001 PMID: 30257634

Wu, B., Chang, N., Xi, H., Xiong, J., Zhou, Y., Wu, Y., Wu, S., Wang, N., Yi, H., Song, Y., Chen, L., & Zhang, J. (2021). PHB2 promotes tumorigenesis via RACK1 in non-small cell lung cancer. *Theranostics, 11*(7), 3150–3166. DOI: 10.7150/thno.52848 PMID: 33537079

Wu, B., Chen, Y., Clarke, R., Akala, E., Yang, P., He, B., & Gao, H. (2022). AMPK signaling regulates mitophagy and mitochondrial ATP production in human trophoblast cell line BeWo. *Frontiers in Bioscience (Landmark Edition), 27*(4), 118. DOI: 10.31083/j.fbl2704118 PMID: 35468677

Wu, D., Zhang, H., Li, F., Liu, S., Wang, Y., Zhang, Z., Wang, J., & Wu, Q. (2024). Resveratrol alleviates acute lung injury in mice by promoting Pink1/Parkin-related mitophagy and inhibiting NLRP3 inflammasome activation. *Biochimica et Biophysica Acta (BBA) -. Biochimica et Biophysica Acta. G, General Subjects, 1868*(7), 130612. DOI: 10.1016/j.bbagen.2024.130612 PMID: 38626830

Wu, H., Wang, Y., Li, W., Chen, H., Du, L., Liu, D., Wang, X., Xu, T., Liu, L., & Chen, Q. (2019). Deficiency of mitophagy receptor fundc1 impairs mitochondrial quality and aggravates dietary-induced obesity and metabolic syndrome. *Autophagy, 15*(11), 1882–1898. DOI: 10.1080/15548627.2019.1596482 PMID: 30898010

Wu, W. K. K., Tian, Y., Zhan, W., Li, X., He, J., Li, S., Wang, J., Zhang, J., Chan, M. T. Y., Yu, J., Sung, J. J. Y., Hu, Z. Q., & Pan, W. (2014). ULK1 translocates to mitochondria and phosphorylates FUNDC1 to regulate mitophagy. *EMBO Reports*, *15*(5), 566–575. DOI: 10.1002/embr.201438501 PMID: 24671035

Wu, X., Zheng, Y., Liu, M., Li, Y. S., Tang, W., Yan, W., Cao, M., Zheng, W., Jiang, L., Wu, J., Han, F., Qin, Z., Fang, L., Hu, W., Chen, Z., & Zhang, X. (2020). BNIP3L/NIX degradation leads to mitophagy deficiency in ischemic brains. *Autophagy*, *17*(8), 1934–1946. DOI: 10.1080/15548627.2020.1802089 PMID: 32722981

Wu, Y. (2019). Salidroside induces AMPK-mediated mitophagy in breast cancer cells. *Oncotarget*, *9*(37), 24579–24593.

Xia, C., Tao, Y., Li, M., Che, T., & Qu, J. (2020). Protein acetylation and deacetylation: An important regulatory modification in gene transcription [Review]. *Experimental and Therapeutic Medicine*, *20*(4), 2923–2940. DOI: 10.3892/etm.2020.9073 PMID: 32855658

Xiao, D., Zhang, L., & Wang, J. (2019). The role of parkin-mediated mitophagy in cardiovascular diseases. *International Journal of Sciences*, *8*(05), 25–29. DOI: 10.18483/ijSci.2049

Xiao, H., Zheng, Y., Ma, L., Tian, L., & Sun, Q. (2021). Clinically-Relevant ABC Transporter for Anti-Cancer Drug Resistance. *Frontiers in Pharmacology*, *12*, 648407. Advance online publication. DOI: 10.3389/fphar.2021.648407 PMID: 33953682

Xie, C., Zhuang, X., Niu, Z., Ai, R., Lautrup, S., Zheng, S., Jiang, Y., Han, R., Gupta, T., Cao, S., Lagartos-Donate, M., Cai, C., Xie, L., Caponio, D., Wang, W., Schmauck-Medina, T., Zhang, J., Wang, H., Lou, G., & Fang, E. (2022). Amelioration of Alzheimer's disease pathology by mitophagy inducers identified via machine learning and a cross-species workflow. *Nature Biomedical Engineering*, *6*(1), 76–93. DOI: 10.1038/s41551-021-00819-5 PMID: 34992270

Xie, Y., Liu, J., Kang, R., & Tang, D. (2021). Mitophagy in Pancreatic Cancer. *Frontiers in Oncology*, *11*, 616079. DOI: 10.3389/fonc.2021.616079 PMID: 33718171

Xin, J. (2023). Critical signaling pathways governing colitis-associated colorectal cancer: Signaling, therapeutic implications, and challenges. *Digestive and Liver Disease*, *55*(2), 169–177. DOI: 10.1016/j.dld.2022.08.012 PMID: 36002360

Xi, Y., & Xu, P. (2021). Global colorectal cancer burden in 2020 and projections to 2040. *Translational Oncology*, *14*(10), 101174. DOI: 10.1016/j.tranon.2021.101174 PMID: 34243011

Xu, B. W., Li, S. S., Ding, W. L., Zhang, C., Rehman, M. U., Tareen, M. F., Wang, L., & Huang, S. C. (2025). From structure to function: A comprehensive overview of polysaccharide roles and applications. *Food Frontiers*, *6*(1), 15–39. DOI: 10.1002/fft2.490

Xue, D., Pan, S. T., Zhou, X., Ye, F., Zhou, Q., Shi, F., He, F., Yu, H., & Qiu, J. (2020). Plumbagin Enhances the Anticancer Efficacy of Cisplatin by Increasing Intracellular ROS in Human Tongue Squamous Cell Carcinoma. *Oxidative Medicine and Cellular Longevity*, *2020*, 5649174. DOI: 10.1155/2020/5649174 PMID: 32308804

Xu, H. M., & Hu, F. (2022). The role of autophagy and mitophagy in cancers. *Archives of Physiology and Biochemistry*, *128*(2), 281–289. DOI: 10.1080/13813455.2019.1675714 PMID: 31596150

Xu, Y., Shen, J., & Ran, Z. (2020). Emerging views of mitophagy in immunity and autoimmune diseases. *Autophagy*, *16*(1), 17–3. DOI: 10.1080/15548627.2019.1603547 PMID: 30951392

Xu, Z., Zhao, G., Zhang, L., Qiao, C., Wang, H., Wei, H., Liu, R., Liu, P., Zhang, Y., Zhu, W., & You, W. (2024). Tong-Xie-Yao-Fang induces mitophagy in colonic epithelial cells to inhibit colitis-associated colorectal cancer. *Journal of Ethnopharmacology*, *334*, 118541. DOI: 10.1016/j.jep.2024.118541 PMID: 38992403

Yahanda, A. M., Alder, K. M., Fisher, G. A., Brophy, N. A., Halsey, J., Hardy, R. I., Gosland, M. P., Lum, B. L., & Sikic, B. I. (1992). Phase I trial of etoposide with cyclosporine as a modulator of multidrug resistance. *Journal of Clinical Oncology*, *10*(10), 1624–1634. DOI: 10.1200/JCO.1992.10.10.1624 PMID: 1403040

Yalchin, M., Baker, A.-M., Graham, T. A., & Hart, A. (2021). Predicting colorectal cancer occurrence in IBD. *Cancers (Basel)*, *13*(12), 2908. DOI: 10.3390/cancers13122908 PMID: 34200768

Yamashita, S. I., Arai, R., Hada, H., Padman, B. S., Lazarou, M., Chan, D. C., Kanki, T., & Waguri, S. (2025). The mitophagy receptors BNIP3 and NIX mediate tight attachment and expansion of the isolation membrane to mitochondria. *The Journal of Cell Biology*, *224*(7), e202408166. DOI: 10.1083/jcb.202408166 PMID: 40358358

Yamashita, S., Sugiura, Y., Matsuoka, Y., Maeda, R., Inoue, K., Furukawa, K., Fukuda, T., Chan, D., & Kanki, T. (2024). Mitophagy mediated by BNIP3 and NIX protects against ferroptosis by downregulating mitochondrial reactive oxygen species. *Cell Death and Differentiation*, *31*(5), 651–661. DOI: 10.1038/s41418-024-01280-y PMID: 38519771

Yan, C., Luo, L., Guo, C., Wang, H., & Jin, J. (2017). Doxorubicin-induced mitophagy contributes to drug resistance in cancer stem cells from HCT8 human colorectal cancer cells. *Cancer Letters*, *388*, 34–42. DOI: 10.1016/j.canlet.2016.11.018 PMID: 27913197

Yan, F., Cao, X. X., Jiang, H. X., Zhao, X. L., Wang, J. Y., Lin, Y. H., Liu, Q. L., Zhang, C., Jiang, B., & Guo, F. (2010). A novel water-soluble gossypol derivative increases chemotherapeutic sensitivity and promotes growth inhibition in colon cancer. *Journal of Medicinal Chemistry*, *53*(15), 5502–5510. DOI: 10.1021/jm1001698 PMID: 20684596

Yang, X., Pan, W., Xu, G., & Chen, L. (2019). Mitophagy: a crucial modulator in the pathogenesis of chronic diseases.. Clinica chimica acta; international journal of clinical chemistry.

Yang, A., Rajeshkumar, N. V., Wang, X., Yabuuchi, S., Alexander, B. M., Chu, G. C., Von Hoff, D. D., Maitra, A., & Kimmelman, A. C. (2014). Autophagy is critical for pancreatic tumor growth and progression in tumors with p53 alterations. *Cancer Discovery*, *4*(8), 905–913. DOI: 10.1158/2159-8290.CD-14-0362 PMID: 24875860

Yang, C., Singh, P., Singh, H., Le, M. L., & El-Matary, W. (2015). Systematic review: Thalidomide and thalidomide analogues for treatment of inflammatory bowel disease. *Alimentary Pharmacology & Therapeutics*, *41*(11), 1079–1093. DOI: 10.1111/apt.13181 PMID: 25858208

Yang, J., Shay, C., Saba, N. F., & Teng, Y. (2024). Cancer metabolism and carcinogenesis. *Experimental Hematology & Oncology*, *13*(1), 10. DOI: 10.1186/s40164-024-00482-x PMID: 38287402

Yang, P., Shuai, W., Wang, X., Hu, X., Zhao, M., Wang, A., Wu, Y., Liang, O., & Wang, G. (2025). Mitophagy in Neurodegenerative Diseases: Mechanisms of Action and the Advances of Drug Discovery. *Journal of Medicinal Chemistry*, *68*(4), 3970–3994. DOI: 10.1021/acs.jmedchem.4c01779 PMID: 39908485

Yang, Q. E. (2021). Human cancer xenografts in immunocompromised mice provide an advanced genuine tumor model for research and drug development-A revisit of murine models for human cancers. *Biochimica Et Biophysica Acta (BBA) -. Biochimica et Biophysica Acta. G, General Subjects*, *1865*(8), 129929. DOI: 10.1016/j.bbagen.2021.129929 PMID: 33991617

Yang, S., Wang, X., Contino, G., Liesa, M., Sahin, E., Ying, H., Bause, A., Li, Y., Stommel, J. M., Dell'Antonio, G., Mautner, J., Tonon, G., Haigis, M., Shirihai, O. S., Doglioni, C., Bardeesy, N., & Kimmelman, A. C. (2011). Pancreatic cancers require autophagy for tumor growth. *Genes & Development*, *25*(7), 717–729. DOI: 10.1101/gad.2016111 PMID: 21406549

Yang, X., Xiong, H., Guan, Z., Okai, I., Ye, D., Song, Y., Li, X., Wang, L., Liu, L., Du, S., Lin, D., & Shao, S. (2012). Higher expression of Caveolin-1 inhibits human small cell lung cancer (SCLC) apoptosis in vitro. *Cancer Investigation*, *30*(6), 453–462. DOI: 10.3109/07357907.2012.675384 PMID: 22545709

Yang, X., Zhu, J., Wu, J., Huang, N., Cui, Z., Luo, Y., Sun, F., Pan, Q., Li, Y., & Yang, Q. (2018). (−)-Guaiol regulates autophagic cell death depending on mTOR signaling in NSCLC. *Cancer Biology & Therapy*, *19*(8), 706–714. DOI: 10.1080/15384047.2018.1451277 PMID: 29611762

Yang, Y., Ma, F., Liu, Z., Su, Q., Liu, Y., Liu, Z., & Li, Y. (2019). The ER-localized Ca2+-binding protein calreticulin couples ER stress to autophagy by associating with microtubule-associated protein 1A/1B light chain 3. *The Journal of Biological Chemistry*, *294*(3), 772–782. DOI: 10.1074/jbc.RA118.005166 PMID: 30429217

Yao, N., Wang, C., Hu, N., Yao, M., Li, H., Zhang, L., He, C., Wang, H., & Zhou, Q. (2019). Inhibition of PINK1/Parkin-dependent mitophagy sensitizes multidrug-resistant cancer cells to B5G1, a new betulinic acid analog. *Cell Death & Disease*, *10*(3), 232. Advance online publication. DOI: 10.1038/s41419-019-1470-z PMID: 30850585

Yao, X., Cao, Y., Lu, L., Xu, Y., Chen, H., Liu, C., Chen, D., Wang, K., Xu, J., Fang, R., Xia, H., Li, J., Fang, Q., & Tao, Z. (2022). Plasmodium infection suppresses colon cancer growth by inhibiting proliferation and promoting apoptosis associated with disrupting mitochondrial biogenesis and mitophagy in mice. *Parasites & Vectors*, *15*(1), 192. DOI: 10.1186/s13071-022-05291-x PMID: 35668501

Yau, W. W., Wong, K. A., Zhou, J., Thimmukonda, N. K., Wu, Y., Bay, B. H., Singh, B. K., & Yen, P. M. (2021). Chronic cold exposure induces autophagy to promote fatty acid oxidation, mitochondrial turnover, and thermogenesis in brown adipose tissue. *iScience*, *24*(5), 102434. DOI: 10.1016/j.isci.2021.102434 PMID: 34027318

Ye, D., Zhu, J., Su, S., Yu, Y., Zhang, J., Yin, Y., Lin, C., Xie, X., Xiang, Q., & Yu, R. (2025). Natural small molecules regulating the mitophagy pathway counteract the pathogenesis of diabetes and chronic complications. *Frontiers in Pharmacology*, *16*, 1767–1773. DOI: 10.3389/fphar.2025.1571767 PMID: 40308774

Ye, L. Y., Hu, S., Xu, H. E., Xu, R. R., Kong, H., Zeng, X. N., Xie, W. P., & Wang, H. (2017). The effect of tetrandrine combined with cisplatin on proliferation and apoptosis of A549/DDP cells and A549 cells. *Cancer Cell International*, *17*(1), 40. DOI: 10.1186/s12935-017-0410-1 PMID: 28360820

Ye, M., Wang, S., Wan, T., Jiang, R., Qiu, Y., Pei, L., Pang, N., Huang, Y., Huang, Y., Zhang, Z., & Yang, L. (2017). Combined inhibitions of glycolysis and AKT/autophagy can overcome resistance to EGFR-targeted therapy of lung cancer. *Journal of Cancer*, *8*(18), 3774–3784. DOI: 10.7150/jca.21035 PMID: 29151965

Yessenkyzy, A., Saliev, T., Zhanaliyeva, M., Masoud, A. R., Umbayev, B., Sergazy, S., Krivykh, E., Gulyayev, A., & Nurgozhin, T. (2020). Polyphenols as Caloric-Restriction Mimetics and Autophagy Inducers in Aging Research. *Nutrients*, *12*(5), 1344. DOI: 10.3390/nu12051344 PMID: 32397145

Yin, J., Guo, J., Zhang, Q., Cui, L., Zhang, L., Zhang, T., Wang, C., Liu, Y., & Wang, H. (2018). Doxorubicin-induced mitophagy and mitochondrial damage is associated with dysregulation of the PINK1/parkin pathway. *Toxicology In Vitro*, *51*, 1–10. DOI: 10.1016/j.tiv.2018.05.001 PMID: 29729358

Yin, K., Lee, J., Liu, Z., Kim, H., Martin, D. R., Wu, D., Liu, M., & Xue, X. (2021). Mitophagy protein PINK1 suppresses colon tumor growth by metabolic reprogramming via p53 activation and reducing acetyl-CoA production. *Cell Death and Differentiation*, *28*(8), 2421–2435. DOI: 10.1038/s41418-021-00760-9 PMID: 33723373

Yin, Z., Zhang, J., Chen, L., Guo, Q., Yang, B., Zhang, W., & Kang, W. (2020). Anticancer Effects and Mechanisms of Action of Plumbagin: Review of Research Advances. *BioMed Research International*, *2020*(1), 6940953. DOI: 10.1155/2020/6940953 PMID: 33344645

Youle, R. J., & Narendra, D. P. (2011). Mechanisms of mitophagy. *Nature Reviews. Molecular Cell Biology*, *12*(1), 9–14. DOI: 10.1038/nrm3028 PMID: 21179058

Yuan, J., & Yankner, B. A. (2000). Apoptosis in the nervous system. *Nature*, *407*(6805), 802–809. DOI: 10.1038/35037739 PMID: 11048732

Yuan, Y., Zheng, Y., Zhang, X., Chen, Y., Wu, X., Wu, J., Shen, Z., Jiang, L., Wang, L., Yang, W., Luo, J., Qin, Z., Hu, W., & Chen, Z. (2017). BNIP3L/NIX-mediated mitophagy protects against ischemic brain injury independent of PARK2. *Autophagy*, *13*(10), 1754–1766. DOI: 10.1080/15548627.2017.1357792 PMID: 28820284

Yu, L., Chen, Y., & Tooze, S. A. (2018). Autophagy pathway: Cellular and molecular mechanisms. *Autophagy*, *14*(2), 207–215. DOI: 10.1080/15548627.2017.1378838 PMID: 28933638

Yu, L., Qin, J., Zhang, M., Gao, Y., & Zhao, Y. (2024). Research Progress on the Anti-Liver Cancer Mechanism and Toxicity of Rhubarb Anthraquinone. *Drug Design, Development and Therapy, 12*, 6089–6113. DOI: 10.2147/DDDT.S489377 PMID: 39717199

Yu, M., Nguyen, N. D., Huang, Y., Lin, D., Fujimoto, T. N., Molkentine, J. M., Deorukhkar, A., Kang, Y., San Lucas, F. A., Fernandes, C. J., & Jimenez, C. R.. (2019). Mitochondrial fusion exploits a therapeutic vulnerability of pancreatic cancer. *JCI Insight, 5*(16), e126915. DOI: 10.1172/jci.insight.126915 PMID: 31335325

Yu, Y., Zhao, Y., Choi, J., Shi, Z., Guo, L., Elizarraras, J., Gu, A., Cheng, F., Pei, Y., Lu, D., Fabbri, M., Agarwal, S., Zhang, C., Jung, S. Y., Foster, J. H., & Yang, J. (2022). ERK Inhibitor Ulixertinib Inhibits High-Risk Neuroblastoma Growth In Vitro and In Vivo. *Cancers (Basel), 14*(22), 5534. Advance online publication. DOI: 10.3390/cancers14225534 PMID: 36428626

Zafar, A., Wang, W., Liu, G., Wang, X., Xian, W., McKeon, F., Foster, J., Zhou, J., & Zhang, R. (2021). Molecular targeting therapies for neuroblastoma: Progress and challenges. *Medicinal Research Reviews, 41*(2), 961–1021. DOI: 10.1002/med.21750 PMID: 33155698

Zage, P. E., Whittle, S. B., & Shohet, J. M. (2017). CD114: A New Member of the Neural Crest-Derived Cancer Stem Cell Marker Family. *Journal of Cellular Biochemistry, 118*(2), 221–231. DOI: 10.1002/jcb.25656 PMID: 27428599

Zamanian, M. Y., Golmohammadi, M., Yumashev, A., Hjazi, A., Toama, M. A., AbdRabou, M. A., Gehlot, A., Alwaily, E. R., Shirsalimi, N., Yadav, P. K., & Moriasi, G. (2024). Effects of metformin on cancers in experimental and clinical studies: Focusing on autophagy and AMPK/mTOR signaling pathways. *Cell Biochemistry and Function, 42*(4), e4071. DOI: 10.1002/cbf.4071 PMID: 38863255

Zhang, H., Bosch-Marce, M., Shimoda, L. A., Tan, Y. S., Baek, J. H., Wesley, J. B., Gonzalez, F. J., & Semenza, G. L. (2008). Mitochondrial autophagy is an HIF-1-dependent adaptive metabolic response to hypoxia. *The Journal of biological chemistry, 283*(16), 10892–10903. (Retraction published J Biol Chem. 2023 Aug;299(8):105125)DOI: 10.1074/jbc.M800102200

Zhang, C., Liu, Z., Bunker, E., Ramamoorthy, S., Rodrigues, L. O., Djaballah, H., & Pfeiffer, S. (2017). Sorafenib targets the mitochondrial electron transport chain complexes and ATP synthase to activate the PINK1–Parkin pathway and modulate cellular drug response. *The Journal of Biological Chemistry, 292*(36), 15105–15120. DOI: 10.1074/jbc.M117.783175 PMID: 28673964

Zhang, D., Gao, C., Li, R., Zhang, L., & Tian, J. (2017). TEOA, a triterpenoid from *Actinidia eriantha*, induces autophagy in SW620 cells via endoplasmic reticulum stress and ROS-dependent mitophagy. *Archives of Pharmacal Research*, *40*(5), 579–591. DOI: 10.1007/s12272-017-0899-9 PMID: 28211011

Zhang, G., Hou, J., Shi, J., Yu, G., Lu, B., & Zhang, X. (2008). Soluble CD276 (B7-H3) is released from monocytes, dendritic cells and activated T cells and is detectable in normal human serum. *Immunology*, *123*(4), 538–546. DOI: 10.1111/j.1365-2567.2007.02723.x PMID: 18194267

Zhang, H., Yin, C., Liu, X., Bai, X., Wang, L., Xu, H., Li, F., Zhang, J., & Zhao, Q. (2020). Prohibitin 2/PHB2 in parkin-mediated mitophagy: A potential therapeutic target for non-small cell lung carcinoma. *Medical Science Monitor*, *26*, e923227. DOI: 10.12659/MSM.923227 PMID: 32320388

Zhang, J., & Ney, P. A. (2009). Role of BNIP3 and NIX in cell death, autophagy, and mitophagy. *Cell Death and Differentiation*, *16*(7), 939–946. DOI: 10.1038/cdd.2009.16 PMID: 19229244

Zhang, J., Xiang, H., Liu, J., Chen, Y., He, R. R., & Liu, B. (2020). Mitochondrial Sirtuin 3: New emerging biological function and therapeutic target. *Theranostics*, *10*(18), 8315–8342. DOI: 10.7150/thno.45922 PMID: 32724473

Zhang, K., Zhang, D., Wang, J., Wang, Y., Hu, J., Zhou, Y., Zhou, X., Nie, S., & Xie, M. (2022). Aloe gel glucomannan induced colon cancer cell death via mitochondrial damage-driven PINK1/Parkin mitophagy pathway. *Carbohydrate Polymers*, *295*, 119841. DOI: 10.1016/j.carbpol.2022.119841 PMID: 35989033

Zhang, Q., Wang, X., Cao, S., Sun, Y., He, X., Jiang, B., Yu, Y., Duan, J., Qiu, F., & Kang, N. (2020). Berberine represses human gastric cancer cell growth in vitro and in vivo by inducing cytostatic autophagy via inhibition of MAPK/mTOR/p70S6K and Akt signaling pathways. *Biomedicine and Pharmacotherapy*, *128*, 110245. DOI: 10.1016/j.biopha.2020.110245 PMID: 32454290

Zhang, R., Gu, J., Chen, J., Ni, J., Hung, J., Wang, Z., Zhang, X., Feng, J., & Ji, L. (2017). High expression of PINK1 promotes proliferation and chemoresistance of NSCLC. *Oncology Reports*, *37*(4), 2137–2146. DOI: 10.3892/or.2017.5486 PMID: 28259921

Zhang, R., Jiang, W., Wang, G., Zhang, Y., Liu, W., Li, M., Yu, J., Yan, X., Zhou, F., Du, W., Qian, K., Xiao, Y., Liu, T., Ju, L., & Wang, X. (2024). Parkin inhibits proliferation and migration of bladder cancer via ubiquitinating catalase. *Communications Biology*, *7*(1), 245. DOI: 10.1038/s42003-024-05935-x PMID: 38424181

Zhang, R., Lu, J., Pei, G., & Huang, S. (2023). Galangin rescues Alzheimer's amyloid-β induced mitophagy and brain organoid growth impairment. *International Journal of Molecular Sciences*, *24*(4), 3398. DOI: 10.3390/ijms24043398 PMID: 36834819

Zhang, T., Liu, Q., Gao, W., Sehgal, S., & Wu, H. (2021). The multifaceted regulation of mitophagy by endogenous metabolites. *Autophagy*, *18*(6), 1216–1239. DOI: 10.1080/15548627.2021.1975914 PMID: 34583624

Zhang, X. Y., Zhang, M., Cong, Q., Zhang, M. X., Zhang, M. Y., Lu, Y. Y., & Xu, C. J. (2018). Hexokinase 2 confers resistance to cisplatin in ovarian cancer cells by enhancing cisplatin-induced autophagy. *The International Journal of Biochemistry & Cell Biology*, *95*, 9–16. DOI: 10.1016/j.biocel.2017.12.010 PMID: 29247711

Zhang, X., Chen, L. X., Ouyang, L., Cheng, Y., & Liu, B. (2012). Plant natural compounds: Targeting pathways of autophagy as anti-cancer therapeutic agents. *Cell Proliferation*, *45*(5), 466–476. DOI: 10.1111/j.1365-2184.2012.00833.x PMID: 22765290

Zhang, X., Wang, J., & Luo, J. (2019a). Berberine induces mitophagy and apoptosis in liver cancer. *Cancer Cell International*, *19*, 98. DOI: 10.1186/s12935-019-0802-9

Zhang, Y. (n.d.). Lycopene regulates mitophagy in breast cancer cells: Experimental and computational evidence. *Journal of Cellular Physiology*, *233*(5), 3671–3681.

Zhang, Y., Goldman, S., Baerga, R., Zhao, Y., Komatsu, M., & Jin, S. (2009). Adipose-specific deletion of autophagy-related gene 7 (atg7) in mice reveals a role in adipogenesis. *Proceedings of the National Academy of Sciences of the United States of America*, *106*(47), 19860–19865. DOI: 10.1073/pnas.0906048106 PMID: 19910529

Zhang, Y., & Liu, J. (2020). Epigallocatechin gallate-induced mitophagy contributes to cancer cell death. *Nutrition and Cancer*, *72*(5), 789–799. DOI: 10.1080/01635581.2019.1659958

Zhang, Y.-M., Miao, Z.-M., Chen, Y.-P., Song, Z.-B., Li, Y.-Y., Liu, Z.-W., Zhou, G.-C., Li, J., Shi, L.-L., Chen, Y., Zhang, S.-Z., Xu, X., He, J.-P., Wang, J.-F., Zhang, L.-Y., & Liu, Y.-Q. (2024). Ononin promotes radiosensitivity in lung cancer by inhibiting HIF-1α/VEGF pathway. *Phytomedicine*, *125*, 155290. DOI: 10.1016/j.phymed.2023.155290 PMID: 38308918

Zhang, Y., Yan, H., Wei, Y., & Wei, X. (2024). Decoding mitochondria's role in immunity and cancer therapy. *Biochimica et Biophysica Acta (BBA) -. Revisiones en Cáncer*, *1879*(4), 189107. DOI: 10.1016/j.bbcan.2024.189107 PMID: 38734035

Zhang, Z. (2019). Quercetin-induced mitophagy suppresses breast cancer growth. *Molecular Carcinogenesis*, *54*(9), 1014–1026.

Zhang, Z. J., Zheng, Z. J., Kan, H., Song, Y., Cui, W., Zhao, G., & Kip, K. E. (2011). Reduced risk of colorectal cancer with metformin therapy in patients with type 2 diabetes: A meta-analysis. *Diabetes Care*, *34*(10), 2323–2328. DOI: 10.2337/dc11-0512 PMID: 21949223

Zhang, Z., Chen, Z., Liu, R., Liang, Q., Peng, Z., Yin, S., Tang, J., Gong, T., & Liu, Y. (2020). Bcl-2 Proteins Regulate Mitophagy in Lipopolysaccharide-Induced Acute Lung Injury via PINK1/Parkin Signaling Pathway. *Oxidative Medicine and Cellular Longevity*, *2020*, 2020. DOI: 10.1155/2020/6579696 PMID: 32148654

Zhao, B., Li, H., Xia, Y., Wang, Y., Wang, Y., Shi, Y., Xing, H., Qu, T., Wang, Y., & Ma, W. (2022). Immune checkpoint of B7-H3 in cancer: From immunology to clinical immunotherapy. *Journal of Hematology & Oncology*, *15*(1), 153. DOI: 10.1186/s13045-022-01364-7 PMID: 36284349

Zhao, W., Chen, Z., Fu, W., Ye, C., Fu, H., Xu, T., Wu, B., Chen, L., & Shan, S. J. (2025). Induction of apoptosis and hypoxic stress in malignant melanoma cells via graphene-mediated far-infrared radiation. *BMC Cancer*, *25*(1), 620–628. DOI: 10.1186/s12885-025-14031-0 PMID: 40197161

Zhao, Y., Han, J., Hu, W., Dai, Y., Wu, X., Liao, X., Zhou, H., & Nie, K. (2024). Xiao-Ban-Xia decoction mitigates cisplatin-induced emesis via restoring PINK1/Parkin mediated mitophagy deficiency in a rat pica model. *Journal of Ethnopharmacology*, *318*, 116882. DOI: 10.1016/j.jep.2023.116882 PMID: 37422100

Zheng, J., Jiang, S., Lin, X., Wang, H., Liu, L., Cai, X., & Sun, Y. (2024). Comprehensive analyses of mitophagy-related genes and mitophagy-related lncRNAs for patients with ovarian cancer. *BMC Women's Health*, *24*(1), 37. DOI: 10.1186/s12905-023-02864-5 PMID: 38218807

Zheng, R., Yao, Q., Xie, G., Du, S., Ren, C., Wang, Y., & Yuan, Y. (2015). Tat-odd-p53 enhances the radiosensitivity of hypoxic breast cancer cells by inhibiting parkin-mediated mitophagy. *Oncotarget*, *6*(19), 17417–17429. DOI: 10.18632/oncotarget.4002 PMID: 26025927

Zheng, Y., Liu, P., Wang, N., Wang, S., Yang, B., Li, M., Chen, J., Situ, H., Xie, M., Lin, Y., & Wang, Z. (2019b). Betulinic Acid Suppresses Breast Cancer Metastasis by Targeting GRP78-Mediated Glycolysis and ER Stress Apoptotic Pathway. *Oxidative Medicine and Cellular Longevity*, *8781690*, 1–15. Advance online publication. DOI: 10.1155/2019/8781690 PMID: 31531187

Zhou, H., He, L., Xu, G., & Chen, L. (2020). Mitophagy in cardiovascular disease.. Clinica chimica acta; international journal of clinical chemistry

Zhou, H., Zhang, Y., Hu, S., Chen, S., Zhu, P., Ma, Q., & Chen, Y. (2017). Melatonin protects cardiac microvasculature against ischemia/reperfusion injury via suppression of mitochondrial fission-vdac1-hk2-mptp-mitophagy axis. *Journal of Pineal Research*, *63*(1), e12413. DOI: 10.1111/jpi.12413 PMID: 28398674

Zhou, J., Li, G., Zheng, Y., Shen, H.-M., Hu, X., Ming, Q.-L., Huang, C., Li, P., & Gao, N. (2015). A novel autophagy/mitophagy inhibitor liensinine sensitizes breast cancer cells to chemotherapy through DNM1L-mediated mitochondrial fission. *Autophagy*, *11*(8), 1259–1279. DOI: 10.1080/15548627.2015.1056970 PMID: 26114658

Zhou, P., Ma, Y. Y., Zhao, X. N., & Hua, F. (2023). Phytochemicals as potential target on thioredoxin-interacting protein (TXNIP) for the treatment of cardiovascular diseases. *Inflammopharmacology*, *31*(1), 207–220. DOI: 10.1007/s10787-022-01130-8 PMID: 36609715

Zhou, W. T., & Jin, W. L. (2021). B7-H3/CD276: An Emerging Cancer Immunotherapy. *Frontiers in Immunology*, *12*, 701006. DOI: 10.3389/fimmu.2021.701006 PMID: 34349762

Zhou, Y., Tao, L., Qiu, J., Xu, J., Yang, X., Zhang, Y., Tian, X., Guan, X., Cen, X., & Zhao, Y. (2024). Tumor biomarkers for diagnosis, prognosis and targeted therapy. *Signal Transduction and Targeted Therapy*, *9*(1), 132. DOI: 10.1038/s41392-024-01823-2 PMID: 38763973

Zhou, Y., Wang, D., & Yan, W. (2023). Treatment effects of natural products on inflammatory bowel disease in vivo and their mechanisms: Based on animal experiments. *Nutrients*, *15*(4), 1031. DOI: 10.3390/nu15041031 PMID: 36839389

Zhu, Y., Massen, S., Terenzio, M., Lang, V., Chen-Lindner, S., Eils, R., Novak, I., Dikic, I., Hamacher-Brady, A., & Brady, N. R. (2013). Modulation of serines 17 and 24 in the LC3-interacting region of Bnip3 determines pro-survival mitophagy versus apoptosis. *The Journal of Biological Chemistry*, *288*(2), 1099–1113. DOI: 10.1074/jbc.M112.399345 PMID: 23209295

Zimmermann, A., Madeo, F., Diwan, A., Sadoshima, J., Sedej, S., Kroemer, G., & Abdellatif, M. (2024). Metabolic control of mitophagy. *European Journal of Clinical Investigation*, *54*(4), e14138. DOI: 10.1111/eci.14138 PMID: 38041247

Zong, Y., Li, H., Liao, P., Chen, L., Pan, Y., Zheng, Y., Zhang, C., Liu, D., Zheng, M., & Gao, J. (2024). Mitochondrial dysfunction: Mechanisms and advances in therapy. *Signal Transduction and Targeted Therapy*, *9*(1), 124. DOI: 10.1038/s41392-024-01839-8 PMID: 38744846

Zou, Y., Li, H., & Chen, W. (2020). Resveratrol promotes mitophagy in cancer cells by activating the PINK1-Parkin pathway. *Biomedicine and Pharmacotherapy*, *128*, 110312. DOI: 10.1016/j.biopha.2020.110312

Zühlke, M. K., Schlüter, R., Mikolasch, A., Henning, A. K., Giersberg, M., Lalk, M., Kunze, G., Schweder, T., Urich, T., & Schauer, F. (2020). Biotransformation of bisphenol A analogues by the biphenyl-degrading bacterium Cupriavidus basilensis-a structure-biotransformation relationship. *Applied Microbiology and Biotechnology*, *104*(8), 3569–3583. DOI: 10.1007/s00253-020-10406-4 PMID: 32125477

Сухоруков, В., Воронков, Д., Баранич, Т., Mudzhiri, N., Magnaeva, A., & Иллариошкин, С. (2021). Impaired mitophagy in neurons and glial cells during aging and age-related disorders. *International Journal of Molecular Sciences*, *22*(19), 10251. DOI: 10.3390/ijms221910251 PMID: 34638589

About the Contributors

Ashok Kumar Pandurangan is an Associate Professor working (August 2017 onwards) in the School of Life Sciences, B.S. Abdur Rahman Crescent Institute of Science and Technology, Vandalur, Chennai, India. Recently, he has been listed three times as one of the Top 2% of Scientists (2020-2022) in the field of Oncology and Toxicology by Stanford University, USA. He completed his Ph.D. in the Department of Biochemistry, University of Madras, Chennai, India, from 2006-2011. Later, he worked as a postdoctoral fellow in the Centre for Cancer Research, Children's Hospital Oakland Research Institute (California, USA), in the field of S1PLyase deficiency in colitis-associated cancer. Then he worked as a postdoctoral fellow in the Department of Nutrition and Dietetics, Universiti of Putra Malaysia (UPM), Serdang, Malaysia. Further, he worked as a Visiting Research Fellow in the Department of Pharmacology, University of Malaya, Kuala Lumpur, Malaysia. He published over 67 research and reviewed articles in peer-reviewed journals 5 books, and 27 book chapters. He received a Teachers Associateship Research Excellence (TARE) grant from SERB, India, in 2018 and several grants in Malaysia.

***

Erdi Can Aytar is currently a Research Assistant in the Department of Horticulture, at Usak University, Türkiye. He received her Master of Science degree in biology from Gazi University in 2016, and her Ph.D. in biology from Ondokuz Mayıs University in 2024. He has research experience in Antioxidant and antimicrobial activity, cancer, isolation of organic compounds, plant physiology and germination. He has worked on national and international projects. He has published several research articles.

Yasmin Banu C is a Research Scholar pursuing her Ph.D. in Bio-technology from the School of Life Sciences, B. S. Abdur Rahman Crescent Institute of Science and Technology, Chennai. She has completed her Masters in Biotechnology from B. S. Abdur Rahman Crescent Institute of Science and Technology, Chennai. She is currently working in the field of ulcerative colitis and colitis-associated cancer, with a primary focus on conducting in vivo studies to understand disease mechanisms and evaluate therapeutic interventions.

Odangowei Inetiminebi Ogidi is a Lecturer, Acting Head, Department of Biochemistry and Sub-Dean, Faculty of Basic Medical Sciences, Bayelsa Medical University, Yenagoa, Bayelsa State, Nigeria. He holds a Bachelor of Science degree in Biochemistry, Master of Science and Doctor of Philosophy degrees in Biotechnology. He has also served as a Lecturer, Head of Departments of Science Laboratory Technology and Biochemistry, and Deputy Director, Centre for Continuing Education in Federal Polytechnic Ekowe, Bayelsa State. He has authored over 80 peer-reviewed academic articles in reputable local and international journals, published over 50 book chapters and presented over 40 conference papers. He is a member of various Journal Editorial Boards. He is indexed in World Scientist and University Ranking.

Saabira Banu Sahubar Sadik did her schooling in M.W.A Matriculation and Higher Secondary School, Gopalapuram, Chennai. She completed her Masters in Food Biotechnology at school of Life Sciences, B.S. Abdur Rahman Crescent Institute of Science and Technology, Chennai, India. Her research interests include Cancer, Food technology and Molecular pathology.

Ronisha Shankar Rao was born in Mysore and completed her studies at Kendriya Vidyalaya Meenambakkam in Chennai. She is currently pursuing an undergraduate B.Tech in Biotechnology at B.S. Abdur Rahman Crescent Institute of Science & Technology. Her areas of interest include bioinformatics, computational biology, and molecular cell biology. Additionally, she is passionate about art and dance. Ronisha is also an active member of several academic and cultural clubs at her institute, where she hones her leadership and teamwork skills. She has published two articles.

Charuwan Thanawiroon is an Assistant Professor at Ubon Ratchathani University in Thailand, specializing in Pharmacy and Pharmaceutical Chemistry. She earned her PhD in Medicinal and Natural Product Chemistry from the University of Iowa, USA. Dr. Thanawiroon has dedicated her career to advancing the field of pharmaceutical sciences, focusing on the analysis of synthetic drugs, medicinal compounds, and pharmaceutical care. Her expertise significantly enhances both research and education in pharmaceutical chemistry, establishing her as a key figure in her academic community.

Manish Kumar Verma, Assistant Professor in the Department of Veterinary Pharmacology & Toxicology. He contributes to both academic and research, focusing on practical knowledge in animal health and pharmaceutical sciences. His work focuses on understanding drug interactions and toxicological effects in animals, aiming to improve treatment efficacy and safety standards in animal care. He published several research articles, review articles and case study.

Bancha Yingngam is working as Associate Professor (Pharmaceutical Sciences and Technology) in the Faculty of Pharmaceutical Sciences at Ubon Ratchathani University, Ubon Ratchathani, Thailand. He received his B.Pharm. and Ph.D. (Pharmaceutical Sciences) at the Ubon Ratchathani, and postdoctoral fellowship at Institute of Pharmaceutical Sciences, University of Graz, Graz, Austria. His areas of interest include artificial intelligence, optimization methods, green chemistry, natural product chemistry, pharmacology, cosmeceuticals, and pharmaceutical nanotechnology. He has authored and co-authored many scientific papers published in international journals, and proceedings of international and national scientific conferences. He has also authored more than 30 book chapters and edited five textbooks.

Index

A

B

C

D

E

F

H

I

M

N

P

T

U

www.ingramcontent.com/pod-product-compliance
Lightning Source LLC
LaVergne TN
LVHW080117011026
849160LV00013B/1125